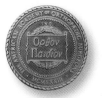

American Academy of Orthopaedic Surgeons

OKU
Orthopaedic Knowledge Update:

Spine

2

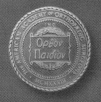

American Academy of Orthopaedic Surgeons

OKU

Orthopaedic Knowledge Update:

Spine

2

Edited by
David F. Fardon, MD
Steven R. Garfin, MD
Jean-Jacques Abitbol, MD
Scott D. Boden, MD
Harry N. Herkowitz, MD
Tom G. Mayer, MD

Developed by the
North American Spine Society

Published 2002
by the American Academy of Orthopaedic Surgeons
6300 North River Road
Rosemont, Illinois   60018
1-800-626-6726

The material presented in *Orthopaedic Knowledge Update: Spine 2* has been made available by the American Academy of Orthopaedic Surgeons for educational purposes only. This material is not intended to present the only, or necessarily best, methods or procedures for the medical situations discussed, but rather is intended to represent an approach, view, statement, or opinion of the author(s) or producer(s), which may be helpful to others who face similar situations.

Some drugs or medical devices demonstrated in Academy courses or described in Academy print or electronic publications have not been cleared by the Food and Drug Administration (FDA) or have been cleared for specific uses only. The FDA has stated that it is the responsibility of the physician to determine the FDA clearance status of each drug or device he or she wishes to use in clinical practice.

The U.S. Food and Drug Administration (FDA) has expressed concern about potential serious patient care issues involved with the use of polymethylmethacrylate (PMMA) bone cement in the spine. A physician might insert the PMMA bone cement into vertebrae by various procedures, including vertebroplasty and kyphoplasty. Orthopaedic surgeons should be alert to possible complications.

PMMA bone cement is considered a device for FDA purposes. In October 1999, the FDA reclassified PMMA bone cement as a Class II device for its intended use "in arthroplastic procedures of the hip, knee and other joints for the fixation of polymer or metallic prosthetic implants to living bone." The use of a device for other than its FDA-cleared indication is an off-label use. Physicians may use a device off-label if they believe, in their best medical judgment, that its use is appropriate for a particular patient (e.g., tumors).

The use of PMMA bone cement in the spine is described in Academy educational courses, videotapes and publications for educational purposes only. As is the Academy's policy regarding all of its educational offerings, the fact that the use of PMMA bone cement in the spine is discussed does not constitute an Academy endorsement of this use.

Furthermore, any statements about commercial products are solely the opinion(s) of the author(s) and do not represent an Academy endorsement or evaluation of these products. These statements may not be used in advertising or for any commercial purpose.

Second Edition
Copyright © 2002
by the American Academy of Orthopaedic Surgeons

ISBN 0-89203-258-8

Acknowledgments

Editorial Board, OKU: Spine 2

David F. Fardon, MD
Orthopedic Surgeon
Knoxville Orthopedic Clinic
Knoxville, Tennessee

Steven R. Garfin, MD
Professor and Chair
Department of Orthopaedics
University of California, San Diego
San Diego, California

Jean-Jacques Abitbol, MD
California Spine Group
San Diego, California

Scott D. Boden, MD
Associate Professor
Department of Orthopaedics
Emory University School of Medicine
Director, The Emory Spine Center
Atlanta, Georgia

Harry N. Herkowitz, MD
Chairman, Orthopaedic Surgery
William Beaumont Hospital
Royal Oak, Michigan

Tom G. Mayer, MD
Clinical Professor, Orthopaedic Surgery
University of Texas Southwestern Medical Center
PRIDE and PRIDE Research Foundation
Dallas, Texas

North American Spine Society

Board of Directors, 2001

Volker K.H. Sonntag, MD
President
Jean-Jacques Abitbol, MD
Thomas J. Errico, MD
Tom Faciszewski, MD
Richard Fessler, MD, PhD
Harry N. Herkowitz, MD
Stanley A. Herring, MD
Neil Kahanovitz, MD
Eric J. Muehlbauer
Joel Press, MD
Robert Watkins, MD
David A. Wong, MD

American Academy of Orthopaedic Surgeons

Board of Directors, 2001

Richard H. Gelberman, MD
President
Vernon T. Tolo, MD
First Vice President
James H. Herndon, MD
Second Vice President
E. Anthony Rankin, MD
Secretary
Andrew J. Weiland, MD
Treasurer
Peter C. Amadio, MD
S. Terry Canale, MD
Robert D. D'Ambrosia, MD
Stephen P. England, MD
Maureen Finnegan, MD
Gary E. Friedlaender, MD
David A. Halsey, MD
Darren L. Johnson, MD
Lowry Jones, Jr, MD
Thomas P. Sculco, MD
James N. Weinstein, DO
William W. Tipton, Jr, MD,
(Ex Officio)

Staff

Mark Wieting
*Vice President,
Educational Programs*
Marilyn L. Fox, PhD
*Director, Department
of Publications*
Lisa Claxton Moore
Senior Editor
Joan Abern
Senior Editor
Mary Steermann
Manager, Production and Archives
Sophie Tosta
Assistant Production Manager
David Stanley
Assistant Production Manager
Kathleen Anderson
Editorial Assistant
Courtney Astle
Production Assistant
Karen Danca
Production Assistant

Contributors

Albert J. Aboulafia, MD
Assistant Professor of Orthopaedic
    Surgery
University of Maryland
Division of Orthopaedic Oncology
Sinai Hospital of Baltimore
Baltimore, Maryland

Todd J. Albert, MD
Associate Professor and Vice Chairman
Department of Orthopaedics
Thomas Jefferson University
Rothman Institute
Philadelphia, Pennsylvania

Howard S. An, MD
The Morton International Professor of
    Orthopaedic Surgery
Rush Presbyterian St. Luke's
    Medical Center
Chicago, Illinois

David F. Apple, Jr, MD
Medical Director
Shepherd Center
Atlanta, Georgia

Michael A. Ashburn, MD, MPH
Professor of Anesthesiology
Director of Pain Management
    Center
University of Utah
Salt Lake City, Utah

Qi-Bin Bao, PhD
Vice President
Research and Development
Disc Dynamics Inc.
Minnetonka, Minnesota

Gordon R. Bell, MD
Vice Chairman, Department of
    Orthopaedic Surgery
Head, Section of Spinal Surgery
Cleveland Clinic Foundation
Cleveland, Ohio

Edward C. Benzel, MD
Director, Spinal Disorders
Cleveland Clinic Foundation
Cleveland, Ohio

Oheneba Boachie-Adjei, MD
Associate Clinical Professor of
    Orthopedics
Hospital for Special Surgery
Weill Medical College of Cornell
    Medical Center
New York, New York

K. Craig Boatright, MD
North Carolina Spine Center
Chapel Hill, North Carolina

Scott D. Boden, MD
Associate Professor
Department of Orthopaedics
Emory University
    School of Medicine
Director, The Emory Spine Center
Atlanta, Georgia

David Borenstein, MD
Clinical Professor of Medicine
Arthritis and Rheumatism
    Associates
Department of Medicine
The George Washington
    University Medical Center
Washington, DC

Douglas C. Burton, MD
Assistant Professor
Section of Orthopedic Surgery
University of Kansas
    Medical Center
Kansas City, Kansas

Jens R. Chapman, MD
Associate Professor of
    Orthopaedic Surgery and
    Neurological Surgery
Department of Orthopaedic
    Surgery
Harborview Medical Center
University of Washington
Seattle, Washington

Patrick J. Connolly, MD
Associate Professor of
    Orthopaedic Surgery
Department of Orthopaedic
    Surgery
State University of New York
Upstate Medical University
Syracuse, New York

Bradford L. Currier, MD
Associate Professor
Department of Orthopaedics
Mayo Medical School
Mayo Clinic
Rochester, Minnesota

Paul Dreyfuss, MD
Associate Clinical Professor
Department of Rehabilitation Medicine
University of Texas Health Sciences
    Center
San Antonio, Texas

Sean Dudeney, MD
Fellow, Spine Surgery
Department of Orthopaedics
Cleveland Clinic Foundation
Cleveland, Ohio

Frank Eismont, MD
Vice Chairman, Department of
    Orthopedic Surgery
Professor of Orthopedic Surgery
University of Miami School
    of Medicine
Miami, Florida

Thomas J. Errico, MD
Chief, Spine Service
Department of Orthopedics
New York University
Hospital for Special Surgery
New York, New York

Tom Faciszewski, MD
Chairman, Department of
    Orthopedic Spinal Surgery
Marshfield Clinic
Marshfield, Wisconsin

David F. Fardon, MD
Orthopedic Surgeon
Knoxville Orthopedic Clinic
Knoxville, Tennessee

Michael G. Fehlings, MD, PhD,
    FRCSC
Professor of Surgery
R. O. Lawson Chair and Head
    Spinal Program
Division of Neurosurgery
University Health Network
Toronto, Ontario, Canada

Jeffrey S. Fischgrund, MD
William Beaumont Hospital
Royal Oak, Michigan

Bruce E. Fredrickson, MD
Professor of Orthopaedic Surgery
Department of Orthopaedic
    Surgery
State University of New York
Syracuse, New York

Robert J. Gatchel, PhD
Professor of Psychiatry
University of Texas Southwestern
    Medical Center
Dallas, Texas

Federico P. Girardi, MD
Instructor, Orthopedics
Spinecare Institute
Assistant Attending Surgeon
Hospital for Special Surgery
Weill Medical College of
    Cornell University
New York, New York

Munish C. Gupta, MD
Assistant Professor of
    Orthopedic Surgery
Department of Orthopedic Surgery
University of California, Davis
Sacramento, California

Richard D. Guyer, MD
Associate Clinical Professor
The University of Texas Southwest-
    ern Medical Center at Dallas
Director, Spine Fellowship
Texas Back Institute
Plano, Texas

Scott Haldeman, MD, PhD
Clinical Professor
Department of Neurology
University of California at Irvine
Irvine, California

Hamilton Hall, MD, FRCSC
Professor
Department of Surgery
University of Toronto
Toronto, Ontario, Canada

R. H. Haralson III, MD, MBA
Associate Clinical Professor
Southeastern Orthopedics
University of Tennessee Center
    for the Health Sciences
Knoxville, Tennessee

John G. Heller, MD
Professor of Orthopaedic Surgery
Emory University School of
    Medicine
Spine Fellowship Director
Emory Spine Center
Atlanta, Georgia

Stanley A. Herring, MD
Team Physician, Seattle Seahawks
Puget Sound Sports and Spine
    Physicians
Seattle, Washington

Richard J. Herzog, MD, FACR
Chief, Teleradiology Section
Department of Radiology and
    Imaging
Hospital for Special Surgery
New York, New York

Paul Hudoba, MD
Illinois Spine and Sports Care Ltd.
Bloomingdale, Illinois

Eric L. Hurwitz, DC, PhD
Assistant Professor In-Residence
Department of Epidemiology
University of California at Los
    Angeles School of Public Health
Los Angeles, California

Sidney M. Jacoby, BA
Medical Student
Jefferson Medical College
Thomas Jefferson University
Philadelphia, Pennsylvania

David Jacofsky, MD
Department of Orthopedics
Mayo Clinic
Rochester, Minnesota

Michael G. Johnson, MD, FRCSC
Spine Fellow
New York University
New York, New York

Safdar N. Khan, MD
Research Associate
Spinal Surgical Service
Hospital for Special Surgery
Weill Medical College of Cornell
    University
New York, New York

Kenneth J. Kopacz, MD
Clinical Assistant Professor
Department of Orthopaedics
New Jersey Medical School
Newark, New Jersey

Francis P. Lagattuta, MD
Medical Director
LAGZ Spine and Sportscare
Santa Barbara, California

Joseph M. Lane, MD
Professor of Orthopaedic Surgery
Assistant Dean of Medical Students
Hospital for Special Surgery
Weill Medical College of Cornell
    University
New York, New York

Casey K. Lee, MD
Clinical Professor
Department of Orthopaedics
New Jersey Medical School
Newark, New Jersey

Alan M. Levine, MD
Director of the Alvin and Lois
    Lapidus Cancer Institute
Division of Orthopaedic Oncology
Sinai Hospital for Baltimore
Baltimore, Maryland

Isador H. Lieberman, BSc, MD,
    FRCSC
Orthopaedic and Spinal Surgeon
Department of Orthopaedics
The Cleveland Clinic Foundation
Cleveland, Ohio

Randall T. Loder, MD
Chief of Staff
Shriners Hospital for Children
Minneapolis, Minnesota

Robert R. Madigan, MD
Associate Clinical Professor of
    Orthopedics
Knoxville Orthopedic Clinic
University of Tennessee Medical
    Center
Knoxville, Tennessee

James Kimbro Maguire, Jr, MD
Knoxville Orthopedic Clinic
Knoxville, Tennessee

Rex A.W. Marco, MD
Assistant Professor
Department of Orthopaedic
    Surgery
University of Texas
M.D. Anderson Cancer Center
Houston, Texas

Tom G. Mayer, MD
Clinical Professor, Orthopaedic
    Surgery
University of Texas Southwestern
    Medical Center
Medical Director
PRIDE and PRIDE Research
    Foundation
Dallas, Texas

Robert F. McLain, MD
Staff Surgeon
Director, Spine Research
    Program
Department of Orthopaedic
    Research
The Cleveland Clinic Foundation
Cleveland, Ohio

Srdjan Mirkovic, MD
Assistant Clinical Professor of
    Orthopedic Surgery
Department of Orthopedic Surgery
Northwestern University
Chicago, Illinois

Sohail K. Mirza, MD
Associate Professor of Orthopaedic and
    Neurologic Surgery
Harborview Medical Center
Department of Orthopaedic Surgery
University of Washington
Seattle, Washington

Peter O. Newton, MD
Director, Scoliosis Service
Children's Hospital, San Diego
Assistant Clinical Professor
Department of Orthopaedics
University of California, San Diego
San Diego, California

Kjell Olmarker, MD, PhD
Associate Research Professor
Department of Orthopaedics
University of Gothenburg
Sahlgren Hospital
Gothenburg, Sweden

Manohar M. Panjabi, PhD
Professor
Department of Orthopaedics and
    Rehabilitation
Yale University School of Medicine
New Haven, Connecticut

Bernard A. Pfeifer, MD
Clinical Assistant Professor of
    Orthopedic Surgery
Boston University School of
    Medicine
Orthopedic Surgery
Lahey Clinic
Burlington, Massachusetts

Christian W. A. Pfirrmann, MD
Fellow, Musculoskeletal Imaging
Department of Radiology
University of California, San Diego
Veterans Affairs Health Care System
San Diego, California

Donald L. Resnick, MD
Professor of Radiology
Department of Radiology
University of California, San Diego
Veterans Affairs Health Care System
San Diego, California

Peter B. Polatin, MD
Assistant Professor of Pain
    Management
Department of Anesthesiology
    and Pain Management
University of Texas Southwestern
    Medical Center
Dallas, Texas

Randall W. Porter, MD
Division of Neurological Surgery
Barrow Neurological Institute
Phoenix, Arizona

Christopher J. Rogers, MD
Assistant Clinical Professor
Department of Orthopaedics
University of California, San Diego
San Diego, California

Björn Rydevik, MD, PhD
Professor
Department of Orthopaedics
University of Gothenburg
Sahlgren Hospital
Gothenburg, Sweden

Kurt P. Schellhas, MD
Director of Neuroimaging and
    Spinal Injection Procedures
Center for Diagnostic Imaging
St. Louis Park, Minnesota

Jerome Schofferman, MD
Director, Research and
    Education
San Francisco Spine Institute
Spine Care Medical Group
Daly City, California

Lali H.S. Sekhon, MB, BS, PhD,
    FRACS
Staff Specialist, Neurological
    Surgery
Department of Neurosurgery
Royal North Shore Hospital
University of Sydney
Sydney, Australia

Tamara A. Shawver, MA
Media and Publications
    Coordinator
Community and Family Medicine
Dartmouth Medical School
Hanover, New Hampshire

T. Samuel Shomaker, MD, JD
Senior Associate Dean
Department of Anesthesia
University of Utah School of
    Medicine
Salt Lake City, Utah

Volker K.H. Sonntag, MD
Vice Chairman
Director, Residency Program
Chairman, Spine Section
Divisions of Neurological Surgery
Barrow Neurological Institute
Phoenix, Arizona

Kevin F. Spratt, PhD
Head Methodologist and
    Statistician
Department of Orthopaedic
    Surgery
University of Iowa
Iowa City, Iowa

David W. Strausser, MD
Clinical Assistant Professor
Department of Orthopedic Surgery
Baylor College of Medicine
Houston, Texas

Bobby K-B Tay, MD
Assistant Professor
Department of Orthopaedics
University of California,
    San Francisco
San Francisco, California

Brett A. Taylor, MD, Major, USAF
Assistant Chief, Orthopedic
    Spine Surgery
Department of Orthopedic Surgery
Wilford Hall Medical Center
Lackland Air Force Base, Texas

Alexander R. Vaccaro, MD
Professor
    Co-Director of the Delaware
    Valley Regional Spinal Cord
    Injury Center
Co-Chief, Spinal Surgery
Thomas Jefferson University and
    the Rothman Institute
Philadelphia, Pennsylvania

Andrew E. Wakefield, MD
Clinical Fellow
Department of Neurosurgery
The Cleveland Clinic Foundation
Cleveland, Ohio

Sidney L. Wallace, MD
Clinical Professor of Orthopedics
Knoxville Orthopedic Clinic
University of Tennessee Medical
    Center
Knoxville, Tennessee

James N. Weinstein, DO, MS
Director, The Spine Center
Medical Director, The Shared
    Decision-Making Center
Principal Investigator, SPORT
Dartmouth-Hitchcock Medical
    Center
Lebanon, New Hampshire

Stuart M. Weinstein, MD
Consulting Physician
Puget Sound Sports and Spine
    Physicians
University of Washington Sports
    Medicine Program
Seattle, Washington

Dennis R. Wenger, MD
Clinical Professor of Orthopedic
    Surgery
University of California, San Diego
San Diego, California

Augustus A. White III, MD, PhD
Professor of Orthopaedic Surgery
Harvard Medical School
Boston, Massachusetts

David A. Wong, MD, MSc, FRCSC
Assistant Clinical Professor
University of Colorado
Denver Orthopedic Specialists
Denver, Colorado

Michael J. Yaszemski, MD, PhD
Associate Professor of Orthopedic
    Surgery and Biomedical
    Engineering
Department of Orthopedic Surgery
Mayo Medical School
Mayo Clinic
Rochester, Minnesota

Hansen A. Yuan, MD
Professor of Orthopedic and
    Neurological Surgery
State University of New York, Upstate
    Medical University
Syracuse, New York

Jack E. Zigler, MD
Clinical Professor of
    Orthopaedic Surgery
VSC School of Medicine
Texas Back Institute
Plano, Texas

Table of Contents

Section 2: Nonsurgical Care

Section Editor: Tom G. Mayer, MD

Section 3: Surgical Care

Section Editor: Harry N. Herkowitz, MD

Section 4: New and Future Developments
Section Editor: Scott D. Boden, MD

Preface

The second edition of *Orthopaedic Knowledge Update: Spine* updates and expands the very successful first edition, published in 1997. The first edition was a successful cooperative venture between the American Academy of Orthopaedic Surgeons (AAOS) and a society composed of physicians of many different specialties whose interests are focused on spine care, the North American Spine Society (NASS). First edition successes were marked by widespread use of the text by students, residents, those preparing to take specialty boards, fellowship trainees, and practitioners wishing to keep current their knowledge of spine care. Increasingly, the text also has served as a source of core information for spine care disciplines other than orthopaedics.

The scope of this text includes all aspects of spine care, but the depth of coverage is not intended to be exhaustive. The authors have assumed that most readers will be engaged in graduate education and/or medical practice and know the basics of spine care. For context and to reaffirm concepts that have withstood recent testing, a certain amount of fundamental information is essential, but as an update, the text focuses on new information and current understandings.

Spine care as a subspecialty has many unique features. Specialists include those who spend most of their time in the operating room, those who do no surgery at all, and many who balance surgical and nonsurgical care. In the surgical arena, separate paths traditionally taken by orthopaedic surgeons and neurologic surgeons have coalesced progressively through shared organizations, literature, and courses. Increasingly, knowledge of nonsurgical care is shared between physiatrists and other nonsurgical specialists and surgeons. Communication between spine radiologists and clinicians has improved through agreements on language and shared participation in societies and educational venues.

In spite of such ecumenism, agreement has not been reached upon what spine care specialists are, how they should be trained, what they should know, how they should be tested, and what they should do. The most basic of those issues, a core curriculum of what spine care physicians should know, has been addressed best, many educators feel, by the first edition of *OKU:*

Spine. With that as a laudable goal, the second edition broadens the spectrum of authors, topics, and viewpoints to increase its multidisciplinary appeal.

Improved understanding and treatment of spinal disorders, made possible by advanced communication, has stimulated a proliferation of information available to the student of spine care. The challenge is not so much being able to find information as being able to sort through the plethora of data available. The goal of *OKU: Spine 2* is to bring the judgment of seasoned experts to the task of selecting what needs most to be learned and to present it in a concise, easily accessible format. An advisory tone results from the text of each chapter being stated by the authors without running reference notations. Following the text of each chapter are annotated recent references and listings of classic references.

While the goals and style of the second edition carry on those of the first, the presentation has been reorganized substantially and many new topics have been introduced. Sections have been changed from disorder-oriented to care-oriented divisions: Evaluations, Nonsurgical Care, Surgical Care, and New and Future Developments. Imaging coverage has been expanded to three chapters. Age-specific aspects of spine care have been added, with one chapter on the aging spine and three devoted to pediatric care. A new chapter is devoted to the spine in sports. Consideration of social and organizational issues has been broadened to include chapters on outcomes and guidelines, impairment and return to work evaluation, and nomenclature and coding. The coverage of nonsurgical methods has been considerably broadened. Coverage of neurologic disorders has been expanded to include chapters on spinal cord injury rehabilitation and primary spinal cord disorders. Two new chapters deal with surgical complications.

The surge of information and technology makes "current mainstream" almost an oxymoron. *OKU: Spine 2* is meant to provide reliable, mainstream information supplied by authors of recognized authority and judgment. It also is meant to be current. However, the speed of progress makes it impossible to cover topics of valid current interest without stepping a bit out of the mainstream. We have undertaken to do that in the new section, New and Future Developments, in which topics of importance that have not yet been evaluated sufficiently are treated.

The section editors were chosen because of their authority, their stature in the spine care community, and because of their long records of devotion to educational endeavors. Likewise, the authors were chosen because of the authority and judgment they could bring to their topics and because they possessed the communications and organizational skills needed to fulfill the mandates of their tasks. We are grateful for the time, devotion, energy, and patience that the section editors and authors have brought to this effort. Many of the authors are not orthopaedic surgeons and some belong to neither of the organizations sponsoring this work; to them we are especially grateful for broadening the scope for the rest of us and because their work was particularly selfless.

We acknowledge all who worked on the first edition of this text for establishing a successful formula and for setting such a high standard. We wish to thank the Boards of AAOS and NASS for entrusting us with the task of updating and expanding upon the first edition. Eric Muehlbauer of NASS provided important coordination of administrative support. Marilyn Fox, PhD, the AAOS Director of Publications, and Joan Abern and Lisa Moore, Senior Editors of the AAOS Publications Department, accomplished in a timely manner the enormous task of bringing piles of manuscripts into a coherent, readable text. And, we wish to thank, in advance, the members of the spine care community for using this text and for providing feedback to guide development of the third edition.

David F. Fardon, MD
Steven R. Garfin, MD

Section 1

Evaluations

Section Editor:
Jean-Jacques Abitbol, MD

Chapter 1

History and Organizations of Spine Care

Sidney L. Wallace, MD

History

Striking advances in spine care have occurred in the 1900s, but the seeds of spine care were sown millenia earlier. Almost 5,000 years ago, Imhotep recorded observations on spinal disease that were preserved in the Edwin Smith papyrus. Hippocrates, however, probably should be considered as the father of modern spine surgery, because he provided early descriptions of spinal curves and the blood supply to the spine; listed spinal diseases including tuberculosis, spondylitis, posttraumatic kyphosis, concussions, dislocations of the vertebrae, and fractures of the spinous process; and devised traction devices for reducing displaced vertebrae. Galen, a Greek physician who also practiced in Rome, contributed to naming deformities of the spine, such as lordosis, kyphosis, and scoliosis, and attempted to achieve active correction of such deformities.

From the period of Greek culture, a curtain fell across medicine in Europe and it was not until the Renaissance that new contributions to medicine and spine care became publicized. Contributions of Vesalius to anatomy and Paré to surgery paved the way for advancement in clinical observations of spinal disorders. Potts, an English physician, provided a description of the tuberculous nature of certain spinal deformities that remains the standard. Pasteur, Lister, Semmelweis, and Halsted contributed greatly toward aseptic surgery, reducing infection. Without Roentgen's 1895 discovery of the Roentgen tube, spine care would have been delayed for decades. Before the end of the 19th century, x-ray machines were in many places in both Europe and the United States. Dandy used air for myelography in 1918 for study of brain lesions only. Sicard, a neurosurgeon in France following World War I, utilized the technique of myelography with lipiodol, a material subsequently supplanted by water-soluble materials for myelograms and other contrast studies. Discography reported by Lindblom in 1948 has been used widely although indications remain controversial.

Important developments in spine care were the introduction of the CT scan and later MRI. The CT scan was introduced in Europe by Radon and Bracewell, but was never appreciated and developed until the 1970s following the work of an American physicist, Cormick, and an English engineer, Hounsfield, who shared the 1979 Nobel Prize in medicine for the CT. In 1952, Purcell and Bloch received the Nobel Prize for their work in developing the concept of nuclear magnetic resonance. The first MRI for imaging was patented in 1972 by Damadian, an American, followed by refinements that have improved and diversified its uses. Electromyography and somatosensory evoked potentials have played roles in not only diagnostic, but also therapeutic situations for monitoring the spinal cord during spinal surgery.

Many individuals of various specialties have contributed to the development and improvement of spine care throughout the 1800s and 1900s. An early orthopaedic specialist who proposed specialized spine care was Joel Goldthwaite, author of works discussing tuberculosis and nontuberculous diseases of the spine, including descriptions of disc herniations. Osler, whom many consider the father of modern medicine, published a 1910 treatise on diseases of the nervous system, discussing spine problems. New information about the anatomy of the spine was published by Small in the 1920s and 1930s and by Batson in 1940. Batson described the venous drainage of the spine, leading to the development of tables and frames for posterior spine surgery.

The discovery of the herniated intervertebral disc as the cause of sciatica and its cure by disc excision, described by Mixter and Barr in 1934, heralded the rapid dissemination of knowledge that has occurred during the latter part of the 1900s. As Mixter and others have reviewed in historic perspectives on this discovery, theirs was a completion of understanding and thoroughness of the description of a phenomenon previously recognized. Holdsworth was the first to analyze and describe the pathology of spinal fractures. Frankel later devised a grading system for the functional levels of paralysis. Dennis proposed a three-column concept of spine stability that has been a keystone in the management of spinal fractures. McNabb's classic work on whiplash injuries of the neck influenced development of the head rest by the automotive industry. King published a classification for scoliosis with risk factors for surgery that aided the surgeon in planning treatment for the patient. White and Panjabi analyzed the mechanics of spine stability, establishing criteria to delineate stable and unstable spine situations. Kirkaldy-Willis described the degenerative cascade enabling a better understanding of the aging process and the surgical management of some of the sequelae such as spinal stenosis.

Spine care has evolved through the centuries, but the most important contributions have burgeoned rapidly since World War II, making it almost impossible to list all of the contributors in this explosion of knowledge. Risser and Harrington were early contributors to the care of the scoliosis patient with the development of the Risser cast and the Harrington rod for spine stabilization. Among the many contributions of Wiltse was the classification that described the etiology and the treatment of spondylolisthesis. Cloward, in 1952, described a circular graft for stabilization of the spine in anterior cervical fusion, and Robinson and Smith, in 1955, established their technique of concomitant anterior cervical discectomy with fusion for cervical radiculopathy.

The lumbar spine has become increasingly important in the last century with emphasis on improved surgical techniques, instrumentation, and diagnostic measures. In 1911, Albee and Hibbs described the technique of spinal fusion using autologous grafts to improve the success rate of fusion. Many types of internal fixation were developed, each technique paving the road for improvement in the materials and instruments for spine stabilization. Roy-Camille promoted the use of pedicle screws using plates for stabilization. Anterior and posterior interbody fusion became popular in the latter part of the 1900s, and graft positioning was enhanced by use of the cage and implants for spine stabilization. With the emergence of endoscopic techniques, techniques using video fluoroscopy, and early robotic surgery, it would seem that there is unlimited potential for continued improvement and research in the constant pursuit of better spine care.

The nonsurgical management of acute and chronic back pain has always been challenging. The use of back schools for education of the patient, newer physical therapy techniques, and development of functional restoration programs, such as that described by Mayer, have been shown to reduce the impact of back pain disability in the workplace and to improve the day-to-day lives of patients.

Organizations

Spine organizations were formed to address specific issues in spine care, to serve the interests of subgroups within specialties, and to provide interchange about spine issues among diverse specialties. These societies provide their members with forums, discussions, meetings, and exchange of written information to develop guidelines for management of patients, to develop protocols for outcome studies, to guide research and continuing education, and to respond to public need.

The Scoliosis Research Society (SRS) was founded in 1966, the Cervical Spine Research Society (CSRS) in 1973, the International Society for the Study of the Lumbar Spine (ISSLS) in 1974, and the American Spinal Injury Association (ASIA) in 1975. Each of these organizations was formed to address certain aspects of spine care.

The North American Spine Society (NASS), formed in 1984, incorporated a multidisciplinary approach to spine care encouraging interchange on all spine-related topics by all medical specialists contributing in spine care. NASS's sister organization, the National Association of Spine Specialists, takes a public advocacy role in issues of spine care.

Other significant spine-related organizations include the Physiatric Association for Spine Sports and Occupational Rehabilitation (PASSOR) of the American Academy of Physical Medicine and Rehabilitation (AAPMR) founded in 1938, the Joint Section on Disorders of the Spine and Peripheral Nerves of the American Association of Neurological Surgeons (AANS), founded in 1931 as the Harvey Cushing Society (in 1966, it became AANS), the Congress of Neurological Surgeons (CNS), and the American Academy of Orthopaedic Surgeons (AAOS) founded in 1933. In 1995, the Council of Spine Societies (COSS) was established as a forum for all major spine societies to discuss issues of mutual interest. Currently the group is discussing the feasibility of a combined Spine Congress as part of the Bone and Joint Decade.

All major specialty societies that include spine care in their training programs regard their members as competent to provide spine care within the limits of their training. Although there are many spine fellowships, some of which are governed by a review board, there is no current certificate of added qualification or subspecialty board certificate in spine that is recognized by any of the major societies. Fourteen spine fellowships are accredited by the Council for Graduate Medical Education (ACGME). The first subspecialty peer review journal published was *Spine* in 1976, and it is the official journal of several American and international spine societies.

Current Status 1995-2000

Change is not a slow continuum of events, but can be sudden in direction and in concepts. These dynamics lend themselves to the constant improvement in spine care discoveries and in the management of patients. The status within the 5 years between 1995 and 2000 has been remarkable in that events and discoveries have increased in tempo. Research and academic pursuits have paved the way for exciting and new methods of improving patient care. Efforts to reduce discogenic pain by electrothermal treatment of the anulus; reduction of tissue trauma by coblation technology; enhancement of fusions by genetically enhanced proteins; provision of prosthetic replacement for discs, computer-assisted observation, robotics, and endoscopic advancements; stimulation of red cell replacement; improved antiadhesion and dural repair gels; vertebroplasty of compression fractures; new injection techniques for diagnosis and treatment; better drugs and protocols for control of pain, inflammation, and osteoporosis; and improved epidemiologic assessment and dissemination of information are all measures in advanced stages of evaluation at the dawn of the 21st century.

Annotated Bibliography

Boden SD, Zdeblick TA, Sandhu HS, Heim SE: The use of rhBMP-2 in interbody fusion cages: Definitive evidence of osteoinduction in humans. A preliminary report. *Spine* 2000;25:376-381.

This is the report of a human clinical pilot trial to determine the feasibility of using rhBMP-2 to substitute for autogenous graft in an interbody fusion cage.

deTribolet N, Porchet F, Lutz TW, et al: Clinical assessment of a novel anti-adhesion barrier gel: Prospective randomized, multicenter, clinical trial of ADCON-L to inhibit postoperative peridural fibrosis and related symptoms after lumbar discectomy. *Am J Orthop* 1998; 27:111-120.

This study demonstrated that an antiadhesive gel barrier was effective in reducing peridural scarring.

Eysel P, Rompe J, Schoenmayr R, Zoellner J: Biomechanical behaviour of a prosthetic lumbar nucleus. *Acta Neurochir (Wien)* 1999;141:1083-1087.

Using an artificial nucleus (PDN device) with a hydrogel core, cadaver discs were replaced. Motion studies before and after PDN injection demonstrated restoration of segmental mobility.

Guyer RD, Ohnmeiss DD: Lumbar discography: Position statement from the North American Spine Society Diagnostic and Therapeutic Committee. *Spine* 1995;20: 2048-2059.

This comprehensive review of the literature resulted in guidelines for indications for using discography.

Jensen ME, Evans AJ, Mathis JM, Kallmes DF, Cloft HJ, Dion JE: Percutaneous polymethylmethacrylate vertebroplasty in the treatment of osteoporotic vertebral body compression fractures: Technical aspects. *AJNR Am J Neuroradiol* 1997;18:1897-1904.

The technique of vertebroplasty as used over a 3-year period demonstrated successful relief of pain in osteoporotic spinal fractures and allowed early mobilization of patients.

Kornblum MB, Wesolowski DP, Fischgrund JS, Herkowitz HN: Computed tomography-guided biopsy of the spine: A review of 103 patients. *Spine* 1998;23: 81-85.

This retrospective study of 103 computer-guided spinal biopsies indicated this was an important tool in determining the etiology of spinal lesions.

Lane NE: Pain management in osteoarthritis: The role of COX-2 inhibitors. *J Rheumatol* 1997;24(suppl 49):20-24.

This discussion of nonsteroidal anti-inflammatory drugs (NSAIDs) and their side effects compared with COX-2 inhibitors shows that COX-2 inhibitors do not inhibit COX-1 isoenzyme activity, eliminating many of the side effects of NSAIDs.

Regan JJ, Yuan H, McAfee PC: Laparoscopic fusion of the lumbar spine: Minimally invasive spine surgery. A prospective multicenter study evaluating open and laparoscopic lumbar fusion. *Spine* 1999;24:402-411.

These studies were performed at eight centers as investigational clinical trials. The surgical approach, technique, and results were described.

Saal JS, Saal JA: Management of chronic discogenic low back pain with a thermal intradiscal catheter: A preliminary report. *Spine* 2000;25:382-388.

This is a prospective nonrandomized clinical trial of patients with chronic low back pain who met the criteria for interbody fusion surgery.

Sculco TP: Blood management in orthopedic surgery. *Am J Surg* 1995;170(suppl 6A):60S-63S.

This is a review of the options for surgeons in blood conservation. Several methods were discussed and recombinant hormone erythropoietin (epoetin olfa) was found to have a role in elective procedures with significant blood loss.

Classic Bibliography

Denis F: The three column spine and its significance in the classification of acute thoracolumbar spinal injuries. *Spine* 1983;8:817-831.

Frankel HL, Hancock DO, Hyslop G, et al: The value of postural reduction in the initial management of closed injuries of the spine with paraplegia and tetraplegia. *Paraplegia* 1969;7:179-192.

Holdsworth F: Fractures, dislocations, and fracture-dislocations of the spine. *J Bone Joint Surg Am* 1970;52: 1534-1551.

King HA, Moe JH, Bradford DS, Winter RB: The selection of fusion levels in thoracic idiopathic scoliosis. *J Bone Joint Surg Am* 1983;65:1302-1313.

Kirkaldy-Willis WH, Wedge JH, Yong-Hing K, Reilly J: Pathology and pathogenesis of lumbar spondylosis and stenosis. *Spine* 1978;3:319-328.

Le Vay D (ed): *The History of Orthopaedics: An Account of the Study and Practice of Orthopaedics From the Earliest Times to the Modern Era*. Park Ridge, NJ, Parthenon Publishing Group, 1990.

White AA III, Panjabi MM (eds): *Clinical Biomechanics of the Spine*, ed 2. Philadelphia, PA, JB Lippincott, 1990.

Wiltse LL: The etiology of spondylolisthesis. *J Bone Joint Surg Am* 1962;44:539-560.

Wiltse LL: The history of spinal disorders, in Frymoyer JW, Ducker TB, Hadler NM, Kostiuk JP, Weinstein JN, Whitecloud TS III (eds): *The Adult Spine: Principles and Practice*. New York, NY, Raven Press, 1991, pp 3-41.

Zimmerman LM, Veith I (eds): *Great Ideas in the History of Surgery*. San Francisco, CA, Norman Publishing, 1993.

Chapter 2

Anatomy of the Spine

Rex A.W. Marco, MD

Howard S. An, MD

Introduction

Knowledge of anatomy is the first step toward better understanding of spinal pathology, imaging studies, and surgical approaches. Understanding normal spinal alignment is critical in the planning and execution of various surgical procedures. Normal thoracic kyphosis is in the range of 20° to 50° (mean, approximately 35°), and normal lumbar lordosis is about 40° to 80° (mean, approximately 60°). The thoracolumbar region between T10 and L2 is almost straight with approximately 5° of kyphosis from T10 to T12 and 3° of lordosis from T12 to L2. Most (60% to 70%) of the lumbar lordosis occurs between L4 and S1 (Fig. 1). The vertebral end plates and pedicles of L3 are usually parallel to the floor in the upright position and perpendicular to the plane of the floor in the prone position. Thoracic kyphosis increases with age, and lumbar lordosis decreases with age. In stance, the normal sagittal vertical axis (sagittal plumb line) falls from the odontoid process through the C7-T1 intervertebral disc and anterior to the thoracic vertebrae (Fig. 2). The axis then crosses the spinal column at the T12-L1 intervertebral disc and falls posterior to the lumbar spine before crossing the spine at the posterosuperior corner of the S1 vertebral body.

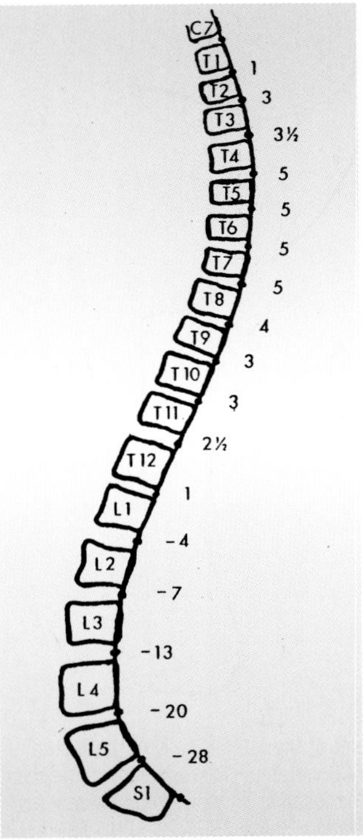

Figure 1 Mean segmental sagittal angulations in the thoracic and lumbar spine. *(Reproduced with permission from Bernhardt M, Bridwell KH: Segmental analysis of the sagittal plane alignment of the normal thoracic and lumbar spines and thoracolumbar junction.* Spine *1989;14:717-721.)*

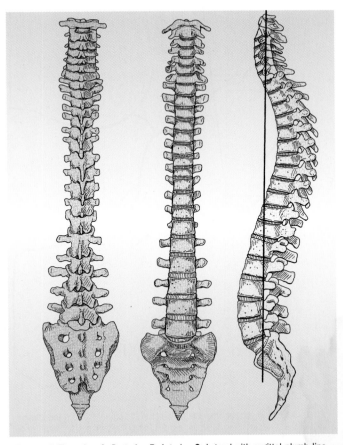

Figure 2 The spine. **A,** Posterior. **B,** Anterior. **C,** Lateral with sagittal plumb line. *(Reproduced with permission from An HS: Anatomy of the spine, in An HS (ed): Principles and Techniques of Spine Surgery. Baltimore, MD, Williams & Wilkins, 1998, pp 1-30.)*

Blood Vessels

The blood vessels supplying the spinal cord are derived from branches of the vertebral, deep cervical, intercostal, and lumbar arteries. The arteries of the spinal cord include the anterior spinal artery, which lies in the anterior median fissure, and the two posterior spinal arteries, which run along the posterolateral sulci. These vessels are reinforced by segmental or radicular arteries.

The anterior spinal artery in the cervical spine arises from the vertebral artery, which originates from the subclavian arteries. The vertebral artery usually enters the C6 transverse foramen and then courses cephalad within the transverse foramen of each vertebra, ultimately winding around the lateral mass and posterior arch of the atlas before passing through the posterior atlanto-occipital membrane into the foramen magnum. The mean distances between the vertebral arteries pro-

gressively increase from C3 to C6. The distance between the lateral aspect of the uncinate process and the medial border of the transverse foramen increases from a mean of 1.7 ± 0.8 mm at C4 to 3.3 ± 1 mm at C6. Vertebral veins are located medial to the arteries in most cases and will thus be injured more frequently than vertebral arteries during anterior cervical surgery. Preoperative CT scans accurately assess the distances between the transverse foramina, thus facilitating orientation during anterior decompressive procedures.

Posteriorly, the lateral aspect of the vertebral foramen is located 9 to 12 mm from the midpoint of the lateral mass at a 5° to 6° medially directed angle in the C3 to C5 vertebrae. The angle is laterally directed 5° to 6° at C6. Knowledge of this anatomy can help prevent injury to the vertebral artery during posterior fixation procedures (Figs. 3 and 4).

The vertebral artery emerges from the transverse foramen of C2 and then courses medially on the anterior portion of the superior surface of the posterior C1

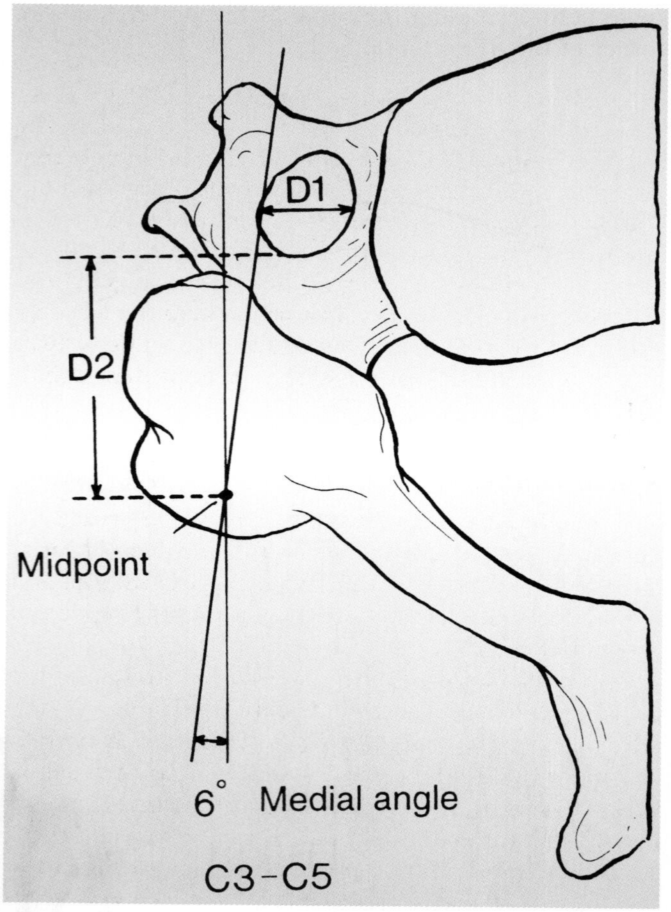

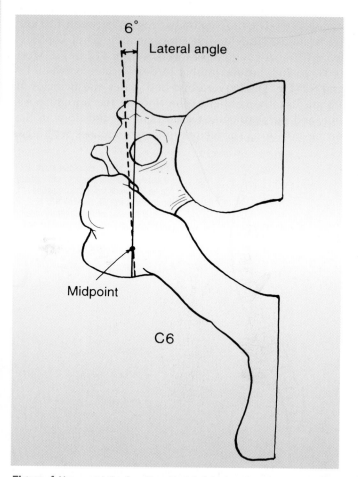

Figure 3 Mean angulation from the midpoint of the lateral mass to the lateral aspect of the vertebral artery foramen in the C3 to C5 vertebrae. D1 = width of the vertebral artery foramen measured at the midpoint; D2 = vertical distance between the posterior midpoint of the lateral mass and the vertebral artery foramen. *(Reproduced with permission from Ebraheim NA, Xu R, Yeasting RA: The location of the vertebral artery and its relation to posterior lateral mass screw fixation. Spine 1996;21:1291-1295.)*

Figure 4 Mean angulation from the midpoint of the lateral mass to the lateral aspect of the vertebral artery foramen in the C6 vertebra. *(Reproduced with permission from Ebraheim NA, Xu R, Yeasting RA: The location of the vertebral artery and its relation to posterior lateral mass screw fixation. Spine 1996;21:1291-1295.)*

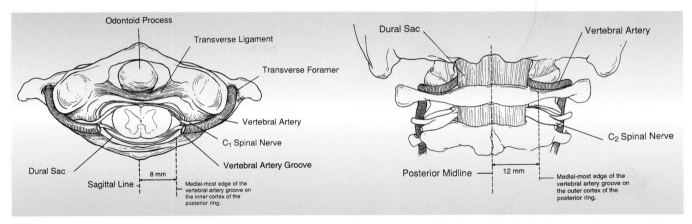

Figure 5 Course of the vertebral artery on the C1 vertebra. *(Reproduced with permission from Ebraheim NA, Xu R, Ahmad M, Heck B: The quantitative anatomy of the vertebral artery groove of the atlas and its relation to the posterior atlantoaxial approach. Spine 1998;23:320-323.)*

ring in the vertebral artery groove. The distance from the midline of C1 to the medial aspect of the vertebral artery groove ranges from 12 to 23 mm on the posterior aspect of the ring and from 8 to 13 mm on the superior aspect of the ring in adult vertebrae. Dissection on the posterior aspect of the ring should thus remain within 12 mm lateral to the midline, and deep dissection on the superior aspect of the posterior ring should stay within 8 mm of the midline to minimize risk of injury to the vertebral artery (Fig. 5).

Radicular arteries enter the vertebral canal through the intervertebral foramina and divide into anterior and posterior radicular arteries. The anterior radicular arteries supply the anterior spinal artery and the posterior radicular arteries contribute blood to the posterior spinal arteries. The most significant radicular artery to the cervical cord is an artery originating from the deep cervical artery, accompanying the left C6 spinal nerve

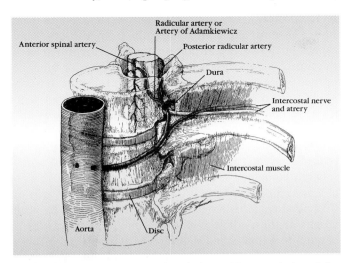

Figure 6 The radicular artery arises from the intercostal or upper lumbar arteries and enters the intervertebral foramen accompanied by the nerve root. *(Reproduced with permission from Lu J, Ebraheim NA, Biyani A, Brown JA, Yeasting RA: Vulnerability of great medullary artery. Spine 1996;21:1852-1855.)*

root. Other medullary feeders to the cervical cord are commonly present at C3 from the left and C5 and T1 from the right. The radicular artery of Adamkiewicz makes a major contribution to the anterior spinal artery and provides the main blood supply to the lower spinal cord. It originates from the left side in 80% of people and usually accompanies the ventral root of T9, T10, or T11, but can originate anywhere from T5 to L5. The artery of Adamkiewicz usually originates from a segmental artery at the level of the costotransverse joint and then enters the intervertebral foramen (Fig. 6). Ligation of segmental vessels over the midportion of the vertebral body will help minimize the risk of injury to the artery of Adamkiewicz. Dissection near the foramen and disarticulation of the costotransverse and costovertebral joints can injure the artery or important collateral vessels.

Spinal Nerves

The spinal nerve roots include 8 cervical, 12 thoracic, 5 lumbar, 5 sacral, and 1 coccygeal. The dorsal and ventral roots join to form the spinal nerve. The ventral root and the dorsal root ganglion are within the intervertebral foramen.

Within the neural foramen, the anterior portion of the cervical root lies anteroinferiorly adjacent to the uncovertebral joint, and the posterior portion is close to the superior articular process. The neural foramen is bounded superiorly and inferiorly by pedicles; anteriorly by the uncinate process, the posterolateral aspect of the intervertebral disc, and the inferior portion of the vertebral body above the disc level, and posteriorly by the facet joint and superior articular process of the vertebral body below. Degenerative changes of these structures may compromise the spinal nerve.

The cephalad and caudal nerve roots are nearly equidistant from the midpoint of the lateral mass. A lateral

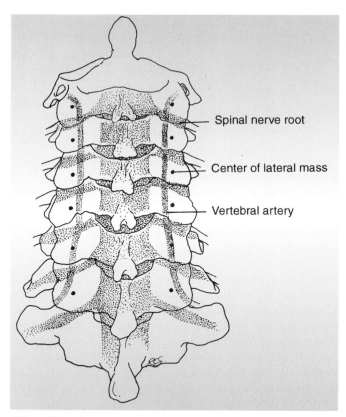

Figure 7 Posterior cervical spine overlay on the spinal cord, nerve roots, and vertebral arteries. *(Reproduced with permission from Xu R, Ebraheim NA, Nadaud MC, Yeasting RA, Stanescu S: The location of the cervical nerve roots on the posterior aspect of the cervical spine. Spine 1995;20:2267-2271.)*

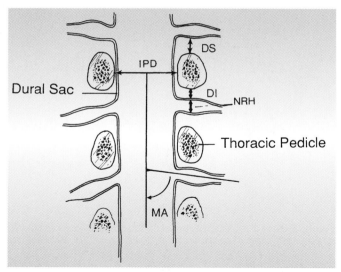

Figure 8 Relationship of the thoracic dura and nerve roots to the pedicles. DS = distance from pedicle to nerve root superiorly; DI = distance from pedicle to nerve root inferiorly. *(Reproduced with permission from Ebraheim NA, Jabaly G, Xu R, Yeasting RA: Anatomic relations of the thoracic pedicle to the adjacent neural structures. Spine 1997;22:1553-1557.)*

mass screw aimed 10° to 15° cephalad in the sagittal plane and 20° to 30° laterally in the horizontal plane should avoid nerve root and vertebral artery injury from C3 to C6 (Fig. 7).

In the thoracic spine, there is a potential space between the pedicles and the dural sac. The mean distance from the thoracic pedicle to the superior nerve root ranges from 1.97 to 3.9 mm from T1 to T12, while the mean distance to the inferior nerve root ranges from 1.7 to 3.7 mm. There is usually more than 1.3 mm from the superior and inferior aspect of the pedicle to the nerve roots above and below the thoracic pedicles (Fig. 8).

The angle formed by each pair of spinal nerve roots and the dural sac becomes gradually more acute in the lower lumbar region. The angles formed by the L1, L2, L3, L4, L5, and S1 nerve roots are about 40°, 32°, 30°, 27°, 27°, and 18° respectively. The dorsal root ganglion usually lies within the upper, medial part of intervertebral foramen. The S1 dorsal root ganglion is more frequently located intraspinally. The mean distance between the pedicle and dural sac in the lumbar spine is 1.5 mm. After exiting from the dural sac, the lumbar nerve root runs obliquely between the inferomedial corner of the upper pedicle and the superolateral corner of the lower pedicle. The mean distances from the lumbar pedicle to the adjacent nerve roots superiorly and inferiorly in the lumbar spine are 5.3 and 1.5 mm, respectively (Fig. 9). Disruption of the medial or inferior pedicle cortex with pedicle instrumentation should be avoided to minimize risk of injury to the dura or nerve roots.

Osseous Structures and Articulations

The width and depth of the vertebral surfaces average 17 and 15 mm, respectively, from C2 to C6 and increase to about 20 and 17 mm, respectively at C7. Vertebral height on the posterior wall in the midsagittal plane ranges from 11 to 13 mm. Projecting laterally from the cephalad aspect of the vertebral body is the anterior tubercle of the transverse process, which joins the posterior tubercle of the transverse process. The pedicles project posterolaterally from the vertebral body at a 30° to 45° angle and join the lamina to form the vertebral arch. The spinal canal or vertebral foramen is triangular in shape with rounded angles, and the lateral width of the canal is significantly greater than the AP depth at all levels. Normal sagittal diameters of the cervical spine are 17 to 18 mm at C3 to C6, and 15 mm at C7. The cross-sectional area of the spinal canal is largest at C2 and smallest at C7. The height of the pedicle is about 7 mm, and the width is about 5 to 6 mm with a slight increase from C3 to C7. As mentioned before, the C2 pedicle is larger with a height of 10 mm and width of 8 mm.

The cervicothoracic junction is a transition region with C7 having similar anatomic characteristics as T1

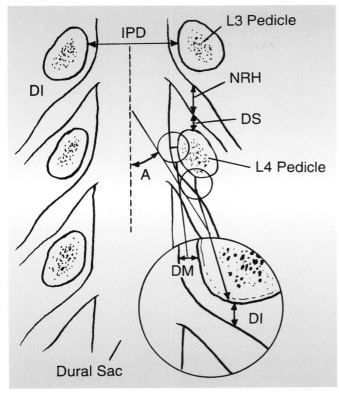

Figure 9 Relationship of the lumbar dura and nerve roots to the pedicles. DM = distance from the pedicle to the dural sac medially; DS = distance from pedicle to nerve root superiorly; DI = distance from pedicle to nerve root inferiorly. *(Reproduced with permission from Ebraheim NA, Xu R, Darwich M, Yeasting RA: Anatomic relations between the lumbar pedicle and the adjacent neural structures. Spine 1997;22:2338-2341.)*

and T2. The dimensions of the vertebral body are larger at C6 and C7 as well as the sizes of the transverse processes and spinous processes. Additionally, dimensions of the spinal canal decrease at C6 and C7, representing a distinct transition to the thoracic region. The articulating facet joint between C7 and T1 resembles the thoracic facet joint. A pedicle screw is an alternative to a lateral mass screw at C7 because the lateral mass of C7 is thinner and the pedicle is wider than the more cephalad cervical vertebrae. Inner diameters of the pedicles at C7, T1, and T2 in the medial to lateral plane average 5.2, 6.3, and 5.5 mm, respectively. Medial angulations of the pedicle are 34°, 30°, and 26° at C7, T1, and T2, respectively.

The height of thoracic vertebrae pedicles measures about 10 mm at T4 and 14 mm at T12, and the width measures about 4.5 mm at T4 and 7.8 mm at T12. The pedicles incline anteromedially ranging from 0.3° at T12 to 13.9° at T4. The pedicle wall is two to three times thicker medially than laterally.

The transverse pedicle width averages 18 mm at L5 and becomes smaller in the upper lumbar spine, averaging 9 mm at L1. The medial angulation or transverse

pedicle angle is about 30° at L5 and only 12° at L1.

Patient specific measurements, including the width of the pedicle and the AP dimensions from the posterior aspect of the pedicle to the anterior aspect of the vertebral body, can be obtained from axial images (CT or MRI). Pedicle angulation in the sagittal plane can be obtained from a lateral radiograph or fluoroscopy. Treatment of individual patients requires a careful review of all available imaging studies and an appreciation of the effect of the disease process on the relevant anatomic structures. Intraoperative radiographics often provide additional useful information.

Lumbar Surgical Anatomy

Dividing each lumbar vertebra into axial and parasagittal subdivisions can facilitate localization of spinal pathology (Fig. 10). The first level in the axial plane is suprapedicular, while the second and third levels are pedicular and infrapedicular. The last level is discal. Knowledge of the relationship of the six posterior elements (superior facet, inferior facet, lamina, spinous process, pedicle, and transverse process) to the different axial levels improves intraoperative orientation and localization. The pedicle and transverse process are the only posterior elements that reside entirely within one level. The remaining posterior elements straddle two or three levels. The superior facet, for example, is located primarily within pedicular level but also overlies the suprapedicular and discal levels. Similarly, the inferior facet spans the same levels, while the lamina spans three to four levels.

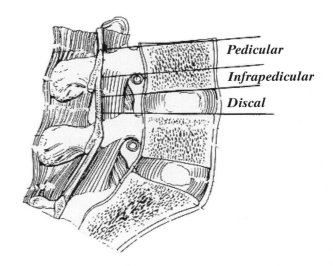

Figure 10 Three-storied anatomic segment. The first story is the discal level, the second story is the infrapedicular level, and the third story is the pedicular level. *(Reproduced with permission from McCulloch JA, Young PH: Musculoskeletal and neuroanatomy of the lumbar spine, in McCulloch JA, Young PH (eds): Essentials of Spinal Microsurgery. Philadelphia, PA, Lippincott-Raven, 1998, p 250.)*

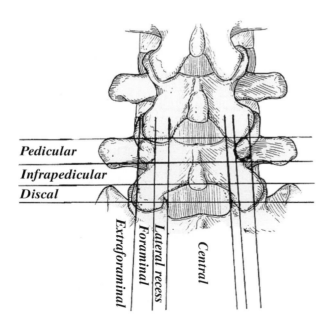

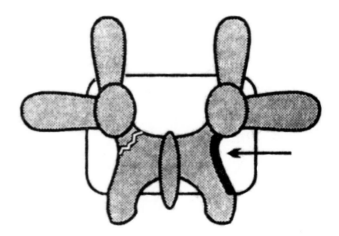

Figure 12 Pars interarticularis (*arrow*). Isthmic defect through the lamina and pars. (*Reproduced with permission from McCulloch JA, Young PH: Musculoskeletal and neuroanatomy of the lumbar spine, in McCulloch JA, Young PH (eds): Essentials of Spinal Microsurgery. Philadelphia, PA, Lippincott-Raven, 1998, pp 249-292.*)

Figure 11 A single anatomic segment consists of the disc and the cephalad vertebra. The anatomic house concept can be used to identify and localize pathologic processes. Further subdivision of the anatomic house into central, lateral recess, foraminal and extrapedicular zones is helpful. (*Reproduced with permission from Riew KD, McCulloch JA: Microdiscectomy: Technique and utility in lumbar disc disease, in Riew KD, McCulloch JA (eds): Seminars in Spine Surgery. Philadelphia, PA, WB Saunders, 1999, pp 119-137.*)

Parasagittal subdivisions of the posterior elements on the AP radiograph provide further localization of intracanal pathology (Fig. 11). The central zone contains the thecal sac and refers to the area underlying the lamina that is medial to the medial aspect of the inferior articular facet. The lateral recess (subarticular zone) contains the superior nerve root and is bounded posteriorly by the overhang of the superior articular facet, laterally by the pedicle, and anteriorly by the vertebral body. The intervertebral foramen (foraminal or pedicular zone) contains the dorsal root ganglion and is bounded superiorly and inferiorly by the cephalad and caudad pedicles, posteriorly by the pars of the cephalad vertebra and the superior articular process of the caudal vertebra, and anteriorly by the vertebral body and disc. The spinal nerve is in the extraforaminal zone and is located lateral to the pars.

The pars interarticularis is the concave lateral part of the lamina (viewed posteriorly) that connects the superior and inferior facets. It is an important landmark for the nerve root anteriorly and the posterior branch of the lumbar radicular artery laterally. The lateral aspect of the superior articular facet is cephalad to the pars, whereas the inferior articular facet is caudal. There is stress concentration at the cephalad portion of the pars where it joins the base of the superior articular facet because the inferior articular process of the cephalad

vertebra abuts the lamina just medial to this portion of the pars. A defect in the cephalad portion of the pars combined with a defect in the lamina medial to the superior articular facet is called an isthmic defect (Fig. 12).

Laminar overlap within the lumbar spine decreases from L1 to S1. An L5-S1 discectomy, thus requires less bone removal during the laminotomy than a discectomy at a more cephalad level. At L2, L3, and L4 the medial border of the pedicle is in line with the lateral aspect of the pars. At L5, the lateral border of the pars is in line with the middle of the pedicle.

Bone Graft Anatomy

The superior gluteal artery and vein enter the sciatic notch above the piriformis and penetrate the gluteus maximus. Injury to the superior gluteal vessels and cluneal nerves can occur during bone graft harvesting from the posterior iliac crest. The average distance from the posterior superior iliac spine to the superior cluneal nerves is 68.8 mm (ranging from 64 to 78 mm), while the average distance to the superior gluteal artery is 62.4 mm (ranging from 58 to 68 mm) (Fig. 13). For posterior iliac crest bone harvesting, the incision should therefore stay within 68 mm from the posterior superior iliac spine (Fig. 14). An incision made parallel to the cluneal nerves and perpendicular to the iliac crest can decrease the morbidity associated with graft harvesting.

The lateral femoral cutaneous nerve (LFCN) has a relatively high risk of injury during anterior iliac crest bone graft harvesting in 50% of individuals. In these individuals, the LFCN either crosses over the iliac crest at or proximal to the anterior superior iliac crest (ASIS) (41%) rather than under the inguinal ligament or it

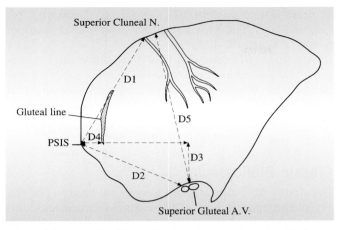

Figure 13 Relationship of the superior cluneal nerves and superior gluteal neurovascular bundle to the posterior superior iliac spine. *(Reproduced with permission from Xu R, Ebraheim NA, Yeasting RA, Jackson WT: Anatomic considerations for posterior iliac bone harvesting. Spine 1996;21:1017-1020.)*

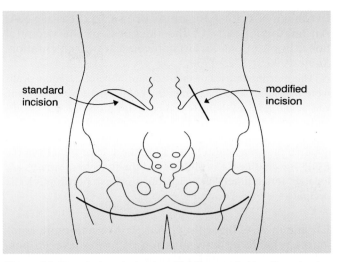

Figure 14 Diagram of standard and modified iliac crest incision. *(Reproduced with permission from Colterjohn NR, Bednar DA: Procurement of bone graft from iliac crest: An operative approach with decreased morbidity. J Bone Joint Surg Am 1997;79:756-759.)*

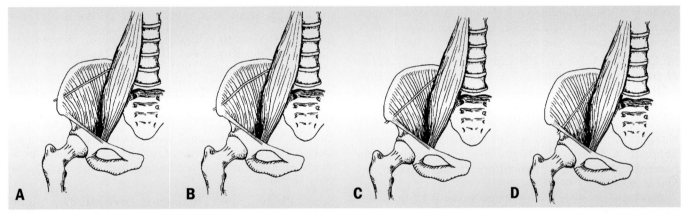

Figure 15 Four positions of the lateral femoral cutaneous nerve in relation to the ASIS. Type A nerves cross over the iliac crest more than 2 cm posterior to the anterior superior iliac spine **(A)**; type B nerves cross over the iliac crest within 2 cm posterior to the ASIS **(B)**; type C nerves cross at the ASIS **(C)**; and type D nerves cross under the inguinal ligament and anterior to the ASIS **(D)**. *(Reproduced with permission from Murata Y, Takahoshi K, Yamagata M, Shimada Y, Moriya H: The anatomy of the lateral femoral cutaneous nerve, with special reference to the harvesting of iliac bone graft. J Bone Joint Surg Am 2000;82:746-747.)*

travels across the iliacus muscle within 3 cm of the iliac crest at a point 5 cm posterior to the ASIS (9%). Maintaining a 2 cm working distance from the ASIS and dissecting on the outer cortex of the ilium should decrease the risk of injury to the LFCN because only a few individuals (2%) have a LFCN that crosses the ilium more than 2 cm posterior to the ASIS (Fig. 15).

Annotated Bibliography

An HS (ed): *Principles and Techniques of Spine Surgery.* Baltimore, MD, Williams & Wilkins, 1998.

This comprehensive text updates the scientific data and principles of spine surgery in one volume.

Cinotti G, Gumina S, Ripani M, Postacchini F: Pedicle instrumentation in the thoracic spine: A morphometric and cadaveric study for placement of screws. *Spine* 1999;24:114-119.

The morphometry and bony landmarks for pedicle screw placement were evaluated on 99 thoracic vertebrae. Thirty to 68% of the pedicles from T4 to T8 were smaller than 5 mm. An entry point located at the intersection between the superior border of the transverse process and the lateral one third of the superior facet had fewer episodes of medial pedicle wall disruption than a more medial insertion point.

Ebraheim NA, Lu J, Biyani A, Brown JA, Yeasting RA: An anatomic study of the thickness of the occipital bone: Implications for occipitocervical instrumentation. *Spine* 1996;21:1725-1730.

The morphometrics of the occipital bone of 52 adult skulls were measured. The maximum thickness of the occipital bone was at the level of the external occipital protuberance (EOP) and ranged from 11.5 to 15.1 mm in males and from 9.7 to 12.0 mm in females. The occipital bone remained thicker than 8 mm in the area lateral to the EOP for at least 2 cm from the EOP. The confluence of sinuses and the transverse sinuses are located immediately beneath the thickest portions of the occiput.

Ebraheim NA, Inzerillo C, Xu R: Are anatomic landmarks reliable in determination of fusion level in posterolateral lumbar fusion? *Spine* 1999;24:973-974.

The ability to determine the appropriate fusion level by observation and palpation of intraoperative anatomic landmarks was evaluated. The correct level was identified in 95% of patients (76 of 80) undergoing posterolateral fusion of the lumbosacral spine. Routine intraoperative lateral radiographs are recommended to help identify the correct fusion level.

McCulloch JA, Young PH (eds): *Essentials of Spinal Microsurgery*. Philadelphia, PA, Lippincott-Raven, 1998.

This text provides invaluable insight into the anatomy and techniques of microsurgery of the spine.

Nakamura S, Takahashi K, Takahashi Y, Morinaga T, Shimada Y, Moriya H: Origin of nerves supplying the posterior portion of lumbar intervertebral discs in rats. *Spine* 1996;21:917-924

Resection of bilateral sympathetic trunks at L2-L6 in Wistar rats resulted in disappearance of the dense nerve network on the posterior portion of the lumbar discs. These results suggest that discogenic pain may be transmitted by sympathetic nerves.

Tanaka N, Fujimoto Y, An HS, Ikuta Y, Yasuda M: The anatomic relation among the nerve roots, intervertebral foramina, and intervertebral discs of the cervical spine. *Spine* 2000;25:286-291.

The disc is located on the shoulder or directly anterior to C5 nerve roots, and in the axilla of 70% to 90% of C6 and C7 nerve roots. The C8 nerve root was located above the disc in 78% of the specimens. Intradural rootlets below C5 traverse with increasing obliquity to reach their respective intervertebral foramina, which can lead to compression at one disc above the corresponding foramina. Approximately 50% of the dorsal rootlets have intradural connections between C5, C6, and C7 segments. The nerve root obliquities and the intradural connections may explain the clinical variation of symptoms resulting from nerve root compression.

Winter RB, Lonstein JE, Denis F, Leonard AS, Garamella JJ: Paraplegia resulting from vessel ligation. *Spine* 1996;21:1232-1234.

A retrospective review of 1,197 consecutive anterior procedures via a thoracotomy or thoracolumbar approach was performed to determine the risk of paraplegia associated with vessel ligation. No patient developed paralyses as a result of vessel ligation.

Classic Bibliography

Bernhardt M, Bridwell KH: Segmental analysis of the sagittal plane alignment of the normal thoracic and lumbar spines and thoracolumbar junction. *Spine* 1989;14: 717-721.

An HS, Gordin R, Renner K: Anatomic considerations for plate-screw fixation of the cervical spine. *Spine* 1991;16(suppl 10):548-551.

Bogduk N, Twomey LT (eds): *Clinical Anatomy of the Lumbar Spine*, ed 2. Melbourne, Australia, Churchill Livingstone, 1991.

Garfin SR, Vaccaro AR (eds): *Orthopaedic Knowledge Update: Spine*. Rosemont, IL, American Academy of Orthopaedic Surgeons, 1997.

Lee CK, Rauschning W, Glenn W: Lateral lumbar spinal canal stenosis: Classification, pathologic anatomy and surgical decompression. *Spine* 1988;13:313-320.

Panjabi MM, Duranceau J, Goel V, Oxland T, Takata K: Cervical human vertebrae: Quantitative three-dimensional anatomy of the middle and lower regions. *Spine* 1991;16:861-869.

Scoles PV, Linton AE, Latimer B, Levy ME, Digiovanni BF: Vertebral body and posterior element morphology: The normal spine in middle life. *Spine* 1988;13: 1082-1086.

Stagnara P, De Mauroy JC, Dran G, et al: Reciprocal angulation of vertebral bodies in a sagittal plane: Approach to references for the evaluation of kyphosis and lordosis. *Spine* 1982;7:335-342.

Vaccaro AR, Rizzolo SJ, Allardyce TJ, et al: Placement of pedicle screws in the thoracic spine: Part I. Morphometric analysis of the thoracic vertebrae. *J Bone Joint Surg Am* 1995;77:1193-1199.

Xu R, Nadaud MC, Ebraheim NA, Yeasting RA: Morphology of the second cervical vertebra and the posterior projection of the C2 pedicle axis. *Spine* 1995;20: 259-263.

Younger EM, Chapman MW: Morbidity at bone graft donor sites. *J Orthop Trauma* 1989;3:192-195.

Zindrick MR, Wiltse LL, Doornik A, et al: Analysis of the morphometric characteristics of the thoracic and lumbar pedicles. *Spine* 1987;12:160-166.

Chapter 3

Biomechanics of the Spine

Michael J. Yaszemski, MD, PhD

Augustus A. White III, MD, PhD

Manohar M. Panjabi, PhD

Biomechanically Relevant Anatomy

The human vertebral column, from an engineering perspective, must perform several competing structural functions simultaneously. For example, it must provide enough flexibility within a certain three-dimensional range of motion so that the person can position his or her head and trunk in the variety of configurations necessary to carry out the activities of daily living. At the same time, it must offer strong resistance to motion that is in excess of this range in order to protect the spinal cord and nerve roots. The spine needs to have strong ligamentous interconnections between the vertebrae and strong tendinous attachment points for muscles, so that it can withstand large forces during the performance of strenuous work. Yet it needs to be finely balanced in both the sagittal and coronal planes to minimize the muscular work necessary to maintain an erect posture at rest. These and other functions are addressed by the bony and soft-tissue anatomy of the 32 vertebral segments (or 33, depending on whether there are three or four coccygeal segments) that are discussed in this chapter.

Vertebrae

The basic vertebral structure, with the exception of C1 (atlas) and C2 (axis), is the same from C3 to the last lumbar vertebra. The size and mass of the vertebrae, however, increase from C1 to L5, reflecting the increasing load that each vertebra must bear compared with the vertebra immediately cephalad to it. The anterior part of each vertebra consists of a cylindrical mass of bone that is mostly trabecular and contains a thin cortical shell. Its superior and inferior surfaces are the slightly concave end plates, which are covered with cartilage. The posterior part of the vertebra, the neural arch, consists of paired pedicles and laminae and seven processes that arise from them. These are the paired superior articular, inferior articular, and transverse processes, and the spinous process.

The facet joints are true synovial joints, and their orientation in the different parts of the spine contributes to the kinematics characteristic of the cervical, thoracic, and lumbar spines. In the cervical spine, the plane of the facet joints is midway between the coronal and axial planes. In the lumbar spine, the plane of the facet joints is roughly midway between the coronal and sagittal planes. This plane increases in its distance from the sagittal toward the coronal proceeding from the L1-L2 facet (approximately 25°) down through the L5-S1 facet (approximately 53°). The planes of the thoracic facet joints require two rotations to describe them. First, the axial plane is rotated through 60° of the 90° toward the coronal plane. Second, the coronal plane is rotated through 20° of the 90° toward the sagittal plane. See Figures 1 and 2 for a graphic representation of the cervical, thoracic, and lumbar facet joint planes. The characteristic coupled motions of rotation with lateral bending in the cervical spine are a result of the facet orientation. For example, as a person performs an axial rotation to the right, the left-sided inferior facet of a given cervical vertebra slides up the plane of the superior facet of the vertebra immediately caudal to it. At the same time, the right-sided inferior facet slides down the superior facet of the immediately caudal vertebra. This reciprocal facet widening on the left and narrowing on the right produces an obligatory lateral bending to the right that accompanies (is coupled to) the right axial rotation.

The coupled motions also occur in the thoracic and lumbar spines. The effect is more pronounced in the lumbar spine than it is in the thoracic spine and is also more complex. For example, axial rotation produces an obligatory coupled lateral bending and a coupled sagittal plane flexion. The coupled lateral bending is opposite the applied axial torque at L1-L2 and L2-L3, and it is in the same direction as the applied torque at L4-L5 and L5-S1. This difference may be a reflection of the increasing angle of the lumbar facet joint plane from the sagittal proceeding from L1-L2 to L5-S1. The coupled

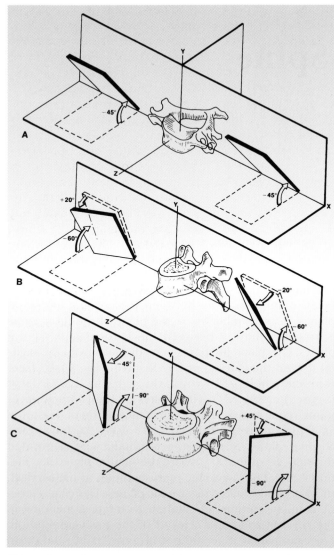

Figure 1 Orientation of cervical **(A)**, thoracic **(B)**, and lumbar **(C)** facet joint planes. *(Reproduced with permission from White AA III, Panjabi MM: Clinical Biomechanics of the Spine, ed 2. Philadelphia, PA, JB Lippincott, 1990, p 30.)*

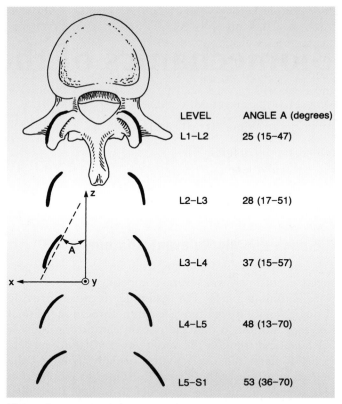

LEVEL	ANGLE A (degrees)
L1–L2	25 (15–47)
L2–L3	28 (17–51)
L3–L4	37 (15–57)
L4–L5	48 (13–70)
L5–S1	53 (36–70)

Figure 2 Variation of lumbar facet joint plane vertical orientation with lumbar level. *(Reproduced with permission from White AA III, Panjabi MM: Clinical Biomechanics of the Spine, ed 2. Philadelphia, PA, JB Lippincott, 1990, p 32.)*

sagittal plane motion is flexion whether the axial rotation is to the right or to the left. In general, the coupled motions are usually less than half of the main motion that produced them. The orientation of the lumbar facet joints imparts an additional mechanical function to them. The nearly vertical orientation of these joints allows them to provide significant resistance to excessive axial rotation in the lumbar spine. Thus, the lumbar facets act in conjunction with the anulus fibrosus to permit axial rotation with little resistance in a physiologic range, and at the same time offer significant resistance to axial motions in excess of the physiologic range. Intact lumbar facet joints limit axial rotation to less than 5° total motion. The function of the anulus fibrosus and

other spinal ligaments in guiding physiologic motion while restricting larger motions is discussed later.

There has been debate regarding the relative contributions of the trabecular core and the cortical shell to the strength of the vertebral body. Earlier studies had indicated that the cortex contributed as much as 65% of the compressive load-carrying ability of lumbar vertebrae. More recent studies have challenged this, and several studies have now demonstrated that the trabecular core of the vertebra carries approximately 90% of the resistance to compressive forces. One anatomic study suggested that the cortex consists of dense trabeculae rather than true osteonal cortical bone. The presence of bone marrow in the trabecular core further increases the compressive strength and energy absorption to failure of vertebral specimens. This enhancement of strength in wet specimens compared with dry specimens has been referred to as a hydraulic cushion effect.

The core of the vertebra consists of connected rods and plates of bone that form a three-dimensional trabecular system. There is an inhomogeneous pattern to the loss of trabeculae that occurs in osteoporosis. The horizontal trabeculae that connect neighboring vertical trabeculae are lost earlier in the course of osteoporosis than are the vertical trabeculae. This results in vertical trabeculae that progressively become both thinner and have a longer unsupported length. According to Euler's column theory, the compressive strength of a column is proportional to the square of its cross-sectional area and inversely proportional to the square of its unsupported length. Thus, the preferential loss of horizontal trabeculae has a profound effect on the compressive strength loss of the vertebral body via both decreases in trabecular diameter and increases in unsupported vertical trabecular length.

Intervertebral Discs

Each intervertebral disc must support, in conjunction with the facet joints, the entire compressive load on the spine at its level. This specialized articulation consists of three parts: the anulus fibrosus, the nucleus pulposus, and the cartilaginous end plates. From an anatomic perspective, the disc is classified as a symphysis. The anulus occupies the outer boundary of the disc and has concentric rings of collagen fibers. In each ring, the fibers are parallel to each other and are inclined 30° from the plane of the disc. Neighboring rings are inclined in opposite directions, so that the collagen fibers in any given ring are arranged at an angle of 120° from the rings that are immediately deep and immediately superficial to it. The collagen fibers in the more superficial rings attach directly to the vertebral body bone via Sharpey's fibers. The fibers in deeper rings attach to the cartilaginous end plates. The alternating arrangement of the fibers in the concentric rings provides resistance to torsional forces in both left and right axial directions and resistance to tensile forces that would tend to separate the vertebrae from each other.

The nucleus pulposus consists of a matrix of collagen, proteoglycans, and mucopolysaccharides. It contains two types of cells: remnants of the fetal notochord, very few of which remain after the second decade of life, and chondrocyte-like cells. The nucleus occupies 30% to 50% of the total disc cross-sectional area in the lumbar spine, and has a water content that ranges from 70% to 90%. The nucleus is in a space whose volume is limited by the anulus and the neighboring cartilaginous end plates. It provides resistance to compressive spinal loads by generating increasing hydrostatic pressure as the applied load attempts to decrease the disc's volume. The cartilaginous end plates, which form part of the nucleus pulposus' boundary and serve as partial attachment sites for the annular collagen fibers, consist of hyaline cartilage.

The discs undergo an age-dependent wear process that is the analog of osteoarthritis in synovial joints. This process, in the discs, is called disc degeneration, and typically begins to appear in the second decade of life in men, and the third decade in women. The degeneration process includes thickening of the anulus collagen fibers and the steady encroachment of those fibers on the space initially occupied by the nucleus pulposus. The nucleus undergoes a decrease in its concentration of mucopolysaccharides and proteoglycans and becomes less effective at retaining water. Osteophytes form at the vertebral margins, and the disc height decreases. This height decrease contributes to a decrease in the space available for the nerve roots in the vertebral foramen. These changes occur in concert with the osteoarthritic changes in the vertebral facet joints, and the two processes of disc degeneration and facet arthritis together constitute spondylosis. The facet osteophytes encroach the spinal canal and contribute to both central and lateral recess stenosis.

The degree of disc degeneration affects the load-bearing characteristics of the spine. In the nondegenerated state, a compressive load causes a pressure increase in the nucleus, and tension in the annular fibers. Most of the load is concentrated uniformly over the end plate via the pressurized nucleus. In a degenerated disc, however, the compressive load is transmitted through the thickened annular fibers without generating a hydrostatic pressure increase in the relatively less hydrated nucleus. The anulus occupies more of the disc cross section, and most of the load is now concentrated on the peripheral parts of the end plate.

Like most biologic materials, the discs are viscoelastic. That is, their mechanical properties are dependent on the rate of loading. This relationship between the load-deformation behavior and the rate of load application changes as the disc degenerates. The greater the degree of disc degeneration, the less viscoelastic the disc. Consider, as an example, the viscoelastic phenomenon of creep, which is the deformation of a material under the influence of a constant load. If the same load is applied to both degenerated and nondegenerated disc specimens, the nondegenerated disc will undergo a smaller total deformation, and take a longer time to reach it, than will the degenerated disc. Thus, the degenerated disc has less ability to attenuate and evenly distribute applied loads to the cartilaginous end plates. These loads can rise to levels of approximately three times the body weight, depending on the position of the person and the task he or she is performing. These large compressive loads represent the reaction forces generated in the disc in response to the tension in the erector spinae and other posteriorly positioned muscles necessary to balance the torso and upper extremities in different body positions and during different tasks.

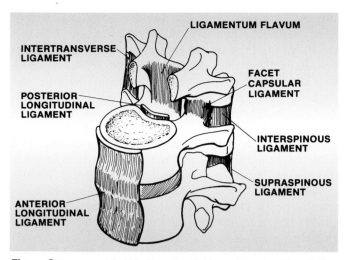

Figure 3 Ligaments of the FSU. *(Reproduced with permission from White AA III, Panjabi MM: Clinical Biomechanics of the Spine, ed 2. Philadelphia, PA, JB Lippincott, 1990, p 20.)*

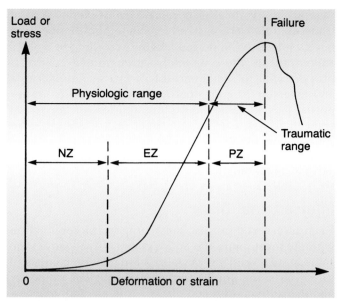

Figure 4 Load-deformation curve characteristic of a ligament or an FSU. *(Reproduced with permission from White AA III, Panjabi MM: Clinical Biomechanics of the Spine, ed 2. Philadelphia, PA, JB Lippincott, 1990, p 21.)*

Spinal Ligaments

The ligamentous connections between adjacent vertebrae from C2 through the sacrum follow a consistent pattern, such that there are seven ligaments that link each vertebra-disc-vertebra complex. This complex is the smallest spinal unit from which mechanical information may be generalized to the entire spine. It has been named either the functional spinal unit (FSU) or the spinal motion segment and will be discussed in the next section. The seven spinal ligaments are the anterior longitudinal ligament (ALL), the posterior longitudinal ligament (PLL), the paired intertransverse ligaments, the paired facet joint capsules, the ligamentum flavum (yellow ligament), the interspinous ligament, and the supraspinous ligament (Fig. 3).

The spinal ligaments, like all ligaments, function as uniaxial structures. Their parallel collagen fibers resist tensile forces, but they do not resist compressive forces. The direction of each of the seven spinal ligaments is such that they are oriented parallel to the direction of motion that they must resist. In addition, their load-deformation behavior is nonlinear. That is, they must offer very little resistance to motions whose magnitude is in the physiologic range and simultaneously offer strong resistance to motions in excess of that range. Thus, a typical load-deformation curve for the spinal ligaments has a toe region in which the slope is low, and a second region in which the slope increases significantly (Fig. 4). This load-deformation curve pattern is also typical of the FSU as a whole and will be discussed in greater detail later.

The ALL begins at the anterior aspect of the basion of the occipital bone and attaches to the anterior surfaces of the atlas and all the vertebrae, including part of

the sacrum. The ALL attaches firmly to the vertebral body edges and is less firmly attached to the anterior fibers of the anulus fibrosus. The PLL arises from the posterior aspect of the basion, covers the dens and the transverse ligament, and extends over the posterior surfaces of all the vertebral bodies down to the coccyx. The PLL has a firm connection to the posterior fibers of the anulus fibrosus, and is wider at the level of the discs than it is at the level of the vertebral bodies. This is different than the ALL, which is wider at the level of the vertebral bodies and narrower at the level of the discs. The material properties of the ALL and PLL are similar. However, the ALL is twice as strong as the PLL because it has about twice the cross-sectional area of the PLL. The ALL offers significant resistance to extension moments applied to the spine that would cause motion in excess of the physiologic range.

The intertransverse ligaments connect neighboring transverse processes to each other and have connections to the deep paraspinal back muscles. From a surgical perspective, these ligaments serve as a guide to preparation of the bone graft bed in a posterolateral lumbar fusion. Dissection to the level of the intertransverse ligaments provides an area free of extraneous soft tissue onto which bone graft can be placed to span adjacent transverse processes. The preservation of the intertransverse ligament mitigates against injury to the nerve roots, which lie in close proximity to its anterior surface as they exit the intervertebral foramina.

The capsular ligaments are oriented perpendicular to the plane of the facet joints. In the lumbar spine, the capsular ligaments work together with the bony facet anatomy to resist axial rotation. These ligaments, at the medial aspect of the facet joint, transition into the lateral aspect of the ligamentum flavum. The thickening of the capsular ligaments and ligamentum flavum that accompanies arthritis of the facet joints contributes to the compression of the nerve roots and thecal sac in the lateral recesses that are part of degenerative spinal stenosis. In the cervical spine, the capsular ligaments resist flexion moments and thus contribute to stability in that direction.

The ligamentum flavum, also called the yellow ligament, extends in a cephalocaudal direction between adjacent laminae, and, as mentioned previously, extends in a lateral direction from one facet capsule, across the midline, to the facet capsule on the opposite side. The description of this ligament in anatomy texts usually indicates that it attaches to the cephalad vertebra in the FSU about one half the distance up the anterior surface of the lamina. The attachment to the caudad lamina of the FSU is usually described as occurring on the cephalic leading edge of that lamina. There are data that suggest these descriptions may not be universally accurate. In some specimens, the yellow ligament may attach further up the anterior surface of the cephalad lamina, while at the same time extending for a distance down the anterior surface of the caudad lamina of the FSU. The ligament exists as a bilayer, with the superficial portion attaching to the leading cephalic edge of the lamina of the FSU's caudal vertebra. The deep layer attaches to the anterior surface of this lamina and may extend for several millimeters in this direction. Many of the specimens, when viewed intact, did not have the midline cleft that is frequently described, but were continuous across the midline, and had connections to the base of the interspinous ligament. The yellow ligament has the highest percentage of elastic fibers of any tissue in the body. In the resting (neutral) position of the FSU, the ligament is in a state of tension and exhibits a prestrain of about 10% over its resting length. The mechanical consequence of this prestrain is that, as the FSU undergoes extension from its neutral position, the yellow ligament shortens about 10% of its neutral length before further spinal extension might cause shortening of the ligament and the potential that it could buckle into the spinal canal.

The interspinous ligament extends between spinous processes. It blends into the yellow ligament on its deep edge, and into the supraspinous ligament on its superficial edge. It resists flexion moments applied to the spine. The supraspinous ligament connects to tips of adjacent spinous processes. It also resists flexion moments and has a better mechanical advantage in doing so than either the interspinous ligament, the yellow ligament, or the facet joint capsules. It is further from the FSU flexion axis of rotation than any of these other ligaments. In addition, it is stronger than the yellow ligament, and its fibers are oriented in a better direction to resist flexion moments than those of the facet joint capsules.

The spinal ligaments, by virtue of their location, composition, and directions, function together with the bony vertebral anatomy to permit FSU motion within the physiologic range and protect the neural elements from excessive degrees of motion. The nomenclature and kinematics pertinent to the FSU will be presented next.

The Functional Spinal Unit

The FSU, or the spinal motion segment, as described previously, is the smallest segment of the spine that exhibits biomechanical characteristics similar to those of the entire spine. The FSU consists of two adjacent vertebrae, the intervertebral disc, and the spinal ligaments. The costovertebral articulations are included in the thoracic spine. Although the FSU is the smallest segment that can be used to make general conclusions regarding spine mechanical behavior, there is often good reason to test multisegmental spinal units (MSUs). For example, certain structures, such as the ALL and PLL, are continuous across many FSUs. Studies of their effect in various loading situations might best be carried out using MSUs. Certain types of investigations, as, for example, those involving instrumentation systems, by their nature must include MSUs.

The scientific evaluation of spine biomechanics necessitates that investigators have a consistent system for communicating results. The use of three mutually perpendicular axes for describing positions in three-dimensional space, and the use of this same orthogonal system for describing all the possible loads, moments, translations, and rotations about those axes, seems to have been adopted by most investigators. Figure 5 demonstrates this system. In the figure, the origin of the coordinate system has been placed at the center of the upper vertebral body of the FSU. Any motion of the upper FSU vertebra with respect to the lower vertebra can be completely described by some combination of a translation along one or more of the three axes and a rotation about one or more of the three axes. Similarly, any loading condition may be completely described by some combination of a force along one or more of the three axes and a moment about one or more of the three axes. Thus, there are six possible descriptors for any vertebral motion: three translations along each of the x, y, and z-axes, and three rotations about those same axes. These descriptors of motion constitute the six degrees of freedom that each FSU has available for movement.

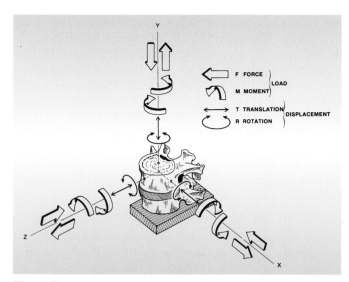

Figure 5 Three-dimensional orthogonal coordinate system for FSU. *(Reproduced with permission from White AA III, Panjabi MM: Clinical Biomechanics of the Spine, ed 2. Philadelphia, PA, JB Lippincott, 1990, p 54.)*

The load-deformation curve that describes FSU motion has similarities to the load-deformation curve for individual ligaments in that it is nonlinear and biphasic. Figure 4 is thus a representative load deformation curve of either a single ligament or an FSU. The term biphasic refers to the fact that this graph has a section (or phase) at low deformation, where the slope is low, and a second distinct section at higher deformations, where the slope is much greater. The first phase represents the FSU's neutral zone (NZ). Motion in the NZ occurs near the resting position of the FSU and is accomplished with very little resistance from either the bony or soft-tissue components of the FSU. When applied loads cause deformations that exceed the NZ limits, the resistance to deformation offered by the facets, disc, and ligaments increases sharply. This is the second phase of the biphasic load deformation curve, and is called the elastic zone (EZ). The total physiologic range of motion (ROM) of the FSU is the sum of the NZ and the EZ. Applied loads to the FSU that cause deformations in excess of the physiologic ROM result in damage to the bone or soft tissue of the FSU, up to the point of failure. This part of the FSU's load deformation behavior is the plastic zone and represents the traumatic ROM. The term nonlinear applies to the FSU's mechanical behavior because, in each of the phases of the graph (NZ and EZ), the tracing is not a straight line. This implies that the flexibility of the FSU, which is defined as the ratio of the displacement observed to the load applied at any position along the graph, is not constant in either of the phases. The spine's nonlinear, biphasic mechanical behavior assumes an even greater degree of complexity because the spine is

also a viscoelastic structure. That is, the load-deformation behavior is dependent on the rate of load application. As mentioned earlier, creep testing of lumbar FSUs demonstrated that the degree of disc degeneration affected the viscoelastic behavior of the specimens. The more degenerated FSUs exhibited more initial deformation and approached their equilibrium deformation more rapidly than the nondegenerated specimens.

Kinematic testing of FSUs shows that axial rotation is different with respect to FSU flexibility than the other rotatory motions (lateral bending and flexion-extension). Flexibility in axial rotation is characteristically less than that in either of the other motions. Two motion combinations are most dangerous to the disc with respect to their propensity to cause disc herniation. These are axial rotation plus lateral bending and the application of sudden compression to an FSU that is positioned in flexion and lateral bending. The T12-L1 FSU has the lowest flexibility among spinal FSUs. The thoracolumbar junction is thus a site of high stress concentration, which is a contributing factor to the observed higher incidence of fractures at this level of the spine.

The various anatomic elements discussed previously contribute to form the vertebral column, which can move in flexion, extension, left and right lateral bending, and left and right axial rotation from a neutral posture to place the torso in an optimal position for accomplishing a variety of activities of daily living. The next section will discuss the biomechanics of that neutral posture, that is, coronal and sagittal plane balance.

Biomechanics of Spinal Balance

The concept of spinal balance needs to be considered from both a static and dynamic perspective and in both the coronal and the sagittal plane. This section will focus on the analysis of static balance and provide a basis for consideration of the more complex topic of spinal balance during movement. Humans need to expend energy in the form of continuous muscular tension to maintain a static standing posture. The optimum standing posture is one in which this muscular effort is at a minimum. This energy minimum occurs in a position characterized by having the torso center of gravity positioned midway between the hip centers in the coronal plane and directly over a line connecting the hip centers in the sagittal plane. For purposes of this discussion, the torso consists of the thorax, abdomen, head, and upper extremities. The location of the torso center of gravity on a lateral radiograph would be difficult to identify. Thus, radiographic analyses of sagittal balance usually use the center of the C7 vertebral body as a convenient, reproducible reference point. Coronal balance can be affected by structural deformities of the spine or the pelvis and lower extremities. For example, leg length discrepancies or hip contractures can position the pelvis obliquely in the coronal plane and force the lumbosacral junction into a position such that the L5-S1 disc is not perpendicular to the gravity line. In this situation, there would need to be compensation in the form of a scoliosis to achieve coronal balance. Of course, in the presence of a level pelvis, a structural scoliosis can be the cause of coronal imbalance, and in such a situation there needs to be an additional compensatory scoliotic curve or curves to provide coronal balance.

The term "structural curve" refers to a curve that exists because of an abnormality in the shape of the vertebral body or a curve that was initially compensatory and flexible, but has stiffened over time as the soft tissues contracted. Structural curves based on misshapen vertebrae may have developed from either failures of formation or failures of segmentation. Failures of formation include hemivertebrae, and failures of segmentation include unsegmented bars and block vertebrae. From a mechanical perspective, the combination most likely to show a progressive deformity is the hemivertebra with a contralateral unsegmented bar.

In contrast to the coronal plane, the normal spine has curves in the sagittal plane. These are the thoracic and sacral kyphoses and the cervical and lumbar lordoses. The sacral and thoracic sagittal curves are structural. In the sacrum, the fixed kyphosis results from the fused sacral segments. The thoracic kyphosis has contributions from the trapezoidal shapes of the thoracic vertebrae, from the intervertebral disc positions, and from the stiffening effect of the ribs and sternum. The cervical and lumbar vertebrae have rectangular projections in the sagittal plane, and both the cervical and lumbar kyphoses result from the positions of the intervertebral discs. The reported normal values for the thoracic kyphosis in the literature ranges from 20° to 50°. The reported range for normal lumbar lordosis is from 20° to 70°.

Radiographic assessment of sagittal balance usually is made with the patient standing, with his or her arms flexed 90° forward and supported on a bar. It is recorded on a 36-in cassette. Several reference points regarding this technique have appeared in the literature, and there is significant variation in the relationship that these reference points have to each other in normal subjects. These reference points include a plumb line through the center of the C7 vertebral body, vertical lines through either the posterosuperior corner of the sacrum or the anterosuperior corner of the sacrum, and a vertical line through the hip axis. The hip axis is located by constructing a line through the center of both

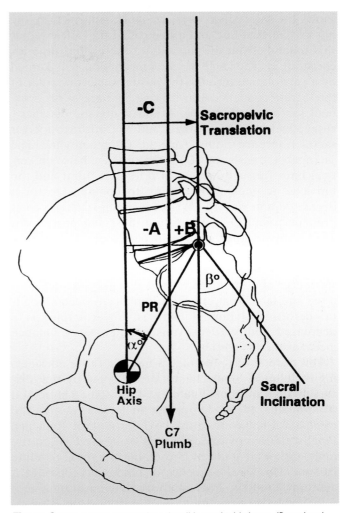

Figure 6 Radiographic constructions describing sagittal balance. *(Reproduced with permission from Jackson RP, Kanemura T, Kawakami N, Hales C: Lumbopelvic lordosis and pelvic balance on repeated standing lateral radiographs of adult volunteers and untreated patients with constant low back pain. Spine 2000;25: 575-586.)*

femoral heads and identifying its midpoint. Figure 6 demonstrates some of these reference points. Average values for these measurements are that the C7 plumb line lies 32 ± 32 mm posterior to the anterosuperior corner of S1 in middle-aged adults and 56 ± 35 mm posterior to this landmark in adolescents and young adults. A vertical line through the anterosuperior corner of S1, which is not drawn in Figure 6, is easier to locate on radiographs of patients with degenerative changes than is the posterosuperior corner of S1. The C7 plumb line has also been found to lie 38 ± 21 mm anterior to the posterosuperior corner of S1, and 39 ± 21 mm posterior to the hip axis. These values vary with the degree of lumbar lordosis, which, along with the sagittal rotation of the pelvis around the hip axis, can vary as one of the compensatory mechanisms to maintain sagittal balance.

Compensatory sagittal pelvic rotation can be described using the pelvic radius technique. Figure 6 shows the sacropelvic angle, α, which is formed by the hip axis vertical line and a line called the pelvic radius that extends from the hip axis to the posterosuperior corner of S1. The angle of sacral inclination, β, is formed by a vertical line through the posterosuperior corner of the sacrum and a line drawn along the back of the proximal sacrum. In Figure 6, A and B are the distances, respectively, of the hip axis and the posterosuperior sacral reference point from the C7 plumb line. The sacropelvic translation (C) is the distance between vertical lines through the sacral reference point and the hip axis. A person attempting to compensate for a decreased lumbar lordosis (as, for example, after a compression fracture), would rotate the pelvis posteriorly. This compensatory change in pelvic position can be described as either an increase in α, the sacropelvic angle, or C, the sacropelvic translation. One of the consequences of normal age-related changes (disc degeneration and facet joint arthritis), lumbar fusion, and sagittal deformity (spondylolisthesis, for example) is a decreased ability to use this compensatory balance mechanism.

This chapter has presented a framework for considering the clinical biomechanics of the spine by first discussing the functional anatomy of the spine's structural components, then progressing to an analysis of the mechanical behavior of the FSU (or motion segment). Finally, the discussion expanded from the FSU to the multisegmental spine by presenting the topic of static balance. This same sequence of functional component anatomy analysis, FSU analysis, and multisegmental spine analysis can be used to address, in a logical manner, topics relevant to the clinical care of people with spine disorders.

Annotated Bibliography

Adams MA, Dolan P: Could sudden increases in physical activity cause degeneration of intervertebral discs? *Lancet* 1997;350:734-735.

The authors hypothesize that discs, unlike bone, do not strengthen in response to sustained loading increases because their low metabolic rate prevents them from keeping pace with adaptive remodeling changes in adjacent tissues. Thus, large and abrupt increases in a person's level of physical activity may leave the lumbar discs the weak link in a strengthening spine.

Iatridis JC, Kumar S, Foster RJ, Weidenbaum M, Mow VC: Shear mechanical properties of human lumbar annulus fibrosus. *J Orthop Res* 1999;17:732-737.

The authors tested the hypothesis that the shear material properties of the anulus fibrosus are affected by the amplitude and frequency of shearing, applied compressive stress, and degenerate state of the tissue. The dynamic shear modulus, G^*, ranged from 100 to 400 kPa, and depended on the experimental conditions and disc degeneration level.

Jackson RP, Kanemura T, Kawakami N, Hales C: Lumbopelvic lordosis and pelvic balance on repeated standing lateral radiographs of adult volunteers and untreated patients with constant low back pain. *Spine* 2000;25:575-586.

This study presents a radiographic method to assess sagittal spinopelvic alignment. The authors discuss the C7 plumb line, sacral reference point, lumbar lordosis, pelvic rotation about the hip axis, and pelvic radius measurement technique as they relate to sagittal spinal balance.

Kaigle AM, Holm SH, Hansson TH: 1997 Volvo Award winner in biomechanical studies. Kinematic behavior of the porcine lumbar spine: A chronic lesion model. *Spine* 1997;22:2796-2806.

Disc degeneration and facet arthritis models were created in porcine lumbar spines in vivo. The range and pattern of motion during subsequent dynamic kinematic testing, and the ability of the muscles to provide stabilization, were both adversely affected by the presence of these spondylotic lesions.

Ogon M, Bender BR, Hooper DM, Spratt KF, Goel VK, Wilder DG, Pope MH: A dynamic approach to spinal instability: Part II. Hesitation and giving-way during interspinal motion. *Spine* 1997;22:2859-2866.

This study assesses the dynamic response of FSUs to pure applied moments in both the intact and unstable (discectomy plus unilateral facetectomy) conditions. Decelerations during periods of increasing FSU velocity (hesitations) and accelerations during phases of decreasing velocity (giving way) were both observed whether the FSU was intact or unstable.

Solomonow M, Zhou BH, Baratta YL, Harris M: 1999 Volvo award winner in biomechanical studies: Biomechanics of increased exposure to lumbar injury caused by cyclic loading. Part 1: Loss of reflexive muscular stabilization. *Spine* 1999;24:2426-2434.

Creep was induced in vivo by cyclic loading of the feline lumbar multifidus. This viscoelastic response of the spine resulted in dramatically diminished muscular activity prior to the onset of muscular fatigue. This decreased muscular stabilization renders the spine susceptible to instability and injury.

Takeuchi T, Abumi K, Shono Y, Oda I, Kaneda K: Biomechanical role of the intervertebral disc and costovertebral joint in stability of the thoracic spine: A canine model study. *Spine* 1999;24:1414-1420.

This canine in vitro study demonstrated that the thoracic FSU neutral zone and range of motion increased after sequential removal of one half the intervertebral disc, the ipsilateral costovertebral joint, and the ipsilateral costotransverse joint.

The coupled motions of lateral bending and axial rotation increased significantly after unilateral partial discectomy and rib head resection.

Vedantam R, Lenke LG, Keeney JA, Bridwell KH: Comparison of standing sagittal spinal alignment in asymptomatic adolescents and adults. *Spine* 1998;23: 211-215.

   The authors determined the relationship of the C7 plumb line to the sagittal vertical axis in asymptomatic adolescents. They compared this and other indices of sagittal alignment to those previously determined in adults. The adolescents tend to stand with the C7 plumb line further posterior than their adult counterparts.

White AA III, Panjabi MM: *Clinical Biomechanics of the Spine,* ed 2. Philadelphia, PA, JB Lippincott, 1990.

   This is a comprehensive textbook that first presents the basic science of spine biomechanics and then discusses treatment options with reference to those biomechanical principles for various spine conditions.

Windhagen H, Hipp JA, Hayes WC: Postfracture instability of vertebrae with simulated defects can be predicted from computed tomography data. *Spine* 2000;25: 1775-1781.

   The authors used CT data to calculate the axial rigidity of cadaveric vertebrae that contained a defect to simulate metastatic disease. The vertebrae were then loaded to failure, and their postfailure rigidity was measured. The noninvasive CT determination of prefracture rigidity correlated somewhat with postfracture stability.

Classic Bibliography

Farfan HF, Cossette JW, Robertson GH, Wells RV, Kraus H: The effects of torsion on the lumbar intervertebral joints: The role of torsion in the production of disc degeneration. *J Bone Joint Surg Am* 1970;52: 468-497.

Hirsch C: The reaction of intervertebral discs to compression forces. *J Bone Joint Surg Am* 1955;37:1188-1196.

Nachemson A, Morris JM: In vivo measurements of intradiscal pressure: Discometry, a method for the determination of pressure in the lower lumbar discs. *J Bone Joint Surg Am* 1964;46:1077-1092.

Nachemson AL, Schultz AB, Berkson MH: Mechanical properties of human lumbar spine motion segments: Influence of age, sex, disc level, and degeneration. *Spine* 1979;4:1-8.

Panjabi MM, Brand RA, White III AA: Mechanical properties of the human thoracic spine as shown by three dimensional load displacement curves. *J Bone Joint Surg Am* 1976;58:642-652.

Panjabi MM, Krag MH, White III AA, Southwick WO: Effects of preload on load displacement curves of the lumbar spine. *Orthop Clin North Am* 1977;8:181-192.

Panjabi MM: The stabilizing system of the spine: Part II. Neutral zone and instability hypothesis. *J Spinal Disord* 1992;390-397.

Schultz AB, Benson DR, Hirsch C: Force-deformation properties of human costo-sternal and costo-vertebral articulations. *J Biomech* 1974;7:311-318.

White III AA, Hirsch C: The significance of the vertebral posterior elements in the mechanics of the thoracic spine. *Clin Orthop* 1971;81:2-14.

White III AA, Johnson RM, Panjabi MM, Southwick WO: Biomechanical analysis of clinical stability in the cervical spine. *Clin Orthop* 1975;109:85-96.

Chapter 4

Bone Physiology

Joseph M. Lane, MD

Safdar N. Khan, MD

Federico P. Girardi, MD

Bone is a composite material that has a unique ability to renew itself. Its many functions include that of an internal structure on which the muscles are arrayed to propel the body, that of a metabolic unit in which 98% of the calcium is maintained, and that of a housing in which most of the blood-forming elements are formulated. Bone consists of a mineral phase of hydroxyapatite and an organic phase, which is approximately 90% collagen plus a series of minor proteins, such as osteopontin, osteocalcin, and osteonectin, that have very significant processing roles.

Bone is arrayed in a cortical lamellar format that provides strength and stability to the skeleton, and it has an intramedullary component consisting of cancellous bone arrayed in a trabecular fashion. Woven bone is the first bone produced at the epiphyseal plate and normally is found during fracture healing. When seen in other circumstances, woven bone represents pathologic bone formation. Cancellous bone is set out in plaques with interconnections; it has a much lower modulus than cortical bone, which has a clearly oriented collagen bias. Cortical bone has a large bone mass and very little surface area. Cancellous bone has a much lower density and a much larger surface area. Because bone turnover is a surface phenomenon, trabecular cancellous bone is, in fact, more rapidly removed and replaced. Cortical bone requires penetration with cutting cones led by osteoclasts and has a much lower rate of turnover. Cortical bone is highlighted by a series of osteons in which there are central haversion canals that contain blood vessels, including the artery and the vein, and a single neural agent. Surrounding this is a series of lamellar circles that form the core of the osteon. Trabecular bone is covered by cellular elements that can be either inactive bone or bone-forming osteoblasts. Resorption is carried out by multinucleated osteoclasts. Osteoblasts that get trapped within the matrix become osteocytes; they have a very rich series of canaliculi that interconnect the osteocytes and provide contact to the surface. Rapid ionic exchange is carried out within these particular cells.

The major cellular elements of bone include osteoclasts, osteoblasts, osteocytes, bone-lining cells, the precursors of these specialized cells, cells of the marrow compartment, and an immune regulatory system that supplies the precursor cells and regulates bone growth and maintenance.

Mature bone cells, osteoblasts and osteocytes, originate from local mesenchymal cells, whereas osteoclasts arise from precursors of the macrophage lineage within the bone marrow. Differentiated bone cells, in close apposition to bone matrix, are responsible for creating, maintaining, and remodeling bone. Hormones produced outside and inside the bone regulate the bone cells throughout their growth and differentiation. These small molecules as well as mechanical, electrical, and chemical stimuli regulate the synthesis, repair, and removal of matrix substances.

Cellular Control of Bone Metabolism

Osteoblasts and Osteocytes

Osteoblasts are bone-forming cells that synthesize and secrete the mineralized bone matrix (osteoid), participate in calcification and formation of bone, and regulate the flux of calcium and phosphate. Bone formation occurs in two stages, organic matrix formation followed by mineralization. This process occurs at the interface between osteoblasts and osteoid. Extracellular mineralization occurs at the junction of osteoid and the new bone.

Preliminary studies demonstrate that a select population of osteoblasts expresses specific receptors for hormones, such as parathyroid hormone (PTH), that affect calcium metabolism. This suggests that cell-to-cell signaling can occur within bone cell precursors. The production and release of paracrine substances (locally produced and locally active hormones such as the prostaglandins and cytokines), as well as calcitrophic hormones, are thought to be responsible for the coupling of osteoblast and osteoclast function. Protein factors produced by the osteoblast directly control the formation and inhibition of osteoclast differentiation from osteoclast progenitor cells within the marrow.

The more differentiated osteoblasts, located where bone formation occurs, are very active cells that synthesize and release organic matrix elements of bone such as type I collagen and osteonectin. Different endocrine, paracrine, and autocrine regulators influence metabolically inactive cell areas within the bone. Osteoblasts produce alkaline phosphatase, collagenase inhibitors, plasminogen activators, interleukin-1, and prostaglandin E_2. Lining cells, along with the entrapped osteocytes, are connected through a network of slender cell processes that traverse the microcanaliculi of bone and form gap junctions. Rapid fluxes of bone calcium induced by PTH are thought to be mediated by these cellular elements.

Activation of mature osteoblasts and osteocytes to states of high metabolic activity can result from a variety of physical and chemical signals. Activation of osteoblasts at specific bone sites is believed to occur after disruption of the lining-cell layer that covers the bone surface. This intracellular gap exposure of the matrix may be caused by shrinkage of the lining cells, which could be hormonally mediated by PTH or prostaglandin E_2. Subsequent molecular alteration of the underlying matrix may result from osteoblast release of collagenase or enzyme release by mononucleated or multinucleated phagocytic cells (monocytes and osteoclasts) lining the matrix. After cell activation, signal molecules, which have mitogenic, differentiating, and chemoattractant properties, modulate cellular events at the specific region of bone. Other unreleased matrix molecules serve as anchoring molecules to which effector cells attach and effect local remodeling of bone.

The complete life cycle of an osteoblast includes the following: birth from a precursor cell; differentiation; matrix formation; extracellular mineralization; and, ultimately, either reentry into the proosteoblast pool, transformation to bone-lining cells, burial as osteocytes, or death. Once an osteoblast becomes surrounded by bone matrix it becomes an osteocyte.

Osteocytes are located within areas called lacunae and do not have the ability to divide. These cells may help to stabilize mineral content, in collaboration with bone-lining cells, by controlling the efflux of calcium ions. Osteocytes have extensive cell processes that project through the canaliculi and establish contact and communication between adjacent osteocytes and central canals of osteons via gap junctions. Osteocytes play important roles in homeostatic, morphogenetic, and restructuring processes that regulate the mineral content and architecture of the bone mass.

The Bone-Lining Cells

Bone-lining cells are believed to originate from osteoblasts that have become inactive. They occupy most of the adult bone surface. These cells are capable of forming bone, without prior bone resorption, in response to anabolic agents and they may regulate mineral homeostasis with the complex of osteoblasts and osteocytes.

Osteoclasts

Osteoclasts are multinucleated giant cells that resorb bone. These cells develop from the hemopoietic compartment, the granulocyte-macrophage colony-forming unit, under direct control of proteins released by the adjacent osteoblasts or T-cell population.

Osteoclasts differ from other mononuclear phagocytes in their specific affinity for bone and unique enzyme profile (ie, tartrate-resistant acid phosphatase). Monocytes or osteoclasts are attracted to bone regions in which there is a gap in lining cells and molecular or macroscopic disruption of the matrix envelope has occurred.

Once a defect has occurred, after breaking the collagen lining of bone, macrophages coalesce and form a well-recognized multinucleated osteoclast. The osteoclasts are bound to the exposed surface and create resorption cavities known as Howship's lacunae. The osteoclasts effectively isolate these cavities from the rest of the environment, and the cavity environment is made acidic by the carbonic anhydrase system. The acidity dissolves away the hydroxyapapite and exposes the proteins, then acidic proteolytic enzymes are released that can dissolve away the collagen, penetrating a significant depth into the bone. The osteoclasts then move gently along the surface until eventually an extended cavity is created. When this process is applied to cortical bone, the osteoclasts create a cutting cone that penetrates deeply into the bone. Following the resorption of bone activity, the osteoclast declines, releasing it from the surface of the bone. The resorption cavity is then able to attract a new group of cells, the osteoblasts, to come in and reestablish the bony structure. When a person is young, all of the resorbed bone is replaced. In older persons, the driving force appears to abate prematurely, leaving a small deficit for every cycle of bone resorption followed by formation.

Bone Remodeling

The specific coupling of bone resorption followed by bone formation, as described previously, begins when osteoclasts are called into action at the defect site, leading to removal of a large segment of bone. The process continues with rapid bone formation by the osteoblasts. There appears to be a biologic coupling between the osteoblast and the osteoclast. Newer data indicate that components such as PTH have receptors on the activated osteoblasts.

When a defect occurs, the osteoblasts set off a signal and release factors that will lead to the recruitment of osteoclasts to the defect site. The osteoclasts will arrive in large numbers and initiate the remodeling phase. The exact signal that calls the osteoblasts into the constructed Howship's lacunae is not clearly identified. A number of hormones play a role in this process, most notably the PTH that is bound by the osteoblasts, and secondarily calls forth the osteoclasts. Calcitonin is another hormone that appears to turn off osteoclastic activity and decrease the number of osteoclasts. The 1,25-dihydroxyvitamin D, which is the active vitamin D metabolite, facilitates the macrophage stimulation and production of a large number of cells that could become available as osteoclasts. A number of growth factors, such as the cytokines and prostaglandin, play a role in this process.

Bone Matrix

Bone matrix consists of a combination of collagen, other inorganic proteins, and the mineral phase of hydroxyapatite. This is a composite material with a very close interrelationship between the collagen and the crystal. Its compressive strength is provided by the hydroxyapatite, and its tensile strength is provided by the collagen. Small amounts of water and a number of inorganic proteins are captive. Bone usually fails in tension because its compressive strength is superior to its tensile strength.

Inorganic Matrix

The primary inorganic matrix of bone consists of calcium, phosphate, and calcium hydroxyapatite material, which contains a number of substitutions, including carbonates, fluoride, and trace metals that can be picked up from the environment. The crystals vary in calcium:phosphate ratio, crystal size, and crystal perfection. Older crystals are larger and have a higher calcium:phosphate ratio.

Organic Matrix

The organic phase is formed mostly (90%) by type I collagen. The rest is composed of noncollagenous proteins and lipids. Collagen is synthesized inside the cell, and processing continues in the extracellular area. The composition of this tissue determines the structure and the mechanical and biomechanical characteristics of

bone. Growth factors, cytokines, and other proteins, such as sialoprotein and osteocalcin, play a significant role in the overall function. The collagen molecules are stabilized by cross-links, which can be found in the urine and are commonly used as markers of bone resorption.

The noncollagenous bone proteins, including osteonectin, osteopontin, and osteocalcin, have several functions such as cell binding, mineral regulation, and adhesion. Bone contains a series of growth factors and cytokines in addition to the noncollagenous proteins. These substances include bone morphogenetic proteins (BMPs), which are differentiation factors, and interleukins, insulin-like growth factors, and transforming growth factor-β, which act as mitogens, although their primary role is chemotaxis. The BMPs, which are osteoid inductors, lead to the differentiation of primitive stem cells along the pathway of osteoblasts.

Bone Mineralization

Bone mineralization is a process of depositing hydroxyapatite onto an organic matrix, and it appears to be under direct and indirect cellular control. It involves the initiation of hydroxyapatite crystals at multiple sites and the growth of these areas. It seems that only type I collagens and closely bound phosphoproteins in the collagen hole zone are able to participate in and support mineralization in vitro. There are some promoters, such as bone sialoprotein and proteolipids, that stimulate this process or affect inhibitors. Matrix vesicles, in contradistinction to the situation at the epiphyseal plate, play minor roles in crystal initiation during lamellar bone formation.

Biomechanics of Bone

Bone is an adaptive tissue that is affected by stimuli, such as mechanical and bioelectrical forces, that result in biomechanical homeostasis. The mechanical integrity of bone depends on both the bone mineral, which is believed to account for the compressive strength, and on the organic bone matrix, which is believed to account for the tensile strength.

Reductions in bone density are known to occur with aging, disuse, and certain metabolic conditions. Bone density increases with heavy exercise, as well as after medical treatment. Bone density has been found to correlate inversely with the risk of hip and spinal fractures.

Each year 700,000 vertebral fractures occur in the United States as a result of decreased bone density. Therefore, local mechanical and humeral factors and systemic factors that result in this phenomenon should be better understood to prevent and successfully treat this disease. There is a relationship between fracture risk and different load regimens that occur both during activities of daily living and in response to minimal traumatic events, such as coughing or bending forward.

It is important to understand that bones of equivalent tissue properties, but with different geometries, will display different structural stiffness. To eliminate these geometric effects, force should be divided by cross-sectional area. Thus, the force deformation plot is transformed to a stress relationship that is independent of specimen geometry. This relationship describes only material behavior. The biomechanical performance of bone depends on the rate of loading, the amount of time loads act on the bone, and the age of the bone tissue.

Bone as a material has different elasticity, strength, energy absorption, ductility, and brittleness characteristics and different viscoelastic and creep behaviors, depending on whether it is cortical or cancellous. Furthermore, the strength of a bone depends on whether it is loaded in tension, compression, or torsion. If the energy delivered to the bone is greater than the energy the bone can absorb, a fracture occurs.

The material behavior and structural properties of the skeleton reach a maximum at age 25 years with peak bone mass and then undergo a steady decline with aging for both men and women. The most significant change with aging is probably the reduction in energy absorption, which is thought to increase the risk of fracture. A 25% reduction in bone density, seen in elderly cadaveric vertebrae, results in a 56% decrease in modulus.

Furthermore, the age-related bone properties vary within the skeleton and bone type. Mechanical properties of bone have been correlated with the apparent density, ash density, histology, collagen composition and content, and composition of cement lines. However, the most reliable measurement of bone that correlates with strength is apparent bone density as determined by the bone mineral mass divided by area.

Bone is a living tissue that responds to mechanical load by remodeling and repairing itself. Cyclic loading can lead to cumulative microdamage and fatigue within the structure of both the trabecular and cortical bone. The body responds by recognizing the defect and then mounting a repair through the remodeling process in which resorption precedes formation. The process of failure with repetitive cyclic injury is called the fatigue property of bone. Activities at the physiologic boundaries can lead to fatigue failure and will naturally initiate a state of repair. The important concept is that a fatigue fracture can occur at stress levels that are substantially lower than those at a traumatic injury event. The fatigue strength of cortical bone has been found to be decreased with elevated temperatures.

Vertebral body compression fractures are associated with significant falls (50%) and significant loads (20%). Thirty percent of fractures have no well-documented antecedent injuries and may represent cumulative microdamage, which surpasses the capacity of repair and will ultimately lead to a fracture. Of the 700,000 compression fractures per year, two thirds are asymptomatic and probably represent this phenomenon of microdamage eventually leading to a true fracture of the vertebral body.

A unique feature of trabecular bone is that it can absorb considerable energy for large compressive loads while maintaining a minimum mass. However, the tensile behavior is much different. Areas such as the vertebral end plates have no clear distinction between trabecular and cortical bone.

There is a clear relationship between the architecture of bone and its strength and modulus. Furthermore, the density of the bulk trabecular bone and both the number and mean thickness of the individual trabeculae, such as in the lumbar spine, are closely related to the strength and modulus. Although bone density is not an absolute predictor of spinal fracture, the decrease in bone density is a good predictor of fracture risk.

As the bone loses mass with aging, its density diminishes and the architectural connectivity of the trabeculae declines. The reduction in density is affected by several variables, such as gender and anatomic region.

Bone mineral density is a measurement of bone mass as corrected for area. It represents a combination of cortical and cancellous bone within the areal window. Bones such as the calcaneus and the vertebral body are mostly trabecular bone. Bone such as the diaphysis of the femur and radius are largely cortical bone, but in each circumstance there is some combination of the two bone types. Trabecular bone is biologically more active and is lost more quickly in the face of a condition such as osteoporosis. At the time of menopause women lose bone at a rate of 2% per year, which represents a 0.5% per year loss of cortical bone and an 8% per year loss of trabecular bone. Thus, the vertebral body, which is rich in trabecular bone, will be the primary site of the rapid bone loss following menopause. With time, this rapid loss slows and a more gradual loss occurs. Men never have a rapid bone loss in the vertebral area, but have a gradual loss throughout life, which parallels the bone loss of a woman long after menopause. Thus, areas rich in trabecular bones, such as the vertebral body, are among the first to manifest osteoporosis.

The geometry of the bone, the mechanical properties of the bone, and the location and direction of loads play fundamental roles in fracture occurrence. Fracture prediction in the human spine is very difficult because of the great variability that exists in magnitudes and directions of the imposed loads during typical daily activities. Furthermore, bone density, microstructure, and morphology are significantly heterogeneous.

Numerous studies have indicated a strong correlation between the fracture load and the trabecular bone density within the vertebral body. These parameters have been analyzed according to different daily activities, such as standing, sit-ups, lifting, or bending forward, to show the increase in bone stress caused by these common situations.

Calcium Metabolism and Balance

The equilibrium between the extracellular and intracellular calcium gradient is essential for normal function and life. Very sophisticated endocrine feedback loops exist to prevent dangerous and life-threatening situations. Almost all (99%) body calcium is in the bone. The PTH-vitamin D-calcitonin system actively controls the rest (extracellular 1%), regulating the fluctuation of the calcium ion from the outside to the inside of the cell.

Bone mineral balance is highly regulated by the action of vitamin D metabolites, PTH, and calcitonin. These hormones control the dietary calcium absorption, bone mineral resorption and deposition, and renal secretion and reabsorption of calcium and phosphorus.

Calcium metabolism is complex and is largely under the control of calcitrophic hormones and vitamin D. Vitamin D is made in the skin when exposed to 1 hour of sunlight or during the ingestion of enriched foods. This vitamin D has approximately a 2-month half-life and is then converted in the liver to 25-hydroxyvitamin D, which has a 3-day half-life. This metabolite is also inactive and can be led to degradation by activation of the P450 hydrolase system. Any drug that upgrades that degradative system will also lead to the loss of vitamin D; the classic drug among these would be barbiturates. The moment calcium levels are low, PTH stimulates the conversion of 25-hydroxyvitamin D to 1,25-dihydroxyvitamin D in the kidney. The PTH leads to the retention of calcium. The 1,25-dihydroxyvitamin D initiates a pathway in the intestine leading to increased absorption of calcium across the gut through calcium-binding protein. The 1,25-dihydroxyvitamin D upgrades the macrophage pathway, and in conjunction with PTH, which works directly on the osteoblast and secondarily leads to osteoclastic activation, combines to produce cannibalization of the skeleton, in a release of calcium. Thus, calcium levels can be raised by increased absorption across the gut, cannibalization of the skeleton, and retention in the kidney. Calcium is critical throughout life and particularly so during the period when individuals are trying to achieve peak bone mass. Calcium intake relatively is greatest from the ages of 10 to 25 years, after which peak bone mass is achieved.

In early adolescence, bone undergoes rapid longitudinal growth with moderate increase in mineral content. Therefore, in the time between the onset of puberty and the achievement of skeletal maturity (age 25 to 30 years), dietary habits and hereditary factors play important roles in determining the peak body mineral content. This mineral content stays nearly constant throughout most of adult life. By the fifth decade, bone mass starts to decline, with significant gender differences in the rate of bone loss. Trabecular bone decreases much more significantly in women than in men. This is not the pattern with cortical bone loss.

Metabolic Bone Disease

Metabolic bone diseases represent a family of disorders of bone formation, resorption, and quality. Osteopenia is a nonspecific term that means decreased radiographic bone density; osteoporosis is a specific diagnosis. In osteoporosis, the bone mass per unit volume is decreased but the mineralized bone matrix remains normal. Osteomalacia is bone fragility in which bone matrix mineralization is delayed and impaired.

Osteoporosis

Etiology

Osteoporosis is an age-related process, which occurs most often following menopause in women and in the elderly of both sexes. It is characterized by a decrease in bone mass, microarchitectural deterioration, and fragility fractures. Occasionally, this condition may result secondarily from hypercortisolism, hyperthyroidism, hyperparathyroidism, alcohol abuse, bone marrow tumors, immobilization, or chronic disease, in which cases the osteoporosis is called secondary.

Based on World Health Organization criteria, it is estimated that 15% of postmenopausal white women in the United States and 35% of women older than 65 years of age have frank osteoporosis. Furthermore, 50% of white women will experience an osteoporotic fracture in their lifetime.

Osteoporosis is associated with numerous risk factors, some of which can be prevented and some of which cannot be modified. One major factor that cannot be modified is the history of a low-energy fracture as an adult. Other nonmodifiable factors include white race, advanced age, female gender, dementia, and poor health.

Potentially major risk factors that can be modified are current cigarette smoking and below average body weight. Minor risk factors that can be modified are estrogen deficiency, low calcium intake, alcoholism, impaired eyesight, recurrent falls, and inadequate physical activity. There is also clear evidence of genetic factors. Individuals who have blond hair, red hair, fair skin, freckles, easy bruising, hypermobility, and/or small build are commonly found to have osteoporosis.

The two most important factors that determine the development of osteoporosis are the presence of diminished bone mass and the rate of bone loss. Peak bone mass generally is achieved by the age of 25 to 30 years. Thereafter, bone undergoes gradual loss that depends on several factors, such as aging, estrogen deficiency, and genetic, environmental and nutritional conditions. Nutritional and psychological diseases, such as anorexia, that primarily affect young women are of special interest because they affect women at an early age when bone mass should be reaching its peak.

A rapid spurt of bone loss occurs around menopause. It actually begins several years before the ultimate onset of menopause, but probably represents a gradual decline of estrogen levels starting at the age of 37 years. Thin women who have no alternative source of estrogen, such as body fat, and women who smoke have higher rates of bone loss.

The primary consequence of bone loss is a significant increase in bone fractures, especially in the spine and hip. Inadequate calcium intake and absorption have been identified as key factors in fracture incidence.

Diagnosis

More than 65% of patients who have a compression fracture will be asymptomatic. Any height loss greater than 2 inches should raise suspicion of a compression fracture. The etiology for fractures could be trauma, localized lesion, or underlying metabolic bone disease. The predominant forms of underlying disease other than osteoporosis are bone marrow abnormalities, endocrinopathy, and osteomalacia.

Results of routine laboratory studies are usually within normal limits in the presence of primary osteoporosis. A low hemoglobin level, elevated erythrocyte sedimentation rate, and abnormal immunoelectrophoresis suggest multiple myeloma, a condition that may exist in as many as 1% of patients older than age 65 years who have osteoporosis. Other than early menopause, the major endocrinopathies are Cushing's disease, type 1 diabetes, hyperparathyroidism, and hyperthyroidism.

A 30% decrease in bone mass usually is necessary to be detected by plain radiographs. Noninvasive bone density determination provides information about the density of bone at a specific site. Bone density of the lumbar spine has correlated very well with the incidence of vertebral fractures. However, bone density determination does not give any information regarding bone formation or resorption. This information can be obtained using serum and urine biochemical determinations of bone collagen breakdown products (N-telopeptide, pyridinoline). Baseline and serial bone density measurements are useful in assessing the degree of osteopenia and in monitoring the progress of a specific treatment.

Dual energy x-ray absorptiometry (DXA) is a widely available and accepted method for assessment of integral (cortical and trabecular) bone mineral in the spine, hip, and wrist. DXA results are provided using the age-matched (Z) score or young normal (T) score. The T-score is given in units of standard deviations compared with bones of a healthy 30-year-old. In normal spines the DXA has a 1% to 2% precision. However, readings in the spine can be affected by different artifacts, such as the presence of osteoarthritis of the facet joints, calcification of the vessels, and rotation of the vertebral bodies.

Bone density measurements in the hip have a 2% to 3% precision. The hip is the site of choice when spinal artifacts are present. Bone density of the hip and spine accurately reflect response to treatment.

Ultrasound is attractive because it does not expose the patient to ionizing radiation, it is noninvasive, and it is relatively inexpensive. Ultrasound studies of bone density show some promise. However, they have only a 70% correlation with the density of the spine and are too insensitive to document response to treatment.

Quantitative CT (QCT) represents a CT scan through a focused window in the midst of the vertebral body. This location represents essentially only trabecular bone, and it is sensitive to changes in bone turnover. The difficulty with the QCT scan is that the altered bone marrow fat content can lead to artifacts, and there is poorer precision. The radiation dose from the QCT scan is 20 times higher than that from DXA, and it does not include the data on cortical bone. The relatively poor precision made this into a secondary method of bone mass determination, except in universities where staff are experienced in the methodology.

A new group of biochemical tests have been developed for clinical use in evaluating bone turnover. There are several serum markers of bone formation, including bone-specific alkaline phosphatase and osteocalcin. Bone collagen degradation products in the urine, particularly the cross-linked N-telopeptides and pyridolines, have the highest specificity to bone resorption activity. The N-telopeptide markers (NTx and CTx) appear to be the most specific and responsive markers of systemic osteoclast activity.

Although transilial bone biopsy is an invasive method, it is still a useful technique in understanding metabolic bone disorders. A 5- to 8-mm diameter core is obtained through a small 1-cm biopsy incision under local anesthesia. Time-spaced dynamic tetracycline labeling allows mineralization rates assessment. Three-day pulses of tetracycline are given during the 2 weeks before a biopsy and bind to newly mineralizing osteoid.

Tetracycline labels are usually normal in osteoporosis, in contradistinction to osteomalacia in which the label is smudged. These abnormal patterns of fluorescent label deposition are diagnostic of osteomalacia.

Bone histomorphometry involves the quantitative analysis of undecalcified bone in which the parameters of bone remodeling are expressed in terms of volumes, surfaces, and cell numbers. Clinical and biochemical studies may fail to predict histologic changes.

Fourier Transform Infrared Microspectroscopy (FTIRM) has been used to study the changes in mineral and matrix content and composition in biopsies of human bone. FTIRM spectra provide information on all tissue components including the collagen as well as the mineral phases. This new technology provides additional opportunity to characterize mineral and matrix changes.

Osteomalacia

Osteomalacia and rickets represent a failure of normal mineralization. The osteoblasts are able to produce sufficient amounts of collagenous osteoid, but the mineralization process is hampered through an array of disorders including poor nutrition, drug-induced alteration of calcium metabolism, and hypophosphatemic rickets. When osteomalacia occurs at a young age, while there is still remaining growth potential, there is an arrest of maturation of the growth plate in the hypertrophic zone, and the condition is called rickets.

Osteomalacia is present particularly in individuals who live in the urban northern United States where vitamin D deficiency can occur. The single most common cause of this syndrome is the failure to maintain a calcium-phosphorus serum level sufficient to promote normal mineralization of the newly formed bone. Entities that can alter this balance include nutritional deficiency, gastrointestinal absorption defects, renal diseases such as tubular acidosis or defects (renal phosphate leak), or renal osteodystrophy. Several pharmacologic agents, such as anticonvulsant medication, can cause excessive destruction of the vitamin D metabolite.

The diagnoses of osteomalacia and rickets are made from a combination of serum, urine, and biopsy assays. The classic osteomalacia is associated with low normal calcium, low phosphate, high PTH, low 25-hydroxyvitamin D, and high alkaline phosphatase (bone alkaline phosphatase). When a patient has a fracture, the alkaline phosphatase will ultimately become elevated after 5 days, but if the patient has an elevated alkaline phosphatase level, osteomalacia should be ruled out. Urinary changes would include a low urinary calcium in the usual nutritional forms, and a biopsy demonstrates widened osteoid and altered as well as delayed mineralization properties.

Renal osteodystrophy is the final stage in chronic renal failure and is a relatively common cause of osteomalacia in adults. Glomerular disease, infections such as nephrotic syndrome, diabetic renal disease, vascular renal disease, and hypertensive renal disease are among those that can lead to renal osteodystrophy. There is a high retention of phosphate, and if the combined calcium phosphate product is increased spontaneous mineralization can occur throughout the body. Renal disease is associated with a secondary hyperparathyroidism that can manifest itself through brown tumors, frequent fractures, osteopenia, and scalloping of the ribs and the fingers in response to poor calcium levels. The hyperparathyroidism can be resolved partially by treating the patient with calcium carbonate that will bind the phosphate and keep the calcium levels reasonable. If hyperparathyroidism becomes destructive, particularly in multiple fractures and bone changes, then a parathyroidectomy is warranted. One of the side effects of a parathyroidectomy is underactive bone with cumulative microdamage. Patients with renal failure, particularly those on dialysis, have a higher rate of infection and represent significant risk for surgical intervention.

Endocrinopathies Affecting Bone

Common endocrinopathies other than premature menopause that affect bone include: glucocorticoid excess, type 1 diabetes, hyperparathryoidism, and hyperthyroidism. Adrenal tumors are rare but iatrogenic hypercortisolism and Cushing's disease are common. Sources of cortisone commonly are present in rheumatic diseases, asthma, skin diseases, and bowel inflammatory diseases. Excessive steroids lead to decreased calcium absorption across the gut, increased urinary excretion of calcium, decreased bone formation, and increased bone resorption that partially is related to secondary hyperparathyroidism. Type 1 diabetes is associated with bone loss partially related to negative nitrogen imbalance and frequent calciuria. Hyperparathyroidism leads to significant bony changes including brown tumors, scalloping along the fingers, and subperiosteal resorption. It is also related to increased bone resorption, and it is best measured by a high N-telopeptide level, which is a marker of increased bone turnover, and an intact PTH. Hyperthyroidism can occur spontaneously or can be iatrogenic. Often patients who have been treated for hypothyroidism will gradually increase their doses of thyroid until it becomes excessive. This can best be detected by an elevated thyrotropin-stimulating hormone. The high turnover state leads to a little loss of bone, every modeling unit goes through its full course of activity, and it never replaces the bone that has been lost.

Paget's Disease

In Paget's disease there is a high turnover state of bone, which can occur in one or many locations and leads to deformity and fracture. The etiology of Paget's disease is not clear although there is a high association with viral particles in the osteoclasts. Bone resorption occurs as an initial stage followed by formation. There is a high turnover state with reversal zones leading to a distorted matrix in a mosaic pattern within the bone. Common findings are of an enlarged skull, a deformity of veins in the bone, and stress fractures. The disease usually starts in one end of the bone and progresses to the other. Within the spine, the vertebral body is enlarged and the disease can lead to spinal stenosis and compression fractures. It is recognized by increased amounts of bone collagen breakdown products and a high level of alkaline phosphatase. Paget's disease responds well to antiresorptive therapy. The severe complication of sarcomatous degeneration is extremely rare, occurring in less than 0.1%. Patients with Paget's sarcoma in the axial site have an extremely grim prognosis, whereas patients with Paget's sarcoma occurring in the humerus have a chance of long-term survival approaching 30%.

Current treatments are focused on decreasing osteoclastic activities. This can be achieved with either bisphosphonates or calcitonin. The indications for medical treatment are bone pain, spinal stenosis, prevention of fractures or deformity, or treatment of high-output congestive heart failure.

Bibliography

Cellular Control of Metabolism

Ducy P, Schinke T, Karsentry G: The osteoblast: A sophisticated fibroblast under central surveillance. *Science* 2000;289:1501-1504.

Bone Biomechanics and Microstructure

Martin RB: Toward a unifying theory of bone remodeling. *Bone* 2000;26:1-6.

Myers ER, Wilson SE: Biomechanics of osteoporosis and vertebral fracture. *Spine* 1997;22(suppl 24):25S-31S.

Osteoporosis

Eyre DR: Bone biomarkers as tools in osteoporosis management. *Spine* 1997;22(suppl 24):17S-24S.

Glaser DL, Kaplan FS: Osteoporosis: Definition and clinical presentation. *Spine* 1997;22(suppl 24):12S-16S.

Lane JM, Riley EH, Wirganowicz PZ: Osteoporosis: Diagnosis and treatment. *J Bone Joint Surg Am* 1996;78: 618-632.

Lane JM: Osteoporosis: Medical prevention and treatment. *Spine* 1997;22(suppl 24):32S-37S.

Lane JM, Russell L, Khan SN: Osteoporosis. *Clin Orthop* 2000;372:139-150.

Melton LJ III: Epidemiology of spinal osteoporosis. *Spine* 1997;22(suppl 24):2S-11S.

Paschalis EP, Betts F, DiCarlo E, Mendelsohn R, Boskey AL: FTIR Microspectroscopic analysis of human iliac crest biopsies from untreated osteoporotic bone. *Calcif Tissue Int* 1997;61:487-492.

Paschalis EP, Betts F, DiCarlo E, Mendelsohn R, Boskey AL: FTIR Microspectroscopic analysis of normal human cortical and trabecular bone. *Calcif Tissue Int* 1997;61:480-486

Rodan GA, Martin TJ: Therapeutic approaches to bone diseases. *Science* 2000;289:1508-1514.

Rapuri PB, Gallager JC, Balhorn KE, Ryschon KL: Smoking and bone metabolism in elderly women. *Bone* 2000;27:429-436.

Warren MP, Stiehl AL: Exercise and female adolescents: Effects on the reproductive and skeletal system. *J Am Med Womens Assoc* 1999;54:115-120,138.

Classic Bibliography

Akesson K, Vergnaud P, Gineyts E, Delmas PD, Obrant KJ: Impairment of bone turnover in elderly women with hip fracture. *Calcif Tissue Int* 1993;53:162-169.

Bailey AJ, Wotton SF, Sims TJ, Thompson PW: Biochemical changes in the collagen of human osteoporotic bone matrix. *Connect Tissue Res* 1993;29:119-132.

Patterson BM, Cornell CN, Carbone B, Levine B, Chapman D: Protein depletion and metabolic stress in elderly patients who have a fracture of the hip. *J Bone Joint Surg Am* 1992;74:251-260.

Teitlebaum SL: Bone resorption of osteoclasts. *Science* 2000;289:1504-1508.

Chapter 5

Nerve Root Pathophysiology

Kjell Olmarker, MD, PhD

Björn Rydevik, MD, PhD

Radicular pain syndromes are common and disabling features of various degenerative spinal disorders. Mechanical nerve root compression is identified as one important pathomechanism of radicular pain, however, nerve root compression can exist without pain. Myelographic, CT, and MRI studies have demonstrated that disc herniation and spinal stenosis exist in at least 20% to 30% of individuals without any symptoms of radicular pain. It also has been reported that during spine surgery under local anesthesia, only irritated or inflamed nerve roots elicit radicular pain by mechanical compression or traction. These and other observations indicate not only that mechanical nerve root deformation is related to sciatic pain production, but also that secondary tissue changes are likely to play crucial roles in the pathomechanisms of pain production. Biochemically induced irritation of nerve roots by nucleus pulposus seems to be important in this regard. The literature on peripheral nerve compression cannot be directly extrapolated to spinal nerve root pathophysiology because the anatomic, biomechanical, and physiologic properties of nerve roots are different.

Anatomy

Spinal nerve roots are relatively well protected from external trauma (Fig. 1). Nerve roots are covered only by a permeable, thin membranous structure, the root sheath, and lack both the epineurium and the perineurium of the peripheral nerves. Nerve root collagen content is sparse relative to that of the peripheral nerves. The nerve fibers are parallel in nerve roots, in contrast to the plexiform pattern in the peripheral nerves. These microscopic properties of the nerve roots can be related to their biomechanical characteristics, which also are different from those of the peripheral nerves. In general, nerve roots are more susceptible to mechanical deformation than peripheral nerves, probably because the connective tissue layers of nerve roots are not as well developed.

The position of the dorsal root ganglion (DRG), a structure important to pain production, is not constant; it can be in the spinal canal, in the intervertebral foramen, or outside the foramen. The size of the DRG varies with the vertebral level. The largest are the L5 and S1

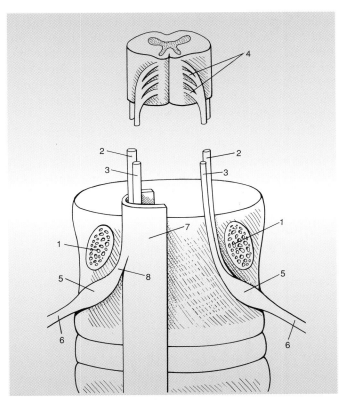

Figure 1 Drawing of the intraspinal course of a human lumbar spinal nerve root segment. The vertebral arches have been removed by cutting the pedicles (1), and the opened spinal canal can be viewed from behind. The ventral (2) and dorsal (3) nerve roots leave the spinal cord as small rootlets (4) that caudally converge into a common nerve root trunk. Just before it leaves the spinal canal, there is an enlargement of the dorsal nerve root, called the DRG (5). Caudal to the DRG, the ventral and dorsal nerve roots mix and form the spinal nerve (6). The spinal dura encloses the nerve roots both as a central cylindrical sac (7) and as separate extensions called root sleeves (8). *(Reproduced with permission from Olmarker K, Hasue M: Classification and pathophysiology of spinal pain syndromes, in Weinstein JN, Rydevik BL, Volker KH, Sonntag VKG (eds): The Essentials of the Spine. New York, NY, Raven Press, 1995.)*

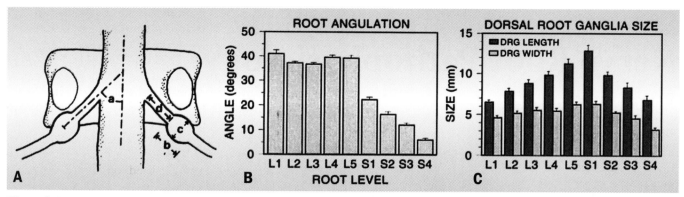

Figure 2 A, Measurement of root takeoff angle (a), DRG length (b), DRG width (c), and distance of proximal ganglia border to root axilla (d). **B,** Relationship of root take-off angle in the coronal plane to vertebral level (mean ± SE, n = 20). **C,** Relationship between DRG length and width and vertebral level (mean ± SE, n = 20). *(Reproduced with permission from Cohen MS, Wall EJ, Brown RB, et al: Cauda equina anatomy: Part II. Extrathecal nerve roots and dorsal ganglia. Spine 1990;15:1248-1251.)*

ganglia, which are about 5 to 6 mm wide and about 11 to 13 mm long (Fig. 2).

Individual variations occur in the degree in which the dura mater and root sleeve are fixed to surrounding skeletal and ligamentous structures. A nerve root that is relatively well fixed to the surrounding tissues, for example, by the Hoffman ligaments, may become stretched and compressed more easily than a nerve root that is more mobile. Blockage of physiologic body movements by a herniated disc or bony entrapment may result in radicular pain and neurologic deficits.

The dura mater and its root sleeve are innervated, especially on the ventral side of the dura. The nerve roots have intrinsic nerves (nervi nervorum) located mainly along the blood vessels, containing both somatic and sympathetic nerve fibers.

Vascularity

Nerve roots receive blood distally from branches of segmental arteries and proximally from branches of the coronal vessels of the spinal cord. The distal arterial branch to the dorsal root forms a ganglionic plexus within the DRG. The vascular network of spinal nerve roots of the cauda equina generally seems not as rich as the vascular supply of peripheral nerves. However, the spinal nerve roots of the cauda equina derive some of their nutritional supply via diffusion from the cerebrospinal fluid (CSF).

In the wall of the endoneurial capillaries of peripheral nerves, there is a diffusion barrier called the blood-nerve barrier, which is similar to the blood-brain barrier of the central nervous system. A corresponding diffusion barrier does not exist in the DRGs because the capillaries of the DRGs are fenestrated. Thus, the permeability of DRG microvessels in the normal state is higher than the endoneurial microvascular permeability of both peripheral nerves and nerve roots. These

anatomic characteristics predispose the DRGs to edema as a result, for example, of mechanical compression.

Physiology

The central and peripheral nervous systems are connected anatomically and physiologically through the spinal nerve roots (Fig. 3). Axonal transport systems, anterograde and retrograde, play important roles in maintaining the functional and structural integrity of the spinal nerve roots and peripheral nerves. The normal DRG can produce spontaneous ectopic discharges and reflected impulses that are similar to mechanically induced discharges. Anatomic variations in the position of the DRGs must be considered in this regard. The normal nerve root does not produce any such discharges. At the nerve endings and synapses in the spinal cord, nociception occurs via complicated mechanisms involving several pain-producing substances and neuropeptides. The DRG is an important site for synthesis

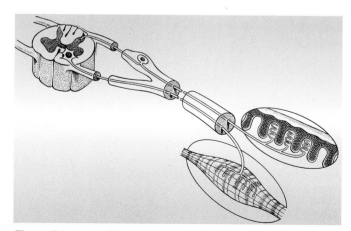

Figure 3 A segment of the spinal cord, the motor (ventral) and sensory (dorsal) nerve roots, the dorsal root ganglion, the spinal nerve, and the peripheral nerve with target organs for the innervation. *(Reproduced with permission from Lundborg G: Nerve regeneration and repair: A review. Acta Orthop Scand 1987;58:145-169.)*

of neuropeptides, such as substance P and calcitonin gene-related peptide, as well as other substances that are transported both centrally and peripherally by the axonal transport systems.

Biomechanics

Compression and stretching of spinal nerve roots affects all tissue components of the roots—nerve fibers, connective tissue, and blood vessels—each of which has distinct mechanical properties and reactions to the mechanical deformation. Nerve roots successfully adapt to mechanical deformation within certain limits; however, if the deformation exceeds those limits, both functional and structural changes may occur. The biomechanics of nerve root deformation in association with spinal stenosis are different from those with disc herniation. Spinal stenosis is generally a slowly developing process during which the nerve roots are compressed in a circumferential manner at slow rate. Moreover, the compression is dynamic and intermittent, varying with posture and often occurring at more than one site along the root. In a dorsolateral lumbar disc herniation, there is more focal compression, flattening of the nerve root, and intraneural tension. Lumbar disc herniation, thus, often is accompanied by both compression and tension of the nerve roots.

To study the mechanics of nerve root involvement in association with central lumbar spinal stenosis, the dural sac and the enclosed cauda equina of human cadaver spines were constricted with a round clamp. Results indicated that the cross-sectional area of the dural sac at the L3-L4 level has to be reduced to about 75 mm^2 (representing 45% of the normal value of approximately 170 mm^2) before constriction results in compression of the cauda equina nerve roots and displacement of the CSF from the dural sac constriction site. A pressure level of about 50 mm Hg among the nerve roots of the cauda equina can be induced experimentally by constricting the dural sac to a cross-sectional area of approximately 65 mm^2. The values reported here, especially the so-called critical area of the dural sac, 75 mm^2, can be used as critical values for the radiologic diagnosis of central spinal stenosis.

In a dog model, the cauda equina was acutely constricted circumferentially to 75%, 50%, or 25% of its normal cross-sectional area. Up to 3 months after surgery, constriction to 75% of the normal area of the dural sac did not cause any neurologic deficits. However, with constriction limited to 50% or 25% of the normal cross-sectional dural sac area, there were changes in both motor and sensory function and structural injuries to the nerve roots.

Spinal nerve root dysfunction is related not only to pressure level and duration of compression, but also to the onset rate of compression. At corresponding compression pressure levels, a rapid onset (0.05 to 0.1 s) causes much more pronounced tissue changes and functional deterioration than does a slow onset (20 s). Moreover, a rapid onset induces more pronounced changes than does a slow onset in terms of nerve root edema, impairment of nutritional transport, and changes in impulse conduction. These rate-dependent physiologic effects are probably based on the viscoelastic properties of the nerve root tissues.

Locally compressed nerve fibers are displaced from the center of the compressed area toward the noncompressed areas. Such longitudinal displacement, maximum at the edges of the compressed segment, is called the edge effect. At the edges where the mechanical deformation is maximum, damage to both nerve fibers and intraneural microvessels is most pronounced. Tissue damage is less likely to occur where the hydrostatic pressure in the nerve tissue is the highest (ie, in the center).

Biologic Effects of Nerve Root Compression

Compression of spinal nerve roots can induce numbness, pain, and muscle weakness. Critical pressure levels have been analyzed in an in vivo compression model of the porcine cauda equina, achieved by an inflatable balloon placed across the surgically exposed spinal canal. The effects of graded compression on blood flow, nutritional supply, and nerve root impulse conduction were analyzed. Even at low pressure levels (5 to 10 mm Hg) compression induced changes in the intraneural microcirculation, especially in terms of reduced venular blood flow. Total ischemia of the compressed nerve root segment occurred at pressure levels close to the mean arterial blood pressure. Compression of the porcine cauda equina at two levels induces ischemia not only at the locations of compression but also in the nerve root segments between the two compressed sites, and functional changes were more pronounced with two-level compression than with one-level compression at corresponding pressure levels.

The intrinsic blood vessels of the nerve roots react to mechanical injury by increased permeability and edema formation, which may increase endoneurial fluid pressure. Such a mechanism has been demonstrated following experimental mechanical compression of the DRG, which led to a miniature closed compartment syndrome.

Effects of experimentally induced graded compression on nerve root impulse propagation have shown an acute pressure threshold for changes in spinal nerve root impulse conduction between 50 and 75 mm Hg.

Higher pressure levels, for example, 100 to 200 mm Hg, lead to more pronounced changes in nerve root function. Function of motor nerve roots recovers more rapidly and more completely than that of the sensory nerve roots after pressure release. Thus, local compression of the cauda equina may injure sensory nerve roots to a greater extent than motor nerve roots. Systemic hypotension may increase the susceptibility of the nerve roots of the cauda equina to compression.

Edema from chronic nerve root compression may cause fibrosis in and around nerve roots, resulting in structural nerve-fiber damage. Chronic nerve root compression may also result in changes in neuropeptides, such as substance P, in the DRG. Experimental chronic nerve-root irritation has also been shown to cause behavioral changes related to neuropeptide dynamics in nerve roots and DRGs as well as *c-fos* gene expression in the spinal cord. These observations may provide a biologic basis for the involvement of the central nervous system in certain chronic nerve root compression disorders.

Acute compression of a nerve root produces only a few seconds of repetitive firing, whereas acute compression of the DRG leads to a general response with many minutes of activity in the axons. Chronically injured dorsal roots, however, are more sensitive and may produce several minutes of repetitive firing in axons of all sizes following acute compression. These observations may explain why irritation of the neural structures is a prerequisite for the occurrence of a neurophysiologic response related to pain.

Radicular pain with a characteristic distribution of pain and neurologic deficit, in the absence of disc herniation, indicates that mechanical compression per se is not the only mechanism underlying pain. This situation suggests that the disc tissue may have some injurious properties of pathophysiologic significance. Experimentally autologous nucleus pulposus can, when applied epidurally, induce inflammatory reactions as well as structural and functional changes in spinal nerve roots. The conduction impairment caused by nucleus pulposus can be completely prevented by intravenous injection of high doses of methylprednisolone, if given within 24 hours of the application of nucleus pulposus. Recently, the presence of the cytokine tumor necrosis factor-alpha (TNF-α) in nucleus pulposus cells was confirmed and TNF-α was suggested to be the main substance mediating the nucleus pulposus effects on nerve roots. TNF-α is known to induce axonal and myelin injury similar to that observed after nucleus pulposus application, and TNF-α has thus attracted interest in this context since its physiologic effects on nerve roots seem to resemble those of nucleus pulposus. Moreover, it has been demonstrated that the nucleus pulposus-induced effects on nerve root function and structure can be prevented by selective pharmacologic inhibition of TNF-α.

Pain Mechanisms

Clinically sequestered disc fragments often are associated with more pronounced radicular pain than covered disc protrusions, and may be more responsive to pharmacologic efforts to control the pain. These observations support experimental data, indicating that nerve root irritation can be induced by nucleus pulposus. However, the detailed mechanism of action underlying the pronounced effects of nucleus pulposus on spinal nerve root structure and function is not known.

Surgical, pathologic, and imaging findings at the lesion site demonstrate that nerve roots can be compressed, deformed, or stretched by disc, facet, pedicle, or ligaments. Congestion and swelling of nerve roots often is identified during decompressive lumbar spine surgery or by MRI. Postmortem studies of nerve roots from patients with lumbar spinal stenosis have demonstrated demyelination, degeneration, and regeneration of nerve fibers as well as atrophy of DRG cells. Experimental studies have demonstrated similar changes. Moreover, edema and inflammatory changes that lead to interstitial and periradicular fibrosis, which probably is associated with disturbed CSF flow, may be related to pain mechanisms.

Clinical and pathoanatomic investigations, including discography, have shown that anatomic pathways frequently exist between the degenerative nucleus pulposus and the adjacent nerve root. Various substances may thus leak from the degenerative disc to the nerve root, causing chemical radiculitis. Venous changes and resultant fibrosis, which possibly are related to defective fibrinolytic activity, may play important roles in the chronicity of sciatic pain syndromes. Nucleus pulposus application on nerve roots has been found to induce pain behavioral changes, particularly in combination with mechanical nerve root deformation.

A nerve root that is compressed or otherwise injured by nucleus pulposus components with resulting nerve fiber changes such as demyelination can produce ectopic discharges that are propagated bidirectionally from the site of the lesion. These discharges result in both central and peripheral sensitization. Central sensitization implies that normally nonpainful afferent impulses could be perceived as pain. Clinically, it has been noted that a nerve root block distal to the lesion or even a peripheral nerve block can be at least temporarily effective in relieving sciatica. These clinical observations are in accordance with experimental findings, which suggest that peripheral afferent impulses are crucial in the pathomechanisms of sciatica.

Annotated Bibliography

Olmarker K, Larsson K: Tumor necrosis factor alpha and nucleus pulposus-induced nerve root injury. *Spine* 1998;23:2538-2544.

This study demonstrates the presence of TNF-α in nucleus pulposus cells.

Olmarker K, Myers RR: Pathogenesis of sciatic pain: Role of herniated nucleus pulposus and deformation of spinal nerve root and dorsal root ganglion. *Pain* 1998; 78:99-105.

Pain behavioral changes are induced by application of autologous nucleus pulposus on nerve roots, particularly in combination with nerve root deformation.

Olmarker K, Rydevik B: Selective inhibition of tumor necrosis factor-alpha prevents nucleus pulposus-induced thrombus formation, intraneural edema and reduction of nerve conduction velocity. *Spine* 2001;26:863-869.

Selective inhibitions of TNF-α can prevent the functional and structural nerve root injury induced by local application of autologous nucleus pulposus.

Classic Bibliography

Cohen, MS, Wall EJ, Brown RB, et al: Cauda equina anatomy: II. Extrathecal nerve roots and dorsal ganglia. *Spine* 1990;15:1246-1251.

Cooper RG, Freemont AJ, Hoyland JA, et al: Herniated intervertebral disc-associated periradicular fibrosis and vascular abnormalities occur without inflammatory cell infiltration. *Spine* 1995;20:591-598.

Cornefjord M, Olmarker K, Farley DB, et al: Neuropeptide changes in compressed spinal nerve roots. *Spine* 1995;20:670-673.

Delamarter RB, Bohlman HH, Dodge LD, et al: Experimental lumbar spinal stenosis: Analysis of the cortical evoked potentials, microvasculature, and histopathology. *J Bone Joint Surg Am* 1990;72:110-120.

Garfin SR, Cohen MS, Massie JB, et al: Nerve-roots of the cauda equina: The effects of hypotension and acute graded compression on function. *J Bone Joint Surg Am* 1990;72:1185-1192.

Jönsson B, Strömqvist B: Symptoms and signs in degeneration of the lumbar spine: A prospective, consecutive study of 300 operated patients. *J Bone Joint Surg Br* 1993;75:381-385.

Kawakami M, Weinstein JN, Hashizume H, et al: Patho-mechanisms of pain-related behaviour produced by intervertebral disc in the rat. *Trans International Society for the Study of the Lumbar Spine.* Helsinki, Finland, 1995, p 53.

Olmarker K: Spinal nerve root compression: Nutrition and function of the porcine cauda equina compressed in vivo. *Acta Orthop Scand* Suppl 1991;242:1-27.

Olmarker K, Blomquist J, Strömberg J, et al: Inflammatogenic properties of nucleus pulposus. *Spine* 1995; 20:665-669.

Olmarker K, Byröd G, Cornefjord M, et al: Effects of methylprednisolone on nucleus pulposus-induced nerve root injury. *Spine* 1994;19:1803-1808.

Olmarker K, Rydevik B: Single- versus double-level nerve root compression: An experimental study on the porcine cauda equina with analyses of nerve impulse conduction properties. *Clin Orthop* 1992;279:35-39.

Olmarker K, Rydevik B, Holms S: Edema formation in spinal nerve roots induced by experimental, graded compression: An experimental study on the pig cauda equina with special reference to differences in effects between rapid and slow onset of compression. *Spine* 1989;14:519-563.

Olmarker K, Rydevik B, Nordborg C: Autologous nucleus pulposus induces neurophysiologic and histologic changes in porcine cauda equina nerve roots. *Spine* 1993;18:1425-1432.

Porter RW, Ward D: Cauda equina dysfunction: The significance of two-level pathology. *Spine* 1992;17:9-15.

Rydevik B, Holm S, Brown MD, et al: Diffusion from the cerebrospinal fluid as a nutritional pathway for spinal nerve roots. *Acta Physiol Scand* 1990;138:247-248.

Saal JS, Franson RC, Dobrow R, et al: High levels of inflammatory phospholipase A2 activity in lumbar disc herniations. *Spine* 1990;15:674-678.

Takahashi K, Miyazaki T, Takino T, et al: Epidural pressure measurements: Relationship between epidural pressure and posture in patients with lumbar spinal stenosis. *Spine* 1995;20:650-653.

Chapter 6

Clinical History and Physical Examination

Robert F. McLain, MD

Sean Dudeney, MD

The Importance of History and Physical Examination

Careful clinical assessment is, potentially, the most valuable service a physician can provide to the patient. A complete examination leads the physician to the correct diagnosis, establishes the magnitude of the problem, and determines appropriate treatment.

With the continuing advances in imaging techniques, clinical examination has been regarded as progressively less important over time. Imaging modalities often are used as a short-cut around the time-consuming process of history taking and physical examination in spite of the knowledge that MRI and CT scanning have a high false positive rate for spinal "disease" and provide no information about the source of pain. Clinicians who depend too heavily on imaging studies are at risk of attributing symptoms to asymptomatic lesions while failing to identify the actual cause of pain. In the absence of careful clinical assessment, MRI may lead to incorrect diagnosis and unnecessary surgery. The history and physical examination determine the nature and extent of care. Radiographic studies should confirm the diagnosis made as a result of the history and physical examination and help guide any surgical treatment proposed.

History

The spinal column can be divided anatomically into the structural spine, made up of vertebrae and joints, and the neurologic spine made up of cord, cauda equina, and nerve roots. Structural symptoms and signs tend to be axial, and neurologic symptoms and signs tend to be peripheral or radicular. In eliciting the patient's chief complaint, it is fundamentally important to find out where the patient feels the pain. Does the patient with a "backache" really have pain in the lumbosacral junction, the thoracolumbar junction, or the buttock and thigh? When a patient complains of leg pain, are the symptoms truly radicular or are they distributed to the buttock or groin? Many patients complain of "sciatica," having no

idea what the term means, then go on to describe purely mechanical back pain with no radicular symptoms at all.

After listening to the patient's description of his or her symptoms, the physician must ask a few screening questions to get an idea of what is the most limiting problem. The physician should ask about the ratio of back pain to leg pain symptoms, and ask the patient to rate pain intensity on a scale from 1 to 10 for both good days and bad days. The physician should also determine functional impairment and whether function is stable or deteriorating, and listen for clues that the patient's primary problem may be confounded by psychosocial issues, such as litigation, job dissatisfaction, or family turmoil. Finally, differentiation between axial and/or peripheral symptoms is required to narrow the differential diagnosis (Tables 1 and 2; and chapter 11).

Axial Symptoms: Back and Neck Pain

The physician should characterize the nature of the pain, noting axial symptoms in terms of location, onset, duration, character, periodicity, and the precipitating, aggravating, and relieving factors of back or neck pain.

Location

Is the patient's pain focal or diffuse, midline or paraspinous, or localized to the occipitocervical, thoracolumbar, or lumbosacral junctions? Midline pain may suggest spondylolisthesis or bony pathology, whereas paraspinous pain suggests muscular pain and spasm. Parascapular pain and sacroiliac joint pain are often of an extraspinal origin. Focal, highly localized pain may be due to a fracture, tumor, infection, or single-level arthrosis or instability. Diffuse symptoms suggest a diffuse process (degenerative disc disease, deconditioning), and chronic, diffuse symptoms are seldom likely to warrant surgical treatment.

Onset

Acute onset of pain suggests an acute injury; the magnitude of any associated trauma suggests the extent of the injury. Insidious onset of pain may be the result of repet-

TABLE 1	The Differential Diagnosis of Back Pain: Spinal Causes of Back Pain

Structural
  Segmental instability
  Discogenic pain, annular tears
  Facet joint arthropathy
  Muscle strain, ligament sprain
  Spondylolisthesis
  Spinal stenosis
  Fracture
  Infection
    Discitis
    Vertebral osteomyelitis
  Inflammatory
    Ankylosing spondylitis
    Rheumatoid arthritis
  Tumors
    Primary
    Secondary, myeloma

Endocrine
  Osteomalacia
  Osteoporosis
  Acromegaly

Hematologic
  Sickle-cell disease

TABLE 2	Extraspinal Causes of Back Pain

Visceral
  Renal calculus, urinary tract infection, pyelonephritis
  Duodenal ulcer
  Abdominal or thoracic aortic aneurysm
  Left atrial enlargement in mitral valve disease
  Pancreatitis
  Retroperitoneal neoplasm
  Biliary colic
  Gynecologic
  Etopic pregnancy
  Endometriosis
  Sickle-cell crisis

Drugs
  Corticosteroids cause osteoporosis and methysergide produces retroperitoneal fibrosis
  Nonsteroidal anti-inflammatory drugs may cause peptic ulcer disease or renal papillary necrosis

Musculoskeletal
  Hip disease
  Sacroiliac joint disease
  Scapulothoracic pain
  Psychogenic

itive trauma, degenerative disease, or a progressive medical disorder. Pain that comes on insidiously but progresses rapidly may indicate a more serious underlying cause. The patient should be evaluated for vertebral pathology, including pathologic fracture caused by tumor, infection, or osteoporosis, and for visceral disease, including pancreatitis and abdominal aortic aneurysm, presenting as low back pain.

Duration
Musculoskeletal pain caused by a sprain or strain usually improves within 6 to 8 weeks of onset. Degenerative disease pain waxes and wanes over a period of years or decades. New pains, or pains that are new to the individual patient with longstanding backache, that last more than 8 weeks warrant full evaluation.

Character
Most backache is experienced as a fairly focal pain, intensified by activity and fatigue and improved by rest. A boring, deep pain, unrelieved by rest or recumbency suggests neoplasia or infection. Sharp, stabbing, incapacitating pain, superimposed on a baseline ache sug-

gests instability, particularly if the patient feels a shift or "catch" with motion. Pain intensified by sitting and vibration exposure (eg, riding in an automobile), flexion-extension, and axial loading is often discogenic. Similar symptoms, of greater intensity, may be seen with discitis or osteomyelitis and are associated with absolute intolerance of motion.

Periodicity
Intense symptoms that come and go every few years suggest recurrent soft-tissue injury. If symptoms recur more frequently, or if the patient is beginning to miss work several times in a given year, the need for further evaluation and more aggressive treatment is apparent.

Factors That Precipitate, Aggravate, or Relieve Pain
Flexion tends to aggravate disc-related symptoms, whereas extension may irritate the facets. Motion may trigger instability, causing acute giving out or stabbing pain. Fatigue can aggravate the muscles, causing spasm and pain. Whole body vibration exposure (operating or riding in a car, heavy equipment, train, or airplane) can precipitate neuropeptide release that can sensitize nerve endings and directly irritate the disc.

    Pain caused by bending, lifting, twisting, or axial loading, and relieved by recumbancy suggests a mechanical disorder. Pain aggravated by flexion, rotation or lateral flexion, or by prolonged sitting or riding in a car tends to be discogenic. Back pain caused by hyperextension may be facet-related, whereas leg pain in extension postures usually is a result of spinal stenosis.

Night pain, or intractable pain unrelieved by rest, suggests tumor or infection. Weight loss, fatigue, malaise, or pyrexia may also be present. Profound morning stiffness, which requires 30 minutes to an hour to "loosen up," suggests inflammatory arthropathy. Inquiries about injury and the circumstances under which pain first appeared are important. Did pain come on immediately after an accident? Was there an examination or radiography at that time? Asking about who the patient feels is to blame for the pain will give an indication of the possibility of litigation.

Specific questions regarding deformity clarify both its onset and progression. Patients with scoliosis may complain of a change in shoulder heights, limb-length discrepancy, a sensation of ribs impinging on the pelvis, or increasing rib prominence posteriorly when they sit against the back of a chair. They also may describe their head as "off to one side" if the deformity is unbalanced in the coronal plane, or rarely, they may describe inability to keep the upper trunk facing forward in the same line as the pelvis. Kyphotic patients may describe increasing deformity as localized pressure at the apex of their curve while sitting against the back of a chair, greater difficulty in looking up or even straight ahead, a sense of vertical compression or shortening of the abdomen, and difficulty with breathing. Because curves tend to be present in more than one plane, a mixture of symptoms may be noted in a given patient.

Peripheral Symptoms: Arm and Leg Pain

Radiculopathy must be characterized precisely. Some regions may be painful; others may be hyperesthetic, numb, tingling, or burning. As with axial pain, radicular symptoms may be focal or diffuse. Focal symptoms occur when a single nerve root is compressed or irritated, sending pain throughout a well-defined anatomic distribution or dermatome. Diffuse symptoms occur when the spinal cord or multiple roots are involved, producing symptoms of pain, numbness, or weakness in multiple dermatomes. Herniated nucleus pulposus typically produces a specific and focal radiculopathy. Central spinal stenosis more often produces a diffuse pattern of symptoms, with bilateral numbness, weakness, and pain.

Thoracic disorders can produce belt-like radicular symptoms, which may be mistaken for intra-abdominal pathology. Well-described radicular pain in the thoracic

and abdominal region also occurs with herpes zoster (shingles), the pain of which is severe and predates the appearance of vesicles. There are a number of less common extraspinal causes of radicular pain (Table 3).

Claudication is quantified by walking distance and may be of either neurogenic or vascular etiology. Patients with neurogenic claudication caused by lumbar spinal stenosis may have leg pain while walking or standing still and usually must stoop or sit to relieve their symptoms. Vascular claudication does not occur while the patient is standing still, but is relieved within 1 or 2 minutes of stopping walking, whether or not the patient sits. Patients with spinal stenosis tend to describe neurologic symptoms, such as numbness, tingling, or heaviness, in addition to pain while walking, and may require longer for relief. Patients who shop will often lean forward over a shopping cart to increase walking tolerance and tend to lean forward on a counter or sink when standing up for normal home activities. Patients with spinal stenosis may have no difficulty pedaling a bicycle or walking uphill, activities that are performed with the spine in flexion; however, they may be rapidly crippled while walking downhill, an activity in which the spine maintains an extended posture.

Radicular pain reproduced by coughing, sneezing, or straining at stool suggests a lesion within the spinal canal. This pain is caused by increased intrathecal pressure, which occurs with those activities. Patients with cervical cord pathology may complain of sudden electric shocks going down the arms and legs with move-

TABLE 3 | Extraspinal Causes of Sciatica

Intrapelvic extraneural compression
  Tumors
  Psoas hematoma
  Endometriosis
  Abscess
  Aneurysms

Extrapelvic extraneural compression
  Gluteal artery aneurysm
  Pseudoaneurysms
  Tumor
  Abscess
  Piriformis muscle syndrome
  Avulsion fractures of the greater tuberosity

Intraneural
  Diabetes mellitus
  Tumors of neural origin
  Fibrosis of the sciatic nerve

ment of the neck (Lhermitte's sign). Arm pain relieved by resting the forearm over the head suggests cervical nerve root tension. Pain in a cervical root distribution suggests cervical disc herniation or foraminal stenosis. Pain in a peripheral nerve distribution suggests an extrinsic lesion. Numbness in the radial three and a half digits and waking up at night because of numbness is suggestive of carpal tunnel syndrome. Shoulder stiffness points toward the shoulder joint as the cause of at least some of the symptoms.

Loss of bowel continence, urinary retention with subsequent overflow, and saddle anesthesia suggest cauda equina syndrome. Such symptoms usually are accompanied by varying degrees of leg weakness, usually bilateral. Spasticity, diffuse lower and upper extremity weakness, and urinary incontinence suggest a spinal cord injury, the level of which is defined by the highest level of neurologic symptoms.

Review of Systems

Respiratory, cardiovascular, gastrointestinal, genitourinary, endocrine, psychological, and other musculoskeletal system reviews may reveal medical contributors to back and leg pain (Table 2). A self-estimate of the patient's personality is helpful. Does the patient tend to be depressed, anxious, obsessive, or easily upset? Answers to these questions establish the patient's capacity to cope with pain and to comply with the rigors of a treatment plan. Ask clearly and plainly about any history of psychological illness or treatment and for details of ongoing treatment.

A family history of back pathology, inflammatory joint disease, or other inflammatory conditions may be relevant. Work history includes the physical tasks performed, particularly with regard to lifting, how much work has been missed, and the patient's relationship with coworkers and supervisors. Social history introduces the patient's spouse or partner and any children. The patient's use of tobacco, alcohol, and pain medications must be quantified. If the patient is smoking, how much? If not, did the patient smoke in the past, and when did he or she quit?

Functional Impairment

Before recommending treatment, the surgeon must know the extent of pain and disability resulting from the spinal disorder. Pain should be quantified in terms of the degree and pattern of pain, rated 1 to 10 at different times during the day. For example, "My typical day is 5 of 10 baseline with 3 hours 8 of 10 usually near the end of the day. The pain goes away when I lie down in bed at night."

Disability is quantified according to the patient's capacity to perform increasing levels of activity. Is the patient missing work, and how much? Is he or she confined to bed, confined to home, able to drive, or to go shopping? How far can the patient walk? Does pain interfere with housework? Can the patient exercise enough to stay fit? Questions tailored to the patient's own activities give an indication of a patient's ability to do what he or she wants or needs to do to stay socially active and employable. It is also important to clarify the limiting factor in a patient's disability. For example, is walking limited by neurogenic claudication or by breathlessness or angina pectoris?

Past History of Spinal Disorders

The past spinal history, which includes previous diagnoses, treatments, and surgeries, begins with determining the first time the patient remembers having back or neck problems. The physician should elicit previous spinal complaints and injuries and characterize them as to onset, duration, treatment, and eventual outcome. Previous surgeries should be reviewed and cataloged according to symptoms before the procedure; the procedure, surgeon, and date; and subjective outcome.

Other treatments, including injections, physical therapy (exercises or modalities), chiropractic treatment, and acupuncture, can be similarly recorded. The response to different classes of medications is recorded with details of their present effectiveness.

Precise determination of the timing of previous nonsurgical modalities relative to current complaints is important. The patient who did not respond to epidural steroids during the posttraumatic recovery period may gain considerable relief of recurrent radicular symptoms when the steroid therapy is tried again a year or so later. It also is necessary to determine the extent to which these modalities have been applied. Many patients who did not respond to physical therapy will, when pressed, reveal that they never had an active exercise program or that they never did the exercises prescribed.

Summary

The history should generate a differential diagnosis for the cause of pain or weakness and estimate the impact of that disorder on the patient. The history should begin to answer these questions: (1) Is there a structural problem? (2) Is there a neurologic problem? (3) How significant are these problems?

Physical Examination

The focus and extent of the spinal examination are guided by the situation and the differential diagnosis derived from the history. The physician may be required to perform a screening examination, or a comprehensive evaluation, depending on the specifics of the examination.

The screening examination is performed in an acute care setting on patients who are in the midst of resuscitation and are headed to the operating room or for further studies. It is a carefully planned and concise evaluation, which provides the most (and most important) information in the shortest time and requires the least cooperation by the injured or obtunded patient. It must identify potentially serious spinal trauma before cord injury occurs or is worsened by subsequent interventions. The screening examination cannot conclusively rule out spinal injury or instability. If it confirms an injury, however, appropriate precautions can be taken and early treatment instituted to protect the neurologic elements.

The comprehensive examination is appropriate for awake and cooperative patients with nonemergent spinal disorders; it is structured to rapidly narrow the differential diagnosis generated by the initial history. It includes "red flag" tests for common, important spinal disorders and attempts to exclude pathology of the hips, knees, sacroiliac joints, and vascular systems as the cause for the patient's back pain. The more subtle aspects are intended for the patient with a complex medical or surgical history and involve specific methods of examination to support or further clarify the putative diagnosis raised in the history. Not all tests are indicated for every patient.

The Screening Examination

The screening examination of the cervical or thoracolumbar spine should rapidly identify spinal injuries or pathology that pose an immediate threat to cord function and spinal stability. The examination can be completed in the emergency room, the radiology suite, or during transport, but is never adequate to diagnose more than the most significant injuries, which are then confirmed by specific radiographs and compensated for during the patient's initial care. When called to assess the injured patient, the spine surgeon must complete a careful, stepwise survey to avoid dangerous oversights and to rapidly identify serious injuries (Table 4). The surgeon should not depend on another physician to do the rectal examination. A general surgeon may have already done this examination but probably was not assessing the same things.

If neurologic function appears intact and the patient can cooperate, longitudinal traction should be maintained while the cervical collar is removed to allow inspection of the neck. The spine surgeon should replace the collar and log roll the patient to visually examine

TABLE 4 | Screening Examination

Rapidly survey airway, breathing, and circulation and initiate resuscitation as necessary.

Immobilize the neck in a collar and the spine on a backboard if not already done.

Obtain history from patient or transport personnel.
Mechanism of injury (fall, motor vehicle accident, speed of collision, ejection from the vehicle).
Neck or back pain, weakness, numbness, or paralysis at time of accident.
Previous illnesses including medications and allergies.
When the patient last ate or drank.

Assess for loss of consciousness, altered mental status, and cooperation.

Examine for facial, head, or neck contusions or lacerations that would indicate a likelihood of cervical spine injury.

Examine for seatbelt marks on the flanks.

Determine neurologic function before directly examining the spine.
Can the patient demonstrate voluntary motion of hands and feet?
Does patient have sensation on each side, at all dermatomes?
Are reflexes normal?
Does rectal examination reveal normal anal tone and perianal sensation?

the thoracic and lumbar spine (Table 5). Because of the large amount of information recorded at the time of formal spinal examination in a patient with cord injury, and because this examination is repeated at regular intervals, a standardized approach to recording this information, as in the ASIA scoring sheets, is recommended (Fig. 1).

Based on the results of the screening examination, plan further testing (radiograph and MRI) and prioritize these examinations relative to other treatments needed to resuscitate and care for the patient. If the patient is intoxicated, head injured, or obtunded, was involved in a high energy trauma, has facial lacerations, multiple distracting injuries, or is going to the operating room emergently for surgery, the cervical spine should not be cleared irrespective of what the radiographs or MRI show. The patient should be reexamined when the confusing factors have resolved and the patient can cooperate fully.

The Comprehensive Examination

The comprehensive spinal examination is intended to delineate which spinal disorders are benign, requiring routine conservative care, which are due to clearly

TABLE 5 | Neurologic Function Determination

Function appears intact

Palpate each interspinous ligament and check for increased interspinous distance or loss of resistance suggesting interspinous ligament rupture.

Inspect the skin for abrasions and inspect/palpate for focal kyphosis.

Evaluate focal pain, spasm.

Note any apprehension the patient may have to motion. A patient in the emergency department with a complete cervical disruption may have the sensation that his or her head is going to fall off if it is not supported with the patient's hands. Never discount the patient's sense of apprehension.

Deficit is found

Determine whether the injury is complete or incomplete, and whether spinal shock is present.

If quadra- or paraplegia is present, evaluate for signs of sacral sparing, signifying an incomplete lesion.

If injury appears complete, confirm presence of spinal shock by testing the bulbocavernosus reflex. The return of the bulbocavernosus reflex (anal contraction on squeezing the glans penis or pulling on the Foley urinary catheter) signifies the end of spinal shock. Only when spinal shock has resolved can a valid assessment be made as to whether a lesion is truly complete or incomplete.

defined and correctable spinal pathology, and which are more complex or ill-defined, warranting more comprehensive evaluation.

Cervical Spine

The comprehensive examination of the cervical spine searches for axial mechanical pathology, radiculopathy, or myelopathy in the upper cord, while excluding other causes of neck and arm pain such as shoulder pathology or peripheral nerve compression at the carpal or ulnar tunnel.

Gait should be examined first. The patient with cervical spine pathology may have a wide based gait caused by loss of proprioception (compression of posterior spinal cord columns). Similar disturbance may be caused by diabetic neuropathy or cerebellar disease. Gait may be jerky or spastic from lateral column cord involvement. Observe the patient's posture for torticollis or cervical kyphosis.

Range of motion should be assessed while the patient is sitting, measuring flexion (normal = 45°), extension (normal = 55°), left and right rotation (normal = 70°), and lateral bending (ear to shoulder) (normal = 40°). The examiner should note the rhythm of motion and presence of pain during or at the extremes of motion and should palpate the neck for paracervical or paraspinous tenderness and for nodes or masses.

Head compression may reproduce radiculopathy. The patient should flex the head slightly laterally and extend slightly before head compression. This Spurling's test should not be confused with Waddell's head compression test used as a simulation test for low back pain. Distraction of the head, simulating traction, may give transient relief of radicular symptoms.

The physician should examine upper limb tone; power; sensation; and biceps, triceps, and brachioradialis reflexes (Figs. 2 through 4). Sensation is tested to determine a pattern of objective or subjective loss. Direct comparison of the two limbs during examination can help patients characterize subtle deficits (feels fuzzy, woody, duller). The physician should test all dermatomes for light touch, using a disposable pin for sharp-dull discrimination and characterizing two-point discrimination in the digits if a deficit is noted.

The determination of the level of the neurologic deficit—spinal cord, nerve root, brachial plexus, and peripheral nerve—is crucial to establishing a final diagnosis in cervical injuries. Motor, sensory, and reflex deficits are correlated to identify the anatomic site of a lesion. Root lesions must be distinguished from peripheral nerve lesions. Tinel's and Phalen's signs always should be assessed to rule out compressive syndromes of the median or ulnar nerves in the carpal or cubital tunnel. If palm numbness is present as a result of compression in the carpal tunnel, the skin over the thenar eminence should be spared because the cutaneous nerve, which is sensory to that area, is a branch traveling superficial to the flexor retinaculum.

Ulnar nerve compression typically occurs at the wrist or at the elbow. In lesions at the wrist, sensory loss to the ulnar one and a half digits is accompanied by motor loss in all the small muscles in the hand except the radial 2 (±1) lumbricals and the muscles of the thenar eminence. With lesions at the elbow, sensory loss extends up the ulnar side of the forearm and power loss occurs in flexor profundus to the ulnar 2 (±1) lumbricals as well as flexor carpi ulnaris.

Myelopathy is suggested by hyperreflexia in upper and/or lower limbs, upgoing plantar responses, and a positive Hoffman's sign. A positive Hoffman's sign is elicited when the middle finger is flicked into extension, and the thumb and other fingers flex briskly in response. Some patients with cervical myelopathy will have a negative Hoffman's sign at rest, but will have a positive sign after repeatedly flexing and extending the neck. In cord compression syndromes, signs are usually bilateral. Unilateral signs suggest root injury or a Guillain-Barré syndrome.

STANDARD NEUROLOGICAL CLASSIFICATION OF SPINAL CORD INJURY

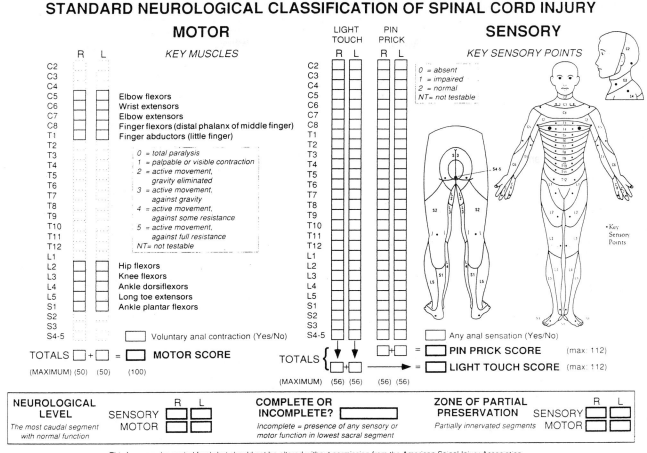

Figure 1 Standard neurologic classification of spinal cord injury. *(Reproduced with permission from the American Spinal Injury Association.)*

Cardinal signs of spinal cord compression and myelopathy include weakness or paralysis with little atrophy (disuse only), hyperreflexia, and Babinski/plantar response. Hyperreflexia is indicated by ankle clonus, patellar clonus, finger flexor clonus (Hoffman's sign), and crossed adductor response. This is tested by tapping the medial femoral condyle with hips slightly abducted. When positive, the test results in adduction of the contralateral lower limb. The test for Babinski/plantar response is performed by scratching a pointed object along the lateral sole of the foot towards the heads of the metatarsals. Before this is done the hallux should be checked for mobility. The noxious stimulus should not reach the head of the first metatarsal or it will mechanically cause the hallux to flex. The reflex response may be normal, in which the hallux plantar flexes with or without fanning of other toes, or pathologic, in which the hallux dorsiflexes with withdrawal response or no response of the other toes. In severe pyramidal loss, Babinski testing can result in involuntary knee and hip

flexion, and rarely, in urinary and fecal incontinence with or without piloerection caused by autonomic outflow. Superficial abdominal and cremasteric reflexes are absent (opposite to deep tendon reflexes).

Myelopathy hand refers to the inability to abduct the ulnar 1 to 3 digits and difficulty with finger extension during rapid, repetitive grip and release. It identifies significant cervical cord compression. In patients with spastic paraplegia and no signs of myelopathy hand, the site of the lesion is likely to be below the C6-7 disc. Ulnar nerve palsy is excluded by demonstrating abduction and opposition of the little finger or active metacarpophalangeal joint flexion in the ulnar digits.

A hyperactive scapulohumeral reflex (SHR) suggests upper motor neuron dysfunction above the C3 vertebral level (C4 cord). SHR is tested by tapping on the spine of the scapula or tip of the acromion in the caudal direction with the patient seated. The reflex is present when the scapula elevates or the humerus abducts.

A sensory level, if present, can define the level of cord

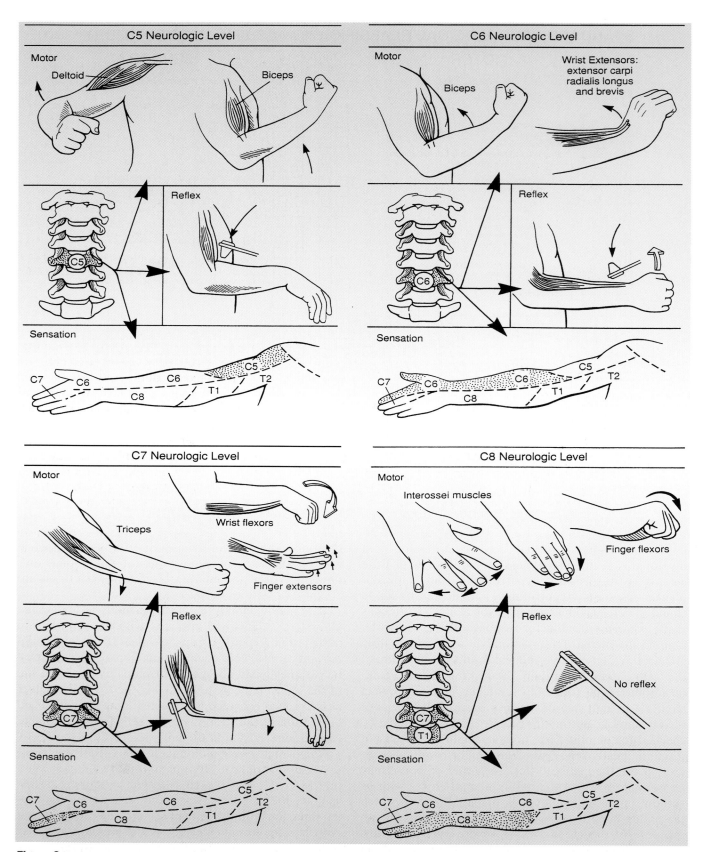

Figure 2 Neurologic evaluation of the upper extremity. *(Reproduced with permission from Klein JD, Garfin SR: History and physical examination, in Weinstein JN, Rydevik BL, Sonntag VKG (eds): Essentials of the Spine. New York, NY, Raven Press, 1995, pp 71-95.)*

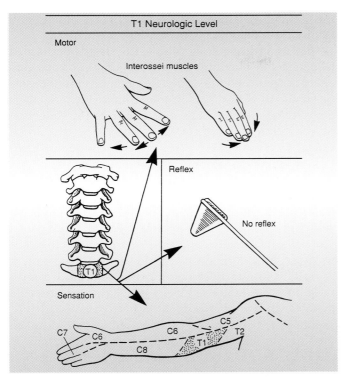

Figure 3 Neurologic examination of the upper extremity, the T1 neurologic level. *(Reproduced with permission from Klein JD, Garfin SR: History and physical examination, in Weinstein JN, Rydevik BL, Sonntag VKG (eds): Essentials of the Spine. New York, NY, Raven Press, 1995, pp 71-95.)*

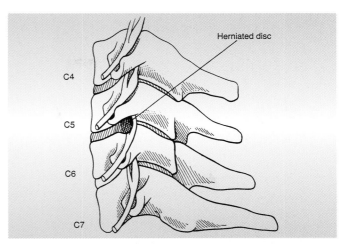

Figure 4 Cervical disc herniation. *(Reproduced with permission from Klein JD, Garfin SR: History and physical examination, in Weinstein JN, Rydevik BL, Sonntag VKG (eds): Essentials of the Spine. New York, NY, Raven Press, 1995, pp 71-95.)*

impairment. If the loss of proprioception extends to the trunk, a tuning fork can be advanced up the spinous processes to identify the level of cord damage indicated on sensory testing. Myelopathy that involves only legs, not arms, is caused by a lesion arising between the T1 and L2 vertebral body levels.

Typical signs of radiculopathy (lower motor neuron lesions) are flaccid paralysis of muscles supplied, severe atrophy of muscles supplied, loss of reflexes of muscle supplied, muscular fasciculation, and muscular contracture of unopposed antagonist muscle group.

Radiculopathy usually involves a specific spinal level, sparing the levels immediately above and below. Bilateral symptoms are uncommon but can occur.

Thoracic outlet syndrome results from compression of the neural and vascular structures between the interscalene triangle and the inferior border of the axilla. It is suggested by a decrease in pulse pressure when performing Adson's maneuver: Palpate the radial pulse at the wrist. Abduct, extend, and externally rotate the arm at the shoulder. The patient then takes a deep breath and holds it, and turns his or her head towards the arm being examined. Compression of the subclavian artery (and, therefore, adjacent brachial plexus) results in a decrease in the palpable pulse. This can also be measured with a sphygmomanometer.

Thoracic and Lumbar Spine

The surgeon should examine gait, posture, and motion as the patient enters the room and moves from chair to examining table and back. A waddling gait may be seen in spondylolisthesis as a result of hamstring tightness associated with flexed hips and knees and a flexed pelvis. Patients with quadriceps (L3, L4) weakness will hyperextend the knee when walking to lock the joint and prevent giving way. Patients with L5 loss may shift weight laterally over the limb in walking as a result of abductor loss (abduction/gluteus medius lurch or Trendelenburg lurch). These patients will also have a positive Trendelenburg sign. Patients with S1 loss may appear to push the pelvis forward and torso backward while standing on the affected limb to avoid using a weak gluteus maximus (extensor/gluteus maximus lurch). A short leg gait can be the result of true or apparent limb-length discrepancy.

Inspection of the patient standing upright and in forward flexion determines the presence of scoliosis or kyphosis. The skin should be examined for cutaneous lesions. Cutaneous neurofibroma, café au lait patches, or axillary freckles are usually present in neurofibromatosis. Surgical scars signify previous surgery. Lumbar range of movement is measured. Schober's test determines the degree of actual excursion in flexion. A line is drawn between the sacroiliac dimples. While the patient is standing upright a point 10 cm superior to this line is marked in the midline. The patient then flexes forward and the distance is remeasured. A 5-cm increase is considered normal.

The sensory examination should be carefully documented, looking for evidence of a dermatomal loss or impairment (Fig. 5). Heel walking, toe walking, and deep knee bend test power in ankle dosiflexors (L4),

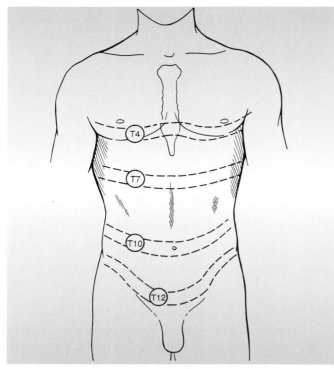

Figure 5 Sensory dermatomes of the trunk. *(Reproduced with permission from Klein JD, Garfin SR: History and physical examination, in Weinstein JN, Rydevik BL, Sonntag VKG (eds): Essentials of the Spine. New York, NY, Raven Press, 1995, pp 71-95.)*

ankle plantar flexors (S1) and the quadriceps (L3, L4) and gluteus maximus (S1) musculature. Sustained flexion of the hip on one side checks hip flexors (L1-L3) on that side, but also abductors (L5) on the other side. The physician should elicit knee and ankle reflexes while

the patient is sitting and test for ankle clonus and Babinski's reflex.

The sitting straight leg raise (SLR) test is performed (Waddell's distraction) while examining hip, knee, and ankle range of motion, for later comparison to the classic supine SLR test. The examiner internally and externally rotates the patient's hips and tests for abduction or adduction limitations. Motor assessment should be repeated through direct testing of quadriceps, hamstrings, tibialis anterior, extensor hallucis longus, and the gastrocnemius-soleus complex (Fig. 6). Results should correlate with functional testing (heel walk, toe walk). Next, with the patient lying supine, the physician should test active and passive straight leg raising. Hoover's test involves putting a hand under the contralateral heel during active SLR testing. If the patient is really trying to raise one leg, the opposite leg must push down into the examiner's hand. This confirms the patient's effort to perform. A positive passive SLR test produces radicular pain, experienced as pain distal to the knee, at less than 70° of passive elevation. Pain in the back, the thigh, or the buttock during SLR does not suggest a positive nerve root tension sign, and these pains are considered signs of a negative SLR. Contralateral SLR should be tested with the patient in the supine position. If the contralateral SLR is positive for radicular pain in the symptomatic leg, this is strongly suggestive of nerve root compression.

While the patient is supine, the examiner should retest hip range of motion to determine if hip motion may produce some component of the patient's back or leg complaints. If there is a restriction to normal motion,

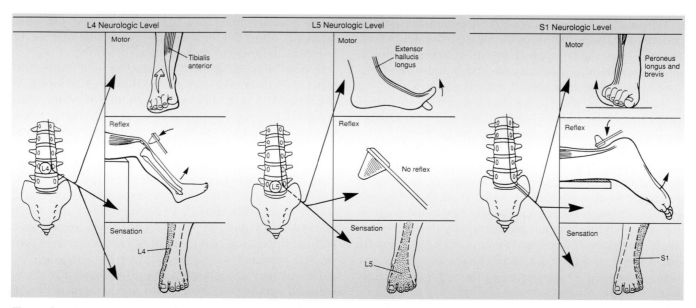

Figure 6 Neurologic evaluation of the lower extremity. *(Reproduced with permission from Klein JD, Garfin SR: History and physical examination, in Weinstein JN, Rydevik BL, Sonntag VKG (eds): Essentials of the Spine. New York, NY, Raven Press, 1995, pp 71-95.)*

pain with rotation or flexion and extension, or start-up pain when the patient first bears weight on the limb, a series of hip radiographs should be obtained to rule out osteoarthritis or osteonecrosis. After checking hip motion, the physician should manually compress the iliac wings to elicit sacroiliac symptoms, and perform a FABER (flexion, abduction, external rotation) figure-of-four test to rule out sacroiliac instability and pain.

The femoral stretch test is less specific than the sciatic straight leg raise. When positive, it reproduces the patient's anterior thigh symptoms. The test is performed while the patient lays prone, flexing the knee and passively hyperextending the hip by pulling up on the foot or front of the thigh. Active extension of the hip joint while prone is the best way to test gluteus maximus function (S1).

Signs of Lumbar Nerve Root Irritation

A variety of different provocative tests have been developed to reproduce leg pain by putting tension on the irritated root through maneuvers of the spine and lower extremities. By applying different tests in series, the consistency and veracity of the patient's complaints can be confirmed (Table 6).

Assessment of Thoracolumbar Deformity

Examination for thoracolumbar deformity must characterize location, magnitude, degree of compensation, and suggest the cause. General examination of the skin and extremities looks for evidence of a systemic cause: cutaneous neurofibroma, café au lait patches, or axillary freckles suggest neurofibromatosis.

Scoliotic deformity warrants specific evaluation. The curve is either static or progressive, based on serial radiographs, and either compensated or decompensated based on standing radiographs and examination. The forward bending test is used to assess rib prominence and paraspinous lumbar prominence. Balance and alignment are determined by evaluating sagittal and coronal plane balance of the standing posture, measured with a plumb line. The flexibility of the curve is determined by evaluating left and right side bending. Relative shoulder heights are measured to determine ribcage iliac crest impingement. The physician should look for pelvic obliquity, which may be due to a suprapelvic cause—spinal deformity, pelvic asymmetry, acetabular dysplasia—or to an infrapelvic limb length discrepancy. Finally, the examiner should evaluate for pain and tenderness over the apex of the curve.

Kyphotic deformities may be postural and correctable, structural and rigid, or acute and progressive, depending on the cause. The physician should assess the severity of the kyphosis, the resulting imbalance, and

TABLE 6 | Provocative Tests	
Test	**Comments**
SLR: sitting and supine	Must produce radicular symptoms in the distribution of the provoked root; for sciatic nerve, that means pain distal to the knee
Lasègue's sign	SLR radiculopathy aggravated by ankle dorsiflexion
Contralateral SLR	Well-leg SLR puts tension on involved root from opposite direction
Kernig's test	The neck is flexed chin to chest. The hip is flexed to 90°, and the leg is then extended similar to SLR; radiculopathy is reproduced
Bowstring sign	SLR radiculopathy aggravated by applying pressure over popliteal fossa
Femoral stretch test	Prone patient; examiner stretches femoral nerve roots to test L2-L4 irritation
Naffziger's test	Compression of neck veins for 10 s with patient lying supine; coughing then reproduces radiculopathy
Milgram's test	Patient raises both legs 3 in off the examining table and holds this position for 30 s; radiculopathy may be reproduced

the degree of functional impairment by determining the patient's sagittal alignment and balance, his or her visual horizon (the ability to look straight ahead or upward while standing), the flexibility of the curve and whether there is evidence of skin ulcers at the kyphos.

For thoracolumbar kyphosis, or lumbar flat-back syndrome, the physician should note the loss of the normal buttocks contour, resulting from the pelvis being flexed upward relative to the spine. The examiner should assess hip flexion contractures, and lumbar range of motion; the patient will have excellent flexion, but will be unable to hyperextend beyond, or even to, neutral lumbar alignment.

Psychosocial Assessment

During the history and physical examination, the physician will often discover facts or signs that are incongruous with the patient's subjective complaints or history. When multiple incongruencies are uncovered, the physician may become skeptical of the patient's motives and veracity. It is always difficult to quantify these intuitive misgivings, but it is important to recognize the value of such insights when it comes to patient selection. To help objectify these otherwise subjective observations, Waddell developed and validated a series of signs and tests that have proved helpful in identifying individuals who are, for one reason or another, magnifying or exaggerating their back and leg pain symptoms.

Waddell's signs include three observations of pain behavior—pain in a nonanatomic distribution, pain out of proportion to stimulus, and exagerrated pain behavior such as grimacing, moaning, and vocalizing or weeping—and four tests or maneuvers. The four tests—skin roll, twist, head-compression, and "flip" tests—are benign maneuvers that simulate provocative maneuvers; they seem like they should produce pain, but in fact, cannot.

The skin-roll test is performed with the patient standing or prone; the physician gently rolls the loose skin over the lower back between the index finger and thumb and asks the patient to report if any radicular symptoms are reproduced. Skin-roll may elicit local dysesthesias caused by dorsal ramus irritation, but should not generate radicular symptoms. The twist test is performed with the patient standing, feet together and hands on hips. Taking the patient's hips in hand, the physician gently rotates the patient's torso to the left and right. This simulates spinal motion, but the shoulders and pelvis move as a unit, with all rotation occurring through the knees, not the back. The head compression test is carried out by applying approximately 5 lb of axial load to the top of the head and asking the patient to report any increase in back pain. This small axial load is not sufficient to generate mechanical pain or instability. Finally, the flip test assesses the consistency of the patient's leg pain symptoms. During the extremity examination, with the patient sitting upright, the symptomatic leg is elevated straight out in front of the patient, creating a 90° SLR. If nerve root compression is present, radicular symptoms should be aggravated. The patient will either complain of the leg pain, or lean back to avoid the SLR effect. The same SLR test is then performed in the traditional supine position. If symptoms are present during supine SLR that were absent during sitting SLR, then the test is positive.

Waddell's incongruency signs do not suggest why the patient is exaggerating pain complaints. A patient may be seeking some secondary gain, or may, after years of ambivalent care, be trying desperately to convince a new doctor of the severity of the pain. It is common for normal patients to have one or two positive Waddell's signs on examination, but patients that manifest three or more incongruencies typically respond poorly to

either surgery or physical therapy unless the underlying cause of the abnormal pain behavior can be corrected first.

Annotated Bibliography

Borenstein DG, Wiesel SW, Boden SD (eds): *Low Back Pain: Medical Diagnosis and Comprehensive Management*. Philadelphia, PA, WB Saunders, 1995.
This is an excellent text that includes detailed accounts of a wide variety of conditions associated with back pain.

McCullough JA, Transfeldt E, McNab I (eds): *Macnab's Backache*, ed 3. Baltimore, MD, Williams & Wilkins, 1997.
This is the most recent version of Macnab's excellent text on the fundamentals of the lumbar spine.

Nitschke JE, Nattrass CL, Disler PB, Chou MJ, Ooi KT: Reliability of the American Medical Association Guides' model for measuring spinal range of motion: Its implication for whole-person impairment rating. *Spine* 1999;24:262-268.
This study shows that measurement of range of movement of the lumbar and thoracolumbar spine in patients with chronic low back pain are subject to considerable intra- and interrater error. Range of movement is therefore of limited value in the assessment of whole person impairment.

Poole GV, Thomae KR: Thoracic outlet syndrome reconsidered. *Ann Surg* 1996;62:287-291.
This study gives an account of the different causes of thoracic outlet syndrome. It identifies history and clinical examination as the most important diagnostic studies and states that careful patient selection with regard to surgery is required for satisfactory results.

Velmahos GC, Theodorou D, Tatevossian R, et al: Radiographic cervical spine evaluation in the alert asymptomatic blunt trauma victim: Much ado about nothing? *J Trauma* 1996;40:768-774.
This study suggests that clinical examination alone can reliably assess all blunt trauma patients who are alert, not intoxicated, and report no neck symptoms.

Vroomen PC, de Krom MC, Knottnerus JA: Consistency of history taking and physical examination in patients with suspected lumbar nerve root involvement. *Spine* 2000;25:91-97.
This study examines the consistency of signs and symptoms of nerve root compression giving rise to leg pain (sciatica). Straight leg raising, crossed straight leg raising, Braggard's sign, and Naffzigger's sign are identified as the most consistent nerve root tension signs.

Classic Bibliography

Hoppenfeld S, Hutton R (eds): *Orthopaedic Neurology: A Diagnostic Guide to Neurologic Levels.* Philadelphia, PA, Lippincott, 1977.

Macnab I, McCullogh JA (eds): *Neck Ache and Shoulder Pain.* Baltimore, MD, Williams & Wilkins, 1994.

Ono K, Ebara S, Fuji T, Yonenobu K, Fujiwara K, Yamashita K: Myelopathy hand: New clinical signs of cervical cord damage. *J Bone Joint Surg Br* 1987;69: 215-219.

Shimizu T, Shimada H, Shirakura K: Scapulohumeral reflex (Shimizu): Its clinical significance and testing maneuver. *Spine* 1993;18:2182-2190.

Waddell G, McCulloch JA, Kummell E, Venner RM: Nonorganic physical signs in low back pain. *Spine* 1980;5:117-125.

Chapter 7

Bone Imaging: Plain Radiography, Computed Tomography, and Radionuclide Bone Scan

Christian W.A. Pfirrmann, MD

Donald L. Resnick, MD

Introduction

Because of significant advances made in the past two decades, it is possible to image the spine with great anatomic detail and in a noninvasive manner to study alterations caused by aging and disease. The present standard assessment of patients with spine symptoms is based on clinical history and physical examination followed by imaging studies to verify the presumed diagnosis. The history and physical examination are crucial in making a preliminary diagnosis, and they dictate further diagnostic evaluation and management. However, they rarely permit identification of the specific spinal structures that give rise to the symptoms.

Recent articles have reported a high rate of abnormal imaging findings in asymptomatic volunteers. These findings make the significance of similar abnormal imaging findings in the evaluation of spinal diseases uncertain. Careful assessment of each new imaging method is mandatory. In addition, concerns about the expanding costs of medical care have increased the demand for scientific evidence for the efficacy of any diagnostic test.

Boos and Lander reviewed 672 articles that focused on the development or application of imaging methods for the assessment of lumbar spinal disorders. They classified the articles according to the following levels of efficacy: technical efficacy, which refers to technical features such as the degree of image resolution and reproducibility; diagnostic accuracy efficacy, which refers to the ability of a test to distinguish between patients with and without disease, usually described in terms such as sensitivity and specificity; diagnostic impact efficacy, which refers to the influence of a test on the diagnosis; therapeutic impact efficacy, which describes the ability of a test to influence the treatment plan or patient management; outcome efficacy, which addresses the issue of whether the test has improved patient outcome and which is the highest level of efficacy; and the cost-effectiveness of a diagnostic test, which is another aspect of the outcome efficacy. The vast majority of the reports (n = 593) evaluated imaging studies for the lumbar spine at the technical efficacy level only. A minor number of the articles (n = 57) focused on the evaluation at the level of diagnostic accuracy. Articles that assessed imaging studies on a higher level of efficacy were sparse (eg, diagnostic [n = 7] and therapeutic [n = 4] impact, patient outcome [n = 9], and cost-benefit analysis [n = 2]). This analysis of the methodologic background revealed frequent biases and flaws in the definition of test populations and patient selection, sample sizes, disease spectrums and comorbidities, and the choice of a gold standard.

Reports on the imaging of spines are numerous and technical development is continuing. However, a critical evaluation of these studies is necessary to assess their impact on diagnosis and treatment.

Plain Radiography

Despite advances in cross-sectional imaging techniques, plain film radiography remains the first step in the imaging evaluation of the spine. Plain radiography provides the highest spatial resolution of all the available imaging methods routinely applied to the spine. Furthermore, important findings are often depicted better in plain radiographs than with CT or MRI. For example, it is clinically and preoperatively important to know the number of lumbar vertebral bodies and to know about transitional variations of the lumbosacral junction. This information is often difficult or impossible to determine with CT or MRI. The lateral masses of the sacrum and the sacroiliac joints usually are not included in the region of assessment with routine MRI and CT of the lumbar spine. Plain films of the lumbar spine provide an overview of the sacrum and the sacroiliac joints, which can be important in accurately diagnosing patients with low back pain caused by such disorders as sacroiliitis and sacral insufficiency fractures. Small syndesmophytes and erosions of the discovertebral junction in ankylosing spondylitis or other seronegative spondylarthropathies also are better depicted with plain films than with CT or MRI. For example, the vacuum phenomenon is a very helpful sign because it virtually excludes infectious processes in the disc. The vacuum phenomenon of the vertebral interspace is easy to identify on plain films, whereas the MRI signal characteristics of the vacuum phenomenon often are very confusing.

The technique for plain radiography has remained fairly stable for many years. AP and lateral views are considered a basic requirement for imaging of the spine. Special views for the odontoid process as well as oblique views of the cervical and lumbar spine usually are helpful for better depiction of the spinal anatomy. A coned, angled, lateral view of the lumbosacral junction might be required in conjunction with the lateral view of the entire lumber spine.

Some studies have questioned the usefulness and efficacy of additional oblique radiographs in the initial evaluation of the lumbar spine. However, in a prospective study of 500 consecutive spinal radiographs, Gehweiler and Daffner showed that in 12% of patients, abnormalities were found in oblique radiographs that were not apparent in AP and lateral views. These abnormalities included degenerative changes of the facet joints in 6%, spondylolysis in 4%, and unusual conditions, including benign tumors, in 2%. These oblique views provide the best depiction of facet joint configuration, subluxation, and osteophyte formation.

Abnormalities in spinal motion have been emphasized as a causative factor in a variety of degenerative spinal processes. Using functional views, especially for diagnosing lumbar segmental instability, is controversial; also, a valid and uniformly acceptable definition of instability is not available. Hayes and associates examined angulatory and translational lumbar spine motion using flexion-extension radiographs in 59 asymptomatic persons undergoing routine preemployment examinations. Their results indicate that 7° to 14° of angulatory motion is present in the lumbar spine but that a large range of normal values exists. Two to 3 mm of translational motion is present in the lumbar spine at each intervertebral level. Twenty percent of asymptomatic subjects in this study had 4 mm or more translational motion at the L4-5 interspace, and at least 10% of subjects had 3 mm or more motion at all levels except L5-S1. In a study of 56 asymptomatic volunteers examined by flexion-extension radiographs, Thallroth and associates found that translational motion of more than 5 mm was observed in 14% of subjects at the L3-4 level and in 29% at the L4-5 level, while more than 4 mm of translation was present in 21% of subjects at the L5-S1 level. In the absence of a valid definition of segmental instability, no substantial data can be found in the literature to assess the diagnostic efficacy of imaging studies to differentiate symptomatic and asymptomatic persons in terms of segmental instability.

Diagnosing degenerative disc disease at the lumbosacral junction compared with other levels is often difficult on the basis of findings derived from routine radiographs. Cohn and associates established criteria for the diagnosis of degenerative disc disease at the lumbosacral junction. One hundred lumbar plain films were analyzed using MRI as the reference standard. Plain film measurements included the anterior and posterior disc heights (ADHs, PDHs); the Farfan ratio, which is the sum of ADH and PDH divided by the measured AP length of the inferior end plate of L5; and the lumbosacral angle. There was a statistically significant difference between normal discs and degenerative discs on radiographs using the parameters of PDH and the Farfan ratio; there was no statistically significant difference regarding ADH or lumbosacral angle. Diagnostic accuracy by visual inspection was not significantly altered using the quantitative data for interpretation of degenerative disc disease (68% correct before quantitative data were provided, 69.5% correct after). The authors believed that the PDH is the most reliable and easily used criterion for detection of degenerative disc disease at the lumbosacral junction. A PDH ≤ 5.4 mm on routine lateral film indicates degenerative disc disease; a PDH ≥ 7.7 mm indicates the absence of degenerative disc disease.

Vertebral end plates can have a variety of curvatures, some related to disease and some that are considered normal variants. The Cupid's bow contour refers to a parasagittal curvature predominantly in the inferior end plates of the lumbar vertebral bodies with an appearance on an AP radiograph similar to a Cupid's bow (Fig. 1). Notochord remnants or mechanical stress applied to a weakened end plate have been emphasized as possible causes of this contour. Chan and associates recently investigated the Cupid's bow contour by means of bone densitometry and imaging-histopathologic correlation. Dual-energy x-ray absorptiometry and radiography of 406 healthy subjects, as well as radiographs and sections of 64 cadaveric thoracolumbar spines, were examined for the presence or absence of the Cupid's bow contour. No relationship between lumbar bone density, body height and weight, and the presence of Cupid's bows was found. Histologic examination showed thickened bone in the end plate around the Cupid's bow, with annular fibers inserting into this region. In cadavers, the Cupid's bow contour occurred at multiple lumbar and thoracic levels, with the highest frequency in the lower lumbar spine. Lateral radiographs enabled better detection of the contour change. The authors con-

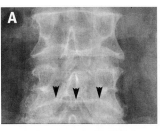

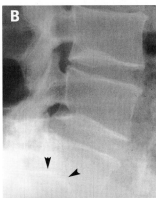

Figure 1 AP **(A)** and lateral **(B)** radiographs of a 72-year-old man. Note the Cupid's bow contour on the lower end plate at the L3 and L4 levels (**A,** arrowheads). On the lateral radiograph, the Cupid's bow contour is characterized by a smooth concave curvature with its center located at the posterior portion of the vertebral end plate and with a steeper slope posteriorly than anteriorly (arrows).

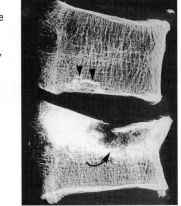

Figure 2 Slab radiograph of the L2-3 level in a 92-year-old man with metastatic disease from adenocarcinoma of the prostate. Osteoblastic metastasis with fracture and Schmorl node formation is seen in cranial end plate of L3 (curved arrow). A Schmorl node without evidence of metastasis is seen in the caudal end plate of L2 (arrows).

cluded that the Cupid's bow deformity is a developmental phenomenon unrelated to osteopenia or mechanical stress on the spine.

Schmorl nodes represent displacement of intervertebral disc tissue into the vertebral body (Fig. 2). Schmorl nodes occur when the cartilaginous plate of the vertebral body has been disrupted. Such disruption can be produced by an intrinsic abnormality of the plate itself or by alterations in the subchondral bone of the vertebral body. Weak areas in the cartilaginous plate include indentation sites left during the regression of the chorda dorsalis, ossification gaps, and previous vascular channels. The subchondral bone can be altered by numerous local and systemic processes, such as osteomalacia, Paget's disease, hyperparathyroidism, infection, neoplasm, and Scheuermann's disease, or by trauma. Pfirrmann and Resnick investigated the frequency and characteristics of Schmorl nodes in an elderly population and correlated the presence and characteristics of Schmorl nodes with degenerative changes of the spine. The anterior portions of the thoracic and lumbar vertebral columns were removed in 100 autopsies. Parasagittal sections were obtained with a band saw and radiographed. On each end plate from T1 to L5, the presence or absence of Schmorl nodes was noted and correlated to the characteristics of the vertebral end plate. The height of each interspace was measured, and the presence of vacuum phenomena and spondylosis was recorded. Schmorl nodes were found in 58 specimens and were multiple in 41 specimens. Two hundred twenty-five of 3,300 vertebral end plates revealed

Schmorl nodes. Schmorl nodes correlated with moderate degenerative changes of the spine, such as the presence of disc space loss. However, there was no correlation with evidence of advanced disc degeneration (ie, marked narrowing of the interspace, vacuum phenomena, or discogenic sclerosis or erosion). Schmorl nodes were associated significantly with claw osteophytes, although no association of Schmorl nodes with traction osteophytes was found. No correlation with the Cupid's bow contour was noted. The authors concluded that Schmorl nodes are a common finding in the elderly spine, with a frequency similar to that reported for a younger population. Schmorl nodes are associated with moderate degenerative changes of the spine. The absence of advanced degenerative disc disease in association with Schmorl nodes and the geometric observations regarding the vertebral end plate support the concept that Schmorl nodes are caused by an abnormality of the discovertebral junction rather than by discogenic factors.

In the assessment of a pars interarticularis defect in the lumbar spine, the 45° oblique lateral radiograph is considered part of the standard imaging. Spondylolysis is seen in 3% to 10% of the adult population. Saifuddin and associates investigated the orientation of the spondylitic defect in 34 patients with 69 defects evident on CT scans. Only 32% of defects were within 15° of the 45° lateral oblique radiographs. Five lesions could not be diagnosed in the oblique radiographs, whereas they could be identified on the lateral or coned lateral views. Therefore, the authors suggest the use of a limited thin-section scan using the reverse gantry angle technique (Fig. 3) rather than oblique radiography when lateral or coned lateral radiographs fail to show a suspected abnormality.

The cervicothoracic junction is difficult to assess with conventional radiography because of frequent nonvisualization of the C7-T1 region. In trauma patients, frac-

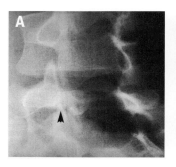
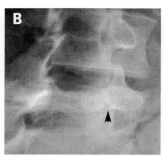
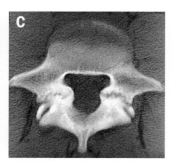

Figure 3 Right **(A)** and left **(B)** oblique radiographs of the lower lumbar spine and **(C)** reverse gantry CT scan of a 24-year-old woman with bilateral pars defects of L5 (**A** and **B**, arrow) *(Courtesy of J. Hodler, MD, Zurich, Switzerland).*

tures in this region are often missed, leading to inappropriate management and worsening of injury. A swimmer's view is often obtained to improve visualization of the C7-T1 anatomy. However, in intoxicated or neurologically impaired patients or those with coexisting upper extremity injury, these views are impossible to obtain. CT is currently used routinely to allow assessment of this region. This approach leads to a significant time delay and to many CT studies with normal findings. Kaneriya and associates compared the cost effectiveness of bilateral oblique radiography with that of CT for excluding C7-T1 injuries in trauma patients. In the first group of patients (n = 196), CT was performed to show C7-T1 anatomy when this region was not adequately revealed on initial three-view cervical spine radiography. In the second group of patients (n = 129), routine three-view radiography was complemented by bilateral oblique views. If these five views failed to reveal C7-T1 anatomy adequately, CT was then performed to show the cervicothoracic junction. In the first group, 26% of patients underwent CT scanning when C7-T1 anatomy was not adequately revealed on routine three-view cervical spine radiography. In the second group, only 13% of patients required CT scanning when five-view radiography failed to reveal C7-T1 anatomy adequately. The cost per completely imaged cervical spine was $92.00 when bilateral oblique radiographs were routinely obtained compared with $116.28 per completely imaged cervical spine when these views were not obtained. The authors concluded that because bilateral oblique radiography appears to be cost effective for the exclusion of cervical spine injuries, it should be used routinely.

Computed Tomography

CT was the first noninvasive imaging method that allowed a clear depiction of both bony and soft-tissue structures in the spine. Although the performance of CT is comparable to that of MRI in the diagnosis of degenerative disorders of the spine, and despite the widespread availability of CT, MRI has increasingly become the standard procedure for cross-sectional imaging of the spine. However, CT offers a higher spatial resolution with lower tissue contrast compared with MRI. Also, CT is usually superior to MRI in the depiction of bony pathology, such as central and lateral spinal stenosis, facet joint arthrosis, calcifications, osteophytes, fractures, and bone destruction by tumor or infection. Recent technical advances in CT include helical and multidetector CT scanning. Significant decreases in examination time and motion artifacts have resulted from these technologies, as well as high-quality multiplanar image reconstructions.

However, CT is not always the examination of choice to evaluate injuries of the cervical spine. In atlanto-occipital dislocations, CT is of limited use because the spatial relationship among the diagnostic landmarks is not seen on axial images. In traumatic spondylolisthesis of the axis (hangman's fracture), plain radiography is almost always sufficient for diagnosis and classification. The key to the stability of these injuries lies in the integrity of the C2-3 disc. Significant disruption of the disc is present when the body of C2 is displaced more than 3 mm with respect to the body of C3 or when the angle between the body of C2 and C3 exceeds 15° on lateral flexion-and-extension radiographs. A teardrop fracture represents a devastating injury to the cervical spine and is typically best seen in the lateral radiograph. Most often C5 and, less frequently, C4 and C6 are affected. In as many as 87% of cases, a sagittal fracture of the compressed vertebral body is present. The frequency of neurologic changes accompanying this injury is very high; no flexion-and-extension radiographs should be obtained. Injuries for which CT is the better imaging method include those to the base of the skull and the craniocervical junction, where overlap interferes with the detection of fractures, such as fractures of the occipital condyles and the Jefferson fracture, and C1-C2 rotatory dislocations.

Plain radiographs are still the best screening examination for acute injuries of the cervical spine. However, it is generally accepted that CT should be performed on patients with suspected cervical injury whose anatomy cannot be adequately revealed by conventional radiography (including the standard three-view examination as well as oblique and other special views, such as the swimmer's view).

Blackmore and associates investigated the cost effectiveness of CT relative to radiography for cervical spine screening in trauma patients. Three cohorts at high risk for cervical spine fracture (focal neurologic deficit, severe head injury, and high-energy trauma in patients older than 50 years), at moderate risk (high-energy trauma in patients younger than 50 years or moderate-energy trauma in patients older than 50 years), and at low risk (moderate-energy trauma in patients younger than 50 years) were studied with plain radiography or CT as a primary screening method. The outcome was measured in terms of the number of cases in which paralysis was prevented, total cost of screening, and cost-effectiveness ratios. In high-risk patients, screening with CT was a dominant cost-effective strategy that lowered the likelihood of paralysis. In moderate-risk patients, screening with CT also was cost effective. In the low-risk group, CT screening helped to prevent cases of paralysis, but the incremental cost-effectiveness ratio was high (more than $80,000 per quality-adjusted life year). The authors concluded that CT is the preferred cervical spine screening method in trauma patients at high and moderate risk for cervical spine fracture.

The second most important application for CT of the spine relates to the postoperative patient with spinal instrumentation. The evaluation of lumbar spinal fusion and pedicle screw placement has become an important indication for CT of the spine. Because of widespread surgical changes and artifacts related to implants, however, imaging of the postoperative spine remains a challenging task.

Herno and associates prospectively investigated the correlation between postoperative CT findings and clinical outcomes 4 years after laminectomy for lumbar spinal stenosis. Postoperative CT performed on 191 patients revealed a high rate of stenosis (64%). The clinical signs, severity of pain, and findings of radiologic instability did not correlate with CT findings. The authors concluded that caution should be exercised in correlating clinical symptoms and signs with postoperative CT findings in patients after surgery for lumbar spinal stenosis.

Plain radiographic evaluation of patients with persistent back pain after lumbar posterolateral or interbody spinal fusion often fails to show accurately the integrity of the bony fusion. Kant and associates investigated the value of plain radiographs in the assessment of instrumented spinal fusion. The fusions included posterolateral fusions or posterolateral and interbody fusions. Autografts, allografts, and a combination of these were

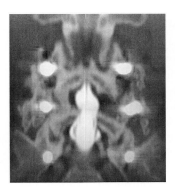

Figure 4 Coronal reformatted CT scan of 44-year-old man woman who had undergone pediculate instrumentation from L4 to S1 and posterolateral fusion with bone grafts. Note the osseous consolidation of the bone graft and incomplete fusion at the L5-S1 level *(Courtesy of J. Hodler, MD, Zurich, Switzerland)*.

also used. Findings with routine radiographs in 75 patients were retrospectively correlated with those of surgical exploration before hardware removal. Correlation between the findings derived from plain films and from surgery was achieved in only 68% of the patients. Fusion at the L4-L5 level was the most difficult to accomplish, and radiographic assessment of this level also was the most difficult. Thus, it appears that in patients with persistent back pain, when nonmechanical causes have been excluded, CT or surgical exploration is the best means of evaluation (Fig. 4).

Weishaupt and associates compared MRI and CT in the assessment of osteoarthritis of the lumbar facet joints. Three hundred eight lumbar facet joints were graded by two radiologists on corresponding CT and MRI using a 4-point scale. The weighted kappa coefficients for MRI versus CT were between 0.61 and 0.49 for readers 1 and 2, respectively. There was agreement (within one grade) between the assessment of MRI and CT in 95% to 97% of cases. With regard to osteoarthritis of the lumbar facet joints, there was moderate to good agreement between findings derived from MRI and those found with CT. The authors concluded that in the presence of an MRI study, CT is not required for the assessment of facet joint degeneration.

Osteoarthritis of the lumbar facet joints, however, is a very common finding, with increasing incidence with advancing age. Radiologic imaging findings are often unable to predict those patients who have pain originating from the facet joints. Schwarzer and associates investigated patients with chronic low back pain to determine whether or not the presence or absence of pain originating from the lumbar facet joints correlated with changes seen with CT. Sixty-three patients with low back pain of more than 3 months' duration underwent CT and injection of local anesthetic in the facet joints. No statistically significant difference in joint scores between those with and without pain originating from the facet joint was found. Thus, CT did not help to identify those facet joints that were painful.

Radionuclide Bone Scan

Radionuclide bone scanning using technetium-labeled phosphonates is a well-accepted method for uncovering a variety of bony lesions, including spinal metastasis and other abnormalities of the spine, such as facet joint arthropathies and pars interarticularis defects or osteoid osteomas, that might be causing spinal pain (Fig. 5). Less frequently used radiotracer-based imaging studies include gallium and labeled white blood cells, mainly for detection of infections.

Single photon emission computed tomography (SPECT) provides cross-sectional images similar to those of CT. Bone SPECT is more sensitive in detecting localized lesions than is planar scintigraphy, with a 20% to 50% higher sensitivity for lesion detection in the lumbar spine. SPECT allows precise localization of a lesion to the vertebral body, disc space, or vertebral arch. This anatomic distinction helps allow accurate diagnosis of the cause of an abnormality. Metastatic tumors commonly involve the posterior portion of the vertebral body, often in combination with a pedicle. Extensive abnormalities involving the vertebral body and vertebral arch, but sparing the pedicles, usually are related to benign causes, as are lesions isolated to articular facets and laminae or disc spaces. In postoperative patients, radionuclide bone scans and SPECT help detect pseudarthrosis and complications following the use of internal fixation devices, including pedicle screws.

A radionuclide bone scan is an effective way to determine the relative biologic activity of a bone lesion. For example, this method is valuable in distinguishing between recent and remote vertebral body fractures. Dutton and associates evaluated the role of SPECT of the lumbar spine in the management of patients with low back pain and suspected spondylolysis. Thirty-three patients with a high clinical suspicion of pars interarticularis defects were included in the study. The results of lumbar radiographs and SPECT bone scintigraphy were compared. Twenty-six of the 33 patients had abnormal findings on lumbar radiographs. Of the 21 patients in whom radiographs indicated spondylolysis, only 6 had abnormal uptake in the pars interarticularis regions with bone scintigraphy.

Gates and associates emphasized the role of SPECT in the evaluation of back pain in patients who had undergone spinal surgery. In 63 patients with back pain and a history of lumbar spinal surgery, the results of SPECT scanning were correlated with surgery, clinical information, and diagnostic radiologic studies. Bone SPECT was negative at the surgical site in 7 of 63 patients. In the remaining patients, the following abnormalities were found: facet joint abnormalities (n = 51), lesions within the disc space (n = 29), pseudarthrosis (n = 20), sacroiliac joint changes (n = 18), and vertebral body lesions (n = 9).

Holder and associates investigated the role of planar radionuclide bone scan and SPECT for detecting symptomatic facet joints. Fifty-eight consecutive patients referred with a diagnosis of possible facet syndrome were imaged. The results were compared with the effect of facet joint injections. Seven patients were diagnosed with the facet syndrome. A high sensitivity (100% SPECT, 71% planar scan) and somewhat lower specificity (71% SPECT, 76% planar scan) were found. The negative predictive value was high (100% SPECT, 93% planar scan). The authors concluded that the high negative predictive value allows radionuclide bone imaging to be used to select patients who might benefit from facet joint injections.

Summary

Imaging of the spine in asymptomatic individuals often reveals abnormal imaging findings that make the significance of such findings uncertain in the evaluation of spinal diseases. Only a few studies have contributed to

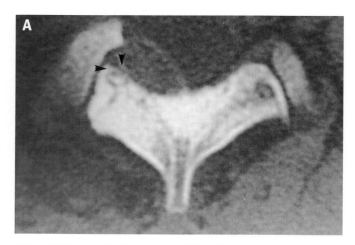

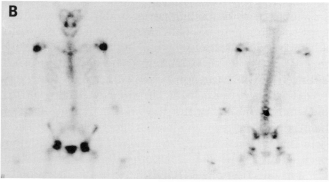

Figure 5 Osteoid osteoma of the spine in a 22-year-old man. **A,** CT scan at the level of the laminae of L3. **B,** Radionuclide bone scan. Nidus with perifocal irregular sclerosis of the right lamina of L3 is shown on CT (**A,** arrowheads). The radionuclide bone scan shows increased uptake in the posterior elements of L3 on the right side (*Courtesy of J. Hodler, MD, Zurich, Switzerland*).

our understanding of the clinical efficacy of imaging studies in the evaluation of spinal disorders. Comprehensive, well-conducted studies investigating the impact of specific imaging methods on the diagnosis and treatment of spinal diseases are needed.

Despite the technical advances in cross-sectional imaging techniques, plain films are still the primary screening method for imaging the spine. These films give a comprehensive overview of traumatic, infectious, and tumorous changes as well as subtle osseous changes that are sometimes not detected with CT and MRI.

Recent advances in CT have led to a significant reduction in examination time, which underscores the usefulness of CT in evaluating of cervical spine injury. However, the choice of a specific imaging method should be tailored to each patient to avoid a high number of negative examinations and increased costs.

Radionuclide bone scans are effective ways to screen the spine and to determine the relative biologic activity of a bone lesion, such as pars articularis defects or facet joint osteoarthritis. SPECT offers higher spatial resolution and better sensitivity than a planar radionuclide bone scan does.

Annotated Bibliography

Boos N, Lander PH: Clinical efficacy of imaging modalities in the diagnosis of low-back pain disorders. *Eur Spine J* 1996;5:2-22.

The authors reviewed 672 articles published from 1985 to 1995 that focused on the development or application of imaging methods for lumbar spinal disorders. The vast majority of reports evaluated imaging studies for the lumbar spine only at the technical efficacy level. Fewer articles focused on evaluation at the level of diagnostic accuracy or assessed imaging studies on a higher level of efficacy.

Plain Radiography

Chan KK, Sartoris DJ, Haghighi P, et al: Cupid's bow contour of the vertebral body: Evaluation of pathogenesis with bone densitometry and imaging-histopathologic correlation. *Radiology* 1997;202:253-256

No clinically important relationships were found between lumbar bone density, body height and weight, and prevalence of the Cupid's bow contour. The Cupid's bow deformity is a developmental phenomenon unrelated to osteopenia or mechanical stress on the spine.

Cohn EL, Maurer EJ, Keats TE, Dussault RG, Kaplan PA: Plain film evaluation of degenerative disk disease at the lumbosacral junction. *Skeletal Radiol* 1997;26: 161-166.

Criteria for diagnosing degenerative disc disease of the lumobosacral junction on plain films were established using MRI as the standard of reference. There was a statistically significant difference between normal discs and increasing severity of degenerative disc disease on radiographs using the parameters of posterior disc height and the Farfan's ratio. Analysis of results indicated that posterior disc height is the most reliable and easily used criterion for detection of degenerative disc disease at the lumbosacral junction.

el-Khoury GY, Kathol MH, Daniel WW: Imaging of acute injuries of the cervical spine: Value of plain radiography, CT, and MR imaging. *AJR Am J Roentgenol* 1995;164:43-50.

This article emphasizes the usefulness of CT and MRI in the diagnosis and management of acute injuries of the cervical spine. The continued importance of conventional radiography is underlined. Specific examples that illustrate the relative merits of plain radiography, CT, and MRI are shown.

Kaneriya PP, Schweitzer ME, Spettell C, Cohen MJ, Karasick D: The cost-effectiveness of oblique radiography in the exclusion of C7-T1 injury in trauma patients. *AJR Am J Roentgenol* 1998;171:959-962.

The authors compared the cost effectiveness of bilateral oblique radiographs with that of CT for excluding C7-T1 injury in trauma patients. Of the first group (196 patients), 26% underwent CT when initial three-view radiography inadequately revealed the cervicothoracic junction. Of the second group (129 patients), 13% underwent CT when routine three-view radiography plus bilateral oblique views were inadequate. The difference was statistically significant ($P < 0.01$). Because bilateral oblique radiographs appeared to be cost effective for the exclusion of cervical spine injuries, the authors suggested that they should be performed routinely.

Pfirrmann CW, Resnick D: Schmorl nodes of the thoracic and lumbar spine: Radiographic-pathologic study of prevalence, characterization and correlation with degenerative changes of 1,650 spinal levels in 100 cadavers. *Radiology* 2001;219:368-374.

In this study, Schmorl nodes correlated with the presence of disc space loss but not with evidence of advanced disc degeneration.

Saifuddin A, White J, Tucker S, Taylor BA: Orientation of lumbar pars defects: Implications for radiological detection and surgical management. *J Bone Joint Surg Br* 1998;80:208-211.

The variation in orientation of spondylolytic lesions was studied by CT in 34 patients with 69 such defects. A wide variation of angles of the defects was found. The authors conclude that lateral oblique radiographs should not be considered as the definitive investigation for spondylolysis. CT scans with reverse gantry angle are suggested for the assessment of spondylolysis.

Computed Tomography

Blackmore CC, Ramsey SD, Mann FA, Deyo RA. Cervical spine screening with CT in trauma patients: A cost-effectiveness analysis. *Radiology* 1999;212:117-125.

Of three cohorts of trauma patients with high, moderate, and low risk for cervical spine fracture studied with plain radiography or CT as a primary screening method, the authors concluded that CT is the preferred screening method in trauma patients at high and moderate risk for cervical spine fracture.

Herno A, Airaksinen O, Saari T, Pitkanen M, Manninen H, Suomalainen O: Computed tomography findings 4 years after surgical management of lumbar spinal stenosis: No correlation with clinical outcome. *Spine* 1999; 24:2234-2239.

In 64% of 191 patients who had postoperative stenosis on CT, clinical signs, severity of pain, and degree of radiologic instability did not correlate with CT findings. The authors conclude that clinical symptoms and CT findings in patients after surgery for lumbar spinal stenosis are rarely correlated.

Kant AP, Daum WJ, Dean SM, Uchida T: Evaluation of lumbar spine fusion: Plain radiographs versus direct surgical exploration and observation. *Spine* 1995;20: 2313-2317.

Plain radiographs of 75 patients were retrospectively correlated with findings at surgical exploration. A correlation was achieved in only 68% of the patients. The authors conclude that, when nonmechanical causes have been excluded, patients with persistent back pain should be evaluated by surgical exploration.

Schwarzer AC, Wang SC, O'Driscoll D, Harrington T, Bogduk N, Laurent R: The ability of computed tomography to identify a painful zygapophysial joint in patients with chronic low back pain. *Spine* 1995;20: 907-912.

In 63 patients with low back pain of more than 3 months' duration who underwent CT and injections of the facet joints, no statistically significant difference was noted between those with and without pain originating from the facet joint.

Weishaupt D, Zanetti M, Boos N, Hodler J: MR imaging and CT in osteoarthritis of the lumbar facet joints. *Skeletal Radiol* 1999;28:215-219.

The agreement between MRI and CT in the assessment of osteoarthritis of the lumbar facet joints was tested, and a moderate to good agreement between MRI and CT was found. When differences of one grade were disregarded, agreement was excellent. The authors conclude that in the presence of an MRI examination, an additional CT examination is not required to assess facet joint degeneration.

Zinreich SJ, Heithoff KB, Herzog RJ: Computed tomography of the spine, in Frymoyer JW, Ducker TB, Hadler NM, Kostuik JP, Weinstein JN, Whitecloud TS III (eds): *The Adult Spine: Principles and Practice*, ed 2. Philadelphia, PA, Lippincott-Raven, 1997, pp 467-522.

A comprehensive overview of imaging the spine with CT is provided.

Radionuclide Bone Scan

Dreyfuss PH, Dreyer SJ, Herring SA: Lumbar zygapophysial (facet) joint injections. *Spine* 1995;20: 2040-2047.

The anatomy, mechanics, pathology, and diagnosis of lumbar zygapophysial joints as a potential cause of back and lower extremity pain are discussed. A critical review of previous studies assessing the role of diagnostic and potentially therapeutic zygapophysial joint injection procedures is presented.

Dutton JA, Hughes SP, Peters AM: SPECT in the management of patients with back pain and spondylolysis. *Clin Nucl Med* 2000;25:93-96.

SPECT bone scans of the lumbar spine were evaluated in the management of patients with low back pain and suspected spondylolysis. Twenty-six of 33 patients had abnormal lumbar radiographs, and only 6 of the 21 patients with radiographs indicating spondylolysis had abnormal uptake in the pars interarticularis regions with bone scintigraphy.

Gates GF: SPECT bone scanning of the spine. *Semin Nucl Med* 1998;28:78-94.

The advantages of SPECT bone scanning are discussed. SPECT provides a far more precise anatomic localization of spinal lesions as compared with conventional bone scans. SPECT allows accurate correlation of a lesion with other cross-sectional imaging techniques such as CT and MRI.

Gates GF, McDonald RJ: Bone SPECT of the back after lumbar surgery. *Clin Nucl Med* 1999;24:395-403.

The results of SPECT scanning were correlated with surgery, clinical information, and radiologic studies in 63 patients. SPECT was negative at the surgical site in only 7 patients, while the others showed facet abnormalities (51), disc space lesions (29), pseudarthrosis (20), sacroiliac joint changes (18), and vertebral body lesions (9).

Holder LE, Machin JL, Asdourian PL, Links JM, Sexton CC: Planar and high-resolution SPECT bone imaging in the diagnosis of facet syndrome. *J Nucl Med* 1995;36:37-44.

Results in 58 consecutive patients with facet syndrome who were imaged with planar and SPECT bone imaging were compared with the effect of a facet joint injection. The sensitivity detecting symptomatic facet joints was high; specificity was somewhat lower; and the negative predictive value was high.

Classic Bibliography

Gehweiler JA Jr, Daffner RH: Low back pain: The controversy of radiologic evaluation. *AJR Am J Roentgenol* 1983;140:109-112.

Hayes MA, Howard TC, Gruel CR, Kopta JA: Roentgenographic evaluation of lumbar spine flexion-extension in asymptomatic individuals. *Spine* 1989;14: 327-331.

Jensen MC, Brant-Zawadzki MN, Obuchowski N, Modic MT, Malkasian D, Ross JS: Magnetic resonance imaging of the lumbar spine in people without back pain. *N Engl J Med* 1994;331:69-73.

Kirkaldy-Willis WH, Farfan HF: Instability of the lumbar spine. *Clin Orthop* 1982;165:110-123.

Resnick D, Niwayama G, Guerra J Jr, Vint V, Usselman J: Spinal vacuum phenomena: Anatomical study and review. *Radiology* 1981;139:341-348.

Resnick D, Niwayama G: Radiographic and pathologic features of spinal involvement in diffuse idiopathic skeletal hyperostosis (DISH). *Radiology* 1976;119: 559-568.

Resnick D, Niwayama G, Goergen TG: Comparison of radiographic abnormalities of the sacroiliac joint in degenerative disease and ankylosing spondylitis. *AJR Am J Roentgenol* 1977;128:189-196.

Resnick D, Niwayama G: Intravertebral disk herniations: Cartilaginous (Schmorl's) nodes. *Radiology* 1978; 126:57-65.

Rhea JT, DeLuca SA, Llewellyn HJ, Boyd RJ: The oblique view: An unnecessary component of the initial adult lumbar spine examination. *Radiology* 1980;134: 45-47.

Schmorl G, Junghanns H, Besemann EF (eds): *The Human Spine in Health and Disease*, ed 2. New York, NY, Grune & Stratton, 1971.

Thallroth K, Alvaranta H, Soukka A: Lumbar mobility in asymptomatic individuals. *J Spinal Disord* 1992;5: 481-484.

Chapter 8

Magnetic Resonance Imaging of the Spine

Richard J. Herzog, MD, FACR

The challenge in imaging the spine lies in the spine's complex osseous and soft-tissue anatomy, along with the myriad disease processes that can afflict it. MRI is but one of the many diagnostic modalities available to the clinician for evaluating patients with pain or dysfunction related to the spinal column or its neural elements. Compared with other radiologic studies currently available to evaluate the spine, MRI provides the greatest range of information. Since the 1970s, when images were first constructed using MRI, there has been a continual stream of new technological innovations in the field of MRI.

The goal of an MRI study is to provide accurate, reliable information concerning the normal and pathologic structures assessed. The value of the information gained from an MRI depends on how it is used (eg, to confirm or to exclude a diagnosis) and on the level of uncertainty of the clinician ordering the study. Before ordering an MRI, the clinician should determine whether the MRI is the appropriate test to provide the information needed and how this information will affect patient care.

MRI Physics and Imaging Protocols

An image of an object can be defined as a graphic representation of the spatial distribution of one or more of its properties. Whereas an image created with an x-ray source is the result of the electron density of the tissue being evaluated, routine magnetic resonance (MR) images represent the spatial distribution of mobile hydrogen atoms in the body. When a body is placed into an external magnetic field, such as an MRI scanner, a very small percentage of the hydrogen atom nuclear dipoles become aligned parallel with the static magnetic field. To create an MR image, radio waves of a specific frequency (RF) are pulsed into the body. The radio waves excite the aligned mobile hydrogen atoms and induce them to change from a lower to a higher energy state. With the termination of the RF pulse, the hydro-

gen atoms emit energy and return to their lower energy state. Images are created by mapping the location of protons that have released energy during their transition from a high to a low energy state. The process of returning from the excited to the equilibrium state is called relaxation and is characterized by two independent time constants, T1 (longitudinal relaxation time) and T2 (transverse relaxation time). T1 and T2 relaxation times are intrinsic physical properties of tissue. The MR signal intensity is mainly dependent on T1, T2, and the proton density, ie, the number of mobile hydrogen ions in the tissue being evaluated. The signal intensity generated by body fluids is also affected by flow.

The imaging techniques for obtaining MRI data are termed pulse sequences. Spin echo (SE), gradient echo (GE), and short tau inversion recovery (STIR) are currently the pulse sequences most often employed. SE pulse sequences are the most commonly used technique and are defined by repetition time (TR) and echo time (TE) values. The TR (time between the application of RF pulses) and the TE (time between the application of the RF pulse and the recording of the echo) are determined at the time of image acquisition. By varying TR and TE, the relative contribution of T1, T2, and the proton density of the tissue being evaluated will determine image contrast. A T1-weighted sequence, which emphasizes the T1 properties of tissue, can be produced with a short TR (400 to 600 ms) and a short TE (15 to 30 ms). A pulse sequence with a long TR (2,000 to 3,000 ms) and a short TE is referred to as a proton density or spin density sequence, and the signal intensity reflects the absolute number of mobile hydrogen ions in the tissue being evaluated. A T2-weighted sequence, which emphasizes the T2 properties of tissue, requires a long TR and long TE. Classic SE sequences have been replaced by fast SE sequences, which significantly reduce scan time.

Contrast resolution depends on the difference in luminance between objects; therefore, differences in signal intensity are critical in contrast resolution. The signal intensity and tissue characterization of normal and abnormal tissue depend on the pulse sequences employed. T1-weighted sequences are ideal for evaluating structures containing fat, subacute hematomas, or proteinaceous fluid because these materials have a short T1 and yield high signal intensity on T1-weighted sequences. T1-weighted sequences, frequently thought of as fat sequences, are excellent for the delineation of normal anatomy and soft-tissue interfaces. The signal intensity on T2-weighted sequences is related to the state of hydration of the tissue imaged. Tissue containing free extracellular water (eg, cerebrospinal fluid, cysts, and necrotic tissue) will yield bright signal intensity on a T2-weighted sequence. Fat saturation facilitates the detection of fluid or edema within tissue on a T2-weighted sequence.

It is not just signal intensity that differentiates normal from abnormal tissue but also tissue and organ configuration. Spatial resolution—the ability to delineate fine detail—is determined by section thickness, field of view, and the size of the acquisition and display matrices. Improved spatial resolution can be achieved using surface coils. Two-dimensional or three-dimensional acquisition techniques are available for specific applications, eg, vascular imaging. High field strength (1.0 to 1.5 T) MRI systems provide higher resolution images compared with low field strength (0.1 to 0.3 T) MRI systems. Low field strength MRI systems are indicated for obese patients or patients with claustrophobia who cannot undergo an examination in a high field strength system. Most open MRI scanners are low field strength MRI systems.

To achieve optimal results from MRI of the spine, characterized by excellent contrast between contiguous structures, maximal spatial resolution, minimal noise and artifacts, minimal acquisition time, and adequate coverage, standardized protocols should be followed. Before undergoing an MRI examination, each patient must be carefully questioned to determine whether any contraindications exist to performing the study. Absolute contraindications include ferromagnetic cerebral aneurysm clips, cardiac pacemakers, and infusion pumps, which can become dysfunctional in external magnetic fields; some heart valves; metallic foreign bodies in the eye or spine; and ferromagnetic cochlear or ocular implants. Relative contraindications that must be handled on an individual basis to determine whether the potential benefit of the study outweighs the risk include pregnancy, recent cardiac or vascular surgery, certain transcutaneous electrical stimulators, and severe claustrophobia. Artifacts can be expected from metallic implants, but artifacts can be reduced with the use of certain pulse sequences (see the section on The Postoperative Spine). The most common cause for degradation of image quality is patient motion, which can be reduced with rapid scan acquisition and patient education and preparation.

The standard MRI protocols for various parts of the spine share certain characteristics. In the sagittal plane, T1-weighted or proton density-weighted sequences are performed along with a T2-weighted sequence. Section thickness is typically 3 mm in the cervical spine, 3 to 4 mm in the thoracic spine, and 4 to 5 mm in the lumbar spine. In the cervical spine, SE or GE axial sequences are preformed with a section thickness of 1 to 3 mm. Thin sections are needed to evaluate the smaller anatomic structures in the cervical compared with the lumbar spine, particularly in the assessment of the neural foramina. In the thoracic spine, T2-weighted or GE axial sequences are performed in the area of a patient's symptoms or at any level where pathologic changes are detected on the sagittal sequences. Axial sequences in the lumbar spine include a T1-weighted or proton density-weighted sequence with a section thickness of 4 mm and an interslice gap of 0.5 mm, along with a fast SE T2-weighted axial sequence with a section thickness of 3 to 4 mm and an interslice gap of 0.5 mm. At least one axial sequence should have contiguous parallel sections from the pedicle of L2 or L3 through the L5-S1 disc level and not merely angled sections through the disc spaces.

The final step in creating an MR image involves image display. Because of the great range of contrast between normal and abnormal tissue, the selection of a single optimal gray-scale representation can be difficult. To evaluate the full gray-scale range of the acquired image, an MR image should optimally be evaluated on high-resolution video display monitors, such as the monitors currently employed in diagnostic workstations. These workstations provide other diagnostic tools to enhance the display of images at the time of interpretation.

Clinical MRI Applications

It is necessary to understand normal spinal anatomy thoroughly before diagnosing pathologic conditions visualized by MRI. An MRI examination provides information about dynamic disease processes, manifesting a spectrum of pathologic changes. Any pathologic change must be understood within the framework of the natural history of the spinal disorder. The transformation of data from an MRI examination into useful clinical information is directly related to the level of expertise of the clinician interpreting the MRI study.

It is important to try to answer the specific clinical question presented at the time of the MRI examination, but this should not preclude a critical analysis of the entire spinal region included in the study. Because clinical bias can impact diagnostic accuracy positively or negatively, each image should be interpreted twice, once with no clinical history made available to the examiner, followed by a second review conducted with the knowledge of results of prior studies and the clinical findings.

Spinal Degenerative Cascade

Degenerative abnormalities of the disc are frequently detected on MRI studies of asymptomatic individuals. These abnormalities do not represent false-positive findings but rather true pathologic changes of spinal structures that are not causing pain or dysfunction. The significance of pathologic changes detected on an imaging study can be determined only by correlating the test results with the patient's clinical presentation.

Both the nucleus pulposus and anulus fibrosus consist of water, collagen, and proteoglycans, with the major differences between the two being the relative amount of these components, level of hydration, and the particular type of collagen that predominates. With MRI, it is possible to delineate different parts of disc architecture. On T2-weighted images, the high signal intensity in the central portion of the disc originates from both the nucleus pulposus and the inner annular fibers. The outer annular fibers demonstrate very low signal intensity, as do the adjacent anterior and posterior longitudinal ligaments. The signal intensity in the disc is related to its state of hydration and to the physicochemical state of the disc tissue. With aging, there is gradual breakdown of proteoglycans in the nucleus, gradual desiccation of the mucoid nuclear material, and loss of anatomic delineation between the nucleus and the inner annular fibers. Past the age of 30 years, an intranuclear cleft, which represents ingrowth of fibrous tissue, can be identified in normal discs on T2-weighted MR images.

Early degenerative changes include annular fissures (tears), which can be oriented horizontally at the insertion of the outer anulus into the ring apophysis, circumferentially in the outer anulus, or radially, extending from the nucleus pulposus to the inner or outer anulus. Annular tears might be present in the periphery of a disc and not communicate with the nucleus pulposus. With MRI, small tears in the outer anulus can be delineated with T2-weighted or gadolinium–diethylenetriamine pentaacetic acid (Gd-DTPA) enhanced T1-weighted images. As a disc ages, coalescence of peripheral tears and delamination of the outer annular fibers might occur and can precipitate a generalized bulge of the disc contour because of the loss of the tensile strength of the outer anulus. A radial annular tear communicating from the nucleus to the outer anulus can be accompanied by progressive collagen disorganization and a reduced nuclear signal intesity on T2-weighted images.

Disc herniations result from the displacement of nuclear, annular, or end-plate material through radial tears. Displacement of the disc material into the region of the outer anulus/posterior longitudinal ligament complex will cause altered morphology of the periphery of the disc, resulting in a focal protrusion of the disc beyond the margin of the vertebral body end plates. A contained disc herniation represents displaced disc material that is still contained by the outer annular fibers and/or the posterior longitudinal ligament. A noncontained disc herniation has extruded through the posterior longitudinal ligament, but the disc material is still in contact with its disc of origin. With the superb soft-tissue resolution with MRI, it might be possible to distinguish between a disc herniation contained by the outer anulus/posterior longitudinal ligament complex versus a herniation that has extruded through this complex. A continuous line of low signal intensity abutting the posterior margin of the disc herniation and bridging the disc space is used by some observers to indicate that a disc herniation is subligamentous or contained. In the largest study to compare this finding on an MRI examination with the results at surgery, an intact or disrupted low signal intensity line posterior to the disc herniation did not predict the type of herniation detected at surgery. Herniated disc material might separate from its disc of origin and become a sequestered fragment. MRI is useful in differentiating between a disc extrusion and sequestration. Sequestered disc fragments usually generate increased signal intensity on T2-weighted images compared with the degenerated disc of origin. When a disc herniation is detected on an MRI study, the information provided on the report should include the size, type, and precise location of the herniated material (Fig. 1) and its effect on the neural structures (Fig. 2). A developmentally small central spinal canal might amplify the degree of neural compression by a herniation (Fig. 3).

Considering the frequency of detection of disc herniations in asymptomatic subjects (approximately 20% to 30% in most studies), specific findings on MRI indicative of a symptomatic herniation would be helpful. Most herniations detected in asymptomatic individuals are protrusions (contained by the posterior longitudinal ligament) and rarely displace or compress nerve roots. There have been reports that symptomatic nerve roots enhance after the administration of gadolinium, but this finding has not been corroborated in a large prospective study. Gadolinium is not routinely administered to a patient with radicular symptoms who has not had prior surgery. Other findings that might be present with a symptomatic disc herniation are enlargement of an impinged nerve root and indistinct margins of the her-

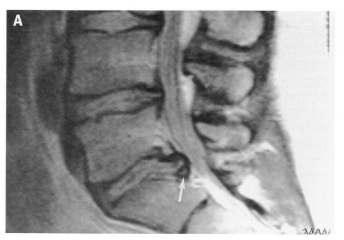

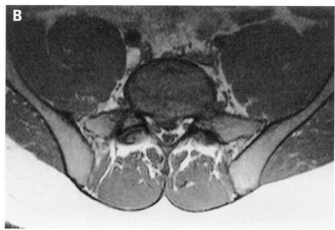

Figure 1 A young weight lifter experienced acute pain during a lift. The sagittal images, proton density-weighted **(A)**, and the axial images, T1-weighted **(B)**, depict a large posterior right paramedian disc protrusion associated with a small bone fragment (limbus vertebra) *(arrow)* displaced from the posterosuperior margin of the S1 vertebral body. The disc protrusion displaces posteriorly and compresses the right S1 nerve root.

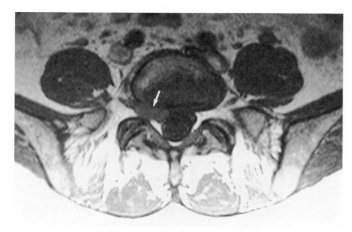

Figure 2 On this T1-weighted axial image, a large lobulated disc extrusion *(arrow)* compresses the right S1 axillary sleeve and impinges on the right L5 nerve root in the neural foramen.

niation caused by the inflammatory reaction in the epidural tissue.

In some patients, the development of annular fissures might lead to internal disc disruption or intervertebral disc resorption without the displacement of disc material. MRI is helpful in the evaluation of these patients because it demonstrates altered signal intensity in the abnormal disc. Unfortunately, detecting discs with decreased T2 nuclear signal intensity in patients who are asymptomatic is common. For this reason, some patients with refractory back pain who have had an MRI study delineating decreased T2 nuclear signal intensity at one or more disc levels are further evaluated with discography. In addition to providing morphologic information, a discogram is a provocative test that demonstrates a patient's pain response when the disc is injected. It is now possible to evaluate the inte-

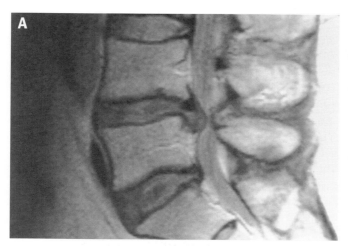

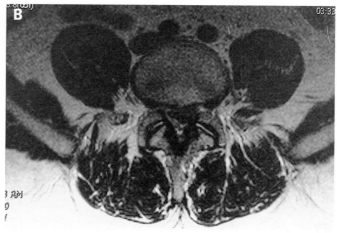

Figure 3 Developmental stenosis of the lumbar central spinal canal. Proton density-weighted sagittal image **(A)** and the T2-weighted axial image **(B)** depict a large posterior left paracentral disc extrusion causing severe thecal sac compression of the left L5 axillary sleeve.

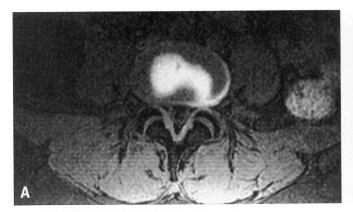

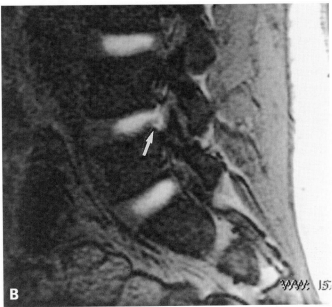

Figure 4 The T2-weighted sagittal images of this iodine-allergic patient with left-sided back pain was normal in the midline and showed a focus of high signal intensity in the outer anulus adjacent to the left neural foramen. On the fat-saturated GE image, the L4-5 disc was normal in the midline sagittal, but on the axial **(A)** and left sagittal **(B)** images, there is a large radial fissure (*arrow*) extending from the nucleus pulposus into the outer anulus adjacent to the left neural foramen along with the appearance of contrast extending circumferentially under the outer annular fibers.

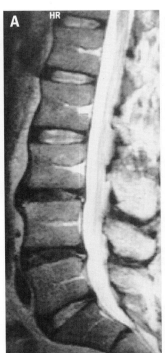

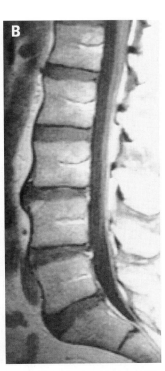

Figure 5 In a patient with midline back pain, the T2-weighted sagittal image **(A)** depicts a focus of high signal intensity in the posterior outer annular fibers in the midline at the L3-4 and L4-5 disc levels, along with reduced nuclear signal intensity (examples of an HIZ). On the T1-weighted sagittal image **(B)** after contrast injection, both posterior outer annular fissures demonstrate enhancement.

rior of the disc by MR discography (Fig. 4), which is not pain provocative, but does not require injection of the disc and therefore is useful in patients who have a history of allergy to iodinated contrast.

If there were a reliable marker for a painful disc on MRI, discography by injection might be eliminated. In evaluating patients with severe chronic debilitating back pain, several investigators have reported on the presence of a focus of high T2 signal in the posterior midline outer annular fibers in discs that precipitated the patient's pain when injected at discography. In addition to having a peripheral focus of high T2 signal intensity, referred to as a high-intensity zone (HIZ), these discs demonstrated low T2 nuclear signal intensity. These fissures contain granulation tissue, and most demonstrate enhancement after the intravenous injection of Gd-DTPA (Fig. 5). Although these investigators reported that an HIZ was a good marker for a painful disc containing an annular tear, other investigators have not found the HIZ to be a reliable marker for a painful disc. In one recent study, outer annular fissures were detected in 11% of asymptomatic individuals younger than 30 years and in 62% of asymptomatic individuals older than 30 years. Recent investigative work has demonstrated that discs with an HIZ demonstrate reduced stiffness with biomechanical testing, especially in response to axial rotation stress. The clinical significance of the MRI-revealed annular fissure requires further investigation.

The natural history of a disc herniation probably depends on the type of material herniated—ie, nucleus, anulus, or end plate—as well as on the size and location of the herniation. MRI has been used to document the resorption of disc herniations in patients treated non-surgically. It is common to see partial or complete resorption of a disc herniation followed over the course of a year. Herniations demonstrating the greatest change in size are disc extrusions or sequestered fragments exposed to the epidural space (Fig. 6). Hernia-

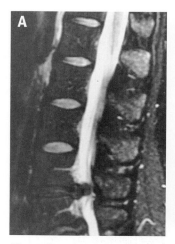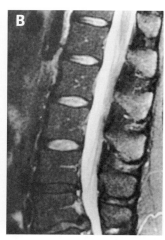

Figure 6 The T2-weighted sagittal image **(A)** depicts a large lobulated disc extrusion at the L4-5 level and large disc protrusion at the L5-S1 level in an aerobics instructor with mild/moderate back pain. After 5 months of therapy that did not include the use of epidural steroids, the patient was pain free. On the 5-month follow-up MRI study, the T2-weighted sagittal image **(B)** shows almost complete resorption of the L4-5 disc extrusion and no change in the size of the L5-S1 disc protrusion.

tions that show peripheral enhancement after the intravenous administration of contrast appear to show a greater decrease in size than do nonenhancing herniations. Herniations that show the greatest decrease in size tend to be associated with better clinical outcomes than the outcomes experienced by patients with herniations that decrease minimally or do not change in size. Reduction in size of disc herniation is caused by resorption from ingrowth of granulation tissue, resolution of any hematoma or inflammatory reaction, and, perhaps, by desiccation.

The degenerated disc usually demonstrates reduced signal intensity on a T2-weighted sequence. In cases of long-standing disc degeneration, fluid-containing fissures might be present in a degenerated disc along with ingrowth of granulation tissue. These pathologic changes can result in increased signal intensity in the disc on T2-weighted images, which should not be confused with an infectious process. Calcification or gas in the disc can be difficult to detect on T2-weighted images because of the decreased signal intensity in a severely degenerated disc and because of the absence of a signal from the calcium or gas. T1-weighted or GE images are more useful in delineating a vacuum phenomenon or disc calcification.

MRI is extremely sensitive to alterations in the vertebral body end plates at a degenerating discovertebral joint. Because of the thinness of the hyaline cartilage, isolated degeneration of the cartilage end plate is difficult to detect. In addition, chemical-shift artifacts might distort the appearance of the cartilage end plate. The vertebral marrow subjacent to a degenerating disc might show altered signal intensity. Type I end-plate

degenerative changes demonstrate reduced T1 signal intensity and increased T2 signal intensity (particularly evident on a fat-saturated sequence) compared with the normal vertebral marrow. The altered signal intensity is caused by the ingrowth of fibrovascular tissue, probably secondary to trabecular failure. Similar end-plate reactive changes are associated with discitis, but with infection, the marrow edema tends to be more extensive, the end plates might be destroyed, and the disc typically demonstrates high T2 signal intensity. The presence of a paravertebral inflammatory mass also helps to differentiate infection from degeneration. Type II end-plate degenerative changes demonstrate altered signal intensity caused by increased fat in the subchondral bone, and type III end-plate degenerative changes represent subchondral sclerosis.

In the cervical spine, because of the paucity of fat in the anterior epidural space, disc herniations projecting into the central spinal canal are easiest to detect on sequences with bright cerebrospinal fluid. Axial sequences provide information on the mass effect of a disc herniation on the thecal sac, nerve root sleeves, or the spinal cord. Herniations causing cord compression might precipitate cord injury detected on MRI as areas of high signal intensity within the cord on T2-weighted sequences. Disc herniations into the neural foramina or lateral to the foramina are easiest to detect on SE T1-weighted or GE sequences. Thoracic disc herniations also are optimally evaluated on sequences with bright cerebrospinal fluid.

Spinal Stenosis

Spinal stenosis has been defined as any type of narrowing of the central spinal canal, nerve root canals (lateral recess), or neural foramina. The narrowing might be caused by osseous or soft-tissue elements. Although plain film radiography is currently the radiologic study initially ordered to evaluate patients with symptoms of spinal stenosis, studies are ongoing to determine whether abbreviated MRI of the spine might be the optimal initial radiologic examination in the algorithm to assess these patients. The goal of MRI and CT with multiplanar reformations (CT/MPR) in the evaluation of patients presenting with neck or back pain, radiculopathy, or intermittent claudication is not just to demonstrate the presence of stenosis but also to define which spinal components are causing the stenosis and which neural structures are affected by the stenotic changes. In the assessment of patients with stenotic symptoms, the advantage of MRI is its ability to depict the soft-tissue structures that can precipitate stenotic symptoms—eg, thickened ligamenta flava, hypertrophied facet capsules, prominent epidural fat, and herni-

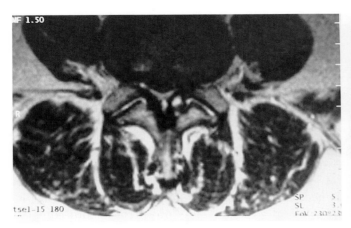

Figure 7 At the L4-5 level on a T2-weighted axial image, there is severe compression of the thecal sac by a posterior midline disc protrusion and hypertrophied ligamenta flava. The left ligamentum flavum contains a small synovial cyst.

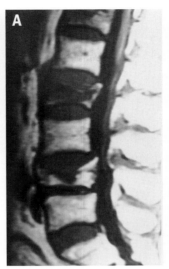 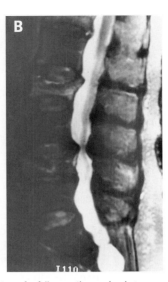

Figure 8 In an elderly patient with a history of a fall currently experiencing neurogenic claudication, the T1-weighted **(A)** and T2-weighted fat-saturated **(B)** sagittal images depict severe central canal stenosis at the L1-2 and L3-4 levels caused by osteopenic compression fractures. Changes from Kümmel's disease are seen in the L2 vertebral body.

ated disc material (Fig. 7)—as well as its excellent depiction of the thecal sac, spinal cord, and spinal nerve roots. Large segments of the spine also are easily evaluated with MRI. The strength of CT/MPR is its depiction of the osseous structures and extent of the bony proliferative changes.

In the lumbar spine, a true midline osseous sagittal diameter measuring between 10 and 12 mm is considered relative stenosis, and a diameter of less than 10 mm is considered absolute stenosis. This diameter is measured from the middle of the posterior surface of the vertebral body to the point of junction of its spinous process and laminae. With developmental stenosis, the reserve capacity of the spinal canal is reduced, thus predisposing the neural elements to impingement or compression by any material encroaching into the central canal. Developmental central canal stenosis might be associated with developmental narrowing of the neural foramina. Acquired stenosis is the narrowing of the central spinal canal, the subarticular lateral recess, or the neural foramina by degenerative changes of the discovertebral joint, facet joints, and ligamenta flava. Acquired stenosis might be superimposed on developmental stenosis. In addition to degenerative osseous changes that can lead to stenosis of the central spinal canal, other osseous abnormalities that might cause stenosis include posttraumatic deformities (Fig. 8), overgrowth of a spinal fusion, Paget's disease, fluorosis, and vertebral hemangiomas. Intraspinal masses (eg, synovial cysts) also might precipitate symptoms of neurogenic claudication.

Central canal stenosis in the cervical spine is typically caused by posterior spondylotic ridges projecting from the vertebral body end plates that narrow the canal and can impinge on the neural elements. The development of a retrolisthesis at a spondylotic level amplifies the

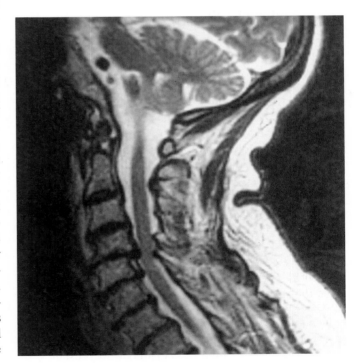

Figure 9 On a T2-weighted sagittal image, spondylotic changes are seen at the C4-5 and C5-6 disc levels, along with an approximate 5-mm retrolisthesis at the C4-5 level, resulting in mild/moderate cord compression. There is no high signal intensity in the cord suggesting myelomalacia.

degree of central canal stenosis because of the decreased distance between the posteroinferior margin of the posteriorly displaced cephalad vertebral body and anterosuperior margin of the lamina of the subjacent vertebra (Fig. 9). This altered spinal alignment, which can cause

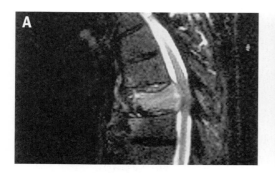

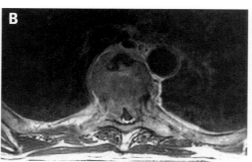

Figure 10 In an elderly patient who presented with the gradual onset of back and leg pain, the T2-weighted fat-saturated sagittal image **(A)** depicts a pathologic compression fracture of the T7 vertebral body, resulting in severe central canal stenosis and cord compression. The postcontrast T1-weighted axial image **(B)** depicts the extension of the tumor into the central spinal canal and the severe central canal stenosis.

cord compression, has been referred to as the "pincer mechanism." Other causes of central canal stenosis include disc herniations and ossification of the posterior longitudinal ligament (OPLL). Detecting early changes of OPLL with standard MRI sequences can be difficult. GE sequences might facilitate the detection of this pathologic condition, but if the precise extent of the OPLL is needed, a high-resolution CT/MPR examination should be performed. The evaluation of stenosis in the cervical spine is more difficult than in the lumbar spine because of the decreased size of the components of the motion segment. Initially, there was great enthusiasm that MRI would delineate the difference between osseous ridges and disc protrusions. The partial volume averaging of disc and ridge, which is seen unless section thickness is approximately 1 to 2 mm, as well as the range of signal intensity present in abnormal disc material and spondylotic ridges, has made the distinction between disc and ridge difficult. Three-dimensional GE volume acquisitions, when successful, might facilitate in making this discrimination. Thin-section (1.0 to 1.5 mm), high-resolution CT studies still provide the greatest information concerning the osseous morphology. Once the stenosis deforms or compresses the thecal sac or spinal cord, MRI is the best noninvasive modality to demonstrate the degree of reduction in the cross-sectional area of the thecal sac as well as the degree of cord displacement or deformation. T2-weighted or STIR sequences are employed to detect any abnormal signal intensity in the cord caused by edema or myelomalacia.

Dynamic MRI scans of the cervical spine are of value in the assessment of patients with traumatic or arthritic conditions (eg, rheumatoid arthritis) who present with C1-2 instability or symptoms of cord impingement. Sagittal fast SE T2-weighted sequences with the patient's neck comfortably positioned in a flexed, neutral, and extended position will demonstrate the extent of the instability and whether there is cord impingement by soft-tissue or osseous structures. Detection of superior subluxation of the dens and subaxial subluxation, as well as measurement of the cervicomedullary angle, can be accomplished on the sagittal sequences. It

is necessary when performing dynamic MRI scans in any patient with instability or potential cord compromise to monitor the study closely, employ fast imaging sequences, and not place the patient in a position that precipitates pain or dysfunction.

Stenosis of the thoracic spine is less common than cervical or lumbar stenosis. Because of the stability of the thoracic motion segments, it is rare to see spondylotic ridges narrowing the central spinal canal. Osteopenic compression fractures and tumor (Fig. 10) are probably the more common causes of thoracic central canal stenosis. Rare causes of stenosis include calcification or ossification of the ligamenta flava or epidural lipomatosis. Whenever stenosis is detected, it is necessary to determine its effect on the spinal cord. Central canal stenosis at the thoracolumbar junction is often related to trauma. Although CT is optimal in evaluating the nature and extent of a fracture and the displacement of fracture fragments, MRI is of value in demonstrating the position and condition of the conus medullaris and assessing the integrity of the spinal ligaments.

Disc degeneration might induce segmental instability and secondary hypertrophy and hyperplasia of the connective tissue elements. In the lumbar spine, degenerative tissue, including posterior bulge of disc-associated end plate remodeling, hypertrophy and bony proliferation of facet joints, and hypertrophy of ligamenta flava and facet joint capsules, might encroach into the central canal, subarticular recess, and/or neural foramina and impinge on, entrap, or compress neural structures (Fig. 11). Degenerative spinal disease is a continuous subclinical process that frequently does not evoke symptoms. As with disc herniations, MRI studies performed on asymptomatic volunteers demonstrate stenotic changes in the cervical and lumbar spine, particularly in older individuals.

Spinal degeneration might be associated with altered spinal alignment, eg, scoliosis or spondylolisthesis. In the lumbar spine, degenerative spondylolisthesis is an important cause of stenosis, most frequently involving the L4-5 segment. Disc degeneration with degenerative changes of sagittally oriented facet joints predisposes

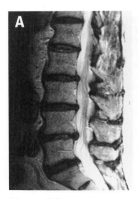
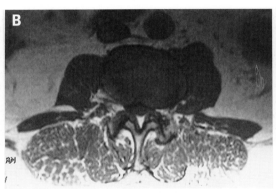
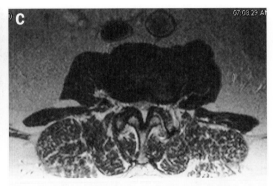

Figure 11 In a patient with neurogenic claudication, the midline T2-weighted sagittal image **(A)** shows multisegmental degenerative changes along with a posterior midline disc protrusion at the L4-5 level. Axial images orthogonal to the central canal are obtained to assess the degree of thecal sac deformation. On the T1-weighted **(B)** and T2-weighted **(C)** axial images at the L2-3 level, mild/moderate right and moderate/severe left facet arthrosis, along with posterior bulge of the disc, result in severe constriction of the thecal sac. Only a minimal amount of cerebrospinal fluid surrounds the cauda equina.

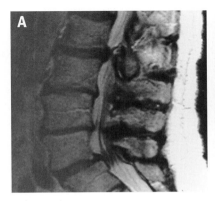
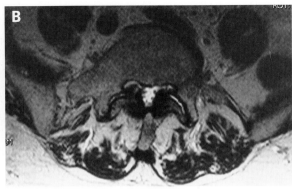

Figure 12 On the T2-weighted sagittal image **(A)** in a patient with back and leg pain, multisegmental central canal stenosis is seen along with a degenerative anterolisthesis at the L4-5 level. On the T2-weighted axial image **(B)** at the L4-5 level, moderate/severe facet arthrosis is causing moderate central canal stenosis along with stenosis of the subarticular lateral recesses and entrapment of the L5 nerve roots.

the motion segment to an anterolisthesis, which rarely progresses beyond a grade I slip because of an intact neural arch. The combination of osseous ridges projecting off the anteromedial margin of the facet joints, hypertrophy of the ligamenta flava, posterior bulge of the disc, and an anterolisthesis can result in severe central canal and subarticular lateral recess stenosis (Fig. 12). If there is asymmetry in the orientation of the facet joints (facet tropism), the anterolisthesis might have a rotatory component causing asymmetrical stenosis of the subarticular lateral recesses. Isthmic spondylolysis associated with an anterolisthesis also might cause central canal stenosis, but the stenosis is typically at the level of the pars defects and not at the level of the disc space, as is seen with a degenerative spondylolisthesis.

With myelography, stenosis is diagnosed by the detection of decreased AP diameter of the thecal sac (typically to less than 11 mm) and by the presence of a partial or complete block of the contrast column. With myelography, it is not possible to determine which components of the central canal are deforming the thecal sac. Precise measurements of the osseous central canal were not possible until the development of cross-sectional imaging studies. In addition, myelography pro-

vides no information concerning the degree of stenosis of the neural foramina. To obtain a true AP diameter of the lumbar central spinal canal with MRI, or to measure the cross-sectional area of the thecal sac, the axial images must be orthogonal to the central canal. Midline sagittal images can be used to measure the developmental size of the canal.

Myelography provides opacification of the thecal sac and a means to assess its dimensions in both the supine and erect positions, including stress views with flexion and extension. Many clinicians prefer myelography and CT-myelography for the assessment of patients with stenosis, particularly when there is a positional component to the patient's symptoms. Although erect myelography provides a more provocative stress examination than supine MRI does, it is unclear whether the information provided on an erect myelogram is unique in predicting patient outcome or is needed in selecting the optimal mode of therapy. Because there is potential morbidity with myelography, the question arises whether the same information can be achieved with MRI. Using a new MRI magnet design, it is now possible to evaluate the lumbar spine with the patient sitting in a neutral, flexed, or extended position. In one recent

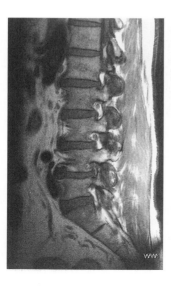

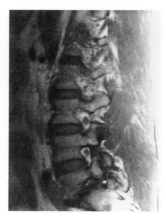

Figure 13 Bulging of the disc and end-plate proliferation results in mild neural foraminal stenosis at the L2-3 and L3-4 levels and moderate stenosis at the L4-5 level. There is impingement of the left L4 nerve root in the neural foramen on the T1-weighted sagittal image.

Figure 14 Proton density-weighted sagittal image in a patient with a grade II isthmic spondylolisthesis at the L5-S1 disc level shows severe cephalocaudal stenosis of the neural foramen and compression of the L5 nerve root between the base of the L5 pars interarticularis and the superior end plate of S1.

study that used this technology, supine and erect MRI (with the patient seated in flexion and extension) was compared with supine and erect myelography in a group of 30 patients, most of whom were being evaluated for stenotic symptoms. There was a high (r = 0.81 to 0.97) correlation between MRI and myelographic measurements and only a small positional difference in dural sac diameters from the supine to the erect positions. The authors concluded that the information gained on the erect MRI study, compared with that of the standard supine MRI examination, was limited.

Neural foraminal stenosis should always be considered as a possible etiology for radicular symptoms. The neural foramen is truly a three-dimensional structure, ie, a canal. Pathologic changes of any structure that borders the neural foramen can impinge or compress the exiting nerve root or dorsal root ganglion. The most

common etiology of neural foraminal stenosis is the presence of osteophytes projecting off the vertebral body end plates (Fig. 13). Degenerative changes of the superior articular process might lead to decreased volume of the posterosuperior compartment of the neural foramen, potentially causing neural compression. Decreased disc height results in cephalocaudal stenosis of the neural foramen, which can be amplified with an anterolisthesis (Fig. 14). Sagittal imaging is mandatory with both MRI and CT to evaluate the neural foramina for the presence of stenosis. Because spondylolysis sometimes is associated with disc degeneration and herniation, MRI can help determine whether radicular symptoms are caused by a disc herniation or from osseous stenosis (Fig. 15). Extraforaminal (far-out) stenosis can occur at the L5-S1 disc level because of the apposition of the base of the transverse process of L5 to the adjacent sacral ala.

In the cervical spine, there is a strong association between degenerative changes of the discovertebral joint and uncinate process hyperostosis (Fig. 16). If axial

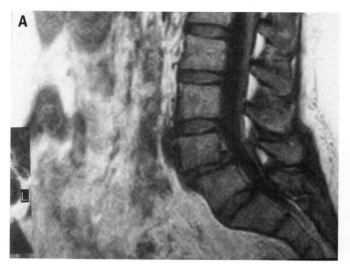

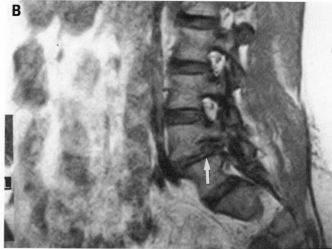

Figure 15 In a large patient with right thigh pain who could not be scanned on a high field-strength MRI system, the midline T1-weighted sagittal image **(A)** and the T1-weighted sagittal image through the right neural foramen **(B)** depict an L4-5 grade I isthmic spondylolisthesis and a disc protrusion (*B, arrow*) projecting into the right L4-5 neural foramen that compresses the right L4 nerve root.

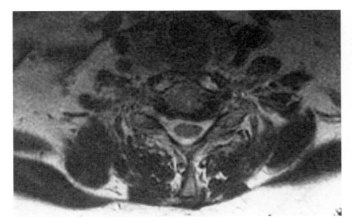

Figure 16 This T2-weighted axial image at the C5-6 level shows degenerative changes of the uncovertebral joints resulting in mild/moderate right and moderate/severe left neural foraminal stenosis.

sequence through the neural foramina. Intravenous injection of Gd-DTPA might help define neuroforaminal pathology by enhancing the extradural and intracanalicular venous channels, nerve root sheaths, and dorsal root ganglia. High-resolution CT studies provide excellent depiction of hypertrophic changes of the uncinate processes, and oblique reformations to assess the neural foramina can be computer generated.

The Postoperative Spine

For patients who have undergone disc surgery and experience recurrent back or leg pain, an MRI study is the optimal imaging examination to evaluate the surgical site and the remainder of the spine. The length of time between surgery and the MRI examination is important in determining the significance of postoperative MRI findings. Several studies have demonstrated no correlation between the immediate postoperative appearance of the spine on an MRI examination and a patient's symptoms. In the first few postoperative months, the changes detected on an MRI study reflect the repara-

and sagittal images in patients with radiculopathy do not demonstrate the cause of the radicular symptoms, additional assessment of the neural foramina can be obtained with an oblique coronal T1-weighted or GE

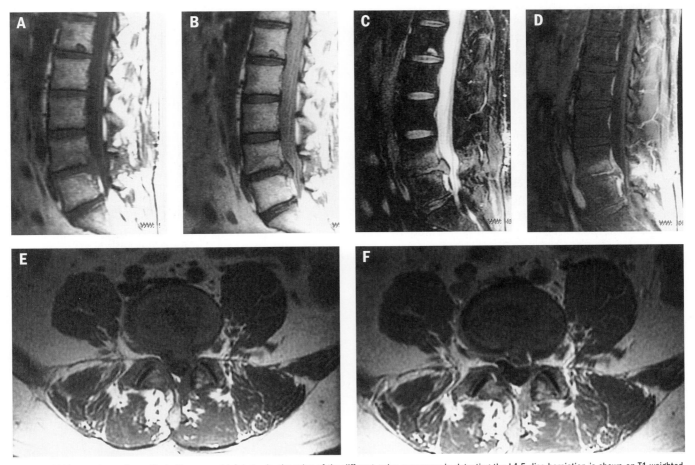

Figure 17 In a postoperative patient with recurrent left leg pain, the value of the different pulse sequences in detecting the L4-5 disc herniation is shown on T1-weighted **(A)**, proton density-weighted **(B)**, fat-saturated T2-weighted **(C)**, and postcontrast fat-saturated T1-weighted **(D)** sagittal images and precontrast **(E)** and postcontrast **(F)** T1-weighted axial images.

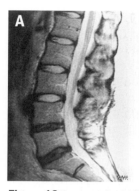
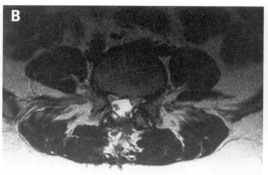
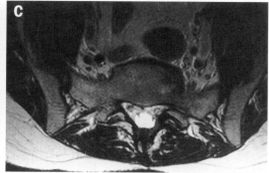

Figure 18 Two years after L4-5 and L5-S1 laminectomies, this patient has bilateral leg dysesthesias. In T2-weighted sagittal images it was difficult to identify the intrathecal nerve roots below L4 **(A)**. A T2-weighted axial sequence was normal at L3-4, showed mild peripheral clumping of the nerve roots at L4-5 **(B)**, and severe peripheral clumping of the nerve roots at L5-S1 **(C)**. The appearance of the nerve roots is diagnostic for arachnoiditis.

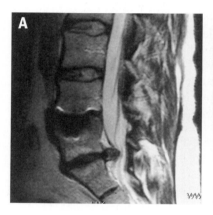
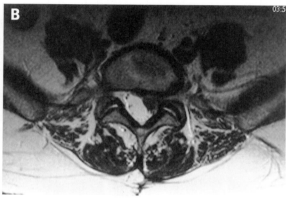

Figure 19 T2-weighted sagittal **(A)** and axial **(B)** images show minimal artifact from threaded titanium fusion cages at L4-5. At the L5-S1 disc level, there is a large posterior left paracentral disc protrusion causing mild/moderate compression of the thecal sac and compression of the left S1 axillary sleeve.

tive response to the surgical procedure. An MRI study in the immediate postoperative period usually does not help to diagnose the etiology of a patient's persistent pain unless there is evidence of a new disc herniation, infection, or complication of the surgical procedure. Even at 1 year after successful disc surgery, an MRI examination might show persistent posterior contour abnormalities of the disc causing mass effect on the thecal sac or nerve roots. One study performed 10 years after treatment for lumbar disc herniations reported that 37% of the patients had a persistent disc herniation, but the presence or absence of a herniation had no significant impact on the outcome.

The value of an MRI study in previously operated-on patients centers on the differentiation between epidural scar and disc herniation. Optimally, at least 2 to 3 months should have transpired since the disc surgery before MRI is performed. Epidural fibrosis is frequently present at the surgical site, and the extent of the fibrosis does not change significantly during the first postoperative year. Recurrent disc herniations are typically contiguous with the disc space, well marginated, and, compared with the disc of origin, isointense or hypointense on T1-weighted images and isointense or hyperintense on T2-weighted images. The intravenous administration of Gd-DTPA is particularly helpful in differentiating disc material from fibrosis (Fig. 17). Potential complications of a surgical procedure must always be considered when interpreting a postoperative study. Immediate postoperative complications include infection and hematoma. Symptomatic thecal sac compression has been reported with the insertion of fat grafts and the use of absorbable materials. Late postoperative complications can include instability and arachnoiditis (Fig. 18).

In the postoperative evaluation of patients decompressed for symptoms of central canal stenosis, the findings on cross-sectional imaging studies, both CT and MRI, have not had a significant correlation with patients' pain patterns, walking capacity, or subjective disability. In one long-term (10-year) postoperative follow-up study in which MRI was used to evaluate patients with lumbar spinal stenosis, there was no significant difference in symptoms between patients whose stenosis had and had not been diagnosed with MRI. Evidence of disc degeneration had a significant association with decreased walking capacity. The poor correlation of MRI with symptoms might have resulted from the lack of quantitative measurements used to characterize the degree of stenosis.

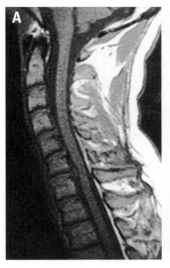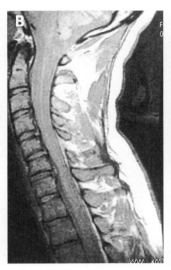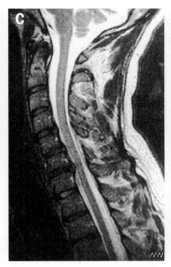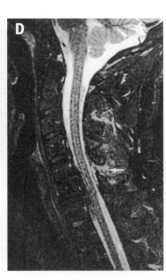

Figure 20 Midline sagittal images in a patient with neck pain 2 weeks postinjury. These images demonstrate the different information provided by different imaging sequences. **A,** T1-weighted. **B,** Proton density-weighted. **C,** T2-weighted. **D,** T2-weighted fat-saturated. The posterior disc protrusions are best depicted on B and C. The disruption of the posterior ligament spanning the base of the spinous process of C5 and C6 is best depicted on B and C. The minimal edema (*D, arrow*) present at the site of ligament disruption is best depicted on D.

A variety of metals and metal alloys have been used in the manufacture of spinal implants. Different metals generate different types of artifacts with MRI. Stainless steel tends to generate prominent artifacts that obscure the site of the implant and the motion segment adjacent to the implant, whereas titanium implants appear as a local signal void and tend not to obscure the adjacent tissue (Fig. 19). Although it is not possible to predict the degree of artifact with a specific implant, employing fast SE sequences (without fat saturation) decreases the amount of artifact created by most implants. GE sequences typically amplify the artifacts from spinal constructs. With MRI, it is possible to assess the integrity of a spinal fusion, but CT/MPR remains the best modality to evaluate the status of a spinal fusion. Sagittal and coronal reformations are needed to demonstrate bridging trabecular bone. In addition, CT/MPR is excellent in demonstrating osseous integration of bone located within an interbody fusion cage or for detecting evidence of cage subsidence, loosening, or displacement. Most cages provide little artifact on a CT study, whereas posterior constructs using pedicle screws can cause marked degradation of a CT image.

Spine Trauma

Plain films are the initial radiologic examinations performed on patients with acute spine injuries. For those with possible instability or fracture, or those with myeloradicular pain or dysfunction, MRI or CT can help elucidate the nature and extent of the soft-tissue and osseous injury. Although MRI provides the greatest amount of information concerning the soft tissues, discs, and spinal cord and can detect evidence of ligament or capsular disruption that might be associated with instability (Fig. 20), thin-section CT is the optimal modality to detect small cortical or laminar fractures and to demonstrate fracture fragment displacement. MRI provides the best assessment of cord impingement or compression by displaced fracture fragments. The distinction between cord hemorrhage and edema, which can be diagnosed with MRI, has predictive value on the outcome of patients after a cord injury. The chances of spinal cord recovery are much greater when only edema or contusion of the cord is detected (Fig. 21) compared with cord hemorrhage, which has a significantly worse prognosis. Patients with developmental stenosis of the cervical central spinal canal or with changes of cervical spondylosis are more prone to traumatic spinal cord injury because of the decreased functional reserve (space surrounding the spinal cord) of their central canals. An increased prevalence of developmental stenosis of the cervical central spinal canal has been reported in athletes who have experienced transient cord neurapraxia or stingers and burners.

Cumulative microtrauma to the spine can result in a spondylolysis of the pars interarticularis, typically at the L5 level. With standard MRI techniques, using a high field-strength MRI system, it is possible to detect pars fractures even when there is no anterolisthesis. Before the development of a complete pars fracture, a stress reaction in the pars might be detected by MRI as a focus of edema in the pars. Fat-saturated T2-weighted or STIR sequences are needed to detect these early changes. Another area of the spine where MRI might

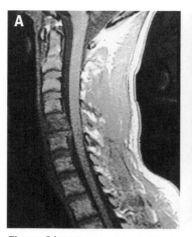
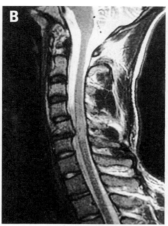
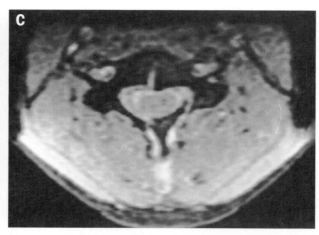

Figure 21 A, T1-weighted and **B,** T2-weighted sagittal images in a young patient after a diving injury depict a compression fracture and posterior displacement of the C5 vertebral body, resulting in stenosis of the central spinal canal. Although spinal cord impingement is minimal, there is increased signal intensity in the spinal cord on the T2-weighted image because of cord edema or hemorrhage. The continuous black line bridging the base of the spinous process represents intact posterior ligaments. **C,** The GE axial image depicts the vertical split fracture of the C5 vertebral body along with the laminal fractures.

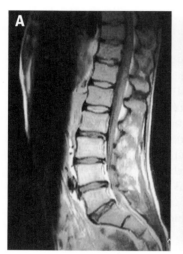
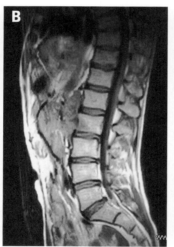
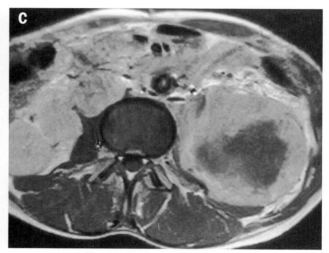

Figure 22 A, To improve the image quality of spinal structures, saturation pulses are applied to the soft tissues anterior to the spinal column, resulting in obscuration of these soft tissues. Because pathology in the retroperitoneum can be the cause of back pain, as in this patient with metastatic testicular carcinoma, the retroperitoneal tissues should be evaluated in the sagittal **(B)** or axial **(C)** plane in at least one sequence.

detect evidence of chronic microtrauma is at the thoracolumbar junction, where repetitive axial loading can cause end-plate irregularity, with edematous changes in the subchondral bone.

Spinal Tumors

MRI is the optimal imaging study to detect and classify a cord tumor. Contrast-enhanced studies are routinely performed in the initial assessment of patients with suspected cord tumors or other processes that might involve the spinal cord, such as multiple sclerosis. Contrast-enhanced MRI is also excellent for detecting intradural-extramedullary lesions such as nerve sheath tumors, meningiomas, or leptomeningeal spread of tumors. With extradural masses, contrast enhancement might be war-

ranted to differentiate between a nerve sheath tumor and a meningeal cyst or a disc fragment. A nonenhanced MRI examination is routinely used to detect osseous metastases. A fat-saturated sequence should be performed in at least one imaging plane to optimize the detection of marrow lesions. Although MRI is very sensitive in detecting marrow abnormalities, it does not provide specific information as to the etiology of the lesion. MRI is the best modality to demonstrate the size of a lesion and to determine whether it is extending into the paravertebral soft tissue, into the central spinal canal, or into the neural foramina. Retroperitoneal tumors can present with back or leg pain, and these masses are easily detected on an MRI study directed to that purpose (Fig. 22). With MR angiography, it is possible to assess

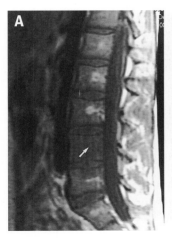 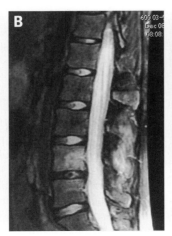 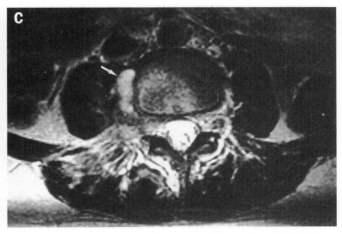

Figure 23 A, T1-weighted sagittal image in an adolescent with unexplained worsening back pain demonstrates loss of the fat signal (*arrow*) surrounding the L4 basivertebral plexus. **B,** On the fat-saturated T2-weighted sagittal image, there is increased signal intensity in the L4 vertebral marrow and reduced signal intensity in the L4-5 disc. **C,** On the T2-weighted axial image, there is a crescentic mass (*arrow*) demonstrating high signal intensity interposed between the vertebral body and the right psoas muscle. Biopsy of the mass and the vertebral body was positive for streptococcus.

the vascularity of tumors in the spine or in the paraspinal tissues.

Spinal Infection

In the adult, infection of the spinal column usually involves the vertebral bodies and intervening disc. The MRI diagnosis of vertebral osteomyelitis is based on the detection of confluent decreased signal intensity in the vertebral bodies and intervertebral disc and indistinct margins of the vertebral end plates on T1-weighted images, increased signal intensity in the disc and the adjacent vertebral bodies on T2-weighted images (detection facilitated with fat saturation), and paraspinal inflammatory masses (Fig. 23). After the initiation of treatment, resolution of the MRI findings can lag behind the clinical improvement in a patient and might persist or even appear to progress while the patient is getting better. The MRI findings in nonpyogenic osteomyelitis, such as tuberculosis or brucellosis, might involve the vertebral body and spare the disc, thus making the diagnosis more difficult. A contrast-enhanced MRI is the optimal examination to detect an epidural abscess; most epidural abscesses are associated with vertebral osteomyelitis.

Conclusion

With its excellent depiction of pathomorphologic and physicochemical abnormalities of the spine, MRI is now the best screening imaging study to assess patients with symptoms related to the spine or its neural elements, although in certain clinical situations (eg, severe scoliosis, the presence of ferromagnetic spinal implants, or for patients with contraindications to an MRI examination), other imaging modalities must be employed for the evaluation of spinal disorders. The complexity of MR technology has outpaced the level of understanding of most clinicians who order and interpret MRI examinations. In contradistinction to the current trend in our national health-care system for more generalists and fewer specialists, perhaps more specialization of radiologists in the field of spinal imaging will help to maximize the information we can obtain from this complex imaging modality.

Annotated Bibliography

Boos N, Rieder R, Schade V, Spratt KF, Semmer N, Aebi M: The diagnostic accuracy of magnetic resonance imaging, work perception, and psychosocial factors in identifying symptomatic disc herniations. *Spine* 1995;20: 2613-2625.

Forty-six preoperative patients with back and leg pain were compared with asymptomatic matched control subjects (age, gender, and occupational risk factors) for the presence of disc pathology. Seventy-six percent of the control subjects had a disc herniation and 13% had disc extrusions. The only substantial morphologic difference between the groups was the presence of neural compromise in 22% of the control subjects (8 of 10 minor) compared with 83% of the patients.

Brant-Zawadzki MN, Jensen MC, Obuchowski N, Ross JS, Modic MT: Interobserver and intraobserver variability in interpretation of lumbar disc abnormalities: A comparison of two nomenclatures. *Spine* 1995;20: 1257-1264.

Two nomenclatures were tested for the assessment of lumbar disc morphology in 98 asymptomatic volunteers and 27 symptomatic patients. The interobserver agreement between two experienced neuroradiologists was 80% for both nomenclatures; intraobserver agreement was 86% for each reader.

Gallucci M, Bozzao A, Orlandi B, Manetta R, Brughitta G, Lupattelli L: Does postcontrast MR enhancement in lumbar disk herniation have prognostic value? *J Comput Assist Tomogr* 1995;19:34-38.

Fifteen patients treated nonsurgically were prospectively evaluated with gadolinium-enhanced MRI. In the 11 of 15 patients who showed peripheral disc enhancement on their initial MRI, all demonstrated marked reduction in the size of their herniation on follow-up MRI examinations.

Herno A, Partanen K, Talaslahti T, et al: Long-term clinical and magnetic resonance imaging follow-up assessment of patients with lumbar spinal stenosis after laminectomy. *Spine* 1999;24:1533-1537.

The MRI findings of 56 patients treated surgically for lumbar central canal stenosis were compared with their clinical outcomes. There was no statistically significant difference in the patients with no stenosis postoperatively versus the patients with stenosis on their MRI scans with respect to severity of pain or walking capacity. The severity of spinal degeneration was more significantly correlated to altered walking capacity than to decreased thecal sac size.

Schmid MR, Stucki G, Duewell S, Wildermuth S, Romanowski B, Hodler J: Changes in cross-sectional measurements of the spinal canal and intervertebral foramina as a function of body position: In vivo studies on an open-configuration MR system. *AJR Am J Roentgenol* 1999;172:1095-1102.

In asymptomatic volunteers, there was a significant position-dependent variation in the size of the neural foramina and the cross-sectional area of the thecal sac; both became smaller in the extended position. The ligamenta flava were thickest in extension and thinnest in flexion.

Silverman CS, Lenchik L, Shimkin PM, Lipow KL: The value of MR in differentiating subligamentous from supraligamentous lumbar disk herniations. *AJNR Am J Neuroradiol* 1995;16:571-579.

Using a 1.5-T MRI system, three MRI criteria for the differentiation between a subligamentous disc herniation versus a transligamentous herniation were tested on 50 patients undergoing first-time lumbar surgery. None of the MRI criteria, including the size of the disc herniation and a continuous low-signal intensity line posterior to the disc herniation, was reliable in diagnosing the type of herniation found during surgery.

Stadnik TW, Lee RR, Coen HL, Neirynck EC, Buisseret TS, Osteaux MJ: Annular tears and disk herniation: Prevalence and contrast enhancement on MR images in the absence of low back pain or sciatica. *Radiology* 1998;206:49-55.

Disc morphology and signal intensity were evaluated on a contrast-enhanced MRI examination in 36 volunteers without back or leg pain. A bulging disc was detected in 81%, annular tears in 56%, a disc protrusion in 33%, and a disc extrusion in 0%. Ninety-six percent of the annular tears enhanced after contrast injection.

Weishaupt D, Schmid MR, Zanetti M, et al: Positional MR imaging of the lumbar spine: Does it demonstrate nerve root compromise not visible at conventional MR imaging? *Radiology* 2000;215:247-253.

Supine and seated flexion and extension MRI examinations were performed on 30 patients with chronic back pain unresponsive to nonsurgical treatment. Seated MRI examinations more frequently demonstrated minor neural compromise than did the supine MRI, and only one case of nerve root compression that was not present on the routine study was identified on a seated study in extension.

Wildermuth S, Zanetti M, Duewell S, et al: Lumbar spine: Quantitative and qualitative assessment of positional (upright flexion and extension) MR imaging and myelography. *Radiology* 1998;207:391-398.

The sagittal dimension of the thecal sac was compared using functional myelography and positional MRI. The quantitative measurements of the two modalities were comparable, and only limited additional information was gained on the erect studies.

Willen J, Danielson B, Gaulitz A, Niklason T, Schonstrom N, Hansson T: Dynamic effects on the lumbar spinal canal: Axially loaded CT-myelography and MRI in patients with sciatica and/or neurogenic claudication. *Spine* 1997;22:2968-2976.

Axial loaded MRI examinations performed on patients with suspected stenosis of the lumbar spine demonstrated a significant reduction in the dural sac cross-sectional area during axial compression in slight extension. Narrowing of the lateral recesses and deformation of nerve roots were estimated but not measured.

Classic Bibliography

Aprill C, Bogduk N: High-intensity zone: A diagnostic sign of painful lumbar disc on magnetic resonance imaging. *Br J Radiol* 1992;65:361-369.

Boden SD, Davis DO, Dina TS, Patronas NJ, Wiesel SW: Abnormal magnetic-resonance scans of the lumbar spine in asymptomatic subjects: A prospective investigation. *J Bone Joint Surg Am* 1990;72:403-408.

Deutsch AL, Howard M, Dawson EG, et al: Lumbar spine following successful surgical discectomy: Magnetic resonance imaging features and implications. *Spine* 1993;18:1054-1060.

Dvorak J, Grob D, Baumgartner H, Gschwend N, Grauer W, Larsson S: Functional evaluation of the spinal cord by magnetic resonance imaging in patients with rheumatoid arthritis and instability of upper cervical spine. *Spine* 1989;14:1057-1064.

Hamanishi C, Matukura N, Fujita M, Tomihara M, Tanaka S: Cross-sectional area of the stenotic lumbar dural tube measured from the transverse views of magnetic resonance imaging. *J Spinal Disord* 1994;7: 388-393.

Paajanen H, Erkintalo M, Kuusela T, Dahlstrom S, Kormano M: Magnetic resonance study of disc degeneration in young low-back pain patients. *Spine* 1989;14: 982-985.

Ross JS, Masaryk TJ, Schrader M, Gentili A, Bohlman H, Modic MT: MR imaging of the postoperative lumbar spine: Assessment with gadopentetate dimeglumine. *AJNR Am J Neuroradiol* 1990;11:771-776.

Ross JS, Modic MT, Masaryk TJ: Tears of the anulus fibrosus: Assessment with Gd-DTPA-enhanced MR imaging. *AJR Am J Roentgenol* 1990;154:159-162.

Tullberg T, Grane P, Isacson J: Gadolinium-enhanced magnetic resonance imaging of 36 patients one year after lumbar disc resection. *Spine* 1994;19:176-182.

Yu S, Sether LA, Ho PS, Wagner M, Haughton VM: Tears of the anulus fibrosus: Correlation between MR and pathologic findings in cadavers. *AJNR Am J Neuroradiol* 1988;9:367-370.

Chapter 9

Pain Imaging: Discography

Kurt P. Schellhas, MD

The radiologic evaluation of spinal pain underwent revolutionary advancement with the advent of MRI. With MRI, one commonly observes degenerative pathology involving multiple spinal structures at multiple levels or segments. The extent of degenerative changes (including disc pathology) that we detect on MRI often far exceeds what can be demonstrated by other imaging modalities. Recent contributions to the spine literature have delineated the concept of spinal disc internal derangement, with or without disc contour abnormality. With the demonstration of such multisegmental disc pathology, the need and demand for provocative spinal testing, such as discography, has increased considerably in recent years.

When evaluating patients with pain of suspected spinal origin, it is vital for the clinician to diagnose accurately the precise origin(s) of pain. Discography has been shown to be a valuable tertiary procedure for precisely this clinical situation (Figs. 1 and 2). Furthermore,

studies have shown that even with the highest resolution MRI scanning, some lumbar disc pathology may completely escape MRI detection, further necessitating the use of discography to determine which disc(s) may or may not relate to clinical complaints. In the cervical region in particular, MRI has been shown to be generally insensitive to the detection of intrinsic cervical disc pathology and clinically significant, pain-producing lesions in the peripheral anulus. MRI sensitivity in the thoracic region is greater than observed in the cervical region, but is still inadequate for a definitive evaluation of discogenic pain. Discography is performed in the lumbar, thoracic, and cervical regions, to evaluate cases of suspected discogenic pain, with or without obvious disc degeneration on preliminary imaging studies. Formal, prospective, controlled investigations of discography in the lumbar, cervical, and thoracic regions, respectively, have demonstrated the following key points: (1) Discs that prove to be anatomically normal at discography

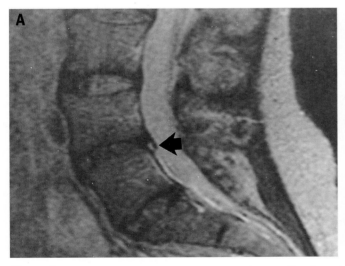
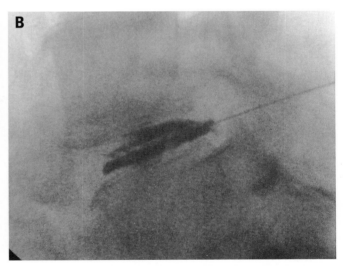

Figure 1 Painful lumbar disc HIZ, demonstrated with high field MRI **(A)** and provoked with discography **(B)**. **A,** Three-millimeter thick sagittal, T2-weighed image of lumbar spine obtained on high field (1.5T) magnet reveals an HIZ lesion (*arrow*) involving the dorsal aspect of the L4-5 disc. **B,** Lateral discography film obtained during injection of same disc. Disc was intensely and concordantly painful during injection.

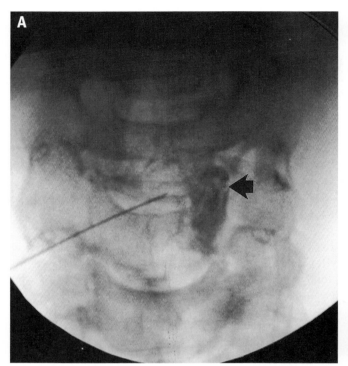

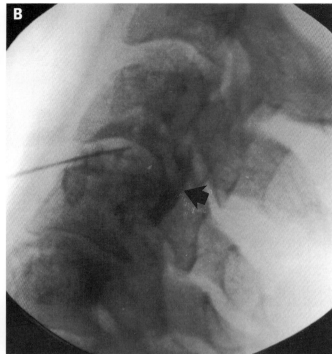

Figure 2 Painfully deranged cervical disc exhibiting full thickness annular tear with extradiscal leakage of contrast. AP **(A)** and lateral **(B)** images during injection reveals needle tip in the center of the disc with contrast leakage (*arrows*).

should be neither painful nor associated with any intense perception when injected to capacity with either contrast or saline. (2) Coincidental, painless annular tears are commonly observed in the cervical and thoracic regions and often are not detectable with state-of-the-art MRI. Such coincidental, painless tears are distinctly less common in the lumbar region. (3) Discs that prove to be intensely painful and clinically concordant (pain identical to and/or closely resembling the pain under investigation) when injected discographically exhibit tears either into or through the outer third of the disc anulus.

It has been demonstrated that discography, when performed by skilled and experienced individuals, with appropriate clinical indications, can significantly improve both surgical and nonsurgical treatment outcomes. Clinical indications for discography include the need for answers to the following: (1) Are spinal disc and/or vertebral body end plate pathologies demonstrated on imaging studies of clinical significance? (2) Is any type of therapeutic intervention needed, and if so, what type (surgical or nonsurgical)? (3) If spinal surgery is being planned, what spinal segments and structures might need to be addressed? (The results of discography will potentially influence the choice of surgical procedure and help answer the question "is a satisfactory surgical outcome possible?") (4) What is the ultimate prognosis?

Technical Considerations

A multidirectional, high-resolution C-arm with a built-in filming device is required to perform state-of-the-art discography. A tilting table facilitates the procedure and is recommended. Although many advocate the routine use of conscious sedation, it has been the experience of others that only rarely is sedation of any kind required. Patients need to be alert and communicative during this procedure.

Lumbar Discography

Clinical investigations of lumbar discography in asymptomatic subjects have revealed that discs that are morphologically normal by discography should not be painful. Coincidental annular tears may exist in normal (pain-free) subjects without pain provocation when injected discographically.

A highly specific MRI marker of high-intensity, concordant with discogenic pain, known as the lumbar disc high intensity zone (HIZ) has been described. A diagnosis of an HIZ must meet stringent criteria, including the use of high field MRI and T2-weighted images. (Fig. 1)

Investigations with pressure-controlled discography have identified both mechanically-sensitive and chemically-sensitive lumbar disc pathologies that are significantly predictive of surgical and nonsurgical outcomes. Mechanically-sensitive discs require annular distention and high-pressure injection to stimulate a response, while the chemically-sensitive discs are sensitive to low pressure and low-volume injection(s).

Cervical Discography

Controlled, prospective study of cervical discography in lifelong asymptomatic subjects and chronic, nonlitigious head and neck pain sufferers has established the validity of this procedure in skilled and experienced hands. MRI has been shown to be insensitive at detecting clinically significant lesions of cervical discs in patients suffering chronic axial and/or radicular pain without neurologic deficit (Fig. 2). The role of upper cervical discs and spinal structures in the pathogenesis of cephalalgia (cervicogenic headache) has been recently investigated and described. Cervical discography performed at all accessible cervical levels (C2-3 through C6-7) may aid the investigation of pain of suspected cervical discogenic origin.

Thoracic Discography

Controlled investigation of discography in the thoracic spine has revealed the limitations of MRI, quite similar to what was found in the cervical region. Discographically normal discs were not painful, and coincidental, painless annular tears were relatively common. Thoracic discography requires considerable operator skill and experience, as pneumothorax and spinal cord injury may result if this procedure is done improperly. This technique should be employed to investigate chronic pain, which may involve the back, rib cage, chest wall, abdomen, or visceral thoracic and/or abdominal compartments, that is suspected to be of thoracic discogenic origin.

In conclusion, discography is an important diagnostic procedure for the investigation of chronic pain of suspected spinal discogenic origin. It is a crucial test in many circumstances when spinal surgery is being either planned or contemplated.

Annotated Bibliography

Derby R, Howard MW, Grant JM, Lettice JJ, Van Peteghem PK, Ryan DP: The ability of pressure-controlled discography to predict surgical and nonsurgical outcomes. *Spine* 1999;24:364-372.

Pressure-controlled discography results were compared, retrospectively, to outcomes for groups of patients treated by nonsurgical means, interbody fusion alone, transverse process fusion alone, and combined fusion. Though there were no significant differences in outcomes across the entire sample, the subset of patients with chemical as opposed to mechanical sensitivity did better with combined fusion than with intertransverse fusion or no surgery.

Donelson R, Aprill C, Medcalf R, Grant W: A prospective study of centralization of lumbar and referred pain: A predictor of symptomatic discs and anular competence. *Spine* 1997;22:1115-1122.

Findings of lumbar discography were compared to responses to McKenzie protocol assessment and posturing in 63 predominantly workers' compensation and litigation-involved patients with low back pain and varying degrees of leg pain. Those whose pain centralized were more likely to have pain on discography and a competent anulus, whereas those whose pain peripheralized had pain and an incompetent anulus.

Ito M, Incorvaia KM, Yu SF, Fredrickson BE, Yuan HA, Rosenbaum AE: Predictive signs of discogenic lumbar pain on magnetic resonance imaging with discography correlation. *Spine* 1998;23:1252-1260.

MRI and discography were used to study 101 lumbar discs in 39 patients. Radial tears were seen commonly by MRI in patients with concordant pain on discography; however, the presence of such tears was not a reliable predictor of pain on discography. Severe loss of nucleus signal and the presence of an HIZ were useful MRI signs in predicting concordant pain at discography.

Milette PC, Fontaine S, Lepanto L, Cardinal E, Breton G: Differentiating lumbar disc protrusions, disc bulges, and discs with normal contour but abnormal signal intensity: Magnetic resonance imaging with discographic correlations. *Spine* 1999;24:44-53.

Two independent observers graded 132 lumbar discs of 45 patients for height, contour, neural compression, MRI signal intensity, and discographically demonstrated degeneration, disruption, and pain provocation. MRI findings of loss of disc height and signal intensity were strongly predictive of discographic findings of disruption of the outer anulus and pain on injection.

Ohnmeiss DD, Vanharanta H, Ekholm J, et al: Degree of disc disruption and lower extremity pain. *Spine* 1997;22:1600-1605.

Discographic findings of the lowest three lumbar discs were compared with pain drawings of 187 patients. Lower extremity pain was as often associated with Dallas grade 2 (disruption of annular fibers with no deformation of the outer annular wall) as with Dallas grade 3 (with deformation of the outer anulus) descriptions, although the grade 3 group reported a greater degree of aching pain.

Saifuddin A, Braithwaite I, White J, Taylor BA, Renton P: The value of lumbar spine magnetic resonance imaging in the demonstration of anular tears. *Spine* 1998; 23:453-457.

For 152 lumbar discs of 58 patients, the authors examined the correlation of an HIZ on MRI with concordant pain provoked by discography, which they took as the gold standard.

They found that the HIZ was highly predictive of pain provocation but cautioned that the usefulness of HIZ is limited by low sensitivity.

Saifuddin A, Emanuel R, White J, Renton P, Braithwaite I, Taylor BA: An analysis of radiating pain at lumbar discography. *Eur Spine J* 1998;7:358-362.

Of 260 lumbar discs injected for discography, 179 were abnormal with 84 posterior annular tears, 15 anteriors, and 45 both anterior and posterior. Isolated posterior tears were associated significantly with concordant radiating pain. Posterior annular tears without neural compression were observed to cause pain radiating into the lower limb.

Schellhas KP, Smith MD, Gundry CR, Pollei SR: Cervical discogenic pain: Prospective correlation of magnetic resonance imaging and discography in asymptomatic subjects and pain sufferers. *Spine* 1996;21:300-312.

Ten asymptomatic volunteers were compared with 10 non-litiginous chronic neck pain patients by MRI and C3-4 through C6-7 discography. Among the asymptomatic volunteers there were 20 discs normal to MRI, of which 17 had annular tears by discography. Among those with symptoms there were 11 discs that were normal by MRI, 10 of which showed tears by discography and two of which had concordant pain with injection. No discographically normal discs were painful.

Schellhas KP, Garvey TA, Johnson BA, Rothbart PJ, Pollei SR: Cervical diskography: Analysis of provoked responses at C2-C3, C3-C4, and C4-C5. *AJNR Am J Neuroradiol* 2000;21:269-275.

Forty patients with suspected upper cervical discogenic pain were examined by discography at C2-3, C3-4, and C4-5. The results were analyzed with particular attention to the value of the procedure for evaluation of C2-3. Concordant head and neck pain was frequently provoked by injection of the C2-3 disc. Fissuring of the C2-3 disc was exceedingly common and did not correspond to the provoked response. Discography demonstrated pathology and pain responses with much more sensitivity than MRI or CT alone.

Wood KB, Schellhas KP, Garvey TA, Aeppli D: Thoracic discography in healthy individuals: A controlled prospective study of magnetic resonance imaging and discography in asymptomatic and symptomatic individuals. *Spine* 1999;24:1548-1555.

Thoracic spines of 10 asymptomatic volunteers and 10 non-litiginous thoracic pain patients were examined by MRI and four-level discography. In the asymptomatic group, 27 of 40 discs were abnormal on discography. Unfamiliar injection pain occurred at sites of Schmorl's nodes in three volunteers. Among the pain patients, 21 of 48 discs were normal on MRI but only 10 of those were normal to discography, and 24 of the 48 injected discs had concordant pain with injection.

Classic Bibliography

Aprill C, Bogduk N: High-intensity zone: A diagnostic sign of painful lumbar disc on magnetic resonance imaging. *Br J Radiol* 1992;65:361-369.

Boden SD, Davis DO, Dina TS, Patronas NJ, Wiesel SW: Abnormal magnetic-resonance scans of the lumbar spine in asymptomatic subjects: A prospective investigation. *J Bone Joint Surg Am* 1990;72:403-408.

Bogduk N, Tynan W, Wilson AS: The nerve supply to the human lumbar intervertebral discs. *J Anat* 1981;132:39-56.

Bogduk N, Windsor M, Inglis A: The innervation of the cervical intervertebral discs. *Spine* 1988;13:2-8.

Brightbill TC, Pile N, Eichelberger RP, Whitman M Jr: Normal magnetic resonance imaging and abnormal discography in lumbar disc disruption. *Spine* 1994;19:1075-1077.

Colhoun E, McCall IW, Williams L, Cassar Pullicino VN: Provocation discography as a guide to planning operations on the spine. *J Bone Joint Surg Br* 1988;70:267-271.

Fraser RD: The North American Spine Society (NASS) on lumbar discography. *Spine* 1996;21:1274-1276.

Sachs BL, Vanharanta H, Spivey MA, et al: Dallas discogram description: A new classification of CT/discography in low-back disorders. *Spine* 1987;12:287-294.

Walsh TR, Weinstein JN, Spratt KF, Lehmann TR, Aprill C, Sayre H: Lumbar discography in normal subjects: A controlled, prospective study. *J Bone Joint Surg Am* 1990;72:1081-1088.

Whitecloud TS III, Seago RA: Cervical discogenic syndrome: Results of operative intervention in patients with positive discography. *Spine* 1987;12:313-316.

Chapter 10

Electrodiagnostics

Francis P. Lagattuta, MD

Paul Hudoba, MD

Neurodiagnostics encompasses electromyography (EMG), nerve conduction studies, somatosensory evoked potentials (SEPs), and motor evoked potentials (MEPs). Recent studies reevaluated the efficacy of neurophysiologic testing in lumbar nerve root lesions. Lesions at the L4 nerve root exhibited EMG abnormalities in 89% of subjects, dermatomal SEP abnormalities in 67%, and abnormal F-wave latencies in 44%. Lesions at the L5 nerve root exhibited EMG abnormalities in 87% of subjects, peroneous SEP abnormalities in 67%, and abnormal F-wave latencies in 66%. Lesions at the S1 nerve root exhibited EMG abnormalities in 55% of subjects, dermatomal SEP abnormalities in 64%, and abnormal F-wave latencies in 24%. Nerve conduction studies were always normal.

Dermatomal SEPs were studied at unilateral L5 and S1 confirmed nerve root lesion levels. The segmental and dermatomal sensitivities for L5 radiculopathy were 70% and 50%, respectively, at two standard deviations. The S1 level for segmental and dermatomal sensitivity was 50% and 10%, respectively. It therefore is important to use EMG in conjunction with SEPs and F-waves to better diagnose nerve root lesions.

Paraspinal muscle mapping recently has been described and refined. In the past, EMG in a nerve root lesion screen included the limb involved and the bilateral paraspinal muscles. In this new technique, five sites on the spine that correspond with the nerve root levels of the multifidus paraspinal muscles are studied and measured to allow for reproducibility. This technique has been found to be more sensitive to upper lumbar root lesions in multiple studies. The paraspinal mapping technique was found to be more sensitive than peripheral EMG studies in diagnosing lumbar radiculopathies as well. A control group had few, if any, abnormalities with the paraspinal mapping technique. Needle EMG studies of the lumbar paraspinal muscles are useful in distinguishing false-positive imaging studies.

Intraoperative monitoring during spinal surgery continues to be an important modality to prevent sensory or motor injury during that surgery. SEPs continue to be used with great success for preventing sensory abnormalities in patients with normal neurologic findings. In large scoliosis studies, intraoperative SEP monitoring had a false positive (or unreliability) rate of 1.6%. SEPs correctly predicted a postoperative deficit in 72% of those patients in whom a deficit was present. Of the 26 false negatives reported, 31% had a nonreversible lesion. In most cases, these were motor deficits. No reliable SEPs were found in 28% of the patients with neuromuscular abnormalities.

MEPs have been used since the late 1980s. The motor cortex is stimulated electronically or by magnetic stimulation. For electrical stimulation of the motor cortex, surface or subdermal needle electrodes are placed on the scalp or placed over the motor cortex. Subdermal needles are placed in the muscles from which the data are to be recorded. Neuromuscular relaxants must be discontinued once testing begins. Another way to stimulate the motor cortex is magnetic stimulation. The spinal cord can be stimulated by using epidural or percutaneous electrodes. When the spinal cord is being stimulated, anesthesia is no longer a concern.

Either myogenic (EMG) or neurogenic (NMEP) responses can be recorded. A myogenic response is a muscle contraction that elicits on EMG. A neurogenic response is the nerve action potential that elicits the contraction in the muscle innervated by that nerve. The myogenic response has a large amplitude and reliable latency. Unfortunately, the effects of anesthesia cause considerable changes to the responses. There is also considerable muscle contraction causing the limbs to move while the patient is on the operating table, causing some interference for the surgeon.

The NMEPs have been found to be more reliable than MEPs in amplitude, latency, and morphology. This finding allows specific criteria to be used to interpret the responses. A 10% increase in latency and 80% decrease in amplitude are significant. There is no movement on the operating table so it can be tested more frequently.

The reliability of MEPs is less than that of SEPs in patients with neurologic deficits. SEPs can be used on a higher percentage of patients with neurologic deficits, yet MEPs, in conjunction with SEPS, will increase the number of patients who will be able to be monitored. Studies of the validity of MEPs and NMEPs have been performed. In one study, there were no false-negative predictions and two true-positive predictions. NMEPs are used most frequently because of reliability and cost. MEP procedures continue to improve as well. At this time, if at all possible, both SEP and NMEP monitoring should be used simultaneously to provide information for both the sensory and motor tracts. The surgeon must be familiar with the protocol in the operating room. The technologists must be well known to the surgeon, the hospital must be committed to the program, and the monitoring must have professional supervision by a physiatrist or neurologist. Last, the anesthesiologist must be consulted regarding specific medication used during the monitoring.

Whether it be diagnostic or intraoperative monitoring, neurophysiologic testing continues to be the best way to monitor nerve function in real time. Neurophysiologic interpretation primarily is done at the time of the patient-physician interface. It is therefore imperative to have a physiatrist or neurologist trained in neurophysiology performing and interpreting these tests.

Recent Bibliography

Braune HJ, Wunderlich MT: Diagnostic value of different neurophysiological methods in the assessment of lumbar nerve root lesions. *Arch Phy Med Rehabil* 1997; 78:518-520.

Dumitru D, Dreyfuss P: Dermatomal/segmental somatosensory evoked potential evaluation of L5/S1 unilateral/unilevel radiculopathies. *Muscle Nerve* 1996;19; 442-449.

Gugino LD, Aglio LS, Segal ME, Gonzalez AA, et al: Use of transcranial magnetic stimulation for monitoring spinal cord motor paths. *Semin Spine Surg* 1997;9: 315-336.

Haig AJ: Clinical experience with paraspinal mapping I: Neurophysiology of the paraspinal muscles in various spinal disorders. *Arch Phys Med Rehabil* 1997;78: 1177-1184.

Owen, Jeffrey H: The application of intraoperative monitoring during surgery for spinal deformity. *Spine* 1999;24:2649.

Padberg AM, Komanetsky RE, Bridwell KH, et al: Neurogenic motor evoked potentials: A prospective comparison of stimulation methods. *J Spinal Disord* 1997;11:21-24.

Classic Bibliography

Dawson EG, Sherman JE, Kanim L, et al: Spinal cord monitoring: Results of the Scoliosis Research Society and the European Spinal Deformity Society Survey. *Spine* 1991;16:S361-S364.

Haig AJ, Talley C, Grobler LJ, LeBreck DB: Paraspinal mapping: Quantified needle electromyography in lumbar radiculopathy. *Muscle Nerve* 1993;16:477-484.

Haig AJ, LeBreck DB, Powley SG: Paraspinal mapping: Quantified needle electromyography of the paraspinal muscles in persons without low back pain. *Spine* 1995; 20:715-721.

Chapter 11

Differential Diagnosis of Spinal Disorders

Richard D. Guyer, MD

Douglas C. Burton, MD

Introduction

The evaluation and treatment of patients with spinal disorders, as in all fields of medicine, begins with a careful history and physical examination. Once this vital step has been performed, a differential diagnosis must be developed. It is crucial to have a differential diagnosis broad enough to include the correct diagnosis. It has often been said that to make a diagnosis, the physician must first think of that diagnosis. This chapter will examine those diagnoses that afflict the spine and those that mimic spinal disorders. General disorders common to the entire spine and specific disorders as they affect the cervical, thoracic, and lumbar spine will be discussed.

General Disorders

General disorders common to the spine include tumor and infection, trauma, seronegative spondyloarthropathies, metabolic bone disease, central nervous system (CNS) disorders, and complex regional pain syndromes.

Tumor and Infection

When evaluating a patient for complaints related to the spine, it is imperative to consider potentially destructive lesions such as tumor or infection. Any patient with unexplained weight loss, fever, chills, night pain, or a history of previous malignancy should arouse suspicion of a destructive lesion or an infection. Routine laboratory studies are helpful, and bone scan is a good screening study of the entire body. The spinal involvement of these diagnoses can be evaluated most carefully with MRI with and without gadolinium contrast enhancement. Fortunately, many of the primary spinal tumors are benign, but often masquerade as a radiculopathy. Neurofibromas (schwannomas), meningiomas, and ependymomas are the most common. Metastatic lesions, however, are more common. If better imaging of the osseous structures is needed, a CT scan can also be of assistance.

Trauma

Most acute spinal trauma is recognized and triaged in emergency departments. However, some patients come to the physician's office for treatment. A careful history and physical examination combined with good quality radiographs usually will identify these patients. Flexion and extension views should be routine, and if any doubt remains, a CT scan of the area in question should be obtained. If the injury is acute and primarily ligamentous, it is possible that plain radiographs, even flexion and extension views, will be negative because of guarding. In this instance, patients with neck injuries should be kept in a collar and reexamined in 10 to 14 days. At this point, the paraspinal spasm should be reduced enough to show abnormal motion on flexion and extension views if an injury exists.

Seronegative Spondyloarthropathies

Any of the seronegative spondyloarthropathies, particularly ankylosing spondylitis (AS), can have spinal involvement. A history of inflammatory bowel disease, urethritis, or psoriasis should lead to further investigation of these disorders, which include Reiter's syndrome, psoriatic arthritis, arthritis of inflammatory bowel disease, and the undifferentiated spondyloarthropathies.

Sacroiliitis is the hallmark of AS, which is strongly associated with HLA-B27. The spinal involvement will exhibit nonmarginal syndesmophytes with squaring of the vertebral bodies and may progress to autofusion or a "bamboo spine" deformity. This condition can lead to kyphotic deformities at any level of the spine and predispose the patient to fracture, often through the calcified disc space, even after seemingly innocuous trauma.

Metabolic Bone Disease

Metabolic bone disease can impact the spine, most commonly in the form of osteoporotic compression fractures. Risk factors for osteoporosis are postmenopausal woman, fair complexion and slight build, as well as cigarette smoking and excessive caffeine or alcohol use, and chronic steroid use. Any patient with risk factors should be evaluated for osteoporosis, even if he or she currently is asymptomatic. Evaluation of patients with discrete spine pain who are suspected of having a compression fracture should include initial plain radiographs. Often the question arises as to whether the fracture is new or old, or whether it is due to osteoporosis or tumor. MRI with gadolinium enhancement can usually distinguish between these entities.

Central Nervous System Disorders

When patients present with neurologic symptoms that wax and wane or with combinations of upper and lower motor neuron lesions, a CNS disorder should be considered. Multiple sclerosis (MS) usually presents as focal or multifocal attacks within the CNS that occur, remit, and then recur. A history of optic neuritis should raise suspicion of MS because up to 40% of patients with MS develop this problem at one point or another. Neurologic dysfunction with both upper and lower motor neuron lesions without sensory deficit is the hallmark of amyotrophic lateral sclerosis (ALS). ALS can easily be confused with cord compression syndromes of the cervical spine and must always be considered when the clinical presentation of myelopathy varies from the usual. Its onset is usually insidious, and it primarily affects patients 40 years of age and older.

Complex Regional Pain Syndromes

Complex regional pain syndromes affecting the upper or lower extremities can mimic spinal disorders and can coexist with them. The distinguishing feature is that radiculopathy and myelopathy do not cause dysesthetic pain or allodynia. However, patients with complex regional pain syndromes can have a compressive lesion in the spine, which may or may not be contributing to their symptoms. These patients should be evaluated with MRI to assess for any central compressive lesion. Cervical ganglion or lumbar sympathetic blocks can also be helpful in the diagnosis and treatment.

Cervical Spine

Radiculopathy

Patients who come to the physician for evaluation of cervical spine disorders typically complain of neck pain, arm pain, generalized neurologic dysfunction, or some combination of these symptoms. Patients with radiculopathy will often complain of pain that radiates in a dermatomal pattern. They also may have weakness or sensory disturbance, and occasionally patients may have a painless radiculopathy. Often neck pain will occur with the radiculopathy and can predominate at times. Radiculopathy is usually the result of either a soft disc herniation or foraminal stenosis that develops secondary to disc-space narrowing and uncinate arthrosis. Patients may come in with their shoulder abducted over their head (SAD sign) or holding their head in their hands, because this "traction" relieves the nerve compression. Provocative tests such as the Spurling maneuver can reproduce the patient's radicular pain. This test is performed by asking the patient to extend and rotate his or her head to the painful side and then applying axial compression. The neurologic examination can be confusing because of a prefixed or postfixed brachial plexus, causing the physical findings to be one level away from that in the imaging studies. In these cases, a selective nerve root block can be helpful in making the diagnosis.

Myelopathy

Patients with myelopathy may or may not complain of neck pain. Often the initial neurologic finding may be subtle, such as problems with balance, difficulty buttoning a shirt, or tingling in the fingers in a nondermatomal distribution. The most frequent complaint is lower extremity weakness. Often these patients will exhibit hyperreflexia in the lower extremities, but they may be hyporeflexic or hyperreflexic in the upper extremities. Myelopathy can occur as a result of a soft disc herniation, but more commonly occurs as a result of cervical spondylosis at one or more levels. Careful assessment of the imaging studies is important because ossification of the posterior longitudinal ligament, more common in patients of Asian heritage, also can cause myelopathy.

Compression Neuropathies

The evaluation of these patients should include a careful peripheral nerve examination because compression syndromes can mimic or even coexist with radiculopathy. The double-crush phenomenon occurs when a nerve is compressed at two levels, such as can happen with a C5-6 disc herniation and an ipsilateral carpal tunnel syndrome.

The median nerve can be compressed at several sites in the upper extremity. The pronator syndrome occurs when the median nerve is compressed proximal to the bifurcation of the anterior interosseous nerve. Symptoms include pain in the volar and proximal portion of the forearm and paresthesias into the median innervated digits of the hand. This compression may be due to the ligament of Struthers and/or an accessory supracondylar process proximal to the elbow, or it may be due to a thickened aponeurotic band of the pronator teres, under which the nerve passes.

The anterior interosseous nerve is a purely motor branch of the median nerve that supplies motor innervation to the flexor pollicis longus, pronator quadratus, and flexor digitorum profundus of the index finger. The deep head of the pronator teres or the tendinous origin of the pronator teres can compress it.

Compression of the median nerve most commonly occurs in the carpal canal. Symptoms include paresthesias of the radial three and one half digits, particularly at night and while driving. Physical examination findings include a positive Tinel sign or Phalen's sign at the wrist.

The ulnar nerve can be compressed in the cubital tunnel as it passes behind the medial epicondyle of the elbow. Symptoms include paresthesias of the ulnar one and one half digits of the hand that are intensified with elbow flexion. Examination findings include a positive Tinel sign at the elbow and reproduction of paresthesias with sustained elbow flexion. Recently it has been shown that elbow flexion with the hand in supination combined with compression of the ulnar nerve has the most sensitivity in patients with electromyography (EMG)-proven cubital tunnel syndrome. Less commonly the ulnar nerve may be compressed in Guyon's canal in the wrist. This compression will affect both the deep and superficial branches of the nerve at this level, causing both sensory and motor findings. It can be differentiated from compression more proximally because the dorsal sensory branch of the ulnar nerve, which supplies the dorsal aspect of the ring and little fingers, is unaffected.

The posterior interosseous branch of the radial nerve can be compressed at any of four sites within the radial tunnel, most commonly the arcade of Frohse. Symptoms include aching pain in the dorsal radial aspect of the forearm. The posterior interosseous nerve has no cutaneous sensory innervation, so there typically are no paresthesias. This condition is frequently confused with lateral epicondylitis, or tennis elbow, so a thorough examination of the lateral epicondyle for tenderness is warranted. The superficial branch of the radial nerve can be compressed as it emerges past the brachioradialis muscle in the forearm (Wartenberg's syndrome or cheiralgia paresthetica).

Rheumatoid Arthritis

Rheumatoid disease in the cervical spine can occur with neck pain, radiculopathy, or myelopathy, although it often can be asymptomatic, particularly at the onset. The disease affects the C1-2 articulation most frequently, also causing basilar invagination and subaxial subluxation. The upper cervical spine should be carefully studied with flexion and extension views. The pos-terior space available for the cord is the most reliable indicator of risk of neurologic progression. Dynamic MRI can also be valuable, particularly the measurement of the cervicomedullary angle. The normal angle is 135° to 175°. An angle less than 135° portends a high likelihood of progression of myelopathy. Less commonly the subaxial cervical spine will be involved, usually with upper cervical lesions as well. Flexion and extension radiographs should be obtained, with 3.5 mm or more of translation or 11° or more of angular change (compared with adjacent levels) being abnormal.

Deformity

The most common reason for deformity of the cervical spine is postlaminectomy kyphosis. This most commonly occurs after a multiple-level laminectomy, particularly in a patient in whom some kyphosis was already present in that region. These patients will complain of neck pain, headache, and can also develop myelopathy because the spinal cord is draped over the posterior portion of the vertebral bodies in a kyphotic segment.

Axial Pain

Neck pain alone can be the patient's primary complaint. In the absence of neural compressive lesions, the facet joints, intervertebral disc, and other soft-tissue structures have been implicated as potential sources of neck pain. These patients will often be given a diagnosis of soft-tissue sprain or strain, although there are no objective measures to validate this designation. Because most patients' symptoms will resolve with time, rest, anti-inflammatory medications, and perhaps physical therapy, a diagnosis of cervical sprain or strain usually will suffice. However, if the patient's symptoms persist, more invasive diagnostic studies can be undertaken. Cervical facet injections can be both diagnostic and therapeutic in the evaluation of these patients, and pain maps have been developed to identify the area of referred pain from the zygapophyseal joints. Discography has been shown to be a safe means of evaluating neck pain. The treatment of discogenic neck pain remains controversial. Studies on the treatment of discogenic neck pain with anterior cervical fusion have shown a success rate between 70% and 80% in appropriately selected patients; however, these were not prospective randomized studies.

Shoulder Disorders

Whereas many patients will complain of neck pain, others will identify the area of the shoulder girdle as the primary source of their symptoms. Many disorders of the cervical spine will have pain referral patterns to this area, but careful examination of the shoulder for intrinsic pathology and an understanding of the myriad disorders that can affect this area are important in determining treatment. The most common pathology is disorders of the rotator cuff. The patient may have a history of injury to this area, but often the onset of pain will be insidious. The pain may radiate down the arm to the elbow and have proximal extension into the trapezial area. Careful examination of the range of motion of the shoulder; palpation of the bony structures, particularly the anterior lateral border of the acromion; and provocative maneuvers such as the impingement test can readily identify rotator cuff disorders. Often these patients will have episodes of giving way that indicate weakness of the deltoid and biceps on manual motor testing because of pain in the shoulder. Care must be taken to not confuse these as signs of radicular weakness.

A rare but frequently overlooked reason for shoulder girdle pain is suprascapular neuropathy. This neuropathy occurs as a result of nerve dysfunction caused by repetitive microtrauma or by a compressive lesion. The compression usually is at either the suprascapular notch or at the spinoglenoid notch, where ganglion cysts are more commonly found. The patient can complain of vague pain in the shoulder, upper arm, or ipsilateral neck. Patients may show weakness and possibly wasting of the supraspinatus and infraspinatus muscles, depending on the site of nerve pathology. EMG will frequently be positive, although because routine EMG will not always be performed this proximally, it must specifically be requested.

Winging of the scapula can also cause vague pain in the shoulder girdle. The cause is either pathology of the long thoracic nerve, causing dysfunction of the serratus anterior muscle, or problems with the accessory nerve (cranial nerve XI), causing trapezial weakness. Long thoracic nerve dysfunction can be caused by surgery, trauma, neuritis, or have a viral etiology. When viewed from the front, the shoulders will be symmetrical, but when viewed from behind, the medial border of the involved scapula will be prominent. If the condition is subtle, winging will be brought about only by fatigue; testing can be done by having the patient perform repeat shoulder flexion, while observing the shoulders from behind. Trapezial weakness resulting from accessory nerve injury is usually less subtle. The patient will have drooping of the affected shoulder and often will give a history of previous surgery in the posterior triangle of the neck.

Thoracic Outlet Syndrome

Thoracic outlet syndrome can cause symptoms of arm and hand paresthesias, neck pain, and headache. The etiology is believed to be dynamic compression of the brachial plexus and/or subclavian artery between the clavicle and a cervical rib or prominent first rib. Often these patients will have scapular ptosis with trapezial wasting. Provocative maneuvers attempt to elicit the dynamic component of the patient's complaint. The Adson's and the Wright's tests both attempt to diminish arterial flow through upper extremity positioning. Recently, the Wright's test has been shown to be more sensitive than Adson's test. The overhead exercise test, in which the patient elevates the arms and repeatedly flexes and extends the fingers, is also very sensitive. The most common motor deficits, when present, are found in the interossei and hypothenar musculature.

Brachial Neuritis

Brachial neuritis, or Parsonage-Turner syndrome, is a benign, self-limiting disease of unknown cause. It commonly occurs as severe pain in the shoulder girdle, with radiation down the arm or into the neck. Movement of the arm intensifies the symptoms, but neck motion usually has no effect. The initial pain usually subsides in the first 2 to 3 weeks, leaving the patient with variable degrees of weakness. The lower motor neurons are affected, and some patients may have a sensory component as well. EMG can be helpful in the diagnosis, and cervical radiculopathy should be ruled out with MRI or CT myelography. The prognosis for recovery is excellent, although full recovery may take up to 3 years and complete return of function is not assured.

Thoracic Spine

Radiculopathy

Thoracic disc herniations (TDH) have been found in up to 11% of presumed asymptomatic individuals in autopsy studies. TDH can be symptomatic, however, causing axial pain, radicular pain, or even myelopathy. Patients may give a history of trauma, such as an axial load or automobile accident. The pain distribution depends on the location of the TDH. Central disc herniations may cause primarily axial pain with intermittent chest wall or even lower extremity paresthesias. Lateral disc herniations are more likely to cause primarily chest wall radicular pain. Radicular-type pain in the absence of a compressive lesion should arouse suspicion of an intrinsic neural lesion, such as activation of latent varicella virus in the form of herpes zoster or shingles.

Myelopathy

Myelopathy can be subtle in these patients, and careful examination of both the upper and lower extremities is mandatory to evaluate for differences in reflexes and tone. Patients may give a history of vague lower extremity disturbance or difficulty with balance and frequent falls. MRI is the imaging study of choice for evaluation of thoracic lesions because excellent images can be obtained in both the sagittal and axial plane and cord signal changes are shown as well.

Deformity

Deformity of the thoracic spine can be found in the pediatric and adult populations and can be readily identified with plain radiographs, preferably 36-in posteroanterior and lateral images. Other findings may be a rib hump, elevated shoulder, or truncal list. Scoliosis in the pediatric population usually is not painful and certainly not disabling. Any patient with severe pain complaints should be carefully examined for other etiologies.

Adult thoracic scoliosis can be painful. The natural history studies that have been reported show that these patients, untreated with surgery, have more pain than age-matched individuals, though it is seldom disabling. Nevertheless, some patients will require surgery as adults because of progression of deformity with imbalance, pain, and for cosmesis. Restrictive disease of the cardiac and pulmonary systems does not occur in curves less than 90°.

In evaluating these patients, care should be taken to examine the sagittal as well as the coronal plane. Scheuermann's hyperkyphosis, as well as other kyphotic disorders, can cause pain as well as problems with balance. Often these patients will complain of pain at the thoracolumbar junction as a result of compensation for their thoracic kyphosis. Scheuermann's hyperkyphosis can also affect the thoracolumbar or lumbar spine, causing pain lower in the spine. Radicular pain in these patients is a result of degenerative changes below the kyphosis, rather than pathology within the affected region.

Patients with fixed kyphotic deformities due to other causes, such as trauma or ankylosing spondylitis, may complain of truncal imbalance. These patients compensate for their hyperkyphosis with increased lumbar lordosis and hip flexion. When examining these patients for sagittal imbalance, it is important to note if they stand in a flexed hip and knee posture. Often they will have hip flexion contractures if their condition has been prolonged. These postural accommodations also place stress on the sacroiliac joints, which should be carefully examined as well.

Axial Pain

Occasionally patients will complain of central thoracic pain without any radicular component. In the upper thoracic spine this pain may be related to cervical spine pathology or shoulder girdle dysfunction, as has already been discussed. In the absence of a cervical or shoulder etiology and without a frank thoracic disc herniation, intrinsic thoracic disc pain is a possibility. Thoracic discography has been shown to be a safe provocative test of pain in the thoracic spine and is the only objective means of identifying the level of discogenic pathology. Treatment of discogenic thoracic pain with arthrodesis is as controversial if not more so than similar procedures in the cervical and lumbar spine.

Another cause of central thoracic pain can be arthrosis of the costovertebral articulation. These patients often can give a history of trauma, particularly to the ribs. This is usually a self-limited disorder, and like many instances of brief thoracic back pain, it is attributed to a thoracic strain or sprain. However, if it persists, fluoroscopic injection with local anesthetic and steroid can be diagnostic and therapeutic.

Visceral Etiologies

The physician should keep in mind that referred pain from disorders within the thoracic and abdominal cavity can also cause thoracic pain. Cholecystitis can often cause back pain with radiation around the right flank, much like a low thoracic disc herniation. Pancreatitis can radiate to the back, as can problems of the esophagus and stomach. Pleuritic pain can also be confused at times with thoracic radicular pain. An aneurysm of the thoracic or abdominal aorta can begin as back pain, and if missed initially, will often result in death. Careful questioning of the patient will usually differentiate these disorders, but it is imperative that these disorders not be overlooked.

Lumbar Spine

Radicular Pain: Herniated Disc

Pain and dysfunction of the lower extremities resulting from compression of the lumbar neural elements usually is caused by intervertebral disc herniation, stenosis secondary to degenerative change of the spine, instability, or a combination of these conditions. Lumbar disc herniation affects approximately 2% of the US population at one time or another. The hallmark is lower extremity pain in a radicular pattern, which is intensified by maneuvers that place tension on that nerve root. If the herniation affects the fifth lumbar root or lower, the sciatic nerve is affected. The straight leg raise, done while seated or supine, will stretch the sciatic nerve and provoke a pain response. Herniations that irritate the second through fourth roots will affect the femoral nerve. The femoral stretch test can be done while standing or prone, with hyperextension of the hip causing tension on the femoral nerve and the affected root.

Patients may complain of sensory and motor disturbance, and may demonstrate deep tendon reflex changes. Occasionally patients can have a painless radiculopathy, although this is infrequent. In these cases, a tumor etiology should be considered as well. Patients with severe canal compromise can have multiple root dysfunction and/or loss of bowel or bladder function, known as a cauda equina syndrome. This condition constitutes a surgical emergency and should be treated as such.

The typical location of a disc herniation is posterolateral. In this position, the traversing root is most commonly affected. Thus an L4-5 disc herniation will not affect the L4 root, which has already exited under the L4 pedicle, but it will displace the L5 root as it travels over the disc toward the L5 pedicle and L5-S1 foramen. This is important to keep in mind, particularly because far lateral disc herniations will have a different effect. Far lateral disc herniations usually will cause dysfunction of the exiting root; that is, an L4-5 far lateral herniation will displace the L4 root in the foramen. After discectomy, these patients may have a period of dysesthetic pain because of manipulation of the dorsal root ganglion, which lies in this area.

MRI is the imaging modality of choice to assess these problems. In patients with previous surgery, gadolinium contrast enhancement allows differentiation between recurrent disc and scar. CT myelography is also very good, although it cannot accurately differentiate scar and recurrent disc. It remains an excellent alternative in the severely claustrophobic patient, although the improvement in open magnet MRI has reduced this indication.

Lumbar Degenerative Disease: Stenosis

Aging of the spine, as with other joints of the body, can bring on bony and ligamentous changes. Narrowing of the disc spaces and hypertrophy of the ligamentum flavum and facet joints are accompanied by narrowing of the spinal canal. Compression can occur in any of three areas: (1) central stenosis, (2) subarticular or lateral recess stenosis, or (3) foraminal stenosis. Symptoms referable to these changes can occur in myriad ways. Some patients may complain of leg pain that occurs in a purely radicular pattern that is often aggravated by activity, and frequently no tension sign will be present. Other patients will have multiple root dysfunction or vague lower extremity complaints. Careful questioning will usually elicit a history of exacerbation with activity or neurogenic claudication. These patients may note improvement in symptoms when leaning forward to walk, as when pushing a grocery cart or walking uphill.

MRI and CT myelography are the studies of choice in evaluating patients with stenosis. In patients with scoliosis or spondylolisthesis, the CT myelogram is often more helpful because it is a dynamic study and can better differentiate bony changes.

Spondylolisthesis

Spondylolisthesis is derived from the Greek words spondylos, meaning spine, and olisthesis, meaning slippage. It can be subdivided into six types: (1) dysplastic, (2) isthmic, (3) degenerative, (4) traumatic, (5) pathologic, and (6) postsurgical. Isthmic, degenerative, and postsurgical etiologies are by far the most common and will be discussed here.

Isthmic spondylolisthesis is caused by fracture or elongation of the pars interarticularis. Although it can manifest itself in childhood or adolescence, it is not congenital; fetal autopsy studies have failed to show its existence. Patients with a history of participation in gymnastics or in football as interior lineman have a higher incidence because of the frequent hyperextension of the spine that those sports require. Patients may come to the physician with complaints of back pain, leg pain, or both. Identification of the pain generator in these patients can be difficult. Often they will have compression of the exiting root beneath the fibrocartilage scar of the pars defect. In the case of an L5-S1 isthmic spondylolisthesis, the L5 nerve root would be affected. Rarely are the caudal roots affected, except in high-grade slips because the defect in the neural arch affords them increased space. Patients with primarily back pain as a result of their disorder need to be carefully evaluated. Often they will have degeneration of the disc above, which may be a source of their pain.

Degenerative spondylolisthesis usually is seen beginning in the fifth decade of life, and L4-5 is the most commonly affected level. These patients typically complain of leg pain with or without back pain that is aggravated by activity. Flexion and extension films are paramount because a supine lateral radiograph may miss the diagnosis. MRI or CT myelogram will show the neural impingement. In contrast to isthmic slips, the traversing rather than the exiting root is affected by degenerative spondylolisthesis.

Postsurgical spondylolisthesis usually occurs in two settings. In the first several months to a few years after decompression, a patient will develop recurrence of leg pain, onset of back pain, or both. These patients develop a segmental instability that is due to the removal of portions of the vertebral elements at prior surgery (or surgeries). It has been shown in biomechanical studies that resection of greater than 50% of the facet joints will render them incompetent. Often, however, the postsurgical spondylolisthesis can be perplexing if only static studies are obtained. Flexion and extension radiographs will usually provide the data needed to make this diagnosis. The second instance of instability occurs in postfusion patients, usually several years after their initial procedure. Facet and ligamentum flavum hypertrophy develops at an adjacent level, often with dynamic instability. This hypertrophy often is called the transition syndrome. Patients may have symptoms of claudication, back pain, or both. MRI or CT myelogram will show the stenosis, while flexion and extension views will demonstrate any instability.

Deformity

Deformity of the lumbar spine, as in the thoracic spine, should be evaluated in both the coronal and sagittal planes. Scoliosis can be a result of idiopathic scoliosis, degenerative disease of the spine, or a combination of the two. Physical examination and radiographs can readily provide sufficient information to make the diagnosis. These patients may have radicular symptoms due to stenosis, particularly on the concave side of the curve. Thirty-six inch films are mandatory to evaluate coronal and sagittal balance. If canal studies are needed, CT myelography is usually more helpful because the deformity makes MRI difficult to interpret. Kyphosis of the lumbar spine can occur as a result of degenerative change of the spine. In the postsurgical setting, particularly after distraction instrumentation of the low lumbar spine, a flat-back deformity can develop. The patient will complain of back pain and fatigue, occasionally with radiation into the proximal thigh. As in the thoracic spine, the patient may flex the hips in an attempt to maintain the head over the pelvis. Stresses transferred to the sacroiliac joint may cause problems there as well.

Axial Lumbar Pain

Low back pain is widespread in the United States, with the lifetime prevalence estimated at 50% to 80%. However, patients rarely receive a specific diagnosis. The symptoms often are diagnosed as a lumbar strain or sprain, and because most occurrences of pain resolve, these diagnoses suffice. After a thorough history and physical examination reveals no neurologic changes and no evidence of trauma, tumor, or infection and radiographs show no evidence of spondylolisthesis or instability, other causes of pain should be examined.

The lumbar facet joints are a potential source of pain. Examination may show pain with lumbar range of motion, and radiographs may show facet arthrosis. Patients may have pseudoradicular or sclerotomal pain that radiates into the thighs or the groin. Diagnostic facet blocks are helpful in making this diagnosis.

The outer third of the anulus of the intervertebral disc is innervated from branches of the sinuvertebral nerve, and the lumbar disc has long been thought to be a source of pain, although this theory remains highly controversial. The diagnosis of discogenic lumbar pain is made with lumbar discography. Lumbar discography is safe, although its efficacy in predicting successful surgical outcomes is unclear. Recently, retrospective studies have suggested that discography that is positive at low pressures may be a better predictor of good surgical outcomes by identifying chemically sensitive discs. As MRI techniques have evolved, attempts have been made to correlate MRI findings with those of discography, particularly the high-intensity zone seen on T2-weighted images in the posterior portion of the anulus. This finding is not universal in patients with positive discography, nor are these discs always painful with discography. Therefore, MRI should not be considered a substitute for discography if a physician is attempting to confirm the diagnosis of discogenic lumbar pain.

Sacroiliac Joint

The sacroiliac (SI) joint is another potential source of low back pain. Patients with SI joint pain will often note discomfort while rising from a seated position. This pain resolves initially with ambulation, but returns with any prolonged activity. The pain may radiate to the upper calf or around the hip and into the groin area, and is often accompanied by trochanteric bursitis. During ambulation the patient may externally rotate the lower extremity on the affected side in an attempt to stabilize the joint. On examination, there may be direct tenderness over the joint, as well as pain on provocative maneuvers. Patrick's test (fabere sign) is often positive, as are the posterior shear and resisted abduction tests. The posterior shear test is performed with the patient supine and the hip and knee flexed to 90°. Posterior force is then directed on the flexed thigh, causing loading of the joint. While the patient still is supine, resisted abduction of the extended lower extremity will also load the SI joint and reproduce pain. Radiographs may or may not show sclerosis of the joint. Fluoroscopic injection of the inferior portion of the joint with contrast can be diagnostic as well as therapeutic.

Coxal Arthrosis

Careful examination of the hips should always be performed during routine lumbar evaluation. Frequently patients with arthritis of the hips are mistakenly believed to have a radicular syndrome. Careful history and physical examination with range of motion of the hips will identify these patients. Hip radiographs are usually diagnostic. If hip films are negative, but the physical examination indicates otherwise, an MRI should be obtained to evaluate for early osteonecrosis of the femoral head.

Meralgia Paresthetica

Patients with radiating pain into the anterior thigh should be examined carefully for an inguinal hernia. Another source of thigh pain can be irritation of the lateral femoral cutaneous nerve, or meralgia paresthetica. This condition can be due to body habitus, tight clothing, or is iatrogenic after a previous inguinal procedure or anterior iliac bone graft harvest done too far distally. A Tinel's sign over the course of the nerve should be positive, and nerve block can be both diagnostic and therapeutic.

Vascular Claudication

The history and physical examination of spine patients should include risk factors for peripheral vascular disease as well as a careful vascular examination. Vascular claudication can mimic neurogenic claudication at first glance. Typically, the pain of vascular claudication will begin more distally, whereas neurogenic claudication begins proximally and spreads distally. Neurogenic claudication typically is worse with extension postures, with patients being able to walk uphill (leaning slightly forward) easier than downhill (extending causing more compression) or being able to walk flexed forward leaning on a shopping cart without significant limitation. Vascular disease may also cause nighttime pain that is relieved by hanging the feet over the edge of the bed. The absence of pedal pulses in any patient warrants vascular consultation.

Annotated Bibliography

Baba H, Maezawa Y, Uchida K, et al: Cervical myeloradiculopathy with entrapment neuropathy: A study based on the double-crush concept. *Spinal Cord* 1998; 36:399-404.

This is a retrospective study of 65 patients with a double-crush phenomenon in the upper extremities. The clinical presentation, order of decompression, and outcomes are reviewed. The authors conclude that cervical decompression should precede addressing the peripheral lesion, particularly in cases of myelopathy.

Bradford DS, Tay BK, Hu SS: Adult scoliosis: Surgical indications, operative management, complications, and outcomes. *Spine* 1999;24:2617-2629.

This is an excellent review of the surgical treatment of adult scoliosis.

Broadhurst NA, Bond MJ: Pain provocation tests for the assessment of sacroiliac joint dysfunction. *J Spinal Disord* 1998;11:341-345.

This is a prospective, randomized double-blind study in which 40 patients who reported pain on each of three sacroiliac joint provocation maneuvers were given a fluoroscopic injection of either lidocaine or saline. The tests were repeated and none of the patients receiving saline had their pain suppressed. The patients receiving lidocaine had substantial suppression of their pain. The authors concluded that this battery of three tests has a specificity of 100% and a sensitivity of 77% to 87% for pain arising from the sacroiliac joint.

Derby R, Howard MW, Grant JM, Lettice JJ, Van Peteghem PK, Ryan DP: The ability of pressure-controlled discography to predict surgical and nonsurgical outcomes. *Spine* 1999;24:364-372.

This is a retrospective review examining the relationship between injection pressure at discography and surgical outcome. The authors conclude that pain at lower pressures may portend a better surgical outcome.

Kuhn JE, Plancher KD, Hawkins RJ: Scapular winging. *J Am Acad Orthop Surg* 1995;3:319-325.

This article reviews the etiology, clinical presentation, and treatment of scapular winging.

Lane JM, Riley EH, Wirganowicz PZ: Osteoporosis: Diagnosis and treatment. *J Bone Joint Surg Am* 1996;78: 618-632.

This is an excellent review of the diagnosis and treatment of osteoporosis.

Leffert RD, Perlmutter GS: Thoracic outlet syndrome: Results of 282 transaxillary first rib resections. *Clin Orthop* 1999;368:66-79.

This is an excellent retrospective review of experience in the surgical treatment of thoracic outlet syndrome. Clinical presentation and common examination findings are reviewed.

McCarty EC, Tsairis P, Warren RF: Brachial neuritis. *Clin Orthop* 1999;368:37-43.

This is a review of the etiology, presentation, and clinical course of brachial neuritis.

Novak CB, Lee GW, Mackinnon SE, Lay L: Provocative testing for cubital tunnel syndrome. *J Hand Surg Am* 1994;19:817-820.

This is a prospective study of patients with EMG proven cubital tunnel syndrome. The authors show that the elbow flexion maneuver with manual compression of the nerve is more sensitive and has a higher positive predictive value than Tinel sign or elbow flexion alone.

Palit M, Schofferman J, Goldthwaite N, et al: Anterior discectomy and fusion for the management of neck pain. *Spine* 1999;24:2224-2228.

This is a prospective, nonrandomized study analyzing the treatment of discogenic cervical pain. The evaluation of these patients is detailed, including comprehensive psychological work-up. At a minimum 2-year follow-up, 79% of patients were satisfied with their outcome.

Plate AM, Green SM: Compressive radial neuropathies. *Instr Course Lect* 2000;49:295-304.

This is a comprehensive review of the anatomy, clinical presentation, diagnostic modalities, and treatment of radial neuropathies.

Preston DC: Distal median neuropathies. *Neurol Clin* 1999;17:407-424.

This is a review article that thoroughly covers median nerve neuropathies at various anatomic sites with a strong review of EMG analysis.

Regan JJ, Ben-Yishay A, Mack MJ: Video-assisted thoracoscopic excision of herniated thoracic disc: Description of technique and preliminary experience in the first 29 cases. *J Spinal Disord* 1998;11:183-191.

This is a prospective study of 29 patients with thoracic disc herniations undergoing thorascopic disc excision. The clinical presentation of these patients was reviewed; seven patients had primarily axial pain, 19 patients had radicular pain, two patients had myelopathy, and one patient had paraparesis.

Romeo AA, Rotenberg DD, Bach BR Jr: Suprascapular neuropathy. *J Am Acad Orthop Surg* 1999;7:358-367.

The authors review the anatomy of the suprascapular nerve and its clinical appearance and treatment in compression syndromes.

Classic Bibliography

Boden SD, Dodge LD, Bohlman HH, Rechtine GR: Rheumatoid arthritis of the cervical spine: A long-term analysis with predictors of paralysis and recovery. *J Bone Joint Surg Am* 1993;75:1282-1297.

Guyer RD, Ohnmeiss DD: Lumbar discography: Position statement from the North American Spine Society Diagnostic and Therapeutic Committee. *Spine* 1995; 20:2048-2059.

Guyer RD, Collier RR, Ohnmeiss DD, et al: Extraosseous spinal lesions mimicking disc disease. *Spine* 1988;13:328-331.

Wiltse LL, Newman PH, Macnab I: Classification of spondylolysis and spondylolisthesis. *Clin Orthop* 1976; 117:23-29.

Chapter 12

The Spine in Sports

Stuart M. Weinstein, MD

Stanley A. Herring, MD

Overview

Whereas spinal pain is common in the general population, it is essentially universal in the athletic population. Specific sports and certain positions and activities within a given sport predispose an athlete to the development of low back or neck pain syndromes. For example, spondylolysis is more common in gymnasts and dancers, in baseball pitchers, and in athletes participating in the throwing events of track and field; "stingers" occur more commonly in wrestlers, particularly with the take-down maneuver, and in football players, especially the defensive backs and offensive linemen. Therefore, a sports medicine physician should have sport-specific knowledge to be a more efficient diagnostician.

The spine is subject to both acute overload and chronic, repetitive overload injuries. The spine and related structures not only are susceptible to injury, they also play integral roles in controlling the normal biomechanics of athletic activity and prevention of injury to key joints (eg, the shoulder) and peripheral nerves (eg, nerve roots). As the core or centrum of motion and function, the spine and related structures are the engines for sports activity. Trunk control and stability are also necessary for any athlete to perform with maximal efficiency and output.

The biomechanical contribution of the spine and trunk in the overhead-throwing athlete serves as a prototypical example of these principles. The spine and trunk are key elements for proper throwing mechanics, including force generation, force transfer, and force attenuation. With complex overhead motions such as the baseball throw, principles of physics demonstrate that the shoulder mechanism alone is incapable of generating the necessary forces to accelerate the shoulder to an angular velocity of more than 7,000° per second and to generate a throwing velocity that is typical of elite athletes. Specifically, it is the larger mass of the trunk that allows it to contribute most of the force (mass × acceleration) and kinetic energy (1/2 × mass × velocity²) to the throw-

ing motion. For example, if the contributions of the lower body and trunk are substantially reduced or eliminated from the throwing motion, such as in the water polo player, the peak throwing velocity is reduced to approximately half that of a professional baseball pitcher.

The spine and trunk also allow transfer of force from the lower quadrants to the throwing arm. Creating a rigid cylinder via muscular tension, they efficiently transform the ground reactive force into rotational force that is transferred to the shoulder mechanism and upper limb. Pure anatomic evidence supports this concept. The latissimus dorsi, which is a prime internal rotator of the upper limb and very active in the acceleration phase of the throwing cycle, has a direct attachment to the free edge of the thoracolumbar fascia, a structure that anchors and stabilizes the lumbar spine. The trunk also acts as a force attenuator, protecting the shoulder from the extreme tensile loads in the follow-through phase of the throwing cycle. As the trunk rotates forward and bends laterally, it reacquires energy, thus dissipating the large distraction forces on the shoulder and associated nerves about the shoulder.

Given the critical role of the spine and trunk in the athlete, specific attention must be given to proper rehabilitation following injury. The athlete may be viewed as the ultimate workers' compensation patient. Time lost from sport is of paramount importance in the elite athlete. A comprehensive and proactive rehabilitation plan is necessary to manage most athletic spine injuries. The initial phase focuses on pain control. While pain usually can be controlled promptly through medication and physical therapy, it is important to realize that absence of symptoms does not imply functional recovery. The process of rehabilitation is ideally sport- and role-specific; however, common principles and practice apply. Maintaining, regaining, or developing core strength is key. This includes strengthening and stabilization of the many muscles and muscle groups that link the lumbar spine through the pelvis to the lower limbs or the cervical spine through the shoulder girdle to the upper limbs. Frequent patterns of muscle imbalances occur and should be recognized. In the lumbar spine, these include tight hip flexors, rotators, and adductors, with weak hip extensors and abductors; in the cervical spine, these include tight suboccipital (capital) extensors, scalenes, and pectoralis minor, with weak scapular stabilizers and thoracic extensors.

Rehabilitation for flexibility, strength, power, agility, and balance are all part of a well-designed plan. Even in the younger athlete, in whom aggressive resistance strengthening may not be appropriate, early emphasis on core strengthening and functional sport-specific tasks may afford protection from additional spine as well as peripheral joint injury. For example, core strengthening of the pelvic and hip girdle musculature in the early adolescent female athlete may reduce the incidence of anterior cruciate ligament injuries by avoiding excessive hip adduction moments through more efficient trunk and hip abductor muscle control. In the throwing athlete, thoracic spinal extensor and scapular stabilizer strengthening may reduce the risk of rotator cuff injury by optimizing scapular positioning and kinematics during the throwing cycle. Finally, repetitive training in this fashion may stimulate neuromuscular development and motor patterning even before the objective development of strength gains.

Cervical Spine

Transient Quadriplegia/Cervical Cord Neurapraxia

In contrast to traumatic spinal cord injury in the general population, the vast majority of spinal cord injuries in athletics involve the cervical spine. Many of these are incomplete injuries, meaning that some neurologic function is preserved. Participants in the following sports are at higher risk for sustaining a cervical spinal cord injury: football (defensive player/tackling), gymnastics (dismounting), soccer (goalie), ice hockey (being checked from behind, or hitting the boards headfirst), diving (hitting the pool bottom). Although the overall incidence of spinal cord injury in the high school and college population appears relatively small at approximately 1 per 100,000 participants per year, when considering that several million young athletes compete at these levels, it is clear that a substantial number of catastrophic spinal cord injuries will occur each year.

By definition, transient quadriplegia/cervical cord neurapraxia (TQ/CCN) is a transient phenomenon. These injuries are distinct from stingers, which are peripheral nerve injuries. The term transient quadriplegia is less specific than cervical cord neurapraxia because loss of sensation may occur with or without loss

of motor function. The clinical distinction between a spinal cord injury and a cervical nerve root injury is based on the number of limbs involved. Whereas specific subsets of spinal cord injury (eg, central cord syndrome) will result in distinct clinical patterns, spinal cord injury universally results in two- to four-limb involvement as opposed to a peripheral nerve injury or radiculopathy, which results in single-limb involvement. Typically, the symptoms and signs of TQ/CCN resolve within 24 hours, although a more prolonged recovery can occur. Extended signs and symptoms following a cervical spinal cord injury would probably not be classified as neurapraxia. The pattern of clinical recovery parallels that of the injury. For example, in a central cord syndrome with preferential involvement of the upper limb spinal tracts, there is greater upper than lower limb motor and sensory deficit, and recovery usually occurs in the lower limbs first, with the hands last to improve.

The cervical spinal cord and dura accommodate a wide range of spinal motion without injury through unfolding of redundant neural tissue as well as elastic deformation of neural tissue. With spine flexion, the spinal canal dimensions widen but the neural contents, including the spinal cord and nerve roots, are maximally stretched and tightened. With spine extension, the spinal cord and nerve roots are slackened, but the spinal canal is narrowed.

There are two primary mechanisms of cervical spinal cord injury in the athletic population, axial load and hyperextension. The axial load mechanism occurs when the cervical spine is slightly flexed; for example, straightening the cervical lordosis, followed by directly impacting an immovable object such as the ground or another player with the crown of the helmet or head. This action results in two possible injuries. In the presence of a central disc herniation or posterior bony bar, transient compression of the anterior cord and anterior spinal artery may occur as the cord is stretched over these fixed structures, resulting in both direct and indirect cord compression and cord ischemia. The other injury results through minimization of the shock-absorbing capacity of the cervical spine as it acts like a segmented column. The momentum of the body against a fixed cervical spine results in progressive breakdown of the passive stabilizers, resulting in fracture-dislocation. This latter injury is more likely to cause a permanent neurologic deficit, especially in the presence of spinal stenosis.

The hyperextension mechanism results in spinal cord injury primarily by narrowing the central spinal canal. Hyperextension causes infolding of the ligamentum flavum, which can result in a transient physiologic stenosis of the central canal even in the absence of true spinal stenosis. However, in the presence of fixed spinal stenosis (congenital or acquired), the spinal cord is at greater risk of direct compressive injury or injury secondary to a vascular insult. In the general population, the presence of premorbid cervical spinal stenosis substantially reduces the chances of neurologic recovery following spinal cord injury.

One of the key elements in the diagnostic evaluation of the athlete with TQ/CCN is the imaging assessment, which ultimately plays an important role in determining return to competition. The goal of the initial radiographic examination is to determine the integrity of the spinal elements, typically assessed by plain radiographs. First, if the athlete is wearing a helmet, a lateral cervical spine radiograph is taken with the helmet left in place; with the helmet off, a full series is administered in a controlled environment such as the emergency department, including flexion and extension views if the athlete is neurologically stable. Advanced imaging, such as MRI or contrast-enhanced CT, evaluates for compromise of the contents of the spinal canal, including the presence of spinal stenosis. However, although the determination of spinal stenosis is very important, the assessment of this condition has been controversial. Ideally, the spinal canal bony dimensions can be measured directly from MRI or contrast-enhanced CT. These tests also allow direct observation of the spinal canal for a soft-tissue disc herniation, posterior bony bar, the shape of the spinal cord, and the amount of cerebrospinal fluid remaining around the cord at multiple levels (the so-called functional reserve). MRI may also allow for dynamic assessment of the spinal canal in both neutral and extension cervical positioning.

Before the widespread availability of MRI, the imaging evaluation of the athlete with a cervical spinal cord injury relied heavily on plain radiographs, in which, unlike MRI or CT, magnification error is a factor. Measurement of the Torg ratio, an indirect measurement of the bony dimensions of the spinal canal using a lateral cervical radiograph, is used to neutralize the magnification error. The Torg ratio is the sagittal diameter of the spinal canal measured from the back of the vertebral body to the corresponding spinolaminar line divided by the AP diameter of the vertebral body at that same level. Although this method of determining spinal stenosis has been found to be highly sensitive (> 90%, thus few false negatives), it has an extremely low positive predictive value (~13%, thus a large number of false positives). The major pitfall of the Torg ratio is that athletes, particularly large athletes, have correspondingly large vertebral bodies so that the ratio is skewed toward a lower number, implying spinal stenosis. Also, the size and shape of the spinal cord, the functional reserve of the spinal canal, and the presence of a disc herniation cannot be assessed by this method. Thus, the Torg ratio should not be considered the standard measurement

following TQ/CCN; instead, an advanced imaging study is necessary.

As a result of the transient nature of TQ/CCN, as opposed to a permanent neurologic injury (complete or incomplete), determination of return to competition becomes very important. The sports medicine physician must provide current and accurate medical information to allow all parties—physician, athlete, family, coach/team, player advisor/agent—to make an educated rather than a solely emotional decision. Whereas there is yet no substantial objective evidence in the athletic population that recurrent concussive injury to the spinal cord results in permanent neurologic damage, due consideration must be given to the potential for the development of myelopathy, particularly if spinal stenosis is present. The only published study of return to competition following TQ/CCN included 110 athletes, 63 (57%) of whom returned to competition. Of those 63 athletes, 35 (56%) sustained at least one additional episode of TQ/CCN. No athlete was described as developing a permanent neurologic injury, even though the number of recurrent episodes of TQ/CCN ranged up to 25 and direct assessment of the spinal canal and spinal cord reportedly revealed a significant correlation between spinal stenosis and the development of recurrent TQ/CCN. There are several design flaws in this study that may limit the validity of the reported conclusion that even in the presence of spinal stenosis, recurrent TQ/CCN does not predispose the athlete to permanent deficits. Because MRI was not performed on all athletes, the relationship between recurrent TQ/CCN and true spinal stenosis cannot be determined. Further, it is not known whether the players with the more severe pathoanatomy on MRI returned to competition. Finally, it is not known whether results from a limited follow-up period can be extrapolated to the long-term outcome.

Therefore, while there may be a greater than 50% chance that an athlete will sustain another episode of TQ/CCN after returning to full competition following the initial episode, the reported absence of risk of developing a permanent spinal cord injury after a subsequent episode of TQ/CCN is less certain. Also, if the development of spinal stenosis is assumed to be in part a degenerative process resulting from chronic repetitive overload to the cervical spine, even in the absence of permanent neurologic deficit, long-term quality of life issues may arise as a result of pain caused by acceleration of these degenerative changes. Similar to other potentially career-ending injuries, various factors are ultimately considered in determining return to competition in these athletes, including medical, psychosocial, and economic issues. The sports medicine physician must provide an objective opinion despite the pressures that undoubtedly will be applied by all the parties involved.

Stingers

In general, athletically induced peripheral nerve injuries are difficult to diagnose, particularly if pain is the initial complaint rather than weakness or sensory disturbance. The stinger is probably the most common yet least understood peripheral nerve injury that occurs in sports. This is a peripheral nerve injury, not a spinal cord injury, despite the frequent misuse of the term stinger to describe the burning hands that often are associated with the central cord syndrome. Historically, there has been a great deal of controversy as to the pathomechanics and pathoanatomy of this injury, including a tensile (or stretch) injury to the upper trunk of the brachial plexus, a tensile injury to the cervical nerve root, a compressive injury to the upper trunk of the brachial plexus, and a compressive injury to the cervical nerve root.

Certain neuroanatomic facts implicate the cervical nerve root–spinal nerve complex (CR-SN) as the primary site of injury. The CR-SN is more susceptible to both tensile and compressive loads than is the brachial plexus. There is also a differential vulnerability of the anterior (motor) root as compared with the posterior (sensory) root. The anterior nerve root lacks the dampening effect of the dorsal root ganglion, has a thinner dural sheath, and directly aligns with the spinal cord, all of which place it at greater risk of injury. It is the CR-SN that is the weak link from the spinal cord to the terminal branches of the brachial plexus and is probably the primary anatomic structure injured, whether the mechanism is compression or stretch.

As with TQ/CCN, accurate diagnosis of a stinger requires an understanding not only of the specific sport but also of the skill level of the athlete. The tensile overload mechanism is more common in the inexperienced or younger athlete because of relative neck and shoulder girdle muscle weakness. The head and involved upper limb move in opposite directions, widening the distance between the shoulder and the mastoid process. With the compressive overload mechanism, the head and neck are forced into the extreme of the posterolateral quadrant ipsilateral to the involved limb, mimicking the typical Spurling's maneuver commonly performed during a routine physical examination. This injury results in neuroforaminal narrowing, with the fifth through seventh CR-SN most susceptible because of the inherent cervical spinal mobility at these levels. This compressive overload mechanism is more typical in the experienced athlete and is often technique related. In football, tackling and blocking are the most common activities that cause stingers, with the tacklers and the blockers usually sustaining the injuries.

The hallmark symptoms and signs of the stinger are as follows: sudden, unilateral pain and dysesthesias in a dermatomal referral pattern, usually C5, C6, or C7; relatively short duration of pain, lasting seconds to minutes; usually fairly quick resolution of sensory disturbance, although occasionally lasting days to weeks; and possibly persistence of weakness, consistent with the neuroanatomic principles of anterior nerve root vulnerability. The development of simultaneous bilateral cervical nerve root injury is very uncommon; therefore, involvement of more than one limb should always prompt the consideration of a spinal cord injury, not a stinger. More often than not, the symptoms and signs associated with a stinger resolve fairly quickly. However, frequent recurrences occur, with each subsequent event more likely to result in persistent motor deficit.

The assessment of the athlete with a presumed stinger requires a careful sideline examination and serial assessments on the sideline, in the locker room, in the training room, and in the office. Because of the noncatastrophic nature of this injury and the relatively quick resolution of pain, the initial sideline examination is often an inadequate, cursory evaluation of hand grip strength. However, assessment of cervical range of motion and local tenderness and a thorough neurologic examination are required. Passive, provocative cervical range-of-motion testing on the sideline should be performed only if the athlete demonstrates full active motion without pain, to avoid exacerbating a potentially unstable spinal condition. The neurologic examination must include motor testing of the C5 through C7 myotomes because these muscle groups are much more likely to be affected than the intrinsic muscles of the hand, which are predominantly innervated by the C8 and T1 nerves. Identifying mild weakness in these athletes may require repetitive testing of any given muscle to fatigue because a single manual muscle test may be unreliable, given the relatively greater baseline levels of strength found in athletes.

The necessity for ancillary testing such as imaging and electrodiagnostics depends on the persistence of symptoms and signs and the number of stingers the athlete has sustained, which is often underreported. Imaging of the cervical spine reveals anatomic abnormalities that may contribute to the development of the stinger, whereas electrodiagnostic testing assesses neurophysiologic function. These studies often complement each other. If the athlete fully recovers within seconds to minutes from a first episode, then no additional testing may be necessary. However, for recurrent episodes or persistent symptoms or signs following an initial stinger, testing should be pursued. Plain radiographs with oblique and flexion-extension views may reveal degenerative changes, neuroforaminal narrowing due to uncovertebral or zygapophyseal joint arthropathy, hypermobility, instability, and frequently, postural dysfunction as evidenced by loss of cervical lordosis (which may be chronic, not necessarily resulting from a single injury). Advanced imaging such as MRI may more readily demonstrate neuroforaminal stenosis and disc abnormalities including herniation and degenerative disc changes. A cervical MRI or contrast-enhanced CT scan should almost always be obtained if an athlete experiences severe, unrelenting pain; if the neurologic examination demonstrates profound weakness; or if there is delayed recovery.

The Torg ratio has been used in the context of the evaluation of the stinger. However, in addition to the inherent limitations of this indirect measure of central spinal canal stenosis described earlier, the underlying principle by which the Torg ratio was designed does not apply to the radiographic evaluation of peripheral nerve injuries such as the stinger. Advanced imaging studies in players who have sustained stingers have revealed substantial degenerative changes, including neuroforaminal stenosis. The degenerative processes that result in these lateral canal changes also contribute to central canal stenosis; therefore, it is not uncommon to observe central and foraminal stenosis in athletes who have sustained a stinger. However, the central stenosis is probably an incidental finding and does not contribute to the pathomechanical or clinical patterns observed in these athletes. Another ratio that may more specifically address the site of pathology is the foramen height, as measured on oblique cervical spine radiographs, divided by the vertebral body height of the vertebra just caudal to the foramen. The usefulness of this ratio has yet to be determined.

If clinical weakness persists for longer than 2 weeks, or if weakness significantly worsens over the first few days postinjury, then electrodiagnostic testing is reasonable. The goals of electrodiagnostic testing are to confirm the diagnosis of cervical nerve root injury versus the less common brachial plexus injury, to quantify the degree of nerve injury (eg, differentiate a neurapraxic root injury from axonopathy), to isolate a specific nerve root level, and to assist with planning appropriate rehabilitation and return to competition. Electrodiagnostics can be performed as early as 7 to 10 days following the onset of symptoms, with electromyography (EMG) being the most sensitive technique for evaluating axonal loss in the presence of continued clinical weakness. However, milder injuries may be difficult to recognize because these injuries typically result in a relatively mild degree of axonal injury and variable degree of neurapraxia. Motor unit recruitment abnormalities in the affected muscles may be the only abnormality identified, therefore requiring careful examination. Although EMG should be able to differentiate a brachial plexus injury from cervical radiculopathy, particularly through exami-

nation of the paraspinal musculature, early re-innervation of the cervical paraspinals following nerve root trauma may preclude identifying these abnormalities.

Well-established return-to-competition guidelines do not exist for the stinger. Return-to-competition decisions should be based on clinical, electrodiagnostic (absence of acute abnormalities), and imaging findings (absence of an acute cervical disc herniation), with additional consideration given to whether the injury is a first time or recurrent problem and other intangible psychosocioeconomic factors. In any case, there must be full recovery of strength in the affected muscle(s). Further, the player should complete a comprehensive rehabilitation program that emphasizes the correction of postural faults, particularly the forward head posture typically associated with the plain radiograph finding of straightening of the cervical lordosis.

A combination of muscular imbalances about the neck and shoulder girdle and areas of segmental spinal dysfunction characterize the forward head posture. The highlights of these postural abnormalities include increased thoracic kyphosis, excessive scapulae protraction and glenohumeral internal rotation, hyperflexion of the lower cervical and upper thoracic segments with relative hypomobility of the zygapophyseal joints, hyperextension of the upper cervical segments with hypomobility, compensatory segmental hypermobility of the midcervical segments (which may contribute to progressive degenerative changes at these segments), and weakening of many muscle groups attributable to either shortening or lengthening with alteration of their normal length-tension relationship. Muscles that are shortened include the capital and cervical extensors, sternocleidomastoid, upper trapezius, levator scapula, pectoralis minor and major, anterior deltoid, subscapularis, serratus anterior, and anterior scalene. Muscles lengthened include the capital and cervical flexors, middle and lower trapezius, rhomboids, thoracic extensors, and latissimus dorsi.

Correction of these postural faults requires skilled manual therapy including joint and soft-tissue mobilization techniques followed by a specific strengthening program, after which the athlete should exhibit balanced flexibility and strength through the cervicothoracic spine and shoulder girdle. Complete correction of the cervical lordosis may not be achievable and should not be considered an absolute contraindication to return to competition.

Finally, return to competition may vary depending on the number of stingers an athlete sustains in one season. As indicated earlier, recurrent stingers are more likely to result in residual neurologic deficit, particularly weakness, so that with multiple stingers the decision to delay returning an athlete to competition is relatively easy in that full clinical recovery has not taken place. If an athlete sustains an initial stinger and demonstrates full recovery within 15 minutes, then return to the same game is allowed. Otherwise, if full recovery occurs within a week, then return to the next game is allowed. Prolonged recovery following a first stinger is relatively uncommon, yet a limited amount of rehabilitation usually is indicated to address specific cervicothoracic stabilization exercises and to provide equipment modification such as pads and rolls to help prevent excessive excursion of the head and neck into the posterolateral quadrant. A general rule is that a player is held from competition for the number of weeks that corresponds to the number of stingers sustained in a given season (eg, 2 weeks for a second stinger). If more than three stingers occur in a season, consideration should be given to ending the season for the player if there is persistent significant weakness, persistent acute abnormalities on EMG (and if necessary, serial EMGs), and cervical disc herniation or significant foraminal stenosis revealed by MRI.

Lumbar Spine

Spondylolysis and Spondylolisthesis

This discussion will be limited to isthmic spondylolysis, which is a defect of the pars interarticularis. The prevalence in the general population is about 3% to 6%, approximately two to three times greater in whites than in blacks and in men than in women. There is a disproportionately higher prevalence of spondylolysis in the athletic population, with certain sports considered to be high risk, such as gymnastics, volleyball, weight lifting, wrestling, dance, rowing, diving, and track and field. Within certain sports, specific activities or positions are also at risk, including the lineman in football, the pitcher in baseball, and those taking part in throwing events in track and field.

The causes of spondylolysis are probably multifactorial, including genetic and mechanical. Pars interarticularis defects are not congenital. The vast majority of pars defects occur at L5, probably because of maximal cyclic loading and repetitive shear at this segment. The pars is the center of force concentration in the lumbar spinal segment. The lower incidence in the adult may be reflective of higher cortical bone density and strengthening of the neural arch with aging. Pars interarticularis fractures are not similar to typical stress fractures elsewhere in the skeletal system for several reasons: pars defects develop at an earlier age, are often pain free, do not frequently demonstrate callus formation or periosteal reaction during healing, and may persist on radiographs after symptom resolution. Spondylolisthesis, or "slip," occurs uncommonly, in up to 10% of indi-viduals with spondylolysis, typically manifesting during the adolescent growth spurt. Slips are more common in girls. Progression of a slip may relate to the degree of slip at primary manifestation but, unlike the development of the pars defect, usually is not correlated to the intensity of the athletic activity.

Several rules apply when evaluating low back pain in the young athlete. First, children are not small adults and do not have adult problems. Second, if the problem is severe enough to cause the child to stop participating in the athletic activity, the symptoms must be taken seriously. Third, lumbar strain is not usually on the differential diagnosis list. A pars interarticularis injury must be considered in any young athlete who complains of new onset low back pain. However, other causes of mechanical low back pain, including anterior column pathology (eg, disc injury, vertebral end plate fracture), posterior column pathology (eg, zygapophyseal joint synovitis, transverse or spinous process fracture), and nonmechanical etiologies of low back pain, including tumor and infection, must be considered.

The symptoms associated with spondylolysis are typically low back pain becoming worse with activities such as running, jumping, and twisting, especially with stress in extension. Radicular pain is unusual, but when present is primarily in an L5 distribution resulting from a mass effect from the spondylitic defect, inflammatory radiculitis, or foraminal stenosis associated with spondylolisthesis. The clinical signs are usually extension-provoked low back pain, accentuated with ipsilateral rotation and single leg extension. This latter sign, although not pathognomonic, is strongly suggestive for a pars defect in the young athletic population. Pain often is relieved with flexion postures. Hamstring inflexibility is frequently present and may represent heightened neural tension as opposed to primary myofascial tightness. Rarely is a true neurologic deficit present, because the intrinsic elasticity of the neural system in these young people is quite forgiving.

Imaging of the pars defect may help to confirm the clinical suspicion of acute spondylolysis. Several questions arise when considering imaging tests. First, will imaging affect treatment? In other words, will the treatment change whether a pars defect is identified or not? Second, will a defect always be identified? Third, if a defect is identified on an imaging study, does that automatically implicate it as the pain generator? And finally, which imaging modality is considered the best for identifying a pars fracture? Four types of imaging modalities, each with pros and cons, are routinely available for evaluating low back pain, including plain radiography, single-photon emission CT (SPECT) bone scan, CT, and MRI.

Plain radiography is clearly the least expensive and

most easily obtainable type of imaging, but it is also the least sensitive and specific. A positive finding does not confirm a pain-generating structure. Depending on the extent and plane of the pars defect, there also may be difficulty identifying it on plain radiograph. Further, the radiation dose is substantial, particularly with oblique and coned-down lumbosacral junction spot views.

A SPECT bone scan is a physiologic study; it is approximately two to three times more sensitive than planar bone scan imaging and is helpful in identifying a specific level of involvement with some anatomic accuracy. However, a SPECT bone scan does not yield detailed images of anatomy, so a positive study does not guarantee that the abnormality is a pars defect (versus, for example, a zygapophyseal joint injury or osteoid osteoma). It also results in a concentrated radiation dose to the gonads as a result of primary renal excretion of the radionuclide and is not practical to monitor healing, in that a SPECT scan may remain hot for 6 months or longer after symptom resolution.

CT is useful as it is relatively easy to obtain and the newer helical scanners are very fast, with limited radiation field scatter. CT may also allow staging of the lesion, which may be useful in determining appropriate treatment. The negative aspects of CT are possible difficulties in determining which level(s) to scan and technical factors such as slice thickness; also, CT does not demonstrate physiologic activity.

Finally, the positive aspects of MRI include the lack of ionizing radiation, the ability to simultaneously evaluate for other spinal pathology, and the possibility of identifying early pars lesions by visualizing bone edema on T2-sagittal imaging. However, the routine use of MRI for confirming symptomatic pars defects is not yet validated.

Thus, there is no single confirmatory imaging study. Current trends include limiting plain radiography to a standing lateral and possibly an AP, and a SPECT bone scan followed by CT with thin, stacked cuts (no greater than 1.5 mm) limited to the abnormal area on the SPECT scan. MRI may prove to be the most sensitive and specific imaging modality and allow for monitoring of healing, but at this time, it is not routinely used for this purpose. If the SPECT scan is normal, it is extremely unlikely that the young athlete's pain is caused by an acute pars fracture.

The natural history of asymptomatic spondylolysis found incidentally on plain radiographs is generally favorable, even with continuation of athletic activity. As indicated earlier, spondylolisthesis is uncommon. Significant progression of a slip is also relatively unusual, even in young athletes, although this risk is, in part, age dependent. If an athlete between the ages of 8 and 13 years comes to the physician with a symptomatic spondylolysis or spondylolisthesis, careful observation is necessary because progression of a slip is more common in this age group, particularly during the growth spurt. It is very important to realize that progressive listhesis can occur in this age group without symptoms, so standing lateral lumbar spine radiographs are indicated twice yearly until the athlete reaches skeletal maturity. Progression is also more common in girls, in the presence of steeper lumbosacral angles, and when the initial slip was at least a grade 1 at initial presentation. For athletes older than 13 years, progression of a slip is unusual, and prognosis is favorable with or without documented bony healing of the pars defect.

Intuitively, the goal of treatment of any acute pars interarticularis fracture is bony healing. However, this may not be a realistic goal, based on the severity (ie, extent of separation, bony maturity, bilateral versus unilateral) of the defect(s). True bony union may be possible if the defect is unilateral, in its early stage of development with minimal separation, and has no sclerotic margins. For this reason, imaging of the young athlete is reasonable to stage the pars lesion and thus set realistic outcome goals. However, if a given treatment program for a presumed acute spondylolysis always includes rest and bracing, then formal imaging may not be necessary unless the athlete does not respond positively.

Historically, treatment options for spondylolysis and spondylolisthesis have included rest, bracing, activity modification, lower quadrant flexibility and core strengthening, epidural steroid injections for radicular pain and possibly pars injections for axial pain, and surgery. The use of rigid bracing has been debated. In fact, the use of a rigid brace may increase motion at the L5-S1 motion segment. Bracing may simply be an anchor, keeping the athlete from continuing to participate in athletic activity. The required duration of activity modification or limitation to achieve maximal bony healing of the pars fracture is unclear. If bony union is the goal, however, a longer period of rest probably is warranted.

From a practical perspective, the following algorithm probably is reasonable. If there is a strong clinical suspicion for an acute spondylolysis in a young athlete, a lateral radiograph should be taken to determine if a spondylolisthesis is present. The next imaging step would be a SPECT bone scan, followed by a thin-section, limited CT if a hot area is present on the SPECT scan, to observe the pars defect(s). If the SPECT scan is normal, consideration should be given to a lumbar MRI to rule out another potential pain generator. An MRI would also be reasonable before the SPECT scan if the radiograph already demonstrates a spondylolisthesis.

If a partial or early fracture without sclerosis is identified by CT, then the athlete is advised to rest from the offending activity and other overload activities for at least 12 weeks. Bracing is optional; if used, a lumbosacral corset may be just as effective and certainly less expensive and cumbersome than a rigid brace. If pain relief cannot be obtained by rest alone, then a brace or corset should be a requirement at least during waking hours. The safe amount of physical activity to be allowed during this convalescent period is unknown. Once the athlete is pain free, even if before 12 weeks, it is probably reasonable to begin some rehabilitation measures such as passive lower extremity flexibility, nonloading aerobic activity such as deep water running, and early trunk stabilization exercises in a neutral position. A follow-up limited CT may be useful in documenting bony union. The decision to return to competition should be based on clinical recovery, extent of bony healing, degree of slip, age of the athlete, the particular sport, and completion of a comprehensive rehabilitation program. If the athlete is younger than 13 years and returns to competition, twice-yearly standing lateral lumbar radiographs are necessary to assess for progression of a slip unless there is evidence of bony healing. Surgical fusion should be considered if significant progression or progression to grade 2 or more occurs, particularly if radicular symptoms develop. It also should be considered even with axial pain only and possibly even without pain if the athlete is young enough that continued slippage is likely. Return to competition following a fusion may be reasonable if all criteria are met. Ultimately, this decision rests with the athlete and his or her family.

Lumbar Discogenic Syndromes: Axial and Radicular

The physical demands of sport lead to very high compressive and shear forces often several times greater than body weight, across the three-joint complex. A normal intervertebral disc is generally more tolerant of compressive than shear force, with the potential for outer anulus disruption occurring at greater than 3° of segmental rotation. Quick and sudden alterations in the direction of force vectors, typical of many athletic activities, increase the risk of overload failure of the disc. Disc degeneration, with or without injury, will affect the intrinsic stability of the segment, leading to perturbation of the instantaneous axis of rotation, increasing the susceptibility to overload injury.

Youth does not protect a person from developing lumbar disc abnormalities, although genetic predisposition may lead to relatively early disc degeneration in the young adolescent or teenage athlete. Disability from sports because of low back injury is common. While not all low back pain is disc related, the anulus of the disc is innervated and thus is potentially a pain generator.

Although first-time low back pain may resolve spontaneously and quickly, there is a high recidivism rate, with a propensity toward chronicity. The intervertebral disc often is implicated as the source of this recurrent or persistent pain. Thus, given the physical demands of athletic activity, early diagnosis and management is necessary, whether the treatment is surgical or nonsurgical.

In the young athlete, if acute spondylolysis is ruled out, then an acute disc injury must be considered. Sudden onset of axial low back pain is typical of an acute annular tear, central disc herniation, or end plate herniation. The clinical appearance of athletes with discogenic low back pain syndromes may be obvious, but not infrequently variation from the typical symptoms and signs occurs. For example, acute annular tears or central disc herniations may not have the classic symptom of pain provocation with flexion maneuvers; instead, pain may be provoked by extension and even relieved by flexion postures. Radicular pain is not always in a typical dermatomal distribution, with isolated hamstring or Achilles-area pain often the only clinical manifestation. Further, given the extreme flexibility of some athletes, the range of a positive dural tension sign may need to be substantially increased to beyond the usual 70°. Noncompressive radiculitis mediated through biochemical pathways may also be more common in the young athlete.

The principles of the rehabilitation program for athletes with discogenic low back pain syndromes are similar to those for the general population, but usually the process is more aggressive and comprehensive to achieve safe return to competition as quickly as possible. Although the natural history of most radiculopathies attributable to a herniated disc is favorable, early surgical intervention to relieve the referred leg pain may be considered in the athlete to accelerate the rehabilitation process. Several factors contribute to this decision including age of the athlete, level of competition, and time of the season. Reasonable expectations must be discussed with the athlete and team representatives at the outset of treatment. With or without surgery, it should be emphasized that the key to successful long-term return to competition following a low back injury is ongoing management in which the athlete is an active participant.

The rehabilitation program should be comprehensive and eclectic. The goals of rehabilitation generally can be divided into acute and subacute phases. The acute phase is primarily passive and includes protection of the injured tissue, control of pain and inflammation, and prevention of secondary soft-tissue and joint stiffness. The duration of this phase varies, but the intent is to progress quickly to the more active subacute phase. The key to achieving a rapid progression in the exercise program is successful early management of pain. A common treatment flaw in the acute phase is undermedication, resulting in poor pain control and sleep regulation. This flaw can not only delay functional progression but also may lead to excessive pain behavior that can complicate the recovery process. Intervention with epidural steroid injections may be indicated earlier in the acutely injured athlete with discogenic pain than in the general population. Failure to control radicular pain during this acute phase may indicate the need for surgical consultation. Successful elimination of radicular pain through surgery does not negate progression through the next phase of rehabilitation.

The emphasis during the subacute phase is to regain full, pain-free range of motion of the spine and associated pelvic and lower limb structures, to optimize strength and endurance of the trunk and lower extremities, to optimize balance and coordination, to facilitate return to normal athletic activity, and to prevent further injury and recurrences. Normal biomechanics can be restored through targeted manual therapy techniques. Early controlled loading of healing tissue can influence the alignment of collagen during remodeling. Core strengthening through trunk and pelvic stabilization exercises can begin with neutral spine postures, advancing to more challenging postures and positions in which the athlete must recruit key muscles to provide more support and stability. Emphasis is directed to the muscles that attach directly to the thoracolumbar fascia, including the abdominal obliques, gluteus maximus, transversus abdominus, and latissimus dorsi.

Tight and hypertonic muscles reciprocally inhibit weaker agonist muscles, and attempting to strengthen weak muscles first will lead to substitution patterns. For example, abdominal and gluteal muscle weakness usually is associated with tightness of the hip flexors, adductors, and rotators. Recognition of these typical patterns of muscular imbalance about the spine and pelvis facilitates expansion of movement boundaries. Recruitment and sequencing patterns may be more important than absolute strength development. Neuromuscular reorganization is the key to balance training, which is probably one of the most overlooked components of the functional rehabilitation program. The end point of the rehabilitation program depends on the needs of each individual athlete and includes sport-specific movements and targeted strengthening and conditioning. A comprehensive in-season and out-of-season program should be designed with the long-term goal of injury prevention and activity maintenance.

Annotated Bibliography

Overview

Young JL, Casazza BA, Press JM, Herring SA: Biomechanical aspects of the spine in pitching, in Andrews JR, Zarins B, Wilk KE (eds): *Injuries in Baseball.* Philadelphia, PA, Lippincott-Raven, 1998, pp 23-35.

This comprehensive discussion of the role of the spine/trunk in each phase of the throwing cycle emphasizes the assessment and rehabilitation of the kinetic and kinematic chain.

TQ/CCN

Cantu RC: Sports medicine aspects of cervical spinal stenosis. *Exerc Sport Sci Rev* 1995;23:399-409.

Three case presentations highlight the clinical and imaging factors that contribute to return to play decision making with emphasis on the concept of functional spinal stenosis.

Torg JS, Corcoran TA, Thibault LE, et al: Cervical cord neurapraxia: Classification, pathomechanics, morbidity, and management guidelines. *J Neurosurg* 1997;87:843-850.

The authors of this prospective study of 110 athletes with documented transient quadriplegia/cervical cord neurapraxia concluded that spinal stenosis is a significant risk factor for development of recurrent episodes, but not permanent spinal cord injury.

Stingers

Kelly JD IV, Aliquo D, Sitler MR, Odgers C, Moyer RA: Association of burners with cervical canal and foraminal stenosis. *Am J Sports Med* 2000;28:214-217.

The authors describe a new ratio method that focuses on foraminal stenosis rather than central stenosis as the significant pathoanatomic feature of the stinger or burner.

Levitz CL, Reilly PJ, Torg JS: The pathomechanics of chronic, recurrent cervical nerve root neurapraxia: The chronic burner syndrome. *Am J Sports Med* 1997;25:73-76.

This study emphasizes cervical nerve root injury rather than brachial plexus injury as the pathologic injury of the stinger or burner.

Weinstein SM: Assessment and rehabilitation of the athlete with a "stinger": A model for the management of noncatastrophic athletic cervical spine injury. *Clin Sports Med* 1998;17:127-135.

This is a comprehensive description of the pathoanatomy, pathomechanics, and clinical presentation of the stinger with a detailed review of the rehabilitation and return to competition determination in an athlete with a stinger.

Spondylolysis and Spondylolisthesis

Campbell RS, Grainger AJ: Optimization of MRI pulse sequences to visualize the normal pars interarticularis. *Clin Radiol* 1999;54:63-68.

The authors describe various MRI sequences that may optimally visualize the normal and abnormal pars interarticularis, although MRI has generally not been utilized for the diagnosis of spondylolysis.

Congeni J, McCulloch J, Swanson K: Lumbar spondylolysis: A study of natural progression in athletes. *Am J Sports Med* 1997;25:248-253.

This is a study of 40 athletes with back pain and positive bone scan and normal radiograph. CT study revealed 45% chronic nonhealed pars fracture, 40% acute fractures, and 15% no fracture. Authors emphasize the role of the CT in diagnosis and management of spondylolysis.

Micheli LJ, Wood R: Back pain in young athletes: Significant differences from adults in causes and patterns. *Arch Pediatr Adolesc Med* 1995;149:15-18.

In this retrospective case comparison of 100 adolescent athletes to 100 adults with back pain, the conclusion was that the primary diagnosis differs in each group. Specifically spondylolysis is most common in the younger group and discogenic pain is most common in the older group.

Morita T, Ikata T, Katoh S, Miyake R: Lumbar spondylolysis in children and adolescents. *J Bone Joint Surg Br* 1995;77:620-625.

This is the first study that correlates the stage of the pars fracture (ie, early, progressive, or terminal) with the likelihood of true bony healing, but there is no discussion of clinical outcome.

Muschik M, Hahnel H, Robinson PN, Perka C, Muschik C: Competitive sports and the progression of spondylolisthesis. *J Pediatr Orthop* 1996;16:364-369.

This is a retrospective clinical and radiologic review of 86 athletes with spondylolisthesis with average initial slip of 10%. In 33 athletes, average progression was 10.5% over 5 years, 36 had no change, 7 had a decrease, and 10 were undetermined. No clinical symptoms occurred in any athlete.

Lumbar Discogenic Syndromes: Axial and Radicular

Bronner S: Functional rehabilitation of the spine: The lumbopelvis as a key point of control, in Brownstein B, Bronner S (eds): *Functional Movement in Orthopaedic and Sports Physical Therapy: Evaluation, Treatment, and Outcomes.* New York, NY, Churchill Livingstone, 1997, pp 141-190.

The author provides a very thorough discussion of the rehabilitation progression for low back pain including both practical recommendations and theoretical bases for core strengthening.

Gatt CJ Jr, Hosea TM, Palumbo RC, Zawadsky JP: Impact loading of the lumbar spine during football blocking. *Am J Sports Med* 1997;25:317-321.

This is the report of a small study (5 subjects) measuring compression and shear forces at the L4-5 level in linemen during blocking drills.

Herring SA, Weinstein SM: Assessment and nonsurgical management of athletic low back injury, in Nicholas JA, Hershman EB (eds): *The Lower Extremity and Spine in Sports Medicine*, ed 2. St. Louis, MO, Mosby-Year Book, 1995, pp 1171-1197.

This very comprehensive summary includes a detailed section on low back excercises, spinal injections, and return to play in the low back-injured athlete.

Young JL, Press JM, Herring SA: The disc at risk in athletes: Perspectives on operative and nonoperative care. *Med Sci Sports Exerc* 1997;29(suppl 7):S222-S232.

This is a critical review of current concepts on the management of acute disc injury and sciatica with application to the athletic population.

Classic Bibliography

Bodner RJ, Heyman S, Drummond DS, Gregg JR: The use of single photon emission computed tomography (SPECT) in the diagnosis of low-back pain in young patients. *Spine* 1988;13:1155-1160.

Clancy WG Jr, Brand RL, Bergfield JA: Upper trunk brachial plexus injuries in contact sports. *Am J Sports Med* 1977;5:209-215.

Gracovetsky S: The spine as a motor in sports: Application to running and lifting. *Spine: State of the Art Reviews* 1990;4:267-286.

Herzog RJ, Wiens JJ, Dillingham MF, Sontag MJ: Normal cervical spine morphometry and cervical spinal stenosis in asymptomatic professional football players: Plain film radiography, multiplanar computed tomography, and magnetic resonance imaging. *Spine* 1991;16 (suppl 6):S178-S186.

Poindexter DP, Johnson EW: Football shoulder and neck injury: A study of the "stinger." *Arch Phys Med Rehabil* 1984;65:601-602.

Steiner ME, Micheli LJ: Treatment of symptomatic spondylolysis and spondylolisthesis with the modified Boston brace. *Spine* 1985;10:937-943.

Torg JS, Pavlov H, Genuario SE, et al: Neurapraxia of the cervical spinal cord with transient quadriplegia. *J Bone Joint Surg Am* 1986;68:1354-1370.

Torg JS, Sennett B, Pavlov H, Leventhal MR, Glasgow SG: Spear tackler's spine: An entity precluding participation in tackle football and collision activities that expose the cervical spine to axial energy inputs. *Am J Sports Med* 1993;21:640-649.

Watkins RG: Nerve injuries in football players. *Clin Sports Med* 1986;5:215-246.

Wiltse LL, Widell EH Jr, Jackson DW: Fatigue fracture: The basic lesion is isthmic spondylolisthesis. *J Bone Joint Surg Am* 1975;57:17-22.

Chapter 13

Evaluation of the Pediatric Spine Patient

Robert R. Madigan, MD

When a child undergoes a spinal evaluation, the physician should have a carefully planned strategy so that no significant problems are missed. The demand for more specific and complete documentation coupled with reduced payment schedules and the litigious nature of US society requires detailed and accurate records. Therefore, it is essential to establish an accurate, efficient, and reliable method for evaluating the pediatric spine patient.

Most spine evaluations of children and adolescents are prompted by spinal pain, the presence of real or suspected spinal deformity, and/or asymptomatic spinal abnormalities that have been discovered during unrelated evaluations. An example of the latter would be a hemivertebra noted on a chest radiograph as part of a cardiac evaluation. The evaluation should include a detailed history, physical examination, radiographic evaluation, and appropriate diagnostic imagery and laboratory studies.

Back Pain

The prevalence of low back pain in the middle-aged adult population is reported to be 60% to 80%, and approximately two thirds of those who experience back pain will have recurrences. Reported prevalence of back pain in children and adolescents varies from 11% to 50%. One reason for this wide range is that the prevalence of low back pain changes with the age of the patient; it is minimal before age 7 years, increases to 10% by age 10 years, and peaks at 50% by age 15 years. In addition, longitudinal studies have demonstrated forgetfulness of pain episodes among youth who may well consider them a normal life experience. Although by late adolescence the rate approaches that of the adult population, children and adolescents tend to minimize these episodes; only 2% to 15% will seek medical help for their ailment.

It is useful to categorize the causes when evaluating a child with back pain. The list in Table 1 is only a guide,

TABLE 1 | Back Pain in Children and Adolescents

Developmental
Spondylolysis/spondylolisthesis
Scheuermann's disease (thoracic and lumbar)
Painful scoliosis

Traumatic
Herniated disc
Vertebral apophysis fracture
Fracture
Overuse (strains/sprains)

Inflammatory
Discitis
Vertebral osteomyelitis
Rheumatologic disorders

Neoplastic disorders
Benign (osteoid osteoma, osteoblastoma, aneurysmal bone cyst)
Malignant (leukemia, lymphoma, sarcoma)

Psychosomatic back pain

however, because the categories easily can overlap. For example, a painful scoliosis could be caused by vertebral osteomyelitis or by a herniated disc. Studies from tertiary orthopaedic centers indicate that in half to two thirds of children with back pain, a definable diagnosis can be made.

Although spondylolysis and spondylolisthesis are the most common identifiable causes of back pain in children, tumors ultimately will be found in 5% to 10% of children with back pain. In children younger than age 10 years, discitis and tumor are more common; in children older than 10 years, spondylolysis, spondylolisthesis, Scheuermann's disease, and overuse syndrome will more likely be the cause. Many times an exact diagnosis cannot be made, and it is always advisable to reevaluate the child after a period of observation. Minor ailments will resolve spontaneously, and more serious problems will advance and become more evident.

The problem of painful scoliosis merits emphasis; this is a description of symptoms and signs, not a diagnosis. In general, severe and disabling pain is unusual in children and adolescents with idiopathic scoliosis. Approximately one fourth of patients with adolescent idiopathic scoliosis will complain of back pain, but this is usually mild, nonspecific, nonradiating, and intermittent, and it resolves with rest. Severe and persistent pain, especially when it interferes with activities of daily living or play and sport activities merits a more complete evaluation to establish the etiology.

The parent of a child with back pain frequently asks about the relationship between back pain and heavy school backpacks. Studies have shown that children often carry backpacks that exceed weight limits proposed for much larger adults. It also has been shown that carrying heavy school backpacks on one shoulder significantly alters posture and gait. There currently is no scientific evidence to support the perception among orthopaedic surgeons and families that these heavy school backpacks precipitate back pain. A recommendation to parents would be to reduce the total weight to a level that is practical and to encourage the child to carry the load symmetrically on both shoulders.

The relationship between complaints of pain and possible underlying psychological problems should be explored after meticulous evaluation fails to identify an obvious cause of the pain. Children with complaints of back pain have a higher incidence of other complaints such as recurrent abdominal pain and headaches. This underscores the need to look for these problems in the history and review of anatomic systems. Children whose parents exhibit chronic back pain problems are more likely to have similar complaints. Although they can represent a genetic predisposition such as a greater likelihood of herniated disc, these behaviors may have been learned through observation of parental chronic pain behavior. Thus both aspects should be explored in the family history. Psychological causes of back pain do exist in children and adolescents but at a much lower prevalence than in the adult population. When the orthopaedic surgeon is convinced that this may be the cause, appropriate referral should be considered.

School Screening for Spinal Deformity

The value of school screening programs for the detection of scoliosis is not universally accepted in the western world. At the present time some type of school screening is carried out in all 50 of the United States, with 19 states mandating a school screening program.

The initial universal program in Canada has been mostly discontinued. After studying the problem, Great Britain declined to institute a program. Japan, Sweden, Germany, and Italy have instituted voluntary programs. The concept of school screening for scoliosis currently is recommended by the Scoliosis Research Society and the American Academy of Orthopaedic Surgeons. In 1993 the United States Preventive Services Task Force published a report stating they were unable to make a definite recommendation either for or against scoliosis screening.

The effectiveness of school screening for scoliosis is questionable. Five key principles of effective screening should be evaluated and applied to scoliosis screening programs.

1. The condition screened for is an important health problem. However, the only curves requiring brace or surgical treatment are those of 30° or more, and these constitute only a small percentage of curves (0.25%) discovered in screening programs.

2. An asymptomatic phase of the disease exists during which screening is the only way to identify an affected individual. Smaller curves are not painful and have no functional impairment. Although school scoliosis screening identifies some children who ultimately receive treatment, an excessive number of children are referred who would never require treatment, resulting in unnecessary expense and increased parental and child anxiety.

3. Tests or examinations are simple, reliable, and acceptable to the population screened. The definition of scoliosis suggested by the Scoliosis Research Society is a lateral deviation of 10° or more, combined with a rotational deformity. The scoliometer is an inclinometer specifically adopted to measure the angle of trunk rotation. Its main advantages are low cost and no associated morbidity. The Adams forward bend test is a visual observation of the angle of trunk rotation. Trunk rotation or inclination is a topographic abnormality that is detected by the forward bend test, quantified by the scoliometer, and used to indicate the possible presence of scoliosis. It is possible to have a negative forward bend test and a positive scoliometer measurement; therefore, both should be used in concert. Small physiologic asymmetries of the spine are observed in 20% to 25% of children with no radiographic evidence of scoliosis. The goal in scoliosis screening is to maximize both the sensitivity (ability to identify children with scoliosis) and specificity (ability to identify children who do not have scoliosis). To meet this goal, the current

recommendation is to screen all children at age 10 years using both the Adams forward bend test and the scoliometer with a criterion for referral of 7°. All positive children are rescreened before referral for medical evaluation. This procedure will effectively reduce the number of unnecessary referrals and give an acceptable sensitivity and specificity rate of approximately 85%.

4. There is an accepted and effective nonsurgical treatment for scoliosis. The purpose of school screening is to detect curves when they are small so that treatment can be instituted and surgery avoided. The nihilists in the scoliosis community believe that bracing does not change the natural history of scoliosis. Lack of an effective nonsurgical treatment would obviate a screening tool that detects the problem early. However, two significant developments in recent years have tended to swing the pendulum in favor of screening. First, to evaluate the efficacy of any treatment program the natural history of the disease must be known. There are now sufficient data on the natural history of curve progression to determine what curves will require treatment. Second, the results of a prospective controlled study comparing treated and untreated patients indicated that bracing is more effective than no treatment in reducing curve progression.

5. Benefits from treatment outweigh the costs of the screening. Although this appears to be a simple analysis, it is confounded by the definition of benefits and costs. Benefits and costs to whom— patient, family, society? School screening is a very sensitive tool capable of picking out cases of spinal deformity in the screened population. However, the more sensitive the screen (ability to identify children with scoliosis), the less specific (ability to eliminate children without scoliosis) it becomes. In other words, overgeneration of false positives results in an unacceptable number of unnecessary referrals. The cost includes not only the funding of the screening program, but also the costs of physician office visits, radiographs, and the inherent expenses of patient travel and parental time off from work. Anxiety of the children and their parents about spinal deformity represents another societal cost. In pure dollars and cents, it likely is not possible to justify these programs as cost effective. Many physicians believe that the improved care of patients because of earlier detection justifies the additional expense.

The debate over screening probably will continue indefinitely. Articles in the bibliography promote both sides of the argument. The best compromise may be to continue screening until questions can be answered accurately and scientifically, to continue research on the natural history of idiopathic scoliosis as the benchmark to evaluate treatment programs, to adjust the screening protocols to maximize both the sensitivity and the specificity, to continue to scrutinize all nonsurgical modalities to determine their effectiveness, and to eliminate emotions from decision making.

Pediatric Spinal History

The first step in the evaluation of the child with spinal deformity or back pain is a detailed history. It is essential that all children, even adolescents, be accompanied by a parent to maximize the accuracy and completeness of the history. The history of present illness should be probed in a thorough and unhurried manner. To improve efficiency, a history evaluation sheet can be filled out by the child and parent before the office visit, and the past history, family history, social history, and review of systems can be conducted while the physician does the physical examination. The direction of questions will vary depending on the initial complaint.

For children with a complaint of pain, the physician should attempt to differentiate mechanical from nonmechanical pain. Mechanical pain is aggravated by activity and relieved by position change or rest, whereas nonmechanical pain is unchanged by activity. Mechanical pain usually lies in the realm of the orthopaedic surgeon. Facts to be elicited include: (1) how long the pain has been present; (2) what brings on the painful episodes and what reduces the pain; (3) did the pain begin suddenly as the result of a traumatic event or appear gradually; (4) what part of the spine is painful and does the pain radiate into the extremities; (5) are there associated neurologic symptoms such as numbness or weakness; (6) are there any systemic symptoms such as fever, anorexia, weight change, malaise, or bowel or bladder changes; (7) is the pain present at night and does it awaken the patient from sleep; (8) is the pain changed by coughing or sneezing; and (9) what treatments have been undertaken before the present visit (for example, is the pain relieved by aspirin, nonsteroidal anti-inflammatory drugs, or narcotic analgesics). One of the most important historic facts to be elicited is how the pain has affected the normal activities of the child. If the pain has reduced or eliminated normal play or sports activities, it is significant and needs to be evaluated very thoroughly. To the trained evaluator, each question and its subsequent answer will steer the history into a more precise direction and, finally, lead to formation of a small differential diagnosis outline.

For children with spinal deformity, other specific questions must be asked. How long has the deformity been present? Who first noted the deformity? Has the deformity progressed and how rapidly? Is there pain associated with the deformity? Has there been any previous treatment and was the treatment perceived to be effective? Has the deformity affected the child's social, athletic, or play activities? The child's maturity should be evaluated carefully. Has the girl reached her menarche? Has there been a recent growth spurt or is growth slowing down? For boys, the appearance of axillary hair is equivalent to the menarche and indicates the slowing of growth. The 6 months before and immediately following these markers form the period of most rapid growth and represent the period of greatest risk of spinal deformity progression.

Although uncommon, inflammatory conditions such as juvenile ankylosing spondylitis can be seen in children and adolescents. Often the complaints are of vague spinal pain, symptoms in other joints such as the hips, and vague systemic complaints such as stiffness, fatigue, and decreased stamina. It is significantly more common in boys and almost unheard of in the black population. Complaints of change in gait, change in appearance or function of lower extremities, and bowel or bladder dysfunction suggest intraspinal abnormalities such as spinal dysraphism or neoplasm.

The history should include all surgical events, including fractures; major medical illness, especially if it is ongoing; drug allergies; and medicines taken on a regular basis. The family history is most important to determine diseases with a familial pattern, such as idiopathic scoliosis, inflammatory joint disease, hereditary neurologic disease, a history of back pain, or herniated nucleus pulposus.

The social history is an important source of information about the child's environment. Does the child live in a stable home environment, attend regular school, smoke, or use tobacco products? Does the child participate in regular athletics or physical fitness, and if so, at what level?

Finally, the review of systems focuses on the systems most associated with the information previously obtained. For example, back pain complaints may point to the genitourinary or neurologic system, while spinal deformity may lead to further questions on the cardiorespiratory system.

Additional information will be needed for evaluation of the cervical spine of an infant or small child. Is the deformity congenital or did it develop after birth? Does it appear to affect the child's functions? Has there been any history of trauma? Is the problem progressive or static? Are there any associated problems such as pain, paresthesias, weakness, or change in gait pattern? Was the child's birth difficult or traumatic (suggestive of possible occult trauma)? Are there any associated health problems such as cardiac or renal abnormalities? Who first noted the problem?

In the case of trauma with associated pain and limitation of cervical motion, it is important to document the mechanism of injury, especially the amount of force involved. Is the pain mechanical, what is its severity, what makes it worse, and what makes it better? Is this a first time event or a recurrent problem? Does it affect the child's function in any way? Are there any associated symptoms such as pain radiating into upper extremities, paresthesias or weakness in upper extremities, or headache? At times, the asymptomatic child is referred because of abnormalities noted on other examinations, such as a chest radiograph or presports evaluation in children with Down syndrome, to rule out cervical abnormalities.

Physical Examination

Standing

The examination begins with observation of gait and inspection of the neck, trunk, and limbs for asymmetry. Torticollis may indicate a primary orthopaedic problem or underlying neurologic problem. Trunk asymmetry including uneven shoulders, prominent scapula, hypokyphosis of the thoracic spine, waist asymmetry, and pelvic obliquity, point to a scoliotic deformity. Cutaneous abnormality such as café au lait spots may indicate neurofibromatosis. Midline cutaneous abnormalities including hairy patches, sinuses, dimples, lipomas, or hemangiomas signal underlying spinal dysraphism. The anterior chest wall must be evaluated for abnormalities such as pectus excavatum or pectus carinatum. Tenderness of the posterior spine and sacroiliac joints to fist percussion can indicate infections, trauma, or fracture. Pelvic obliquity is checked posteriorly with the patient in the standing position; if there is pelvic obliquity, scoliosis and leg length inequality must be evaluated. When determining range of motion of the thoracic and lumbar spine in all parameters, the orthopaedist should look for painful or guarded motion and loss of motion.

Inflammatory spondylitis is suggested by loss of lumbar lordosis, stiffness of the lumbar spine, and decreased rib cage excursion with respirations. The loss or decrease in lumbar flexion can be quantified by the Schober test. With the child upright and viewed from the back, a line is drawn parallel to the lumbosacral junction and marks are placed 5 cm below and 10 cm above the line. The distance between the marks is measured with the child standing. On forward bending, the distance between the marks is remeasured; an increase of at least 6 cm is normal. Involvement of the costover-

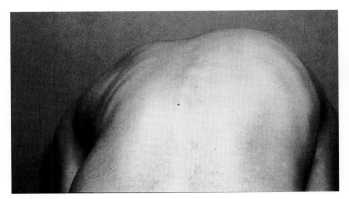

Figure 1 The forward bend test can be performed with the examiner in front of or behind the patient. Asymmetries of different areas of the spine will be better seen by changes in the amount of forward flexion.

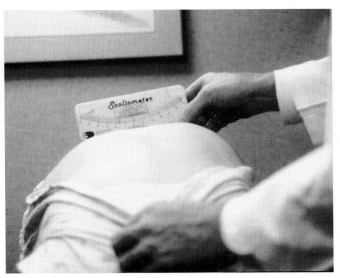

Figure 2 The scoliometer is a hand held inclinometer that measures the ATR. It enables the examiner to quantitate the ATR and is recorded as the maximum reading for each curve.

tebral joints can reduce chest excursion in the midthoracic level. Thoracic excursion measured at the fourth intercostal space (immediately under the axilla) from maximal expiration to maximal inspiration should be at least 5 cm.

Trunk rotation is a topographic abnormality that can be detected by scoliometer measurement or by viewing the posterior thorax from the front or rear position as the patient bends from the waist in the Adams or forward bend test (Fig. 1). A positive test often is associated with scoliosis but does not equate with a diagnosis of scoliosis. Approximately 20% of adolescents may have a trunk asymmetry on the forward bend test but 2% or fewer will have underlying scoliosis. The scoliometer is an inclinometer developed to objectively measure trunk rotation or inclination. Its advantages include minimal exposure, no known associated morbidity, and production of an objective measurement of the angle of trunk rotation (ATR) (Fig. 2). Numerous studies have validated its low interobserver and intraobserver error. Because results of these tests differ in many children (approximately 10%), both examinations are necessary. A scoliometer reading of 7° is an indication for subsequent radiographic evaluation to document the diagnosis of scoliosis.

When trunk asymmetry in the forward bend test is accompanied by deviation to one side (asymmetric muscle spasm), it is an indicator of spinal lesions (eg, bone tumor, spinal cord lesion, infection, asymmetric hamstring tightness, or herniated disc), which require a more complete evaluation. The forward bend test should also be conducted in the sagittal plane. Sagittal abnormalities such as hyperkyphosis can be masked in the heavier individual when standing, but will become more obvious when viewed from the side in the forward flexed position. Hyperkyphosis indicates the need for a more thorough evaluation for Scheuermann's kyphosis,

congenital kyphosis, and scoliosis caused by intraspinal pathology.

With the child still standing, foot deformities are noted, especially underlying cavus foot. Atypical clubfeet, asymmetry of foot size, and progressive foot deformities are clues to the presence of an associated spinal dysraphic state. It is easiest to test plantar flexion power (gastrocnemius-soleus muscle; S1 root) by asking a standing patient to rise and descend on one foot while comparing the two sides; with normal muscle power, 10 single-foot toe raises are possible. Finally, the Gower's sign is a good indicator of weakness in the pelvic girdle muscles, and is elicited by watching the child squat or sit and then rise to a standing position.

Sitting

With the child sitting facing the examiner, the examination proceeds from cephalad to caudad. The physical examination of the cervical spine is similar to the evaluation of the thoracic and lumbar spine. The physician first looks for deformity not only of the neck but also the cranium and facies. Torticollis like scoliosis is a sign and not a diagnosis. When this sign is present, the etiology must be found (Table 2). The range of motion of the cervical spine and associated symptoms such as pain are noted. Tenderness of the anterior and posterior cervical area and upper thoracic muscle tenderness and trigger point pain are sought.

Many syndromes are associated with spinal abnormalities. Lhermitte's sign, the sensation of electricity radiating down the spine or limb on active or passive flexion of the head, has been associated with multiple

TABLE 2 | Differential Diagnosis of Torticollis

Congenital muscular torticollis

Neoplastic (posterior fossa tumors, cervical spine tumors)

Sandifer syndrome (gastroesophageal reflux and torticollis)

Klippel-Feil syndrome

Atlantoaxial rotatory displacement

Basilar impression

Atlanto-occipital anomalies

Unilateral absence of C1

Grisel's syndrome (torticollis and inflammation of adjacent neck tissues)

sclerosis, Pott's disease, cervical tumor, head injury, and cervical cord tumor. A short neck, low hairline, and decreased cervical motion would suggest Klippel-Feil syndrome. Cleft lip and palate is the most common craniofacial anomaly; 13% of these individuals will have cervical spine anomalies. These anomalies, usually spina bifida and vertebral body hypoplasia, are predominantly in the upper cervical spine. Oculoauriculovertebral dysplasia (Goldenhar's syndrome) demonstrates the relationship between facial anomalies and vertebral anomalies. The typical eye defect is an epibulbar dermoid on the conjunctiva and the common ear anomaly is a preauricular fleshy skin tag. Hemivertebrae and block vertebrae are the most common spine anomalies of this syndrome and can occur anywhere along the spine.

Muscle power, sensory responses, and reflexes of the upper extremities are easily checked in the sitting position. Asymmetry of the upper limbs and vascularity are noted, and it is easy to test the patellar (L4) and Achilles (S1) reflexes. The modified or sitting straight leg raise (SLR) test can be performed to corroborate the more traditional supine test or Lasègue's test. With the patient sitting comfortably, the hips and knees are naturally flexed at 90°; as the physician extends the knee to observe the foot, the patient extends the hip and leans backward if true tension signs are present. This test is especially important in the adolescent if any underlying nonorganic problems are suspected.

Supine and Prone

The final element of the spinal examination is performed in the lying position. With the child supine, the abdomen can be examined and abdominal reflexes evaluated. Asymmetrical abdominal reflexes associated with scoliosis indicate possible hydrosyringomyelia. Range

of motion in the hip, knee, and ankle is determined. Hip and spinal disease easily can be confused; both should be examined, even when symptoms suggest only one area of pathology. The physician should understand the Thomas test for hip flexion contracture and the Patrick or Faber test to unmask pathology in the sacroiliac area.

The SLR test and the related measurement of the popliteal angle can separate intrinsic spinal disease from myostatic contracture and primary hip pathology. The SLR is the degree that the leg with an extended knee can be elevated from the horizontal by flexing the hip. An inability to raise the leg toward the vertical position can indicate pathology in a number of areas. Primary hip disease can restrict hip flexion and may be confirmed by range of motion and the Thomas test. Hamstring tightness due to myostatic contracture or spasticity also causes limitation of SLR and is suggested when the test elicits no complaints of pain. Tight hamstrings frequently are associated with Scheuermann's kyphosis and spondylolysis/spondylolisthesis, but also are found in normal children after periods of rapid growth and in poorly conditioned children.

A decreased SLR, especially when accompanied by pain, can indicate nerve root inflammation. Pain produced by raising the straight leg and stretching the sciatic nerve is suggestive of radiculopathy, especially if the pain extends distally past the knee. If there is any question, the knee can be flexed slightly and the foot dorsiflexed (Lasègue's test), again stretching the sciatic nerve and reproducing the patient's pain. A positive contralateral SLR test reproduces pain in the opposite leg, further confirming radicular irritation.

The femoral stretch test with the patient prone or in the lateral position is performed by extending the thigh at the hip with the knee flexed; reproduction of the patient's anterior or anterolateral thigh pain suggests involvement of the more cephalad roots (L2, L3, and L4). Measurement of the popliteal angle (Fig. 3) indicates muscle spasticity or contracture and confirms suspected tension signs. The normal angle varies by individual and with age. In children younger than 3 years, the mean is 6°; from 4 to 10 years it increases (more hamstring tightness) to 25°. A popliteal angle greater than 50° is considered abnormal. The popliteal angle can be asymmetric and result in an apparent sciatic scoliosis on the forward bend test.

The prone hyperextension test is used to determine whether hyperkyphosis noted in the standing or sitting position is fixed or correctable. A patient lying in the prone position with the arm at the side is asked to raise the head and shoulders off the examining table. Correction of the increased kyphosis suggests a flexible spine and indicates a postural kyphosis caused by poor sitting and standing mechanics, not a fixed spinal abnormality

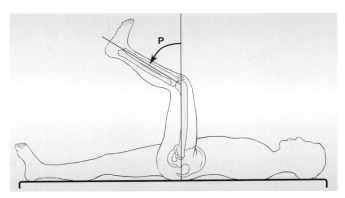

Figure 3 The popliteal angle is measured with the patient supine and the hip flexed to 90°. The tibia is then extended at the knee until maximum resistance is encountered. The angle formed by the tibia and a line extended from the femur is the popliteal angle, and it indicates the degree of hamstring muscle spasm or contracture.

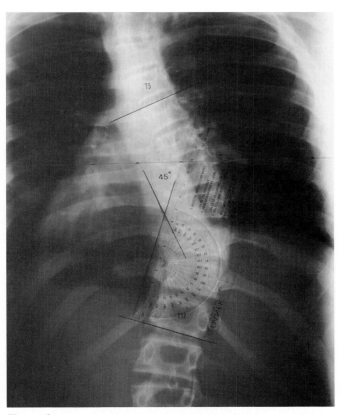

Figure 4 The Cobb method for measuring degree of scoliosis is measured on the standing AP or PA film taken at a 6-ft distance. A line is drawn across the top of the superior end vertebra and across the bottom of the inferior end vertebra. A second set of lines is drawn perpendicular to the end vertebral lines. The intersection of these two perpendicular lines is the Cobb angle.

such as Scheuermann's kyphosis or congenital kyphosis. The remainder of the neurologic examination includes muscle testing, sensory responses, and evaluation for clonus and pathologic Babinski's reflexes. The distal peripheral pulses are palpated, and the lower extremities are evaluated for atrophy and/or cutaneous abnormalities.

The Galeazzi test is conducted with the child supine and the knees and hips flexed 90°. Discrepancy in the relative height of the knees indicates inequality in the femurs if the hip joint is located. In the reverse Galeazzi test, the child is prone and the hips are neutral, with the knees flexed to 90°. The relative height of the heels is noted; a discrepancy indicates inequality in the length of the tibias. This is an easy way to separate pelvic obliquity secondary to leg length inequality from that secondary to lumbar scoliosis.

Plain Radiographs

Disc space narrowing, vertebral end plate irregularities, vertebral scalloping, destructive radiolucent or radiodense lesions, fracture, osteopenia, and pars defects are some of the abnormalities that can be detected by plain radiography. Every child with back pain should have at least an AP and lateral radiograph of the spine in the area of maximum symptoms. Films for suspected instability should include an AP and a standing flexion and extension lateral view. Oblique views can be added if a suspected pars defect is not seen on the lateral view. Plain radiographs will identify approximately one third of patients with pars defects; because of their ready availability, they are the initial evaluation of choice.

The radiographs establish the diagnosis suspected from the history and physical examination. The most common spinal deformity, adolescent idiopathic scoliosis, is diagnosed when a 10° or greater curve with rota-

tion is present. For optimum radiographic evaluation of spinal deformity, specific techniques are necessary. Radiation exposure, especially to the developing breasts and thyroid, is minimized by use of PA projections, fast x-ray film, x-ray tube filtration, beam collimation, and rare earth screens. For the older child and adolescent, a standing PA and lateral radiograph taken at a 6-ft distance on a 36-in film will accurately represent the anatomic spine and is the standard for measurement techniques. The entire thoracic and lumbar spine and the superior pelvis are included to measure the deformity, and to establish the Risser stages of spinal maturity. The curve magnitude is measured by the Cobb method (Fig. 4). Typically the iliac crest apophysis ossifies from anterior to posterior, which appears in a coronal projection as lateral to medial. Risser divided the crest into four quadrants grading the degree of ossification from 1 to 4. A grade of 0 is given if the apophysis is not present and a grade of 5 indicates complete closure of the apophysis with fusion to the iliac crest. Risser grade 0 occurs in the prepubertal or early pubertal stages before the adolescent growth spurt, and Risser grades 1 and 2 are at the beginning of rapid growth.

Risser grades 3 and 4 occur in the more mature adolescent, usually postmenarchal when the child is in the decreasing phase of the growth spurt. Children with Risser grades 0 and 1 have the highest incidence of scoliosis progression.

Radiographic evaluation of vertebral rotation is measured on the coronal film using the system of Nash and Moe. The rotation of the apical vertebra (the most rotated vertebra; the vertebra most deviated from the vertical axis, usually at the center of the curve) is graded from 0 to 4. Zero rotation occurs when the pedicle shadow is symmetric and equidistant from the sides of the vertebral body. In grade 1, the pedicle shadow on the convex side has moved away from the side toward the center. In grade 3, the shadow is in the center of the vertebral body. Grade 2 is intermediate between grades 1 and 3. When the pedicle shadow passes beyond the midline, a grade of 4 is given.

The distance of the apical vertebra from the center axial line is evaluated on the standing coronal film. Significant curves have the greatest magnitude, the most rotation of the apical vertebra, and the greatest lateral shift of apical vertebra from the vertical axis. Bending films used to assess curve flexibility are not needed to make the diagnosis, but are used when treatment (brace/surgery) programs are considered; they should not be ordered routinely.

A supine AP and lateral film will be most valuable in infants, children, and adolescents with limited ability to cooperate, or when bone detail is necessary for suspected congenital curves. For patients in wheelchairs or with leg length inequality, a sitting or assisted sitting film will equate to the standard standing projections and represent the actual effect of gravity loading on both the primary and compensatory curves. Because radiation effects are cumulative and should be minimized, radiographs should be ordered to give the maximum amount of useful information with the least number of films. All young women of childbearing age should be queried about possible pregnancy before taking radiographs.

Radiographic evaluations of the pediatric cervical spine always have been a source of concern for the orthopaedic surgeon because of the confusing and changing anatomy and the infrequency of these studies. A clear understanding of the common normal variation in the child's spine and the parameters that separate normal from abnormal is useful.

The cervical spine approaches adult size by age 8 years, and the vertebral bodies gradually lose their oval or wedge shape and become more rectangular. Because of the orientation of the facet joints and the relative laxity of the ligaments and cartilage elements of the pediatric spine, increased physiologic or normal cervical instability is noted in children younger than age 8 years. Most injuries (90%) that occur in children younger than 8 years are located at C3 or higher. Thus, children in the first decade are unique; older children will have radiographs similar to those of the adult population.

The infant cervical vertebrae ossify from numerous ossification centers that are connected by various synchondroses. The cartilaginous synchondroses have a radiolucent appearance and can be confused with fractures. Synchondroses tend to have smooth margins that are noncongruent until they coalesce with other centers. Fractures tend to be irregular, sharp, congruent, and situated in different locations than synchondroses.

The cervical prevertebral soft tissue, a helpful indicator of cervical spine trauma in adults, is unreliable in infants and children because of wide normal variations of width and configuration. The additive effects of respiration and neck position will alter these normal soft-tissue shadows. Films taken during expiration (crying) and with the neck flexed will give a false impression of a soft-tissue retropharyngeal mass.

The most useful films to evaluate the cervical spine are the open mouth odontoid view, the AP view, and flexion-extension lateral views. Flexion-extension views should always be voluntary and should not be ordered in severe trauma until the static AP and lateral views have been evaluated.

In the normal upper cervical spine, the odontoid, the spinal cord, and free space each occupy one third of the space; this is the so-called rule of thirds. Two measurements made on lateral flexion-extension views are worth committing to memory. The atlas-dens interval (ADI) is the distance between the anterior cortex of the dens and the posterior portion of the ring of the atlas (C1). In children, an ADI of 5 mm or larger as measured on the lateral flexion film is abnormal. The space available for the cord (SAC) is the distance between the posterior cortex of the dens and the anterior cortex of the posterior portion of the ring of the atlas. Applying the rule of thirds in children, cord compression is likely if the SAC is less than the transverse diameter of the odontoid. Increase in the ADI can be seen in trauma and chronic conditions such as rheumatoid arthritis, Down syndrome, and congenital anomalies (Fig. 5).

Because of their general increase in ligamentous laxity, children have increased normal or physiologic laxity on lateral radiographs of the cervical spine. This laxity most often is seen between C2 and C3. To differentiate this pseudosubluxation from pathologic instability, familiarity with the posterior cervical line of Swischuk is useful (Fig. 6). A line is drawn from the anterior cortex of the posterior arch of C1 to the anterior cortex of the posterior arch of C3. Normally, the anterior cortex of the posterior arch of C2 lies posterior to the posterior cervical line in extension and neutral positions. In pseudosubluxation of C2, where the vertebral body of C2 appears anteriorly displaced on the lateral flexion view, the posterior cervical line may (1) touch, (2) pass through, or (3) be 1.5 to 2.0 mm anterior to the anterior cortex of the posterior arch of C2. If the line misses the arch by 1.5 mm, the orthopaedist should be suspicious, but if the distance is 2 mm or more, true dislocation should be assumed.

Atlantoaxial rotatory displacement is one of the most common causes of torticollis in children; it represents a continuum of pathology from mild subluxation to complete dislocation. The plain radiograph of a normal child whose head is rotated into the torticollis position will be similar to that seen in the pathologic condition of fixed rotatory subluxation of C1 on C2. When the problem is suspected on plain radiograph, the diagnosis can be confirmed with a CT scan using dynamic rotation views. On the plain radiograph open mouth view of a child with rotatory displacement, the lateral mass of C1 that has rotated anteriorly appears wider and closer to the dens with decreased space between it and the dens, and the opposite lateral mass appears narrower with increased space between it and the dens. These radiographic findings only indicate the position of C1-C2 at the time of exposure and do not determine if it is a permanent or fixed position.

Orthopaedic surgeons frequently are called on to evaluate athletes with transient radiculopathy, burners, or paraparesis. Measurements on plain radiographs cannot predict congenital cervical spinal stenosis. Normally the width of the body and the width of the canal are equal and would give a ratio of 1. If the ratio between the spinal canal measured on the lateral radiograph and the width of the body at its midpoint is less than 0.8, cervical spinal stenosis should be suspected but MRI is needed to establish the diagnosis.

Spina bifida occulta (SBO) is an isolated disorder of posterior vertebral development in which a failure of posterior vertebral fusion results in absence or dysplasia of the spinous process and at times the lamina. The malformation most commonly affects L5 and/or S1 vertebral levels and is estimated to occur in up to 30% of the population. SBO often will be found on lumbar radiographs. In most cases, SBO is of no clinical significance but its presence should concern the orthopaedist for two reasons. If a surgical procedure with the midline approach is undertaken, the exposed dura should be protected because it is not protected by a complete bony arch. Second, SBO can be associated with other pathologic conditions such as congenital scoliosis, spondylolisthesis, spinal dysraphism, Klippel-Feil syndrome, and lumbar disc herniation.

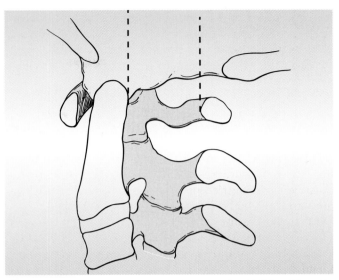

Figure 5 The ADI and SAC are indicators of atlantoaxial or C1-C2 instability and are measured on the flexion and extension lateral cervical films. The instability is generally demonstrated on the flexion-lateral view. ADI is measured from the posterior cortex of the ring of C1 to the anterior cortex of the odontoid process of C2. The SAC is measured from the posterior cortex of the odontoid to the anterior cortex of the posterior ring of C1. Cord compression is suggested if the SAC is equal to or less than the diameter of the odontoid process.

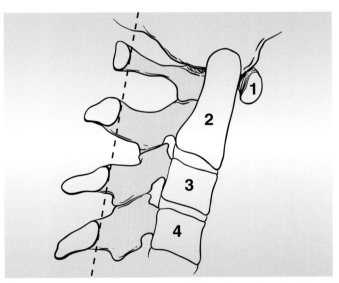

Figure 6 The posterior cervical line of Swischuk is used to differentiate physiologic pseudosubluxation of C2 on C3 from pathologic instability as viewed on the flexion-lateral view of the cervical spine. The line is drawn through the anterior cortex of the posterior arches of C1 and C3. In physiologic pseudosubluxation, the line passes through the anterior cortex of the posterior arch of C2.

Spondylolysis and spondylolisthesis are found in approximately 6% of the population and will be encountered frequently. The isthmic or pars defect frequently is seen on the lateral view, particularly with bilateral defects. Unilateral defects may result in sclerosis of the pars or lamina on the opposite side. This

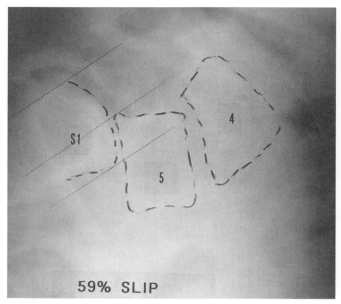

59% SLIP

Figure 7 The percentage of displacement of L5 on the sacrum is measured on the standing lateral lumbar film with the beam centered at L5. A line is drawn parallel to the posterior cortex of the body of the sacrum. A second parallel line is drawn at the posterior inferior corner of the body of L5. A third parallel line is drawn at the anterior superior edge of the sacrum. The distance between the first and second line (amount of slip) is divided by the distance between the first and third line (width of the body of the sacrum) to give the percentage of slip.

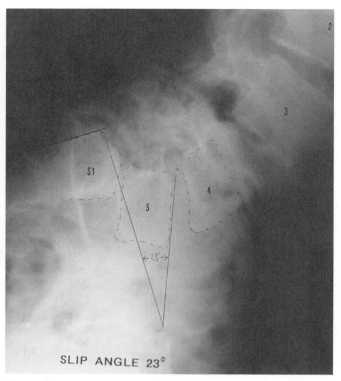

SLIP ANGLE 23°

Figure 8 The slip angle measures the amount of forward tilting of the fifth lumbar vertebra over the sacrum and is calculated on the standing lateral lumbar film. The slip angle is formed by a line drawn parallel to the inferior or superior aspect of the body of L5 and a line perpendicular to the posterior aspect of the body of the sacrum. An angle greater than 55° in the immature patient indicates a high likelihood of progression.

should not be confused with a tumor such as osteoid osteoma; it represents an area of increased stress with subsequent increase in bone formation. When suspected but not seen on the lateral film, a pars defect can be seen on the oblique view with observation of the collar on the Scottie dog. At times, because of continued repair of the isthmic abnormality, there will be an elongation of the pars rather than a defect.

If spondylolisthesis is suspected, standing lateral radiographs should be taken to maximize the amount of instability present. The degree of slip is measured relative to the anterior-posterior diameters of the sacrum and is graded I, 1%-25%; II, 26%-50%; III, 51%-75%; and IV, 76%-100% (Fig. 7). In a skeletally immature patient, the slip angle has been found to be most useful in determining the likelihood of progression. The normal slip angle should be 0° to -10°. Values in excess of 55° correlate with a higher likelihood of progression and should always be measured in the standing lateral radiograph (Fig. 8).

Computed Tomography

CT is not a screening modality but is used to further define pathology noted on plain radiographs or bone scan. CT scanner technology has been improved, especially in areas of image resolution, reduction in acquisition time, and software for three-dimensional (3-D)

reconstruction. CT scanners are readily available, and interpretation of the scan is familiar to radiologists and orthopaedic surgeons.

CT scans can be invaluable in evaluating fractures and bone tumors that have been identified or suspected on plain radiographs or bone scans. Their diagnostic characteristics, exact locations, and real or potential spinal instability can be assessed. If brace or cast immobilization has been used to treat spondylolytic lesions, CT scans can be used to determine if healing has occurred in the pars area. CT is useful to determine the adequacy of spinal fusion. When retained metal implants preclude the use of MRI to evaluate spinal cord and root pathology, myelography coupled with CT imaging will provide the most information.

The use of 3-D CT has significantly improved the ability to understand pathology in complex developmental anomalies of the upper cervical spine and in severe congenital scoliosis/kyphosis. Progressive distortion of vertebral morphology often obscures the presence of bony bars (failures of segmentation) and hemivertebrae (failure of formation) on radiographs, especially in the older child. Reformatted images produced from thin CT sections can help clarify the pathology, but the global morphology of the anomalous segments and their interrelationships are not easily perceived (Fig. 9).

When atlantoaxial rotatory displacement is noted on plain radiographs (open mouth or odontoid view), it is difficult to determine if the subluxation is fixed. Fixed rotatory subluxation of C1 or C2 is confirmed by the dynamic CT scan. Axial cuts are made at the C1-C2 area. In the normal cervical spine, C1 will rotate from side to side around the odontoid as the head is turned. In fixed rotatory subluxation (clinically the child will have torticollis), the axial CT demonstrates subluxation on the initial film. The diagnosis is made if the subluxation persists when the scan is repeated with the head maximally turned in the opposite direction.

Magnetic Resonance Imaging

MRI is the diagnostic modality of choice in evaluating intraspinal and paraspinal soft-tissue abnormalities in infants, children, and adolescents. The key to interpretation of MRI is knowledge of the normal anatomy, which can be particularly difficult in infants and small children. Significant normal changes in children younger than 2 years affect MRI: ossification of the cartilaginous end plates of the vertebrae; change from red to yellow marrow in the vertebrae; weight-bearing stresses on the spine as the infant begins to sit, stand, and walk; and changing water content of the discs. The conus can normally extend to the body of the third lumbar vertebra in infants 3 months old and younger. After 3 months, the conus should lie at the L1-L2 level. Approximately 25% of asymptomatic adolescents will demonstrate MRI evidence of disc degeneration.

One technique to improve resolution on MRI is to suppress voluntary motion by sedating young children and infants. Children younger than 12 years usually require heavy sedation or low-dose general anesthesia, both of which increase the morbidity of the procedure. Gadolinium is a safe intravenous contrast agent, and no major reactions have been reported in infants and children. It is similar to iodinated contrast media in that it penetrates highly vascularized areas and produces an increase in signal intensity in those areas on T1-weighted images. Gadolinium is useful in differentiating edema, cyst formation, and necrosis from actual tumor and, therefore, is helpful in evaluating suspected neoplastic processes.

MRI should be considered to confirm the clinical impression of discitis, epidural abscess, lumbar disc herniations and slipped vertebral apophysis, spinal cord tumor, spinal trauma with neurologic abnormalities, atypical scoliosis, and certain cases of congenital vertebral anomalies. When evaluating atypical scoliosis and congenital vertebral anomalies, the entire spine must be

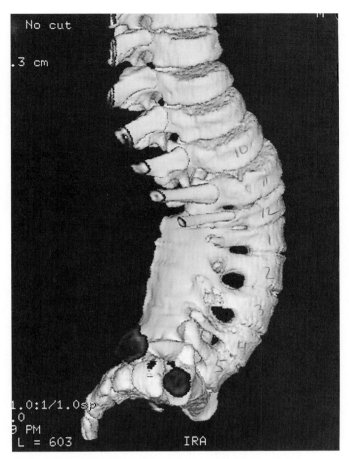

Figure 9 3-D reconstructions of CT can be generated with new software advances. This 5-year-old child has a significant and extensive failure of segmentation of his lumbar spine that results in a rare lordoscoliosis deformity. The extent of the bony bar can be seen on the 3-D CT.

imaged from the posterior fossa to the tip of the sacrum because the pathologic conditions will not necessarily be located at the region of the scoliotic deformity.

MRI is expensive, has a morbidity associated with the use of deep sedation and anesthesia, and should not be used as a screening tool. It should be reserved for patients whose clinical symptoms and signs point to an underlying soft-tissue abnormality or in clinical situations with a high incidence of associated neurologic abnormalities. The yield of correct diagnoses will increase if the orthopaedic surgeon shares his concerns and suspicions with the neuroradiologist who can tailor the technique to obtain the maximum information.

Radionuclide Bone Imaging

Radionuclide scans (scintigraphy) are useful for evaluation of infection, tumor, stress reactions, and fractures. The two studies used for detection of infection are the gallium Ga 67 scan and the indium In 111 labeled white blood cells. In the indium In 111 scan, the radionuclide is incubated with a sample of the patient's blood; the labeled white blood cells are reinjected into the patient and migrate to the area of infection.

By far the most common scan used for evaluation of spine problems is the technetium Tc 99m scan; the delayed bone phase is the most useful to the orthopaedic surgeon. Technetium Tc 99m scintigraphy measures the level of active bone turnover. In addition to a normal amount of background activity, normal increased uptake is noted adjacent to the physis in metabolically active areas. Pathologic areas of heightened turnover are associated with tumors, infection, and fracture. In addition, it is possible to see areas of decreased activity secondary to decreased blood supply; for example, in osteonecrosis. Technetium Tc 99m scintigraphy is significantly more sensitive in picking up areas of bony pathology than plain radiographs and should be used as a screening modality to locate areas of suspected abnormality that then can be further scrutinized with CT or MRI to establish the diagnosis. When problems such as discitis, bone neoplasms, occult fracture, or stress reactions/fractures are suspected, the bone scan should be the next imaging modality selected after the plain radiograph.

One of the most common clinical dilemmas that faces the orthopaedic surgeon is diagnosing suspected stress reaction/fractures in the young athlete with lumbar pain. A good way to conceptualize pars interarticularis abnormalities secondary to repeated microtrauma is as a continuum, from stress reaction of the pars to acute metabolically active stress fracture to chronic established less active stress fractures. Spondylolysis refers to a defect in the pars that can be detected radiographically, whereas a stress reaction is not radiographically apparent and is diagnosed by increased tracer uptake on bone scintigraphy. The current concept is that metabolically active lesions, stress reactions, and recent stress fractures have a good chance of healing with immobilization while the more chronic established lesions are less likely to heal.

Single photon emission CT (SPECT) is a technique that is basically CT of conventional bone scintigraphy. SPECT improves the diagnostic ability of bone scintigraphy by permitting separation of bony structures that overlap in standard planar images, resulting in precise localization of the anatomic area involved. In addition, it is possible to quantify the level of activity by comparing the activity of the affected vertebra to that of a contiguous unaffected vertebra. SPECT is the modality with the highest degree of both sensitivity and speci-

ficity in detecting stress lesions/fractures in the pars interarticularis. Approximately 25% of lesions present in SPECT will be seen on plain radiographs, and planar bone scintigraphy will show only 50%.

Ultrasonography

The most effective use of ultrasonography is in screening for renal tract deformities associated with congenital spinal abnormalities such as congenital scoliosis and Klippel-Feil syndrome. Significant renal abnormalities are present in approximately one fourth of these individuals. Because of its low cost, lack of morbidity, and ready availability, it is the ideal screening tool; all patients with these spinal deformities should have a renal ultrasound examination.

Because sound waves do not penetrate bone, ultrasonography is not effective for spinal cord imaging in the older infant and child. The unossified midline posterior elements of the vertebral column in the neonate and infant (up to 3 to 6 months of age) provide an acoustic window for visualizing the spinal cord, filum terminale, nerve roots, cauda equina, and distal thecal sac. Spinal ultrasound is indicated in infants with physical findings that suggest an underlying dysraphic lesion and infants with caudal regression or anorectal malformations that carry a risk of cord tethering. Intraoperative ultrasonography has gained increased acceptance in the neurosurgical community to accurately measure the extent of cord tumors and cystic lesions.

Laboratory Tests

Although routine laboratory tests are not indicated in the evaluation of pediatric back pain or deformities, they can be invaluable when infectious, inflammatory, or neoplastic etiology is suspected. The initial tests to consider are a complete blood count and erythrocyte sedimentation rate (ESR). Fever, elevated ESR, anemia, and leukocytosis can be seen in infection, inflammatory arthritis, and childhood leukemia or lymphoma. A mild anemia is most suggestive of infection or inflammatory problems, while severe anemia suggests a malignant neoplastic process. Children with juvenile ankylosing spondylitis do not have rheumatoid factors, nor do they have antinuclear antibodies in the serum. The most helpful finding in these patients is the presence of HLA-B27, which is found in approximately 90% of patients with juvenile ankylosing spondylitis.

Annotated Bibliography

Back Pain in Children and Adolescents

Anderson K, Sarwark JF, Conway JJ, Logue ES, Schafer MF: Quantitative assessment with SPECT imaging of stress injuries of the pars interarticularis and response to bracing. *J Pediatr Orthop* 2000;20:28-33.

The authors show how quantification of the SPECT scan intensity by use of the SPECT ratio can be used to select the subgroup most likely to benefit from brace treatment and they demonstrate that reduction in SPECT intensity relates directly to symptom improvement.

Burton AK, Clarke RD, McClune TD, Tillotson KM: The natural history of low back pain in adolescents. *Spine* 1996;21:2323-2328.

These authors present a longitudinal study of a cohort of 216 11-year-old children with a follow-up of 4 years. They present the natural history, show that prevalence increases with age, and that it has a recurrent nature and minimal morbidity.

Evaluation of Spinal Deformity in Children and Adolescents

Dickson RA, Weinstein SL: Bracing (and screening): Yes or no? *J Bone Joint Surg Br* 1999;81:193-198.

This article articulates the arguments against the concept of school screening programs. It is presented by two respected scoliosis surgeons on both sides of the Atlantic. The arguments are presented in a nonemotional and scientific manner with a corresponding bibliography.

Goldberg CJ, Dowling FE, Fogarty EE, Moore DP: School scoliosis screening and the United States Preventive Services Task Force: An examination of long-term results. *Spine* 1995;20: 1368-1374.

This article challenges the validity of school screening. It presents the findings of the United States Preventive Service Task Force, which were published in 1993, and presents the argument against school screening from the viewpoint of the epidemiologist.

Winter RB, Lonstein JE: Editorial: To brace or not to brace: The true value of school screening. *Spine* 1997;22:1283-1284.

This is a straight and brief presentation of the argument in favor of school screening for scoliosis by the fathers of school screening. It lists a good bibliography of the key articles that support the efficacy of bracing for idiopathic scoliosis and, therefore, the benefit of a school screening program.

Classic Bibliography

Bodner RJ, Heyman S, Drummond DS, Gregg JR: The use of single photon emission computed tomography (SPECT) in the diagnosis of low-back pain in young patients. *Spine* 1988;13:1155-1160.

Bunnell WP: Outcome of spinal screening. *Spine* 1993; 18:1572-1580.

King H: Back pain in children, in Weinstein SL (ed): *The Pediatric Spine: Principles and Practice.* New York, NY, Raven Press, 1994, pp 173-183.

McCarthy RE: Evaluation of the patient with deformity, in Weinstein SL (ed): *The Pediatric Spine: Principles and Practice.* New York, NY, Raven Press, 1994, pp 185-224.

Rickard K: The occurrence of maladaptive health-related behaviors and teacher-rated conduct problems in children of chronic low back pain patients. *J Behav Med* 1988;11:107-116.

Chapter 14

The Aging Spine

Jack E. Zigler, MD

David W. Strausser, MD

Introduction

Geriatric related disorders of the spine are becoming an increasingly important concern to the physician practitioner in the United States. This is due to a combination of factors. The elderly are becoming an ever-increasing percentage of the population as the baby boom generation ages. In 1980, 12% of the US population was over 65 years of age. By the year 2020 this percentage will increase to 17%. By 2050 it is estimated to be 22%, or 68 million people. In addition to the increasing numbers of older people, life expectancies continue to rise as medical care and general health knowledge improve within developed countries. According to US Bureau of Census figures, individuals who reach the age of 65 years have life expectancies of 79 years (males) and 83 years (females). As life expectancies continue to increase, so too will the level of activity and demands this segment of the population will place upon itself to continue leading an active and productive lifestyle.

With this increased number of aging patients, practitioners will be presented with an increasing number and array of spine-related disorders. It will become even more important for caregivers to improve their awareness of these disorders and to be able to effectively diagnose and treat them in an appropriate manner.

General Considerations

During the evaluation and treatment of any patient, the practitioner and patient typically have a mutual goal: accurate diagnosis and treatment to eliminate pain, deformity, and physical limitations. However, in the elderly patient, the treatment goal is frequently different from that of the younger patient, who may be more concerned with a return to work or sports activities. As a result of this variance in expectations the desired effect of treatment in the elderly patient must be addressed on a case-by-case basis.

Multiple issues should be discussed with each patient to ensure that both the physician and the patient are mutually aware of what would be considered a treatment success. These issues include pain, functional limitations, deformity, ability to exercise and maintain a healthy lifestyle, and the natural history of the patient's particular disorder.

Pain is typically the primary reason the patient with a spine-related disorder seeks medical attention. Historically, pain has been undertreated in most patients, particularly with respect to chronic pain and/or cancer pain. Undertreatment of pain relates to the physicians' concerns regarding chronic narcotic usage and "addiction" to narcotic medication. As pain management has become more sophisticated and society has become more empowered, the pendulum rapidly is swinging in favor of more adequate treatment. Physician undertreatment now has significant medical and legal repercussions. There is less concern for drug addiction and more concern for patient satisfaction.

Elderly patients can have multiple reasons for spine-related pain. These include degenerative disorders causing axial pain, mechanical instability, neurogenic pain, and osteoporosis-related pain. Frequently these patients will have disorders that are not amenable to surgical treatment and hence, in the surgeon's mind, a "cure." Care must be taken to avoid dismissing the patient's symptom complaints and failing to use other treatment methods, such as appropriate medication (narcotic and nonnarcotic), bracing, physical therapy, and lifestyle/activity modifications. Simply telling the patient to "just learn to live with it" creates both animosity and despair. Medication alternatives include nonsteroidal anti-inflammatory medications. The new COX-2 selective medications may provide a safer medical profile. Acetaminophin and those medications containing acetaminophen can be effective analgesics, but the physician must be vigilant in avoiding daily dosing of greater than 3.5 g/day and in avoiding acetaminophen-containing medications in those patients with liver disorders.

Chronic narcotic medication usage should be considered as a reasonable option in the appropriate elderly patient. Those patients with pain unresponsive to all other treatment remedies who are not surgical candidates may require this last alternative. Physical tolerance to the medication will occur but not to the degree typically expected. Pseudoaddiction may occur in those patients who are undertreated, leading to drug-seeking behavior simply for pain control. True narcotic addiction in elderly patients, with drug-seeking behavior such as medication hoarding and physician manipulation, is infrequent. With increasing age comes an increasing number of medical disorders, and many elderly patients are on several medications. The prescribing physician must be aware of these medications (antihypertensives, cardiac agents, lipid-lowering agents, etc) and possible interactions with those medications prescribed for pain control, inflammation, or muscle relaxation.

The importance of physical activity, regular exercise, and a spine-related exercise regimen should be discussed with the patient. The ability of the individual to participate in such a program obviously depends on his or her overall physical condition. The more physically fit elderly patient may require a more realistic expectation as to what limitations his/her spinal condition will place on physical abilities.

Occasionally patients may present with radicular pain from stenosis or postlaminectomy syndrome, but are not surgery candidates due to underlying medical conditions. These patients may be considered for a trial of dorsal column stimulation as an effective treatment adjunct. This procedure can be performed initially on a trial basis and ultimately, with local anesthetic/intravenous sedation, as an outpatient with minimized medical risk. If effective, it may significantly reduce narcotic usage and dependence and relieve the patient's primary problem, pain.

Ultimately, the patient and practitioner should come to a common understanding and agreement regarding the etiology of the patient's pain and realistic goals for pain relief. Complete relief and cure frequently are not possible. This situation should not be considered a failure. Through appropriate treatment and patient education the goals of pain reduction and increased physical activity and independence can often be achieved.

Medical Considerations

A complete preoperative medical evaluation is critical in the elderly patient before proceeding with surgical treatment. This evaluation should involve a consultation with an appropriate medical specialist prior to surgery. This process should not be centered on simply clearing the patient for surgery. Current treatment for known existing medical disorders must be optimized before the added physiologic stresses of anesthesia and surgical trauma. Diabetes and hypertension should be well controlled. Cardiac and pulmonary function need to be optimized as well. Thorough medical evaluation occasionally may reveal existing underlying medical disorders previously unknown to the patient.

Continued care by the same medical specialist in the immediate postoperative period is ideal. This care provides for doctor-patient familiarity during the hospital stay. The medical physician should have a general understanding of the nature of the planned surgical procedure, including length of surgery, anatomic location, expected blood loss, and anticipated postoperative immobility. Understanding these factors facilitates preoperative evaluation and medical recommendations.

Another important preoperative consideration in the elderly patient, which is typically ignored in the younger patient, is nutritional status. Nutritional status is of particular importance in the elderly patient who smokes, is physically inactive, and who may have underlying metabolic disorders. Poor preoperative nutritional status can lead to increased risk for wound healing, infection, and delayed physical recovery time. Markers of nutritional status are albumin, total protein, and total lymphocyte count. For those elderly patients considering elective spine surgery, early preoperative nutritional status evaluation should be part of the routine workup. Those patients displaying serologic evidence of compromised nutritional status should be evaluated and treated by appropriate nutritional guidance before surgery.

The patient's anticipated level of postoperative physical ability also needs to be considered prior to surgical treatment. The mere presence of a surgical condition on spine imaging studies does not necessarily mean that surgical treatment is indicated. Improving symptoms of neurogenic claudication by lumbar decompression may not be beneficial in the elderly patient who has such significant cardiopulmonary restriction that he cannot ambulate functionally. Surgical treatment must be individualized in the elderly. The overall risk-benefit ratio must be assessed to ensure that the appropriate patient-individualized treatment will ensue.

Anatomy and Biomechanics of the Aging Spine

The degenerative cascade affecting the human spine begins as early as the second or third decade of life. The typical elderly patient is several decades into the degenerative process. Degenerative changes may ultimately affect the mechanical properties of spinal motion and cause instability and pain symptoms.

The earliest lesion of the degenerative process is

thought to occur at the disc level. The normally well-hydrated nucleus pulposus undergoes a process of dehydration secondary to fragmentation and loss of negatively charged glycosoaminoglycans. There is a gradual increase in collagen and a disproportionate loss of chondroitan sulfate compared with keratin sulfate. With these biochemical changes come mechanical alterations in disc function. As the nucleus becomes more inept at load sharing, there is increased stress placed on the anulus, particularly posteriorly. Fissures develop within the anulus, which themselves may cause pain. Disc bulges or nucleus pulposus herniation may occur. With decreased disc height and altered mechanical function of the disc, degenerative changes begin to occur posteriorly in the facet joints.

This degenerative process can lead to localized segment stiffening or instability within different levels of an individual spine. Stiffened levels display decreased disc height, calcification of the ligaments, and osteogenesis of the facet joints, eventually leading to spinal stenosis. Disc bulging along with osteophyte formation, bony facet overgrowth, and decreased disc and foraminal height also contribute to stenosis. Clinical symptoms may be absent or present only as mild stiffness or pain. Stenosis may occur either centrally, causing claudication, or laterally, causing a radiculitis with radiculopathy or root claudication symptoms.

Stiffness of one particular segment may lead to instability or hypermobility of an adjacent segment. Hypermobility and destabilization may cause degenerative spondylolisthesis or kyphoscoliosis. These changes may be discovered radiographically but are frequently asymptomatic. If symptomatology is present, it may be due to localized mechanical pain, muscular fatigue, or neurologic symptoms caused by compression.

Degenerative Disease of the Cervical Spine

The major clinical manifestations of degenerative disease of the cervical spine include axial neck pain, radiculopathy, and cervical myelopathy secondary to stenosis. Facet joint disease may lead to neck pain, crepitus, and decreased range of motion (Fig. 1). Isolated posterior element disease alone rarely causes sufficient foraminal narrowing to cause radiculopathy. Treatment typically consists of anti-inflammatory medications, soft collar, and physiotherapy. Surgery is rarely indicated in the patient with axial neck pain emanating from posterior joint spondylosis. Cervical facet injections may be both diagnostic and therapeutic.

When degenerative disc disease accompanies facet arthropathy, radicular pain may become associated with neck pain. Uncovertebral spurring combined with loss of disc height may lead to foraminal narrowing and

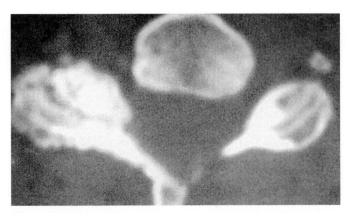

Figure 1 Axial CT image of the cervical spine with severe unilateral facet arthrosis and ipsilateral foraminal stenosis.

nerve root impingement. Those patients with congenital stenosis may also display symptoms of myelopathy. Although most patients respond to conservative treatment, those with persistent radiculopathy may require surgical intervention. Traditionally, orthopaedic spine surgeons have favored anterior decompression with discectomy, decompression, and cervical fusion. This avoids the possible complications seen with laminectomy, such as late instability and deformity. This is the preferred approach for one- or two-level disease, or where cervical kyphosis is present (Fig. 2). Use of allograft combined with plating is becoming a more common approach, thus avoiding the morbidity associated with autogenous tricortical iliac crest. Single-level fusion rates appear to approach that of autogenous graft without plating.

Patients exhibiting clinical signs of myelopathy and cervical stenosis may require decompression (Fig. 3). With disease involving three or more levels, in the lordotic spine, laminoplasty allows for excellent decompression with reduced morbidity and earlier rehabilitation (Fig. 4). There is less surgical morbidity and less postoperative stiffness than in a multilevel anterior decompression and fusion.

Degenerative Disorders of the Lumbar Spine

Lumbar spondylosis is ubiquitous in the elderly population. Most patients will become symptomatic at some point in their adult lives. Degenerative disc disease, facet arthrosis, and muscle deconditioning may all be sources of pain. Low back and radiating proximal leg pain (pseudoradicular pain) may result from disc disease or facet hypertrophy and inflammation. This pain typically responds to traditional conservative treatment. However, with advanced changes, central or foraminal stenosis may occur with subsequent neurogenic claudication or radiculopathy. Foraminal stenosis may occur

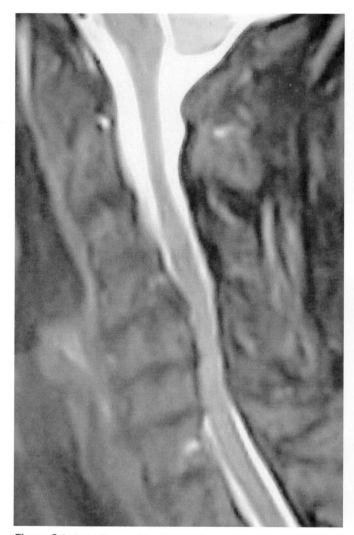

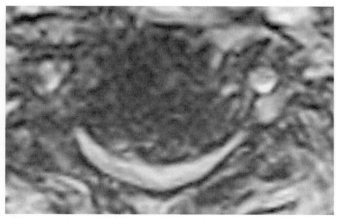

Figure 3 Axial MRI scan of the cervical spine with severe stenosis and flattening of the spinal cord.

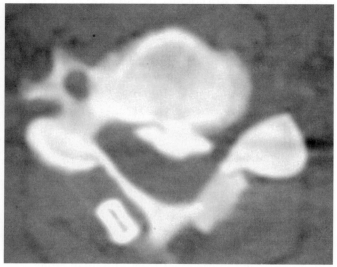

Figure 2 Sagittal MRI scan of the cervical spine revealing midcervical central stenosis with impingement of the spinal cord.

Figure 4 Axial CT scan of cervical spine revealing ossification of the posterior longitudinal ligament. Status after left laminoplasty.

secondary to loss of disc height and accompanying facet hypertrophy. Lateral recess stenosis occurs with hypertrophy of the superior articular process. Congenital stenosis or a trefoil-shaped canal may lead to earlier onset of symptoms.

Surgical decompression may be necessary in those patients unresponsive to conservative treatment (which may include epidural steroid injections). Goals of surgery include central decompression, foraminotomy, and partial facetectomy for lateral recess stenosis. Fusion is recommended for those patients with spondylolisthesis. Instrumentation should be performed for those patients with preoperative dynamic instability, iatrogenic instability due to wide decompression or facet fracture, or associated same-level discectomy. Instrumentation increases the rate of fusion, but does not always lead to improved clinical outcome.

Rheumatoid Arthritis

Surgical treatment of rheumatoid arthritis in the cervical spine in the elderly patient poses many hazards. These include increased infection rates, poor wound healing, frequent skin breakdown, and compromised internal fixation due to osteoporosis. With improving earlier medical management, there is hope that the number of patients with advanced disease requiring surgery will decrease.

Rheumatoid involvement of the cervical spine may cause occipitocervical disease with basilar invagination, C1-C2 instabilty, or subaxial instability (Fig. 5). Basilar invagination may cause proximal cord or brainstem compromise with resulting myelopathy. Diagnosis of myelopathy may be delayed due to rheumatoid involvement in the extremities or peripheral neuropathy mask-

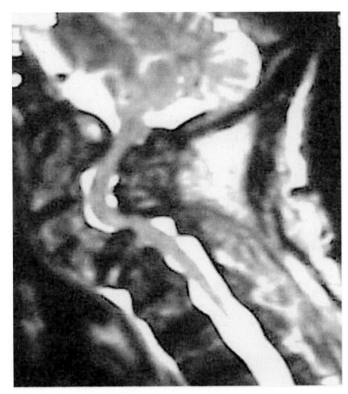

Figure 5 Sagittal cervical MRI scan in a patient with advanced rheumatoid arthritis.

ing typical myelopathic findings. Short-term cervical traction followed by occipitocervical fusion in situ may be performed for spinal cord compromise. Occipitocervical bone grafting and wiring with postoperative halo traction immobilization has been the historic treatment. Newer plate/rod/screw constructs with greater rigidity may allow for elimination of postoperative halo traction.

C1-C2 instability is the most common abnormality seen. Canal and cord compromise occur with increasing instability. Surgical decompression and stabilization is indicated in those patients with a posterior atlanto-dens interval of less than 14 mm, as any progression beyond this leads to a significantly increased risk of paralysis. A cervical MRI study performed in flexion allows for visualization of any pannus and the resultant space available for the cord. Those patients with quadriplegia and a preoperative posterior atlanto-dens interval of less than 10 mm have a poor prognosis for recovery of neurologic function. Before performing fusion for occipitocervical disease, the patient must be evaluated for subaxial instability as well. Extending the fusion to include the levels of questionable instability is preferable to short fusion.

Osteoporosis-Related Disorders

Osteoporosis is a systemic, age-related metabolic disorder affecting the entire axial and appendicular skeleton.

It results in decreased bone mass and an increased incidence of fractures. The bone mass that remains has a normal calcium content and normal bone matrix. Primary osteoporosis is an age-related loss of bone mass. Secondary osteoporosis is loss of bone as a result of an associated endocrinopathy or disease state. As the percentage of the elderly has increased in the United States, so has the incidence of osteoporosis-related disorders.

Primary osteoporosis has been subclassified by Riggs and Melton into type I, postmenopausal osteoporosis, and type II, senile osteoporosis. Type I is six times more common in women than in men and is related to estrogen deficiency with age at onset of 51 to 65 years. It affects primarily trabecular bone mass and is osteoclast mediated. Because of its effect on trabecular bone, vertebral and distal radius fractures are more commonly associated. Type II senile osteoporosis is osteoblast mediated and affects women twice as frequently as men. Cortical bone is primarily affected at age 75 years or older. Fractures of the hip, pelvis, and proximal humerus are more common. Senile osteoporosis is thought to be due to the effects of aging, calcium deficiency, and increased parathyroid hormone.

Peak bone mass occurs in the mid thirties. After achievement of peak bone mass, bone loss begins at a rate of 0.3% per year for men and 0.5% per year for women. With onset of postmenopausal osteoporosis, loss accelerates to 2% to 3% per year for women. After this period of 6 to 10 years, it returns to the premenopausal rate of loss. Estrogen deficiency, either surgical or due to normal maturation, is directly related to postmenopausal osteoporosis.

There are multiple well-identified risk factors for osteoporosis. These include inadequate calcium and vitamin D intake, inadequate weight-bearing exercise, smoking, excessive alcohol use, Caucasian race, chronic steroid use, and early menopause. Metabolic disorders such as hyperparathyroidism, Cushing's syndrome, hyperthyroidism, and vitamin D-related disorders can be secondary causes of osteoporosis.

The incidence of fracture is related directly to the degree of bone mass loss. Therefore, accurate measurement of bone mass is essential to evaluating risk and following treatment. Bone mineral density (BMD) can be measured precisely utilizing dual-energy x-ray absorptiometry (DXA). Measurements may be performed peripherally (wrist or foot) or centrally (lumbar spine and hip). Peripheral measurements are able to diagnose osteoporosis and can be performed with a smaller and less expensive DXA scanner. However, they have only a 70% correlation with hip and spine bone mass. Bone mass measurements within the spine in regions of significant spondylitic changes and osteoarthritis may reveal normal or near normal values despite significant bone loss within the vertebral body itself. This is presumed to be due to inclusion of the dense vertebral osteophytes into the bone mass measurement.

The World Health Society has classified bone density measurements into four levels of bone loss. This classification is based on a comparison with the peak bone mass of a young same-gender normal individual. Those individuals within one standard deviation are considered normal. Those between one to 2.5 standard deviations are considered to be osteopenic. If bone mass loss is greater than 2.5 standard deviations, they are considered to have osteoporosis. Severe osteoporosis is reserved for those with a significant loss of bone mass and an osteoporotic-related fracture.

The best treatment involves prevention early in life, including appropriate calcium and vitamin D intake, regular exercise, and avoiding smoking and excessive alcohol intake. With established bone mass loss, those patients at high risk can be treated with estrogen replacement, calcitonin, a selective estrogen modulator (such as ralixofene hydrochloride), or bisphosphonates (alendronate).

Second-generation bisphosphonates such as alendronate reverse the gradual loss of bone mass. With daily long-term usage there appears to be an increase of bone mass in the spine of approximately 2% to 3% a year and a 50% reduction in the number of spine and hip fractures.

Vertebral Compression/Wedge Fractures

Vertebral body strength and resistance to axial load is significantly dependent on both the quantity and quality of the rich trabecular network within the bone. With loss of bone mass affecting vertebral body trabecular bone, there is a reduction in the size and number of trabeculations, leading to reduced resistance to compression and shear. In addition to this loss, there is a reduction in the connectivity of the individual trabeculations, effectively reducing their load-bearing ability. Vertebral osteoporotic compression fractures typically involve the mid-thoracic or thoracolumbar region of the spine. This involvement is in part due to the kyphotic sagittal alignment, with greater load bearing on the vertebral body with increasing kyphosis. Thoracic fractures typically assume a wedge shape, while lumbar fractures appear to result from vertical axial compression (Fig. 6).

Compression fractures may clinically present along a continuum with respect to the degree of associated pain. These are low-energy insufficiency fractures with either spontaneous onset or occurrence while performing an activity as simple as reaching forward to lift an object. Most clinicians are familiar with the typical presenta-

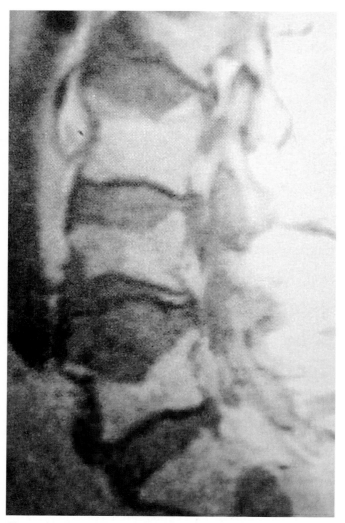

Figure 6 Sagittal lumbar MRI scan revealing multiple level compression fractures.

tion of an acute onset of relatively well-localized pain emanating from the fractured vertebra. However, patients may also present with rather longstanding low-grade local pain or may have evidence of a subacute or chronic healed compression fracture noted incidentally on a chest radiograph. These patients may have no recollection of a painful event. The pathomechanisms believed to be responsible are progressive microfractures that occur within the vertebral body causing minimal or low grade pain. The amount of pain on presentation has not been well correlated with a particular radiographic appearance. In addition, thoracic vertebral wedging in and of itself is not necessarily indicative of a past or present fracture. Thoracic wedge deformities have been associated with thoracic spondylosis as well as osteoporosis and fractures. Therefore, treatment must be individualized based on the patient's history, location of symptoms, and correlation with physical examination and radiographic findings.

A thorough history and physical examination are essential in these patients on presentation. The timing of pain onset, location of pain, and any neurologic symptoms should be determined, and review of systems and other medical disorders should be done. The clinician must be aware of the increased incidence of tumor metastasis and infection as possible etiologies of vertebral fracture in the elderly. Physical examination should involve a diligent attempt to locate the true location of the pain source with respect to the vertebral segment(s) involved. This includes manual palpation and percussion of individual spinous processes to elicit the area of maximum tenderness. This area should be marked with a radiographic marker to identify the verebral body on AP and lateral radiographs. A careful neurologic examination should rule out nerve root or cord compression findings. Neurologic compromise is a rare finding in the patient with a low-energy compression fracture. However, symptoms may worsen later in the fracture period with radiographic evidence of increasing fracture progression and associated deformity.

Plain radiograph findings may reveal a wedge-shaped thoracic fracture or a more vertically oriented fish-mouth-shaped lumbar fracture. Correlation with the physical examination is important. The area of deformity should be classified as appearing acutely fractured, subacute with signs of healing, or chronic (healed or not healed). These patients will often have multiple levels of wedge-shaped deformities or remote chronic healed compression fractures, making radiographic interpretation difficult. The amount of compression in percentage and angulation should be measured to document any progression on future examinations. If there is any concern regarding the presence of neoplasm, infection, or neural compression, MRI with contrast enhancement should be performed. As with plain radiographs, MRI findings suggesting edema, consistent with acute fracture, are not always clinically painful.

It is important to be aware that those patients with a prior insufficiency fracture at any location are at increased risk for subsequent fracture. Women with a preexisting vertebral fracture are thought to have up to a four times greater risk for subsequent vertebral fracture compared to those with no preexisting fracture. Those with other types of a preexisting fracture have a relative risk of two for other combinations of subsequent fracture.

Treatment

Initial treatment historically has been conservative, with the goals of pain control and maintenance of sagittal alignment. Narcotic medication for pain control and use of an external orthosis, such as a Jewett extension brace, are the typical recommended treatments. Frequently, however, body habitus and the patient's reluctance to wear an orthosis will eliminate this form of treatment. Nasal calcitonin can be used both for its antiresorptive effects and analgesic effects on acute insuffiency fractures.

Surgical treatment options for painful osteoporotic fractures are becoming more common in the United States. There are two percutaneously performed techniques being done to reduce the amount of pain and/or restore sagittal alignment of the affected vertebral body. These techniques are typically performed in acute or subacute fractures. The first of these is percutaneous vertebroplasty. This technique involves a percutaneous posterior transpedicular placement of polymethylmethacrylate (PMMA) via needle into the fractured vertebral body. This can be done under conscious sedation using fluoroscopic or CT guidance. PMMA is injected with pressurization via syringe to stabilize the facture and to reduce pain. One study involving 29 patients with 47 fractures with an average injection amount of 7.1 mL of PMMA reported 90% with significant pain relief immediately after the procedure.

The second interventional procedure is vertebral kyphoplasty. Although this is a similar technique with respect to anatomic approach, an inflatable balloon tamp is introduced bilaterally via a catheter into the vertebral body. Each balloon tamp is inflated with saline containing radiographic dye under syringe pressurization and fluoroscopic control to elevate the depressed body. The balloons are then individually deflated and the resultant cavity filled with PMMA (Figs. 7 and 8). The goal is to reestablish vertebral body height in addition to fracture stabilization. Vertebral kyphoplasty is a new technique that currently is undergoing a randomized prospective trial.

At this early stage, both techniques appear to offer a promising option for the patient with severe pain who wishes to avoid the typical 6- to 12-week period of fracture healing and orthosis use. Obviously, both techniques should be performed only by those physicians appropriately trained and able to treat the possible complications such as infection and neurologic injury. These techniques also open the door to possible use of other injectable substances that are skeletally incorporated (such as hydroxyapatite) and remodel with time, rather than PMMA. Adequate trials are necessary to evaluate both effectiveness and complication rates of these procedures.

Surgical Considerations in Elderly People

With improving imaging modalities and surgical technique, increasing numbers of elderly persons are being

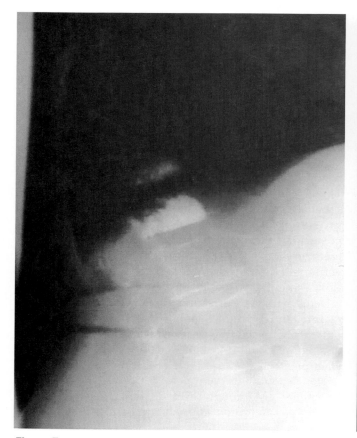

Figure 7 Lateral radiograph of thoracolumbar compression fractures after injection with PMMA.

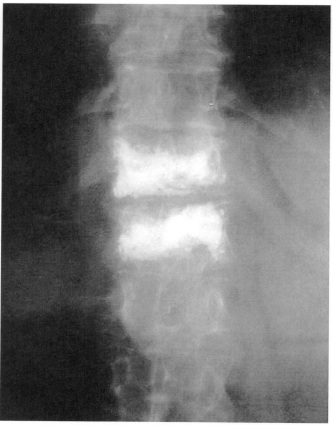

Figure 8 Thoracolumbar compression fractures after injection with PMMA via kyphoplasty technique.

considered candidates for surgical treatment. The ultimate goal of surgically relieving pain and improving quality of life must be counterbalanced with concern for perioperative morbidity and mortality. The patient's age, and more importantly, medical status and existence of comorbid factors, must be taken into account when formulating a surgical treatment plan. As with younger patients, the surgical complication rate increases with the length and extent of surgery, which must be considered in the surgeon's decision to perform a fusion with instrumentation. The surgeon must critically evaluate the risk versus benefit with each additional procedure performed. Surgical complication rates in patients over the age of 70 years range from 6% to 29%. Depending on the extent of the surgical procedure performed, complication rates have varied from equivalent to those of the younger population to significantly higher. In general, those patients requiring limited decompressions or surgery for disc herniations tend to have fewer complications. Overall cost, length of hospital stay, and need for placement in rehabilitation units during recovery are increased in the elderly, and particularly so in the patient undergoing fusion. However, with appropriate patient selection, limited comorbid factors, and atten-

tive perioperative care, significant improvements in function can be obtained with acceptable morbidity.

The effect of osteoporosis on internal fixation must also be considered preoperatively . When considering pedicle screw fixation and/or fusion, preoperative bone densitometry provides accurate information with respect to spine bone mass. In vitro studies have shown that there is a positive linear correlation between BMD and pullout strength. However, this correlation does not automatically doom the patient with osteopenia or osteoporosis to hardware failure or pseudarthrosis. Rather, accurate knowledge of the preoperative degree of osteoporosis heightens the surgeon's awareness of the need for carefully planned instrumentation implantation. Osteoporosis decreases the BMD of the entire pedicle including the trabecular, subcortical, and cortical regions. Thinning of the cortical region of the pedicle, which also occurs, may increase the risk for pedicle fracture during screw placement. To reduce this risk, screw diameter should not exceed 70% of the outer diameter of the pedicle. Placement of pedicle screws using triangulation technique with convergence of the screws will improve the resistance to pullout. Deeper screw insertion provides greater fixation, but penetration through the anterior cortex may place vascular structures at risk. PMMA can also be used during screw insertion for additional strength of fixation. Up to a twofold increase in pullout resistance can be achieved with bone cement augmentation. This may be performed during primary screw insertion in the severely osteoporotic patient or when replacing a failed screw with a similar or larger diameter screw. Care must be taken during bone cement placement to avoid extrusion into the canal or neuroforamen and subsequent nerve injury.

Conclusion

Providing care for the elderly patient with a spine-related disorder requires careful attention to a unique subset of concerns and disorders. Both nonsurgical and surgical care require attention to these issues to provide appropriate care on a patient-individualized basis. With this care and understanding, the goals of decreased pain with improved mobility and quality of life can be achieved while minimizing risk and complications.

Annotated Bibliography

Biomechanics

Halvorson TL, Kelley LA, Thomas KA, Whitecloud TS III, Cook SD: Effects of bone mineral density on pedicle screw fixation. *Spine* 1994;21:2415-2420.

This was a cadaveric study revealing high correlation of pedicle screw pullout with BMD. Utilization of offset laminar hooks in conjunction with pedicle screws at adjacent segments increased the pullout strength to twice the expected value.

Hirano T, Hasegawa K, Takahashi HE, et al: Structural characteristics of the pedicle and its role in screw stability. *Spine* 1997;22:2504-2510.

Osteoporosis leads to thinning of the pedicle cortex along with decreased bone density in the cortical, subcortical, and trabecular region of the pedicle. Approximately 80% of the caudocephalad stiffness and 60% of the pullout strength of the pedicle screw depended on the pedicle rather than on the vertebral body.

Hirano T, Hasegawa K, Washio T, Hara T, Takahashi H: Fracture risk during pedicle screw insertion in osteoporotic spine. *J Spinal Disord* 1998;11:493-497.

This cadaveric study noted a 41% pedicle fracture rate in those vertebrae with a BMD of less than 0.7 g/cm^2 and screw diameter of over 70% of the diameter of the pedicle.

Okuyama K, Sato K, Abe E, Inaba H, Shimada Y, Murai H: Stability of transpedicle screwing for the osteoporotic spine: An in vitro study of the mechanical stability. *Spine* 1993;18:2240-2245.

This study found that the tilting force, cut-up force, and maximum insertion torque correlated with BMD.

Yerby SA, Toh E, McLain RF: Revision of failed pedicle screws using hydroxyapatite cement: A biomechanical analysis. *Spine* 1998;23:1657-1661.

This study evaluated the pullout strength of a 7.0-mm screw placed after pullout of a 6.0-mm screw. A nonaugmented 7.0-mm screw had only 73% of the pullout strength of the 6.0 mm. An augmented 7.0-mm screw had 325% of the strength.

Lumbar Spine Surgery in the Elderly

Ishac R, Alhayek G, Fournier D, Mercier P, Guy G: Results of surgery for lumbar spinal stenosis in patients aged 80 years or more: A retrospective study of thirty-four cases. *Rev Rhum Engl Ed* 1996;63:196-200.

Thirty-four patients underwent lumbar decompression for stenosis. There were only two serious complications, which included a foot drop and a left-sided hemiplegia. The overall result was good in 53% and acceptable in 32%.

Vitaz TW, Raque GH, Shields CB, Glassman SD: Surgical treatment of lumbar spinal stenosis in patients older than 75 years of age. *J Neurosurg* 1999;91(suppl 2): 181-185.

This study contained a total of 65 patients with 79% undergoing fusion for stenosis. There was a 10% serious complication rate and there were no deaths.

Osteoporosis

Bone HG, Greenspan SL, McKeever C, et al: Alendronate and estrogen effects in postmenopausal women with low bone mineral density: Alendronate/Estrogen Study Group. *J Clin Endocrinol Metab* 2000;85:720-726.

This study found a mean increase in BMD at 2 years with treatment with alendronate of 6.0%, conjugated equine estrogen of 6.0%, and combined therapy of 8.3%.

Devogelaer JP, Broll H, Correa-Rotter R, et al: Oral alendronate induces progressive increases in bone mass of the spine, hip, and total body over 3 years in postmenopausal women with osteoporosis. *Bone* 1996;18: 141-150

The authors documented significant and progressive increases in bone mass over a 3-year period of daily 10-mg alendronate. A 7.4% increase in spine BMD was found. Safety and tolerability were compatible with placebo.

Hannan MT, Felson DT, Dawson-Hughes B, et al: Risk factors for longitudinal bone loss in elderly men and women: The Framingham Osteoporosis Study. *J Bone Miner Res* 2000;15:710-720.

Risk factors consistently associated with bone loss in the elderly included thinness, female sex, and weight gain. Weight gain was found to be protective.

Harris ST, Watts NB, Genant HK, et al: Effects of risedronate treatment on vertebral and nonvertebral fractures in women with postmenopausal osteoporosis: A randomized controlled trial. Vertebral Efficacy with Risedronate Therapy (VERT) Study Group. *JAMA* 1999;282:1344-1352.

This was a randomized, double-blind, placebo-controlled trial of patients with a history of a least one vertebral fracture prior to enrollment. Treatment with 5 mg/day, compared with placebo, decreased the incidence of new vertebral fracture by 41% over 3 years. The overall safety profile was similar to that of placebo.

Klotzbuecher CM, Ross PD, Landsman PB, Abbott TA III, Berger M: Patients with prior fractures have an increased risk of future fractures: A summary of the literature and statistical synthesis. *J Bone Miner Res* 2000;15:721-739.

This article was a statistical analysis and summary of the literature. They found a four times greater risk for subsequent vertebral fracture in those with previous fracture. The risk also increases with increasing number of fractures.

Liu G, Peacock M, Eilam O, Dorulla G, Braunstein E, Johnston CC: Effect of osteoarthritis in the lumbar spine and hip on bone mineral density and diagnosis of osteoporosis in elderly men and women. *Osteoporos Int* 1997;7:564-569.

This study revealed the risk of inaccurate spine BMD measurement in those patients with lumbar osteophytes because of osteophyte inclusion during measurement with DXA. There was significantly less effect of hip osteoarthritis on hip BMD measurement.

Nevitt MC, Ross PD, Palermo L, Musliner T, Genant HK, Thompson DE: Association of prevalent vertebral fractures, bone density, and alendronate treatment with incident vertebral fractures: Effect of number and spinal location of fractures. The Fracture Intervention Trial Research Group. *Bone* 1999;25:613-619.

This study found no evidence that the location or number of vertebral fractures should affect the results of treatment with oral alendronate. There was found to be a greater risk of new fracture in the upper rather than lower thoracic spine in those with previous fracture.

Osteoporotic Fractures

Belkoff SM, Maroney M, Fenton DC, Mathis JM: An in vitro biomechanical evaluation of bone cements used in percutaneous vertebroplasty. *Bone* 1999;25(suppl 2):23S-26S.

The authors compared vertebral stiffness before and after compression fracture augmented with transpedicular bone cements. All injected vertebrae were significantly more stiff than nonaugmented.

Cyteval C, Sarrabere MP, Roux JO, et al: Acute osteoporotic vertebral collapse: Open study on percutaneous injection of acrylic surgical cement in 20 patients. *AJR Am J Roentgenol* 1999;173:1685-1690.

The authors found a 75% complete pain relief within 24 hours. One patient had crural pain associated with injection into the psoas muscle.

Heggeness MH: Spine fracture with neurological deficit in osteoporosis. *Osteoporos Int* 1993;3:215-221.

In this small series of patients who developed delayed neurologic changes after benign appearing osteoporotic fracture, there was documented radiographic fracture progression.

Jensen ME, Evans AJ, Mathis JM, Kallmes DF, Cloft HJ, Dion JE: Percutaneous polymethylmethacrylate vertebroplasty in the treatment of osteoporotic vertebral body compression fractures: Technical aspects. *AJNR Am J Neuroradiol* 1997;18:1897-1904.

This was a review of 29 patients with 47 fractures treated with vertebroplasty. Average injection was 7.1 mL per vertebral body. Two patients sustained nondisplaced rib fractures. Ninety percent reported significant pain relief immediately after treatment.

Tohmeh AG, Mathis JM, Fenton DC, Levine AM, Belkoff SM: Biomechanical efficacy of unipedicular versus bipedicular vertebroplasty for the management of osteoporotic compression fractures. *Spine* 1999;24:1772-1776.

This was a cadaveric study, which revealed restoration of vertebral body strength to intact values after unipedicular or bipedicular injection with PMMA.

Classic Bibliography

Boden SD, Dodge LD, Bohlman HH, Rechtine GR: Rheumatoid arthritis of the cervical spine: A long-term analysis with predictors of paralysis and recovery. *J Bone Joint Surg Am* 1993;75:1282-1297.

Deyo RA, Cherkin DC, Loeser JD, Bigos SJ, Ciol MA: Morbidity and mortality in association with operations on the lumbar spine: The influence of age, diagnosis, and procedure. *J Bone Joint Surg Am* 1992;74:536-543.

Ettinger B, Genant HK, Cann CE: Long-term estrogen replacement therapy prevents bone loss and fractures. *Ann Intern Med* 1985;102:319-324.

Greenfield RT III, Capen DA, Thomas JC Jr, et al: Pedicle screw fixation for arthrodesis of the lumbosacral spine in the elderly: An outcome study. *Spine* 1998; 23:1470-1475.

Kirkaldy-Willis WH, Wedge JH, Yong-Hing K, Reilly J: Pathology and pathogenesis of lumbar spondylosis and stenosis. *Spine* 1978;3:319-328.

Lane JM, Russell L, Khan SN: Osteoporosis. *Clin Orthop* 2000;372:139-150.

Quigley MR, Kortyna R, Goodwin C, Maroon JC: Lumbar surgery in the elderly. *Neurosurgery* 1992;30: 672-674.

Chapter 15

Nomenclature and Coding

Tom Faciszewski, MD

Introduction

The subjects of nomenclature and coding have moved from obscurity to among the most commonly discussed, debated, and controversial topics facing spine-care physicians. The spectrum of importance of nomenclature and coding is wide and heavily laden with political, social, and scientific issues.

Why have nomenclature and coding become so important in the practice of medicine? First, physicians must be able to describe accurately diagnoses, treatments, and outcomes in order to discover and provide reliably the most effective advice and treatment for their patients. The diagnosis, which is a name signifying medical knowledge of a given condition, must be defined accurately because it implies the extent and limits of the physician's knowledge of the condition's etiology, pathogenesis, and prognosis. Physicians must define diagnostic nomenclature to describe accurately the specific clinical facets of patients' experiences and the basis for offering a prognosis and for predicting responses to treatment for the diagnosed condition. Without accurately defined terms physicians cannot conduct meaningful clinical research.

Second, nomenclature and coding have become very important for economic reasons. Reimbursement requirements, as well as fraud and abuse issues, have escalated the demand for correct coding. In the United States, changes in federal law have caused a quantum shift in the importance of coding. Similar issues apply throughout the world, although each country has its unique system. These issues respond to political and social concerns and so are, everywhere, subject to frequent change. In this discussion, the example of the current status of these issues in the United States will be explored.

Two recent acts of the US Congress, the Kennedy Kassebaum Health Insurance Portability and Accountability Act 1996 (HIPAA) and the Balanced Budget Act of 1997 (BBA), have created major changes in the practices of US physicians. HIPPA changed the US government's fraud and abuse regulations by increasing civil monetary damages from $2,000 to $10,000, by applying fraud and abuse laws to the private as well as the public sector, by permitting confiscation of personal property for health-care fraud convictions, and by changing health-care frauds from misdemeanors to federal felonies with mandatory prison sentences.

The overall purpose of the BBA was to erase the federal budget deficit and to enable federal regulators to more aggressively attack health-care fraud and abuse, especially as it relates to the anti-kickback statute. Prior to the BBA, the Office of the Inspector General (OIG) had to pursue anti-kickback cases through the Department of Justice, because these cases were considered criminal matters. The BBA allowed the OIG to pursue anti-kickback violations for civil monetary penalties, thereby lowering the standard of proof and obviating the need to go through the Department of Justice. In addition, the BBA requires The Health Care Finance Administration (HCFA) to account for health-care expenditures and to reimburse health-care providers based on documented physician work. HCFA is now required to reimburse physicians for in-office practice expenses based on actual, rather than "assumed" office expenses. In a brief time, these legislative acts served to change the face of the practice of medicine in the United States and pushed to the forefront the demand for precise coding and documentation by physicians and other health-care providers.

Procedure Coding

In the United States, the most commonly used coding for purposes of reimbursement of physicians is Current Procedural Terminology (CPT), which is currently in its fourth edition with the fifth edition scheduled to replace it by 2003. CPT is a systematic listing and coding of procedures and services performed by physicians. There are two main categories of codes contained within CPT. The first is the evaluation and management codes (E/M codes), which describe services performed in broad subcategories, which are then further divided into two or more types of E/M service. For example, there are two types of office visits—new patient and established patient; and two types of hospital visits—initial and subsequent. The second main category is surgical procedures, which is subclassified according to organ system so that, generally, the five-digit codes associated with a given organ system are in the same numbering sequences. In reference to spinal surgery, the majority of the arthrodesis and instrumentation codes are in the 22000 series of codes, and the decompressive procedures such as laminectomy and discectomy are in the 63000 series.

The US government mandates that HCFA have responsible accounting methods for the payments to the health-care industry and physicians. HCFA has relied on the American Medical Association (AMA) to help it to effect these ends. The AMA charges its CPT Editorial Panel and CPT Advisory Committee yearly, to revise the CPT codes. The AMA charges its Relative Value Update Committee (RUC) and the Relative Value Update Committee Advisors to assign relative work values (RVU) for new CPT codes. In general, procedures are valued by determining, from survey information (RUC survey), the sum of the component time, intensity, and the risk of performing the procedure. Physician work value is added to the practice expense value and to malpractice expense to form the total work value for the specific procedure. This total work value (total RVU) is presented to HCFA for approval. For the most part, HCFA has been supportive of the RUC valuations for procedures, but HCFA has authority to disapprove RUC recommendations.

Anyone, including physicians, insurance companies, and suppliers of durable medical equipment, can submit a request for a new code or a coding change. Requests received by the AMA staff, if deemed appropriate, are referred to the AMA CPT Advisory Committee for comment, then to the CPT Editorial Panel for a final decision. If the new code or change to an existing code is accepted, it is next determined whether or not the coding change requires RUC valuation. Specialty societies may then coordinate their efforts to design and collate a RUC valuation survey, for the specific code in question. The recommended survey RVU value for the specific code may be modified by the RUC before it is sent to HCFA for final approval. If approved, the code, with its respective value will be published in the next year's edition of both CPT and the Federal Register.

Procedures, particularly those performed in hospitals and complications of procedures, can also be coded using one of the systems of the International Classifica-

tion of Diseases, Clinical Modification (ICD-CM). ICD-CM is the system used most frequently for coding of diagnosis, and is discussed in detail in the next section.

Diagnosis Coding

The International Classification of Diseases, Ninth Clinical Modification (ICD-9-CM), owned by the World Health Organization (WHO) derives from the Bertillon Classification of Death, first used in 1893. The fifth revision of this classification added causes of morbidity and the seventh revision adopted the name International Classification of Diseases. The Ninth Clinical Modification is in widespread use as of this writing.

ICD-9-CM contains codes related to diagnosis, procedures, and complications. ICD-9-CM provides over 8,000 diagnostic codes, covering the entire scope of clinical diseases. The diagnostic coding section, which is the portion of ICD-9-CM most commonly used by physicians, consists of codes within two general ranges. The first, codes from 001.0 to 999.9, is divided into 17 classifications of diseases and injuries including infectious and parasitic diseases; neoplasms; diseases defined by body systems; congenital anomalies; symptoms, signs and ill defined conditions; and injuries and poisonings. The second, codes from V01.0 to V82.9, describes reasons for patient visits other than disease or injury. V codes may be used when reporting preventive medical treatments, physical examination, postoperative follow-up examinations, physical therapy, radiographs, and laboratory tests.

There have been some limitations in the use of and problems associated with the application of ICD-9-CM. It has been used to form databases for research and to guide public policy, functions for which it never was designed. ICD-9-CM offers no capacity to designate sidedness (eg, is the disc herniation left or right of midline?) and no way to designate acuity or severity (eg, severe life-threatening versus minimally symptomatic spinal cord compression). In spite of its many deficiencies, ICD-9-CM is in general use because it was available at a crucial time in the organization of health care and its acceptance is sufficiently universal to guarantee its perpetuation.

ICD-9-CM diagnosis coding has become increasingly important because of the described governmental changes to health-care policy. The ICD-9-CM diagnosis has come to signify the reason a service was rendered, a test was ordered, or a procedure was performe—functions for which the coding system was not designed.

The WHO planned to replace ICD-9-CM with ICD-10-CM by 1998; however, although ICD-10-CM has been drafted, application has been delayed. Unlike ICD-9-CM, ICD-10-CM contains only diagnosis and no procedural codes. Some of the diffe: include a vastly increased number of categories ies (2033 as compared to 855 in ICD-9-CM); a d it format, a six-digit alphanumeric system with lpha at the beginning and decimal point in middle (eg, C50.333); and more specificity of som²s, sometimes including severity rating and/or side Costs associated with the retooling of compute₁ staff to this new system have delayed its im²ntation. The potential for a greater degree of s city places an additional burden on documentat which must be examined to ensure that it is comp¹sive enough to assign a code.

Because ICD-10-CM contains ₁ocedural codes, HCFA has contracted with Minne Mining and Manufacturing to develop a system of edural coding to be titled ICD-10-PCS. It bears n mblance to CPT. It is an alphanumeric code syste s in ICD-10-CM. However, the two are distinctly rent and the software used to run ICD-10-CM ₁not interface with ICD-10-PCS, because the latter ; alphanumeric system with seven characters with a mixed within the code, not at the beginning as in)-10-CM, and there is no decimal point to delimit code as in ICD-10-CM. A specific date for the im lentation of this system has not been determined wever, the fact that this system exists worries some/sicians because there is a potential for HCFA to im nent the system without the benefit of physician in vement.

Nomenclature

Coding requires translation diagnostic and procedural terms to a system t¹ can be classified and manipulated more easily th standard language. Coding can, therefore, be no m accurate than the terms being translated. An in national committee of anatomists, the Federative C mittee on Anatomic Terminology, has undertaken ₁ arduous task of keeping current an exhaustive list o natomic terms, which provides standards, at least fo what terms are acceptable and how they are spelled, t does not provide definitions and does not include athology.

It has been well docume ed in the field of spine care that some of the most ba₁ diagnostic terms (eg, herniated disc) are not precise defined and are commonly misunderstood in comm¹ications between physicians, patients, insurers, and th e who may influence public policy on matters import t to spine care. The first edition of this text publishe₁ recommendation from a task force of the North An rican Spine Society (NASS), which provided preferr₁ terminology for disc pathology and definitions of t ms related to disc disorders. A revised and expanded ersion, published in 2001, by a

joint task force of NASS and the American Society of Neuroradiology and the American Society of Spine Radiology, has been endorsed by the AAOS and the Joint Section on Disorders of the Spine and Peripheral Nerves of the American Association of Neurological Surgeons and Congress of Neurological Surgeons, as well as by NASS, ASNR, and ASSR. Their work does not include attention to disorders of the vertebral canals (stenosis), disorders of the posterior elements, or procedures.

Research Applications

For physicians trying to do meaningful clinical research, especially when relying on methods that require retrospective retrieval of information or analysis of previously published findings on a subject, the potential for errors introduced by nonstandardized nomenclature and faulty or incomplete coding systems are obvious. The problems may be compounded further, but become less obvious, when the distance from those applying the data to those who collected the data increases, as when data are pooled to guide social policy or administrative decisions.

Information based on the hospital or outpatient patient experience may be abstracted from patients' medical records to form administrative databases, which have been used in attempts to describe many aspects of the delivery and utilization of health care. A variety of conclusions have been drawn from the research performed using administrative databases. These conclusions can have significant and important implications for patients, providers, and society at large, to the extent that such data inform participants in current health-care policy debates.

Although ICD-9-CM data can be used for creating outpatient databases, the most common use of ICD is for the coding of inpatient hospital admissions. The processing of the inpatient medical record information into ICD-coded language follows a typical sequence. First, hospital medical records personnel abstract clinical information in the hospital medical record and discharge summary. The data identified include diagnoses, procedures, and complication data. This information is then converted into ICD code form. Also abstracted are patient demographic data such as age, sex, length of stay, and discharge status. With this patient demographic data and ICD codes, a discharge abstract is constructed. Pooling of discharge abstracts has been referred to as the formation of administrative databases. Administrative databases contain regional discharge abstracts. At the state level, discharge abstracts are received from every hospital within the state. At the federal level, HCFA receives nationwide discharge abstracts relating to Medicare patients. These data are then available for analysis and research questions.

Several studies have been performed to evaluate the accuracy of the data contained within these databases because their usefulness relates directly to the quality of the data contained within them. The limitations of these databases are many, including: nonstandardized nomenclature for labeling diagnoses and procedures; inherent deficiencies of the ICD system; limitations of the coders assigning the codes; institutional differences in coding practices; incomplete data; and inaccurate data.

Annotated Bibliography

Procedure Coding

American Academy of Orthopaedic Surgeons: *Complete Global Service Data for Orthopaedic Surgery, 2000*. Rosemont, IL, American Academy of Orthopaedic Surgeons, 2000.

This text describes the procedure codes that are bundled in parent codes.

American Academy of Orthopaedic Surgeons: *CPT/ICD-9 Cross-Reference for Orthopaedic Surgery, 2000*. Rosemont, IL, American Academy of Orthopaedic Surgeons, 2000.

This text is an excellent reference for cross-referencing of CPT procedure codes to ICD-9 diagnosis codes.

American Medical Association: *CPT 2000: Current Procedural Terminology*, ed 4. Chicago, IL, American Medical Association, 1999.

This text, published yearly, contains current E/M J procedure codes.

Diagnosis Coding

Practice Management Information Corporation: *ICD-9-CM: International Classification of Diseases, 9th revision, Clinical Modification*, ed 5. Los Angeles, CA, Practice Management Information Corporation (PMIC), 1998.

This text presents a guide to ICD-9 coding.

Faciszewski T, Broste K, Fardon D: Quality of data regarding diagnoses of spinal disorders in administrative databases: A multicenter study. *J Bone Joint Surg Am* 1997;79:1481-1488.

This article describes the advantages and shortcomings of ICD-9 coding.

Jones Megman MS, Aaron WS (eds): *St Anthony's ICD-9-Cde Book*. Reston, VA, St. Anthony Publishing, 1

This te guide to ICD-9 coding.

ICD-10 Masy, ed 2. Salt Lake City, UT, Medicode, 2000.

This text ats an introduction to ICD-10 coding.

Nomenclatu

Fardon DF, Ne PC, et al: Nomenclature and classification of thebined task forces of the North American Spine So American Society of Spine Radiology, and the Acan Society of Neuroradiology. *Spine* 2001;26:E93-E

This culminatf a long effort of a combined task force sponsored by NASNR, and ASSR, with members representing various spare specialties, makes an unprecedented effort to standardhe terminology of lumbar disc pathology. The work has endorsed by the sponsoring societies, and by the boards e American Academy of Orthopaedic Surgeons, and the JSection on Disorders of the Spine and Peripheral Nerves o American Association of Neurological Surgeons and Coss of Neurological Surgeons.

Federative Commiton Anatomical Terminology: *Terminologia Anatomiinternational Anatomical Terminology*. Stuttgart, Geny, Georg Thieme Verlag, 1998.

Research Applicatio

Faciszewski T: Spine ate: Administrative databases in spine research. *Spin*997;22:1269-1275.

A scientific study of tadvantages and pitfalls of ICD-9 complication coding is dissed.

Faciszewski T, Johnson Noren C, Smith MD: Administrative databases' coilication coding in anterior spinal fusion procedureWhat does it mean? *Spine* 1995;20:1783-1788.

A scientific study of the vantages and pitfalls of ICD-9 complication coding is discud.

Classic Bibliography

Fisher ES, Whaley FS, Krusit WM, et al: The accuracy of Medicare's hospital clairs data: Progress has been made, but problems remain.*Am J Public Health* 1992; 82:243-248.

Kassirer JP: The quality of car and the quality of measuring it. *N Engl J Med* 1993;32:1263-1265.

Chapter 16

Outcomes Assessment and Guidelines of Care

Bernard A. Pfeifer, MD

David A. Wong, MD, MSc, FRCSC

Major changes in the delivery of health care have occurred during the past decade. Justification of the care selected for a patient always has been a good practice. Analysis of the outcomes of treatment is the basis of judgment of the quality of the care rendered. Selection of the appropriate instrument to measure this health status change is very important to assure correct assessment. In addition, practice variation is still a problem that needs to be addressed. Several studies have shown that the rate of application of a given therapy to a particular problem varies with the location of the care being provided and among providers within the same location. Studies to determine the correct rate of application of a therapy would be powerful. Practice patterns are best modified by presenting data to practitioners and allowing them to find the optimal solution. A system that allows assessment of outcome followed by a standardized approach to a problem with later reassessment is ideal. A discussion of assessment tools currently available will be followed by a discussion of the use of clinical guidelines in practice today.

Outcomes Assessment

Bias can be introduced to assessment of outcomes in many ways. Case or series reports are retrospective collections of convenient samples of patients on which the author-expert bases his or her interpretation of the result. Meta-analyses provide a much higher quality decision by putting a rank order on published reports to assess their strengths and then using that order to support a conclusion. Prospective, randomized, blinded studies are held as the current standard but are very costly and time consuming, and they may be ethically troublesome.

For nonrandom clinical assessment, large numbers of patients may be required. The only practical method to handle this large amount of data is to use a computer to compile results. Computer use requires conversion of the analog results (how the patient feels, how functional the patient is, and so forth) to digital results (scores) that can be analyzed. The construction of these scoring systems is an attempt to find the correct ruler to measure a result. Some scoring systems have been accepted on the basis of historic perseverance. The science of analysis of these instruments marries the psychologist with the statistician, creating the psychometrician.

Descriptions of the methods to be used in the construction of a patient-based instrument are extensive, and the process is costly. The methods should include item generation, either through consensus, panels of experts, or adaptation of other instruments; item reduction, through clinical use or psychometrics; subscale construction; item weighting; pilot testing; and definitive testing for validity, reliability, and sensitivity.

Testing for validity measures the spread of responses to try to avoid effects that are too high or too low and assure the instrument is appropriate for the intended measurement. Reliability testing involves having the same patient retake the test a short time after the original when no change in status is expected. Sensitivity testing involves measuring the ability of the test to assess change in status. Most testing is done through comparison to known tested scales or to expert (clinician) assessment of change.

Patient-Based Instruments Currently Available

Outcomes instruments available today fall into two broad categories: general status and disease specific.

General Status

General status instruments measure the whole person's functional status. One of the best examples is the SF-36 health status questionnaire. This instrument creates eight scales to measure health concepts: (1) physical function, (2) role limitation because of physical health problems, (3) bodily pain, (4) social functioning, (5) general mental health, (6) role limitation because of emotional problems, (7) vitality, and (8) general health perception. The SF-36 probably is the most used and accepted and may be considered a standard. The use of this instrument can best be illustrated in a study of the profile given before and after surgery for four procedures: hip arthroplasty, knee arthroplasty, lumbar discectomy, and scoliosis correction by spinal fusion. The best score improvement was obtained in patients having total hip replacement followed closely by patients who underwent laminectomy for disc herniation. Patients having total knee arthroplasty fared very well; however, the patients with scoliosis correction had lower scores. Although attempts have been made to shorten the SF-36 instrument to 12 items, it appears that this will limit its accuracy and usefulness.

The Sickness Impact Profile is a 136 item instrument that measures ambulation, self-care, emotional function, and household, work, and other activities. The Nottingham Health Profile is shorter and measures similar items. The Duke Health profile of 17 items measures social, psychological, and physical functions.

Disease Specific

Disease-specific functional status measures for the spine patient include the Oswestry Disability Questionnaire, the North American Spine Society (NASS) Instrument, and the Musculoskeletal Outcomes Data Evaluation and Management System (MODEMS). Fairbank and associates at Oswestry created a disability scale of 10 questions related to such events as lifting, carrying, self-care, sleeping, and social functions, with higher numbers on the scale indicating more disability. The NASS expansion of the Oswestry instrument added questions regarding the amount of and how bothersome is the patient's back pain and created neurologic impairment scales. MODEMS inverted the scales and normalized the scale to 100 so that a higher score indicates a better status. The Roland-Morris Disability Scale of 24 questions measures various daily functions, and the Million Instrument of 15 questions measures similar functions.

The McGill Pain Questionnaire of 26 items measures pain and the patient's response to the pain. For chronic pain, the Von Kordoff chronic pain grade may be applicable. Simple visual analog scales are useful but may introduce error depending on the number of scale points and how they are labeled. Pain diagrams are also useful but quantification or digitalization are not yet standardized and may need visual qualitative interpretation. Questions in the MODEMS and NASS instruments assess the amount of pain and neurologic symptoms in either the neck or back.

The Health Interview Survey of three items assesses time lost from work and days spent in bed or with limited activity. The original NASS instrument also has work and compensation status questions.

The Scoliosis Research Society developed an instrument specifically to assess functional as well as cosmetic issues. In a study of its use in evaluating patients' perceptions of results of anterior versus posterior surgery for correction of similar curves, the instrument seemed to function well but the Chronback alpha factor reached only 0.69. For simplicity, the numbers of responses per question available to the subject were limited. Had the number been increased, the Chronback factor would have been higher, pointing out a trade-off in the creation of these instruments: for convenience, limited choices for the patient are preferable; for accuracy, more measurement points are preferable.

Pediatric patients bring additional complexity to the design or choice of outcomes instruments. Does the instrument use the response of the patient, or the parent, or both? At what age does the patient move on to an adult instrument? Another issue is whose report carries more weight?

Measurement of the patient's satisfaction with the process of receiving care may also be incorporated into outcomes research. The HEDIS measure is commonly used by third-party payers and is relatively simple to administer. It measures such parameters as waiting time, courtesy, and so forth.

Among the best series of studies on practice variation and use of outcomes measures to allow physicians to assess their methods are the studies carried out by the Maine Medical Assessment Foundation. Their studies of the care of the patient with herniated disc have shown that patients treated by surgical decompression for a neurocompressive lesion (disc) fared better than those treated nonsurgically. The foundation used nurse reviewers and patient-based questionnaires and analyzed patient status before and after treatment. The project was carefully done but was labor and dollar intensive to assure completeness.

The National Spinal Network (NSN) is a proprietary collaboration of franchised centers, nationwide, that pools outcomes data to assess outcomes of treatment. Baseline results have been published, and follow-up reports should be forthcoming.

The MODEMS project has been an ambitious undertaking by the American Academy of Orthopedic Surgeons (AAOS) to design and test instruments considered appropriate for outcomes research and assessment. In addition, it was to function as a data repository and collator. The large scope of the project, the competitive products available through both manufacturers' value-added services and proprietary entities such as NSN, the cost to the participant clinician, and concerns regarding privacy and data use are factors that have limited success of the project thus far. At the time of publication, MODEMS instruments and scoring algorithms are either near completion of testing or have been validated. They are available from AAOS, NASS, other organizations, and on-line.

Hard Data Analysis

In addition to patient-based outcomes assessment, measurement of so called hard data has to be analyzed. Interobserver reliability refers to the ability of the same observer to come to the same response when measuring the same item. For example, the interobserver error of measure of a scoliosis curve is 5°. Intraobserver error is that between two different observers in ascertaining the same response. For scoliosis curves, this is 10°. In addition, the type of measuring device needs to be appropriate for the study. As one example, Hilibrand and Dina reviewed the appropriate imaging for diagnosis of spinal fusion.

Finally, coupling patient-based data with hard-data outcomes is intriguing. One recent study showed little correlation between the results of radiographic assessment of curve correction and patient scores on the Scoliosis Outcomes Instrument. Another analysis, which reviewed and analyzed cost and result of lumbar fusion, presented summations showing little difference in the patient-perceived result of surgical outcome between those patients who had instrumented fusions compared to those whose fusions were not instrumented. The cost difference is obvious.

Although realization of the goal that outcomes assessments will lead to the ideal of evidence-based medicine has been frustrated by the complexities of formulating and testing outcomes instruments, the ideal remains and the need for better outcomes assessment is compelling. Meanwhile, physicians must apply judgment in the care of their patients, in application of guidelines for care, and in their interpretations of research results based on imperfect data.

Guidelines and Managed Care

Guidelines generally are used by managed care organizations (MCOs) in two forms, each in its own particular area of patient care. The most efficacious use of guidelines by MCOs, seen only recently and too infrequently, has been the application of clinical treatment guidelines as part of a Continuous Quality Improvement (CQI) program to improve the quality of patient care. These clinical treatment guidelines, usually more evidence-based, provide the treatment protocol by which a cohort of similar patients can be treated. Analysis of the outcomes of patients thus treated is subsequently used to refine the treatment guideline to progress towards best care of patients.

The other use of guidelines, which is longest standing and more familiar, is for preauthorization and review of care issues (for example, length of stay). These guidelines are usually proprietary. They generally lack a vigorous development methodology and often represent the opinion of an individual or a small group of healthcare providers. The motivation for the use of these guidelines is often cost containment, rather than quality patient care.

Over the past several years guidelines have been incorporated firmly in the preapproval and review of care (for example, hospital length of stay) processes of MCOs. Most MCOs have embraced systems developed by private entities such as Millman and Robertson and InterQual. These types of proprietary guidelines often have left patients and their physicians frustrated with the process and baffled by a system of hidden or black-box provisions. It often has been apparent that the citing of some specific key words and phrases in the precertification process and in the medical record increases the likelihood of an approval. For example, the words sciatica rather than radicular pain, and numbness rather than decreased sensation, or partial paralysis rather than paraparesis have been more likely to gain approval. This introduces semantic arbitrariness into situations that call for evidence-based medical judgments.

The National Committee on Quality Assurance (NCQA) is an agency that accredits MCOs in much the same way that the Joint Commission for the Accreditation of Health Care Organizations (JCAHO) accredits hospitals. The NCQA recognizes that there has been misuse of guidelines resulting in higher hassle factor for physicians and the denial of appropriate testing, imaging, and treatment. Accordingly, NCQA regulations now include a provision that a member MCO must provide the physician with the reason(s) for a denial of care. The physician must, however, make a formal request for this information. The particular causes of a denial can thus be addressed specifically, rather than the physician and the patient finding themselves in preapproval purgatory or black-box limbo without any knowledge of the reasons for a denial.

Commonly used length-of-stay guidelines are those published by Millman and Robertson. These are optimal recovery guidelines. They presuppose no comorbidity and no complications, a relatively uncommon situation in a spine care patient. In addition, to fit the criteria, every medical evaluation, every investigation, every treatment, and every response to treatment must proceed with maximal time efficiency. Any reasonable or unavoidable delay would, therefore, nullify the guidelines. Furthermore, application of the guidelines assumes a perfectly supportive home environment and availability of home health services or skilled nursing/rehabilitation facilities. In discussions with the American Medical Association (AMA) Council on Scientific Affairs in 1996, and a Task Force of the Practice Guidelines Partnership in 1999, Millman and Robertson officials admitted that they expected their guidelines to apply in only about 10% of patients.

Denial of Care and the Practice of Medicine

In the United States, a number of states have addressed the issue of whether a denial of care constitutes the practice of medicine. The decision has sometimes been made by the state Board of Medical Examiners or in some cases has been specified in a state statute. The review physician or medical director of an MCO could be held to the same standard of care and have the same legal liabilities as the treating physician. Regardless, many treating physicians have found it helpful to point out to a review physician who is denying necessary care that his or her action could constitute the practice of medicine, that the denial will be documented in the patient's chart, and that he or she could be held liable for problems arising from the denial of care.

Guidelines in Managed Workers' Compensation

A number of state and private workers' compensation agencies have adopted treatment guidelines into their managed occupational medicine systems. Physicians have voiced concerns about incorporation of guidelines into workers' compensation because guidelines have been perceived as being aimed at controlling cost without consideration of quality of care. Research has allayed these fears to some extent. Guidelines for the treatment of occupational low back pain were developed in Colorado by a multispecialty task force of physicians and introduced into practice in January 1994. The Colorado State Division of Workers' Compensation subsequently studied treatment costs for a population of patients treated after implementation of the guidelines versus a comparable historic control group treated before the guidelines were introduced. A statistically significant lower cost per patient was found after guidelines implementation without a discernable change in quality of care. However, not all studies of guidelines in managed workers' compensation suggest cost savings. Actual radiograph usage for nearly a thousand patients with a history of low back pain of less than 3 months duration was reviewed. This rate was compared to the number generated by a review of the patient's chart and calculating the rate of radiograph usage based on the recommendations for imaging suggested by the Agency for Health Care Policy and Research (AHCPR) guideline for acute low back pain. If the AHCPR guideline had been followed, radiograph usage would have been

238% higher than actual use.

A major concern in workers' compensation guidelines revolves around the mode of incorporation of the guideline into the system. The alternative approaches are (1) incorporate the guideline itself in a state statute or law, or (2) specify in a statute or law that the operant guideline be the version adopted in the regulations written to govern the implementation of the statute or law. The latter is preferable because treatment guidelines are living documents that can change frequently based on new knowledge or technology. It is much more efficient to modify a regulation than to change a guideline incorporated directly into a statute or law, because even a minor modification of a guideline incorporated in statute requires a complete reengagement of the entire legislative process.

The Future: Continuous Quality Improvement

More than a decade ago, the AAOS assimilated CQI into its strategic plan and began to develop components of a program (Fig. 1). For spine, a Guidelines Committee, a cooperative effort of AAOS and NASS, researched and published treatment algorithms (incorporating evidenced-based medicine where possible) to serve as a common treatment protocol for lumbar pain, herniated disc, and spondylolisthesis. Outcomes instruments, as previously discussed, enable evaluation of the effects of treatment. Clinical evidence, thereby, serves as the agent of change for treatment guidelines. Repeated cycles of this system constitute a CQI program that will lead to better and better quality care for patients (Fig. 1).

The AAOS has funded a pilot study, presently underway in Houston, to help determine whether the AAOS/NASS spine treatment algorithms can be effectively integrated into a managed-care setting. This study will generate data on patient outcomes, as well as usage data for services such as radiographs and MRI. If the

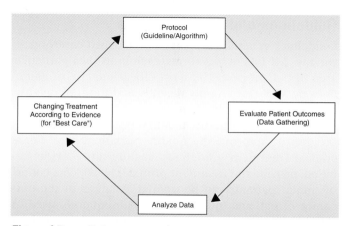

Figure 1 The quality improvement cycle.

algorithms are successfully integrated into managed care in this limited use study, then wider dissemination of the guidelines and the CQI system in managed care probably will follow. The ultimate goal is the best care for patients.

Annotated Bibliography

Outcomes Instruments

Daltroy LH, Cats-Baril WL, Katz JN, Fossel AH, Liang MH: The North American Spine Society lumbar spine outcome assessment Instrument: Reliability and validity tests. *Spine* 1996;21:741-749.

This article describes the formulation and early testing of the NASS low back instrument.

D'Andrea LP, Betz RR, Lenke LG, et al: Do radiographic parameters correlate with clinical outcomes in adolescent idiopathic scoliosis? *Spine* 2000;25:1795-1802.

This is a very nice comparison of patient-perceived clinical outcome with radiologic parameters.

Engelberg R, Martin DP, Agel J, Obremsky W, Coronado G, Swiontkowski MF: Musculoskeletal function assessment instrument: Criteria and construct validity. *J Orthop Res* 1996;14:182-192.

The MFA was developed as a musculoskeletal instrument for both regional and global functional assessment. It was done under a National Institutes of Health (NIH) grant and is a very useful instrument for general (nonspine) orthopaedic problems. This is one of several papers reviewing its construction and use.

Fanuele JC, Birkmeyer NJ, Abdu WA, Tosteson TD, Weinstein JN: The impact of spinal problems on the health status of patients: Have we underestimated the effect? *Spine* 2000;25:1509-1514.

This article describes the use of SF-36 and comorbidities in 17,700 patients to form a Physical Component Summary (PCS) scale that quantifies how patients perceive the impact of their condition on the physical aspects of their daily living. Scores for patients with spinal problems were lower than those for patients with other orthopaedic problems.

Gatchel RJ (ed): *Compendium of Assessment and Research Outcome Instruments for Spinal Disorders.* Rosemont, IL, North American Spine Society, 2000.

This is a comprehensive review of the outcomes instruments currently available with practical application advice. The comments by leaders in the field make this a worthwhile resource. The committee's goal was to be all inclusive.

Haher TR, Gorup JM, Shin TM, et al: Results of the Scoliosis Research Society instrument for evaluation of surgical outcome in adolescent idiopathic scoliosis: A multi-center study of 244 patients. *Spine* 1999;24: 1435-1440.

This article compares the patient perception of anterior versus posterior scoliosis surgery for similar curves. At the same time, it supports the validity of the SRS Outcomes Instrument.

Hozack WJ, Rothman RH, Albert TJ, Balderston RA, Eng K. Relationship of total hip arthroplasty outcomes to other orthopaedic procedures. *Clin Orthop* 1997;344: 88-93.

This is one of several articles presenting this study of the comparison of patient perceptions of outcomes of several procedures. The results are intuitive.

Katz JN: Outcomes instrument development: Basic concepts, in Amadio PC, Wright JG: *Outcomes and Effectiveness in Musculoskeletal Research and Practice.* Course Syllabus, Rosemont, IL, American Academy of Orthopaedic Surgeons, 1996.

This is a review of the methodology for creation of appropriate patient-based outcomes instruments.

Katz JN, Lipson SJ, Lew RA, et al: Lumbar laminectomy alone or with instrumented or non-instrumented arthrodesis in degenerative lumbar spinal stenosis: Patient selection, costs, and surgical outcomes. *Spine* 1997;22:1123-1131

Variation in rates of lumbar fusion by individual surgeons in the same hospital is addressed.

Keller RB, Wennberg DE, Soule DN: Changing physician behavior: The Maine Medical Assessment Foundation. *Qual Manag Health Care* 1997;5:1-11.

The authors describe how rate analysis data simply presented to physicians afforded change in behavior.

Kuntz KM, Snider RK, Weinstein JN, Pope MH, Katz JN: Cost-effectiveness of fusion with and without instrumentation for patients with degenerative spondylolisthesis and spinal stenosis. *Spine* 2000;25:1132-1139.

A meta-analysis of sorts, this article introduces the concept of quality adjusted life years and evaluates it for instrumented and noninstrumented fusions.

Guidelines and Managed Care

American Academy of Orthopaedic Surgeons/North American Spine Society: Draft clinical algorithm on low back pain, in Garfin S, Vaquero A (eds): *Orthopedic Knowledge Update: Spine*. Rosemont, IL, American Academy of Orthopedic Surgeons, 1997, pp A26-A46.

These treatment algorithms were developed by AAOS and NASS.

Blumenthal D: Part 1: Quality of care. What is it? *N Engl J Med* 1996;335:891-894.

This is a good perspective on what quality care means in clinical medicine.

Brook RH, McGlynn EA, Cleary PD: Quality of health care: Part 2. Measuring quality of care. *New Engl J Med* 1996;335:966-970.

The authors discuss how meaningful measures of quality of care might be developed and implemented.

Hyams AL: Practice guidelines and malpractice litigation: A two-way street. *Ann Intern Med* 1995;122:450-455.

The author discusses the legal implications of guidelines and how they can be used by both the defendant and the plaintiff.

Sackett DL: Editorial: Evidence-based medicine. *Spine* 1998;23:1085-1086.

The author outlines the principles of evidence-based medicine and gives a realistic perspective on use of evidence-based medicine in clinical practice.

Shaneyfelt TM, Mayo-Smith MF, Rothwangl J: Are guidelines following guidelines? The methodological quality of clinical practice guidelines in the peer-reviewed medical literature. *JAMA* 1999:281:1900-1905.

The authors further outline the principles of treatment guideline development and review whether the principles are being followed in published guidelines.

Suarez-Almazor ME, Belseck E, Russell AS, Mackel JV: Use of lumbar radiographs for the early diagnosis of low back pain. *JAMA* 1997;277:1782-1786.

In this study of actual radiograph usage compared to that expected when predictions were based on indications from the AHCPR guideline, actual usage was less than the predicted rate.

Wong DA: Developing treatment guidelines, in Mayer T, Gatchel R, Polatin P (eds): *Occupational Musculoskeletal Disorders: Functions, Outcomes, and Evidence*. Philadelphia, PA, Lippincott-Williams & Wilkins, 2000, pp 721-727.

This is a review of the principles of treatment guideline development.

Classic Bibliography

Davis H: Increasing rates of cervical and lumbar spine surgery in the United States, 1979-1990. *Spine* 1994; 19:1117-1124.

Deyo RA, Andersson G, Bombardier C, et al: Outcome measures for studying patients with low back pain. *Spine* 1994;19(suppl 18):2032s-2036s.

Eddy DM: Clinical decision making: From theory to practice. Anatomy of a decision. *JAMA* 1990;263:441-443.

Eddy DM: Clinical decision making: From theory to practice. Designing a practice policy: Standards, guidelines, and options. *JAMA* 1990;263:3077-3084.

Eddy DM: Clinical decision making: From theory to practice. Practice policies: Guidelines for methods. *JAMA* 1990;263:1839-1841.

Fairbank JC, Couper J, Davies JB, O'Brien JP: The Oswestry low back pain disability questionnaire. *Physiotherapy* 1980;66:271-273.

Guyatt GH, Sackett DL, Cook DJ: Users' guides to the medical literature: II. How to use an article about therapy or prevention: B. What were the results and will they help me in caring for my patients? Evidence-based medicine working group. *JAMA* 1994;271:59-63.

Haselkorn JK, Turner JA, Diehr PK, Ciol MA, Deyo RA: Meta-analysis: A useful tool for the spine researcher. *Spine* 1994;19(suppl 18):2076S-2082S.

Hilibrand IS, Dina TS: The use of diagnostic imaging to assess spinal arthrodesis. *Orthop Clin North Am* 1998; 29:591-601.

Keller RB: The methods of outcomes research. *Curr Opin Orthop* 1994;5:86-89.

Melzack R: The McGill Pain Questionnaire: Major properties and scoring methods. *Pain* 1975;1:277-299.

Roos NP, Wennberg JE, McPherson K: Using diagnosis-related groups for studying variations in hospital admissions. *Health Care Financ Rev* 1988;9:53-62.

Ware JE, Jr, Sherbourne CD: The MOS 36-item short-form health survey (SF-36): I. Conceptual framework and item selection. *Med Care* 1992;30:473-483.

Wennberg, JE. Factors governing utilization of hospital services. *Hosp Pract* 1979;14:115-121, 126-127.

Wilson MC, et al: What are the recommendations and will they help you in caring for your patients? *JAMA* 1995;274:1630-1632.

Chapter 17

Evaluating Permanent Impairment of the Spine

R. H. Haralson III, MD, MBA

Introduction

Evaluation of impairment after an injury is sometimes just as important to the patient as the treatment, especially if the patient is unable to return to his or her regular job. Therefore, the treating physician must supply a rating of permanent impairment. However, many physicians are not comfortable rating impairment because it is a complicated process. Thus, it is perfectly reasonable for the treating physician to ask a physician trained in the field to provide the impairment rating. Many jurisdictions require that an impairment rating be provided by a trained and certified evaluator. Several specialty societies provide courses on impairment evaluation, and the American Academy of Disability Evaluating Physicians (AADEP) has an excellent series of training programs. The American Board of Independent Medical Examiners provides certification for impairment rating, and AADEP is presently developing a written and oral examination, the passage of which will eventually be required for fellowship.

Impairment Versus Disability

Impairment is defined as the loss of part of bodily function, whereas disability includes impairment as well as education, motivation, socioeconomic factors, ability to perform activities of daily living, ability to be gainfully employed, and several other difficult-to-measure parameters. Physicians usually rate impairment. Disability usually is rated by vocational counselors who take into account impairment as well as ability to perform certain jobs and the availability of those jobs. Ratings usually are not provided until the patient has reached Maximum Medical Improvement (MMI), meaning that the patient's condition will not change substantially within 1 year. Occasionally, it will be necessary to provide a rating when the patient is not at MMI; for instance, when a patient is still under treatment but has reached a legal temporal deadline. In such cases, the rater should rate the patient as he or she is at the time of the rating but state in the report that change may occur.

In the United States the standard text for evaluating impairment is *Guides to the Evaluation of Permanent Impairment* (AMA Guides) published by the American Medical Association (AMA). Some 40 states either require or suggest use of the AMA Guides and most other states allow its use. Several states, including California, New York, Florida, and Minnesota, have their own systems. Some states specify which edition of the AMA Guides to use, while others require the "most current" edition. Some states mandate parts of the AMA Guides but do not allow the use of other parts. Other texts, such as the American Academy of Orthopaedic Surgeons' *Impairment Rating Guide* are accepted in some jurisdictions. New Jersey does not require that the physician use any text or guide and that the rating be based solely on the rating physician's opinion of impairment. The rating physician must be familiar with the requirements and alternatives in his or her jurisdiction.

The AMA Guides

Because the AMA Guides is the most commonly used text for evaluating impairment, the methods used therein will be discussed in more detail here. The second and third editions and the third edition, revised, of the AMA Guides use only the range of motion (ROM) method for spinal evaluation. The third edition, revised, required use of an inclinometer to measure spinal motion. The diagnosis related estimates (DRE) method was introduced in the fourth edition, published in 1993, and is continued, with some modification, into the fifth edition. The fourth edition intended that the DRE method be used in all cases of spinal injury, but the language describing the requirement is not clear enough and some physicians continued to rely on the ROM method. The fifth edition strengthens the language requiring the use of DRE in all cases involving spinal injury, except for fractures or radiculopathy at multiple levels or recurrent radiculopathy. ROM is used also for evaluation of conditions due to certain diseases and in some cases in which a patient is being evaluated for administrative reasons, such as retirement, when impairment may not be due to one injury but rather the result of many injuries and the effects of aging.

Although controversy remains, many physicians believe that ROM is not a valid method to evaluate spine impairment. Studies have demonstrated a lack of interrater reliability when measuring motion in the spine. Some physicians believe that patients can adversely influence the measurements even though there are maneuvers that check for consistent effort. The goal is to measure the loss of motion in one or more involved motion segments; however, the ROM method measures an entire spinal area. Thus, it theoretically penalizes a patient who has vigorously rehabilitated and regained motion at segments above and below the level of the injury, while rewarding the patient who has allowed his or her spine to remain stiff. The ROM method does not take into account loss of motion for reasons other than injury, such as aging and body habitus. One study demonstrated up to 34% impairment in a series of patients who denied having back pain in the 5 years previous to the study.

Some physicians are still proponents of the ROM method, however. Mayer and associates reported that age, in and of itself, does not necessarily result in stiffness of the spine significant enough to affect impairment rating. The ROM method is easy to use, but does require a thorough review of previous medical records and a complete physical examination, including ROM measurements. Although, intuitively, there does not seem to be a correlation between loss of motion and impairment, some believe further study may prove that loss of motion is a reasonable surrogate for impairment. The fourth edition of the AMA Guides provided no method to adequately assess fractures or radiculopathy at multiple levels or to assess recurrent radiculopathy; therefore, the fifth edition defaults to the ROM method for evaluating patients with those conditions. When the ROM method is to be used it is essential that it be used properly and in its entirety, meaning that the diagnosis component and any neurologic component must be added to the ROM component. Each edition of the AMA Guides provides tables from which the proper values to be combined may be obtained. A physician cannot merely measure the ROM and use that as the sole basis of an impairment rating.

The DRE Method

The DRE method is the preferred way to rate spinal impairment and is required in all cases in which there

has been an injury, except where the patient has fractures or radiculopathy at multiple levels in the same spinal area, or has recurrent radiculopathy. The method is based on placing the patient in one of several categories (eight categories in the fourth edition and five in the fifth edition). Placement in a particular category is determined by the presence of specific objective findings such as muscle spasm, guarding, anatomic numbness or weakness, loss of reflex, loss of structural integrity, loss of bowel or bladder function, or long tract signs. Very specific electromyographic changes that are described in the AMA Guides can also be used to categorize a patient. In addition, the patient may be categorized based on the presence of certain fractures, such as compression fractures or posterior element fractures, that may or may not disrupt the spinal canal.

A major change between the fourth and fifth editions is that in the former, the rating is based on the results of the injury regardless of the treatment, where in the latter, the effects of treatment are considered. Using the fourth edition, the objective findings at any time during the patient's course can be used to categorize a patient, and the resolution or worsening of symptoms with treatment is not considered. Using the fifth edition, the patient is categorized by findings at the time of the evaluation after treatment, and previous findings have less bearing on the rating. The authors of both editions believed that a patient with true radiculopathy would always have some permanent impairment despite resolution of symptoms. Using the fourth edition, a patient with a radiculopathy from a compensable injury was placed in category III and given a 10% to 15% impairment rating even if symptoms abated. Using the fifth edition, the result of the treatment is considered and the patient is rated according to the objective findings that are present at the time of the evaluation, but in no case would a patient who had a definite radiculopathy, confirmed by an imaging study that showed a herniated disc at the proper anatomic site, be rated at zero.

Another change in the fifth edition is that the impairment rating for each category now includes an adjustment of up to 3%. The rating physician may increase a rating up to 3% if there are objective findings that suggest additional impairment. The adjustment should not be increased merely because of a complaint of persistent pain, but should be supported by objective findings.

Loss of Structural Integrity

Loss of structural integrity, which places a patient in category IV of the fifth edition DRE method, has been redefined. As in the fourth edition, there are two methods of determining loss of structural integrity; both use flexion and extension spinal radiographs. The first measures the translation of one vertebra on another. The fourth edition defined loss of structural integrity as greater than 3.5 mm in the cervical spine and 5 mm in the thoracic and lumbar spine; in the fifth edition, the measurements are 3.5 mm in the cervical spine, 2.5 mm in the thoracic spine, and 4.5 mm in the lumbar spine. The second method measures differences in flexion and extension angles of adjacent motion segments. The fourth edition required 11° more angular motion in the sagittal plane at the affected level than at an adjacent level, except that at the lumbosacral level there must be 15° more angular motion than at L4-5. In the fifth edition, loss of motion segment integrity is defined as angular motion greater than 15° at L1-2, L2-3, and L3-4, greater than 20° at L4-5, and greater than 25° at L5-S1. In the cervical spine, it is defined as angular motion that is 11° more than at an adjacent motion segment. The angular method cannot be used in the thoracic spine.

Another significant change in the fifth edition is that the loss of structural integrity includes loss of motion caused by developmental or surgical fusion. If there has been complete or near-complete loss of motion as a result of fracture healing, infection, or a successful or unsuccessful attempt at arthrodesis, the patient is categorized as having loss of structural integrity.

Evaluation of Corticospinal Tract Impairment

In the fourth edition, impairment due to spinal cord injury is determined according to specifications of categories VI, VII, or VIII. Category VI represents cauda equina or cauda equina "like" syndrome without bowel or bladder involvement; category VII is the same with bowel or bladder involvement; and category VIII is total or near-total loss of upper and/or lower extremity function. In addition, the impairment from any of these categories is combined with impairment from categories II through V, as appropriate. Categories VI, VII, and VIII describe the impairment from the injury to the spinal cord or cauda equina, and categories II through V describe the impairment due to local injury such as strain or sprain, radiculopathy, loss of motion segment integrity, or fracture. The final rating is obtained by combining the rating from the local injury with that of the spinal cord injury.

In the fifth edition, injury to the spinal cord is rated using the chapter on neurologic injuries, Chapter 13. The rating physician is referred to Tables 13-15 through 13-21. Table 13-15 represents impairment resulting from gait and station disorders (ie, whether or not a patient can ambulate with or without aids or can stand with or without help). Table 13-16 describes the criteria for rating loss of function of one upper extremity and Table 13-17 describes impairment due to loss of use of both

upper extremities. There is a differentiation based on hand dominance.

Table 13-18 describes impairment from dysfunction of the respiratory system. Tables 13-19 and 13-20 describe impairments resulting from dysfunction of the bladder and rectum, respectively. Table 13-21 describes impairment caused by loss of sexual function. To calculate impairment resulting from corticospinal tract injury, the rating physician should combine values from all of the above appropriate tables with any impairment rating from categories II through V. Tables 13-15 through 13-21 are reproduced as one table, Table 15-6, in the chapter on spinal injuries.

DRE Categories

The following is a description of the DRE categories of the lumbar spine area as described in the fourth and fifth editions. Because the lumbar spine is by far the most common area used when evaluating the spine, it will be described in detail and the differences in the fourth and fifth editions explained.

DRE Lumbar Category I: Complaints or Symptoms

0% Impairment
Category I is for those patients who have sustained a minor back strain that results in no objective findings and no significant structural change. Using the fourth edition, an objective finding at any time during the patient's course places the patient in at least category II, because that edition considers the results of the injury and not the treatment. Using the fifth edition, because the treatment is being considered, findings must be present at the time of the impairment examination of the patient. There are no fractures in this category.

DRE Lumbar Category II: Minor Impairment

5% to 8% Impairment
Using the fourth edition, patients with objective findings at any time during their course were awarded 5% whole-person impairment. Using the fifth edition, because results of treatment are considered, the objective findings must be present at the time of the impairment examination. Most patients in this category should be rated at 5%; however, for patients with unusually severe pain and substantiating objective findings, the physician may award up to an additional 3%. The increase in the award should not be given just because the patient reports pain.

In the fifth edition, this category also includes patients who have had definite radiculopathy, concordant with an imaging study, that has resolved with nonsurgical management. The fourth edition did not require imaging studies to make a diagnosis of radiculopathy. The fifth edition requires an imaging study (MRI, CT/myelogram, or myelogram) that shows a herniated disc at the level and on the same side as would explain the clinical signs. Both editions also include in category II patients who have compression fractures of less than 25% or posterior element fractures that do not disrupt the spinal canal. Patients who have compression fractures at multiple levels in the same spinal area should be rated using the ROM method.

DRE Lumbar Category III: Radiculopathy

10% to 13% Impairment

Using the fourth edition, all patients with significant radiculopathy from disc herniation are in category III with an impairment of 10%, no matter the results of treatment. In the fifth edition, this category includes all patients who have persistent radiculopathy after nonsurgical treatment or radiculopathy that required surgical treatment. Patients with resolution of most symptoms after surgery should be rated lower in the range of 10% to 13%, whereas those with persistent symptoms verified by signs of persistent radiculopathy should be in the upper limits of the range. This category also includes patients with compression fractures that are greater than 25% but less than 50% or with displaced laminar fractures that disrupt the spinal canal.

Using the fourth edition, categories I through III include most patients evaluated for back injuries. However, because the fifth edition considers the result of treatment, patients who have arthrodesis as part of their treatment or who otherwise develop loss of structural integrity because of their injury or treatment may be considered for a higher category.

DRE Lumbar Category IV: Alteration of Motion Segment Integrity

20% to 23% Impairment

Category IV in the lumbar spine is for patients with loss of motion segment integrity, which was defined previously. Loss of motion segment compromise does not include disc space narrowing. In the cervical and thoracic spine, category IV also includes patients with multilevel or bilateral neurologic involvement of nerve roots without evidence of spinal cord injury.

DRE Lumbar Category V: Radiculopathy and Alteration of Motion Segment Integrity

25% to 28% Impairment

This category includes patients with both significant radiculopathy and loss of motion segment integrity. Using the fourth edition, the patient would have to have a translational instability or severe angular deformity as well as significant radiculopathy. Using the fifth edition, this category would include patients who have had an arthrodesis or attempt at an arthrodesis and who also have persistent significant radiculopathy verified by objective findings.

ROM Method

The following is a description of the ROM method in the lumbar area as it appears in the fifth edition. Descriptions of the cervical and thoracic areas are found in the AMA Guides.

The patient must be disrobed except for undergarments. A gown that opens in the back is satisfactory. Chaperones are recommended for opposite sex patients. The use of an inclinometer is required. The single inclinometer method is described in the AMA Guides, however the double inclinometer method, described here, is preferred.

Marks are placed over T12 and S1. With the patient standing in the erect or zero position, after a warm-up period, the inclinometers are centered on the marks and set at zero. The patient is asked to bend forward as far as possible (flexion). It is permissible for the patient to rest hands on knees for comfort. The readings from both inclinometers are recorded. The patient is asked to return to the erect or zero position and to bend backward as far as possible (extension). Again the readings from both inclinometers are recorded. The patient repeats each of these motions three times. The readings from the S1 inclinometer are subtracted from the readings from the T12 inclinometer, resulting in a measurement of true lumbar flexion and extension. With the patient erect again, the inclinometers are placed in the coronal position and zeroed. The patient is asked to bend maximally to the right and then to the left. Again the patient is asked to repeat the maneuver three times and the readings from both inclinometers are recorded. The readings from the lower inclinometer are subtracted from the readings from the upper inclinometer, resulting in measurement of true right and left lateral bending.

All measurements are recorded on a copy of the summary sheet provided in the AMA Guides. The physician then determines the impairment due to loss of ROM by referring to Tables 15-8 and 15-9 and comparing values for true lumbar flexion, extension, and right and left lateral bending. The largest of the three valid (see validity checks below) measurements of true motion is used. In Table 15-8, the impairments for loss of flexion are higher if the patient has loss of sacral flexion. This is because sacral flexion actually represents hip flexion, and a patient with loss of lumbar flexion has a greater impairment if there is a concomitant loss of hip motion.

Validity Checks

One validity check is the consistency measurement. Each of the three measurements of true motion (the result of subtraction of the lower inclinometer from the upper inclinometer) should be within 5° or 10% of the mean of the three measurements. If it is not, the physician should repeat the measurements up to three more times to obtain three consecutive measurements that meet those criteria. If three consecutive measurements that meet the validity criteria cannot be obtained with a total of six measurements, then that part of the ROM evaluation is considered invalid or the patient is asked to return at a later date for reevaluation.

A second validity check, only for the lumbar region, is the comparison of straight leg raising to total sacral motion. The total sacral motion is obtained by adding sacral flexion and sacral extension. Straight leg raising is determined by applying the zeroed inclinometer to the crest of the tibia with the patient in the supine position, then performing straight leg raising to measure and record the angle of maximum comfortable hip flexion. Again, three measurements are obtained and all three should be within 5° or 10% of the median. The total sacral motion is then compared with the tightest straight leg raising. If the tightest straight leg raising is not within 15° of the total sacral motion, the flexion portion of the ROM is considered invalid. The physician has the option of having the patient return at a later date for reexamination. The point of this validity test is that both straight leg raising and sacral, or hip, motion are functions of hamstring tightness and sciatic tension. The inference is that patients who allow straight leg raising more than 15° greater than they will flex their hips by bending are not giving full effort in flexing their spines.

Annotated Bibliography

Cocciarella L, Anderson CBJ (eds): *Guides to the Evaluation of Permanent Impairment*, ed 5. Chicago, IL, American Medical Association, 2000.
    Published in 2000, this replaces the 4th edition, which had become the standard for impairment evaluation.

Andersson GBJ: Diagnostic considerations in patients with back pain. *Phys Med Rehabil Clin N Am* 1998;9: 309-322.
    This describes the full workup of patients with various low back pain patterns including history, physical examination, laboratory tests, and imaging studies.

Andersson GBJ, Frymoyer JW: Joint systems: Lumbar and thoracic spine, in Demeter SL, Andersson GB, Smith GM (eds): *Disability Evaluation*. St Louis, MO, Mosby-Year Book, 1996, pp 277-299.
    This chapter provides a detailed description of physical examination and evaluation of patients with spine problems and describes two classification methods, one based on symptoms and the other on pathoanatomic findings.

Andersson GBJ, Deyo RA: Sensitivity, specificity, and predictive value: A general issue in screening for disease in interpretation of diagnostic studies in spinal disorders, in Frymoyer JW (ed): *The Adult Spine: Principles and Practice*, ed 2. Philadelphia, PA, Lippincott Raven, 1997, pp 305-317.
    This chapter reviews the sensitivity, specificity and predictive value of tests used for screening populations for diseases of the spine and for interpreting test results in a patient who is suspected of having a disease of the spine.

Mayer TG, Kondraske G, Beals SB, Gatchel RJ: Spinal range of motion: Accuracy and sources of error with inclinometric measurement. *Spine* 1997;22:1976-1984.
    This study shows that inaccuracies in measurement of spinal ROM using an inclinometer are due more to lack of training of the physician than to device inaccuracies.

Lea RD, Gerhardt JJ: Range-of-motion measurements. *J Bone Joint Surg Am* 1995;77:784-798.
    The authors present a standardized method to measure and record measurements of ROM of joints including the spine.

Mayer TG, Gatchel RJ, Polatin PB (eds): *Occupational Musculoskeletal Disorders: Function, Outcomes, and Evidence*. Philadelphia, PA, Lippincott-Williams & Wilkins, 2000.
    Chapter 39 provides detailed instructions on how to perform a spine impairment evaluation, using both the DRE and the ROM methods from the AMA Guides.

Classic Bibliography

Alaranta H, Hurri H, Heliovaara M, Soukka A, Harju R: Flexibility of the spine: Normative values of goniometric and tape measurements. *Scand J Rehabil Med* 1994;26:147-154.

Battie MC, Bigos SJ, Fisher LD, et al: The role of spinal flexibility in back pain complaints within industry: A prospective study. *Spine* 1990;15:768-773.

Fitzgerald GK, Wynveen KJ, Rheault W, Rothschild B: Objective assessment with establishment of normal values for lumbar spinal range of motion. *Phys Ther* 1983;63:1776-1781.

Guides to the Evaluation of Permanent Impairment, ed 4. Chicago, IL, American Medical Association, 1993.

Helliwell P, Moll J, Wright V: Measurement of spinal movement and function, in Jayson MIV (ed): *The Lumbar Spine and Back Pain*, ed 4. Edinburgh, Scotland, Churchill Livingstone, 1992, pp 173-205.

Keeley J, Mayer TG, Cox R, Gatchel RJ, Smith J, Mooney V: Quantification of lumbar function: Part 5. Reliability of range-of-motion measures in the sagittal plane and an in vivo torso rotation measurement techniques. *Spine* 1986;11:31-35.

Loebl WY: Measurement of spinal posture and range of spinal movement. *Ann Phys Med* 1967;9:103-110.

Mellin G: Measurement of thoracolumbar posture and mobility with a Myrin inclinometer. *Spine* 1986;11:759-762.

Reynolds PM: Measurement of spinal mobility: A comparison of three methods. *Rheumatol Rehabil* 1975;14:180-185.

Shaffer WO, Spratt KF, Weinstein J, Lehmann TR, Goel V: The consistency and accuracy of roentgenograms for measuring sagittal translation in the lumbar vertebral motion segment: An experimental model. *Spine* 1990;15:741-750.

Waddell G, Somerville D, Henderson I, Newton M: Objective clinical evaluation of physical impairment in chronic low back pain. *Spine* 1992;17:617-628.

Section 2

Nonsurgical Care

Section Editor:
Tom G. Mayer, MD

Chapter 18

Acute Care: Nontraumatic Low Back Pain

Hamilton Hall, MD, FRCSC

Introduction

Most discussions of early intervention for mechanical low back pain stress its complexity and the need for a rapid, precise diagnosis yet offer as treatment a broad mixture of platitudes and nonspecific therapeutic approaches. The management of acute nontraumatic spinal pain fits poorly within a medical paradigm. In many ways the most effective approach is a primarily nonmedical one. The profession's inability to abandon the medical model and instead focus on the issues that are of paramount importance to the patient may partly explain its failure to manage this problem adequately.

The failing is not limited to the lumbar spine. Although this update primarily provides an approach to acute care of the low back, similar problems exist with the medical model for treating nontraumatic pain in the cervical and dorsal spine. The shifts in attitude and practice recommended for the lumbar region have comparable strategies for more cephalad areas. Each site has its own peculiarities, and each requires special assessment and distinct treatment modifications but the basic message is the same. Medicine and its paramedical associates have done a poor job of alleviating spinal pain. Highlights of the pertinent variations follow the main discussion to emphasize, not clutter, the central theme.

The treatment of acute low back pain is neither casual nor unstructured. On the contrary, its intentions are clear and its goals sharply circumscribed. Given that an accurate pathologic diagnosis is rarely possible, treatment is remarkably concise.

Patients come to the practitioner for two overriding reasons. First, they want the pain to stop. Second, they want reassurance that their problem is benign and can be identified. Medicine's response to the first demand is to order a series of fruitless investigations that can, in some cases, prolong or intensify the pain. Its response to the second concern is to provide a differential diagnosis ranging from obscure possibilities to the specter of spinal malignancy. This conventional medical approach neither eliminates the acute pain nor reassures the anxious patient.

In this early, brief, and finite stage at the time of seeking care, the medical model does not apply. Although it sounds like medical heresy, at this initial juncture a conventional diagnosis is not only impossible, it is unnecessary and should be replaced by a rapid, symptom-directed intervention. This replacement is not the assessment of a probable surgical candidate. It is not the treatment of a chronic deteriorating spinal condition. It also is not an approach that every surgeon can accept; it is too foreign to a surgeon's professional training. Low back pain is so ubiquitous it might better be considered a human condition rather than a medical challenge. The increasing popularity of alternative medicine is ample testimony to the inadequacy of the current rigid pathology-based approach.

An effective response fulfills the patient's principal needs: pain control and reassurance. Although the ultimate goal must be the return of function, the short-term objective is simply elimination of the pain that prevents activity. In the acute nontraumatic back, pain elimination can be a brief process measured in hours to days, not weeks to months. The well-established expectation that back pain is inevitably a prolonged and disabling event is wrong. Most acute episodes subside rapidly. Although there is a recognized high recurrence rate, individual episodes can and should be treated independently. For a few patients, chronicity may follow. For far fewer patients, the pain may be the harbinger of a potential catastrophe. These sobering exceptions do not alter the fact that the overwhelming majority of acute nontraumatic spinal pain is benign, self-limiting, and best treated without the delay of making a pathologic diagnosis.

A Clinical Syndrome

Medicine has always used syndromes, a collection of signs and symptoms, to describe conditions for which there is no apparent etiology. Strangely, management of low back pain has evaded this approach. The search for spurious diagnoses and putative physical causes has obscured a simple approach, prolonged interventions, and hindered the rapid provision of relief. The unfounded fear of missing significant pathology has defeated medicine's ability to resolve a common problem.

One alternative is to use a carefully structured history and confirmatory physical examination to identify a clinically relevant pattern of pain. The identified syndrome then forms the basis for initial treatment. Achieving the anticipated outcome confirms the original clinical hypothesis.

Following the Quebec Task Force in 1987, which recognized that clinicians could not reliably differentiate between different pathoanatomic causes of back pain, there has been increased interest in the nonpathologic approach. Several systems of back pain classification have been proposed. Modern sophistication is devolving to a classic approach with which our medical predecessors would have been entirely comfortable. The apparent simplicity of the technique, however, belies its scope and precision.

The four patterns presented here initially were developed 25 years ago and have been modified extensively. They form the basis for clinical recognition and standardized initial management throughout a network of spine rehabilitation clinics that currently assesses over 40,000 new patients annually. Although specific pathology can be inferred, particularly in the two patterns describing leg dominant pain, knowing the precise physical source of the symptoms is not relevant to recognizing the pain pattern or choosing the initial treatment. In fact, separating these syndromes from their presumed pathology heightens the effectiveness of treatment.

The most important step in the initial assessment of a patient with acute nontraumatic spinal pain is determining the location of the dominant pain. Without this precise localization, it is impossible to identify a pattern. Most patients complain of both back and leg pain but the symptoms are rarely of equal intensity. As tedious as it may become, the patient must be required to identify the single site of the most intense or disabling pain. If a direct question fails to elicit an adequate answer, the same information may be obtained by asking, "If I can eliminate only one of your pains, which one would you choose?" or "Of all your pains, which is the one that prevents you from staying active?" With proper questioning the dominant pain site can almost always be established. Allowing patient indecision at this early stage will compromise everything that follows. In these patterns, the buttock is considered a site of back-dominant pain and the line of demarcation between the back and leg is the gluteal fold. Where ambiguity remains, leg pain takes precedence over back pain.

Having identified the location of the pain, the next most important determinant is its consistency. There is perhaps no other item in the history for which it is harder to obtain a clear and unbiased answer. Many patients are reluctant to admit that their symptoms are intermittent because they view this as an admission that their problem is not sufficiently serious to warrant careful medical attention. For those whose pain has already lasted for some time, individual episodes may have blended into an unbroken continuum of pain. Yet the distinction between constant and intermittent is essential. The patient with back-dominant, truly intermittent pain can be virtually certain that the problem is mechanical and benign.

When questioning the consistency of the pain, the examiner must indicate clearly that both responses are important. Before the patient is given an opportunity to answer, it is sometimes helpful for the examiner to acknowledge that although the pain may have stopped occasionally it has always returned and therefore represents a significant problem. Ask if there is a time of day when the symptoms typically wane and if at that time there is any movement or position that can diminish them further. Before finally asking whether or not the pain disappears the examiner may reiterate the understanding that the symptoms will always rapidly return.

The difficulty in obtaining a clear response to this question is increased by the patient's answer to the necessary follow-up question, "When you say the pain disappears, do you mean that it disappears completely?" Having just said that the pain goes away, patients may qualify their response by stating that the pain never stops completely but persists in a reduced form. This description does not constitute intermittent pain. To qualify as intermittent, the pain must be completely absent for an identifiable, albeit transient, period.

The difference between constant and intermittent pain is highly significant. Although the patient need not, and in most cases should not, be party to the examiner's preliminary diagnostic considerations, the presence of constant pain raises several disturbing prospects. The first of these is malignancy. The examiner should weigh the clinical evidence including the patient's age, associated symptoms, and past medical history before deciding to pursue this concern. Constant pain must also be reviewed with reference to the wide range of systemic conditions including rheumatoid disease, ankylosing spondylitis, and enteric disorders in which back pain can play a prominent role. The third possibility with constant pain is the patient with pain-focused behavior who will inevitably report constant pain. Finally, the most common and least threatening presentation of constant pain occurs in the patient who is experiencing constant mechanical symptoms. This pain is clearly responsive to the mechanical factors of position and movement and certain activities will predictably heighten the pain while others will consistently reduce it. The failure to abolish the pain, however, does not necessarily indicate an underlying nonmechanical etiology. More often, it merely indicates a highly irritable local structure that is aggravated by movement or excess load and that remains painful even at rest. Recognizing this possibility allows the examiner to inform these patients that they may recover more slowly than usual and face an increased risk of frequent recurrences but that they have a good chance of final full recovery.

Considering only location and consistency, it is apparent that establishing a clear pattern of pain is not a haphazard activity. Taking the history requires planning and precise execution. The answers have immediate significance and must be accurate and unequivocal.

In constructing the patterns of pain, history takes precedence over the physical examination. The physical assessment should confirm a proposed pattern, not serve as the primary determinant.

The verifying physical examination should include movement testing, principally flexion and extension. Either or both of these movements should reproduce the typical back-dominant pain or aggravate the acute leg pain. Irritative testing should include assessment of the femoral nerve with, for example, the femoral stretch test, and of sciatic nerve irritation using straight leg raising or one of its variants. Basic conductive testing includes appropriate assessments of L4, L5, and S1. The comprehensiveness of the neurologic examination will vary according to the history, but a basic screen should never be eliminated even in patients with clearly back-dominant pain. The final elements of the physical examination must include a test for upper motor involvement, such as the plantar response, and sensory testing in the saddle area between the buttocks to assess low sacral root function.

Although pattern recognition relies primarily on history, the physical examination must be concordant. A significant discrepancy requires reevaluation of the history or a decision that the complaints are not typical, nontraumatic spinal pain and therefore dictate a more intense immediate investigation.

It is impossible for a properly trained health-care professional to completely refrain from a consideration of pathology. Every clinical presentation suggests a probable source of pain, one that links the patient's signs and symptoms to a conventional medical diagnosis. The validity of the correlation, however, is less important than the recognition of the syndrome. Treatment in the acute phase of nontraumatic spinal pain is directed at the rapid resolution of symptoms and must be based on the clinical presentation. A change in the identity of the presumed pain generator will alter neither the observed pattern nor the therapeutic approach it demands. A pathologic model may be helpful to explain the situation to the patient or to reassure a clinician uncomfortable with complete reliance on the history and physical examination, but it will not assist in the management.

Pattern 1

Pattern 1 describes back-dominant pain, pain felt most intensely although not exclusively in the back or buttock (Table 1). Symptoms may be constant or intermittent but are always intensified with forward bending. This fact usually can be gleaned from the history and often is associated with a complaint of increased pain on sitting. Typically, patients with pattern 1 pain would rather walk slowly than stand still, but would rather stand still than sit down.

The physical examination separates pattern 1 into two subsets, fast and slow responders. As the designation implies, these two groups respond differently to the initial mechanical treatment. The fast responder notes that the pain is increased on flexion, verifying the history but experiences some relief of pain with lumbar extension. The slow responder is also worse with flexion, a prerequisite for pattern 1 but is equally or more aggravated by lumbar extension. The remainder of the physical examination including all the neurologic tests is normal or, as in the case of a long-standing absent reflex, noncontributory.

Pattern 1 probably reflects pain arising from the intervertebral disc or the adjacent ligaments including the anulus fibrosus. The specific pathology within the disc, for example annular distortion or internal derangement, does not have to be established to initiate treatment. In fact, the disc need not be implicated at all.

TABLE 1 | Characteristics of Pattern 1

History

Back dominant
    Back
    Buttock

Worse with flexion

Constant or intermittent

Physical examination

Worse with flexion and better with extension = fast responder

Worse with flexion and no change/worse with extension = slow responder

TABLE 2	**Characteristics of Pattern 2**

History

Back dominant
    Back
    Buttock

Worse with extension

Never worse with flexion   -Movement or position
                                 -Loaded or unloaded

Always intermittent

Physical examination

Worse with extension

No effect or better with flexion

TABLE 3	**Characteristics of Pattern 3**

History

Leg dominant—below buttock

Leg pain is affected by back movement/position

Previously or currently constant

Physical examination

Leg pain changes with back movement

Constant leg pain cannot be abolished with movement or position
    Better with specific back position = fast responder
    No change/worse with any back position = slow responder

Must have a positive irritative test (typical) and/or conduction loss

Pattern 2

Pattern 2 refers to the second syndrome of back-dominant pain (Table 2). It is considerably less common than pattern 1 and more tightly circumscribed. The pain in the back or buttock is consistently worse with bending backward and is never intensified with bending forward, either repetitively or in a sustained posture. The back pain is always intermittent.

The physical examination simply confirms the history. The patient's symptoms are aggravated with extension and are either unaffected or improved on flexion. Again, the neurologic examination including irritative and conductive tests is normal or noncontributory.

Pattern 2 can be attributed to pain generators located within the posterior joint complex including the associated capsular and ligamentous structures. Treatment, however, is dictated by the clinical syndrome and does not require anatomic localization of the pain source.

Pattern 3

Pattern 3 defines leg-dominant pain, which is worse below the gluteal fold than in the back or buttock (Table 3). It does not distinguish between dominant pain site above or below the knee. Many patients also report pain in the back. The pattern does not require exclusivity of leg pain, merely dominance. To qualify as pattern 3, the leg pain must be constant either at the time of the examination or, where spontaneous recovery has commenced, in the recent past. Because the leg pain represents a back complaint, it must change with spinal movement or altered position.

As in pattern 1, the physical examination divides patients into two subgroups. Fast responders are those whose leg symptoms can be reduced, though never eliminated, by specific postures. The slow responders either experience no relief or are aggravated by all back movements or positions. The neurologic examination must include either a positive irritative test, such as the femoral stretch or straight leg raise, or demonstrate a newly acquired conduction loss. To be considered positive, the irritative test must reproduce the patient's typical leg-dominant pain described in the history. The production of back pain does not constitute a positive irritative test. Once again the physical examination is used to support, not establish the proposed pattern.

The correlation between the pattern of symptoms and the clinical pathology is more closely linked in patients with leg-dominant pain. Pattern 3 describes true sciatica, radicular leg pain caused by a combination of chemical and mechanical nerve root irritation, the most common cause for which is a recent disc herniation. Providing acute-phase pain control, however, does not require a detailed analysis whether the lesion is contained, partially extruded, or sequestered.

Pattern 4

Pattern 4 represents leg-dominant pain brought on by activity and relieved by rest (Table 4). Pain control is rarely a problem because it can be achieved rapidly by the cessation of activity and assisted by assuming a flexed posture. The leg symptoms are always intermittent and of short duration. Because patients rarely volunteer the change in spinal position required for pain relief, they must be asked specifically. The interviewer's

TABLE 4	Characteristics of Pattern 4

History

Leg dominant—below buttock

Leg symptoms worse with activity

Leg symptoms better with postural change

Intermittent—short duration

Physical examination

No irritative finding

+/- conduction loss

assumption that the pain produced with walking is, in fact, leg pain must be confirmed with a direct query and a request that the patient indicate the precise location of the dominant pain. A description of back-dominant pain, indicating pattern 2, is frequently incorrectly labeled as pattern 4. Nowhere is a careful analysis of the history more critical.

The physical examination is frequently noncontributory. Because pattern 4 pain must be leg dominant, back pain on movement adds nothing to the pattern identification. There are no positive irritative tests. There may be no conduction loss or one may occur transiently only after periods of exertion. In pattern 4 the history may be the only clue.

Pattern 4 designates the symptom complex produced by neurogenic claudication. The commonly used term spinal stenosis is incorrect because the stenosis itself is neither symptomatic nor necessarily pathologic. Anything that disrupts the normal vascular supply, particularly the venous drainage of the nerve roots, can produce the recognizable clinical picture. In the acute phase it is the syndrome, not the precise pathology, that can be identified by history and physical examination, and it is the syndrome, not the pathology that directs choices of treatment.

While three of the patterns recognized in the low back have comparable clinical presentation in the neck, neurogenic claudication is found only in the lumbar spine. Compression of the cervical spinal cord has radically different consequences than pressure on the exiting nerve roots of the cauda equina. Similarities and differences in the presentations will be discussed briefly after analyzing the components of rational management.

Fundamental Elements of Treatment

It surprises some clinicians to discover that in many cases patients offer the best approach for their own pain control. In addition to facilitating pattern recognition, careful questioning about aggravating and relieving factors will offer useful information about the best means of controlling the episode. Once again, the rules of engagement are not those of conventional medical management. Here the primary goal is rapid relief of pain and the elimination of unwarranted fear. In this time-limited phase, the pragmatic view matters more than the theory. For treatment to be effective it need only exceed the normal rate of recovery and offer benefits unobtainable in the natural history. Prolonged therapy for a short-term problem is inappropriate. Addressing underlying issues such as obesity, poor physical condition, or socioeconomic distress may have a role in the long-term treatment of chronic disabling back pain but can delay or hinder management in the acute phase.

Education

Basic
Basic patient education may consist of no more than an answer to the question, "What happened to me?" Most patients in acute distress have little interest in a detailed anatomy lesson or the current theories of chemical irritation. They want only to know that their problem is recognizable, manageable, and finite. An unequivocal statement that the patient's symptoms are common and amenable to rapid treatment may be all that is required.

In many cases, patients suffering a severe back pain episode are more disabled by fear of the unknown than by the mechanical problem itself. Providing a plausible answer coupled with legitimate reassurance is the primary educational goal. In acute nontraumatic back pain, the pathophysiologic diagnosis usually remains speculative so investigation and consultation can delay or even prevent a useful instructive response. Precision becomes the enemy of pragmatic education. Using identifiable clinical syndromes permits immediate positive feedback.

Patients may have already discovered movements or positions that moderate the pain. The challenge is to extract this information from the history then return it to the patient in a structured fashion. The value of the education may be more in reassuring the patient that the clinician is credible and on familiar ground than to offer new information.

Comprehensive
Occasionally, even in the acute episode, a more detailed educational program is helpful. This may take the form of a small group learning session incorporated within

an active physical therapy setting. Useful topics include basic anatomy, simple biomechanics, practical modifications in the activities of daily living, and the acknowledgement that fear is the inevitable companion of back pain.

Infrequently a more formal back school can be used. This approach to back education has enjoyed several waves of popularity separated by periods of skepticism. The literature has not supported the value of group education, although this lack may be less an indictment of the technique than a condemnation of its inappropriate goals. The fundamental purpose of back school is to increase patient understanding, diminish apprehension, and perhaps improve the simple psychomotor skills required to minimize an acute attack. If only these defined short-term goals are measured, the reported results are considerably improved. The designation back school can apply to any formalized educational process and need not entail elaborate or expensive measures. How much education is necessary and how it is delivered is a highly individualized decision. Pamphlets, books, audiotapes, and video presentations have all been tried and have been shown to be effective in limited circumstances.

The important issue is not how the education is delivered or even the particular information conveyed. The primary purpose of back education in the early stages of mechanical back pain is to reduce fear and to promote a positive outlook through a better understanding of the benign self-limiting nature of the acute episode. Incorporating simple physical techniques that promote symptom resolution is a worthwhile secondary goal. The patient with enough knowledge and training to take an active part in the pain-control process has the best chance of success.

Educating the patient to accept back pain as a normal event rather than a debilitating illness may require a major alteration not only in the expectations of the sufferer but also in the attitude of the treating physician. If the instructor remains trapped within an inflexible medical approach, it may be impossible to deliver the pragmatic and optimistic message essential to effective early back education.

Physical Modalities

Professionally Administered
Conventional physical therapy has a limited role in the management of acute nontraumatic spinal pain. Because treatment can be directed solely at the rapid resolution of pain without reference to specific causes, ersatz science inhibits practical success. This early phase of back pain management does not require, indeed cannot possess diagnostic certitude, and selecting a treatment option based on hypothetical pathology is not appropriate. The application of heat, for example, whether through hot packs, ultrasound, or interferential current may be transiently helpful but holds no curative property. The choice of one modality over another can be based entirely on its pain-relieving effectiveness or lack thereof.

Transcutaneous electrical nerve stimulation, traction, acupuncture, and the gamut of therapeutic options should be regarded in the same way. Anything that aborts an acute attack is beneficial. In a condition where the natural history is overwhelmingly favorable, treatment response should be rapid and sustained. Because no modality creates measurable, persistent physical change and none need increase the typical pain, the patient or the practitioner who endures or allows heightened pain in the mistaken belief that a modality takes time to heal completely misunderstands the treatment.

Because an emotional response is an integral part of acute back pain, the placebo effect of any professional treatment is significant. Magnet field therapy, cold laser, craniosacral adjustment, or therapeutic touch have never demonstrated any objective, reproducible physical effect yet all remain popular and all claim to assist the relief of pain. Anecdotal experience is not a substitute for a randomized controlled trial, yet the reputation of this group and other similar therapies rests entirely in the realm of personal reports and testimonials. Acute nontraumatic, nonmalignant back pain normally improves spontaneously. Whether it is the aura of professional competence or just fortuitous timing, an acute attack can subside during a course of almost any treatment, particularly if the duration of that treatment is sufficiently extended. The issue here is not safety but economics and needless dependency.

The place for a back support in the acute episode is similarly difficult to validate. Short-term use does not produce physical weakness or create psychological dependence. If the back brace reduces pain, it is helpful. Patients must be aware that its role is solely symptom reduction; it neither immobilizes nor biomechanically protects the spine. It is not body armor and it cannot prevent further painful episodes. Brace use must be combined with this necessary information and with the understanding that its role should be limited to those periods in the day when it assists in maintaining a more normal level of activity.

Unfortunately, all of these modalities, methods, or materials can be misused. Unless their function is clearly defined, severely limited, and combined with a legitimate transfer of responsibility from the treating professional, early-stage physical treatments may become the prelude to late-stage reliance and loss of control.

Self-Administered

Liniment, massage, a heating pad, or a bag of frozen vegetables can all serve to reduce the pain of an acute episode. Most patients experiencing attacks of low back pain do not seek professional help from a doctor, chiropractor, or physical therapist. The majority of patients rely on their own intuition, the advice of friends and family, or perhaps consultation with a local pharmacist. Counterirritants are widely used and frequently helpful. Lacking professional mystique, their results, while still containing an element of placebo, are straightforward and easier to quantify. If ice relieves the pain then ice will be used again. If liniment exacerbates the situation, it will be discarded. The pragmatism inherent in this approach should be reflected in the medical response. In the absence of a legitimate disease, the patient may know best.

Individualized Pain Control

The following brief descriptions outline the essential elements for each of the four patterns of nontraumatic spinal pain. The strategies used should be determined without regard to presumed underlying pathology and should be judged on their ability to reduce swiftly or to abolish the primary pain. Treatment can be divided into three areas: movement, position, and materials. Each has varying significance for a particular pattern.

Pattern 1

Fast Responder

Fast-responding patients with pattern 1 pain exhibit back-dominant pain aggravated by forward bending and reduced or eliminated by lumbar extension. The key treatment strategy is repetitive movement, particularly repetitive extension (Fig. 1). The most useful technique, described within the McKenzie method of physical therapy, is a prone push-up in which the patient raises the shoulders, arches the back, and avoids lifting the pelvis. A similar but less aggressive stretch can be accomplished with the patient standing, hands on the buttocks and knees locked. To be an effective pain control technique, the extension movement must be repeated frequently. A schedule of 10 repetitions performed hourly is typical.

The ideal position is one that maintains or exaggerates lumbar lordosis. The typical flexed sitting posture will require correction. It is important for the clinician and the patient to differentiate between aggravating the dominant pain and simply being uncomfortable. The former is unacceptable. The latter is unavoidable. Focus attention on the intensity and location of the typical pain. Patients often complain that increasing the arch in the low back is uncomfortable but when questioned

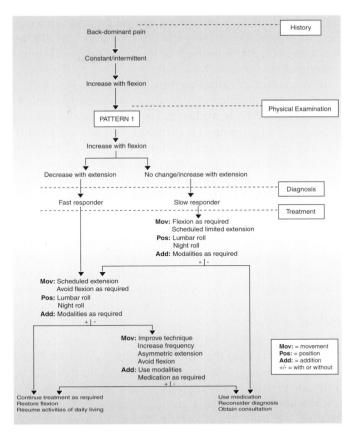

Figure 1 Low back pain treatment algorithm—pattern 1.

closely report that the typical pain has either disappeared or shifted toward the midline. This latter response, called centralization, is accepted as an indicator of a positive prognosis in spite of the fact that the pain may temporarily increase in its new location.

To restore lordosis in sitting requires some form of lumbar support. A soft sponge-rubber roll frequently is recommended. For patients who report that their back pain increases when they are recumbent at night, a rolled towel at waist level often provides relief. The roll helps maintain the spine in a neutral position, presumably minimizing load on the pain-generating structures. Once again it is necessary to clarify the difference between discomfort and exacerbation.

Slow Responder

The slow-responding patient has pain on flexion but also has pain on lumbar extension. Arching backward is often more unpleasant. Although the ultimate goal for all patients in this group is repetitive extension, paradoxically the slow responder will often start with repetitive flexion. Supine knees to chest stretches may initiate pain reduction that can then be continued in extension. For the slow-responding patient, lying prone on a flat surface may prove too uncomfortable to be tolerated, and it may be necessary to lie prone over one or two pillows. By altering the hand position, the sloppy push-up can be modified to create little additional extension.

The amount of initial posture change can be modest. The use of a lumbar roll is still recommended but its size may have to be reduced. The size of the towel roll at night, if night pain is a problem, should remain substantial enough to place the spine in a neutral position.

This subgroup of patients poses a challenge to rapid pain control. Their response is generally more protracted and it is difficult to obtain the proper balance between repetitive flexion and extension. This group also is prone to sudden severe exacerbations of pain if the physical treatment is inappropriate or simply too aggressive. Pattern 1 slow responders demand a meticulously structured program. Both casual instruction and vague reassurance are worthless.

Pattern 2

Pattern 2 describes an uncommon but clearly defined syndrome. Because the back-dominant pain is produced only on extension and is never increased on flexion, the obvious repetitive movement is forward bending (Fig. 2). Frequently this is best accomplished with the patient seated. With the hands on the knees, the arms support the weight of the upper body. Bending the elbows lowers the trunk as close to the thighs as possible. The arms are then used to push the torso up, reducing activity in the paraspinal muscles. As in pattern 1, structured repetitive movement is the goal. The exercise prescription should be specific, detailed, and easily performed.

Because pattern 2 is always intermittent and because most patients in this group have already discovered that bending forward relieves the discomfort, posture correction is seldom required. This illustrates one difference between short-term management and long-term control. Posture correction may well be essential for preventing recurrences and promoting full functional recovery but it is unnecessary and even counterproductive in pain control for pattern 2.

Because increasing lordosis increases pain, a lumbar support is contraindicated. The neutral spinal position achieved by a rolled towel at night, however, may be as effective in this pattern as it is in pattern 1.

Pattern 3

Back-dominant patients respond to repetitive movement. The acute, leg-dominant pain of pattern 3 responds to rest (Fig. 3). Repetitive movement in any direction is generally aggravating. For some, lying prone over a pillow may diminish the leg pain. Others find it best to rest prone, supporting the upper body on the

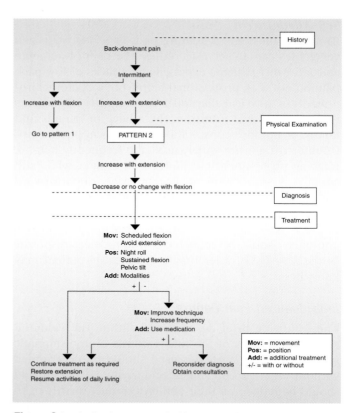

Figure 2 Low back pain treatment algorithm—pattern 2.

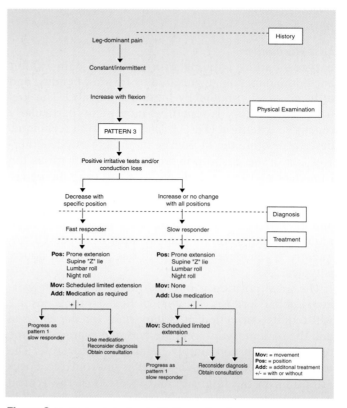

Figure 3 Low back pain treatment algorithm—pattern 3.

elbows like a child watching television. Still others gain partial relief by lying supine with the calves of the legs on the seat of a chair and the knees are drawn up over the abdomen. This "Z" position is the antithesis of lying prone yet one or both orientations may serve as an effective method of reducing the leg-dominant pain, another illustration of the value in treating a clinical syndrome rather than putative pathology. Although the lesion may be the same, the physical mechanism of early pain control varies considerably.

The use of a lumbar support and a night roll may both be beneficial. It is an empiric decision based solely on the patient's report of a decrease in the leg pain.

Few individuals with acute leg-dominant pain are able to carry out their normal daily activities. Although prolonged bed rest is inadvisable, this group of patients requires frequent rest periods. Providing a rigid schedule conveys a reassuring sense of professionalism and understanding. Recommending an efficacious rest position for 15 minutes out of each hour gives the patient a period of pain control while the remaining 45 minutes provides an opportunity to complete the necessary activities of daily life.

Pattern 4

Pain control in pattern 4 usually is not a problem. The disability and the pain are linked to attempts at maintaining normal function. As long as the patient remains at rest or sufficiently confines the level of activity, pain will be controlled. Because symptom control generally is achieved by a flexed posture, sustaining this position while walking can prove an effective method of decreasing the recurrent leg symptoms (Fig. 4). This requires a degree of trunk muscle control and for this reason, pattern 4 is the only pattern in which the initial treatment includes strength and endurance training.

Dating from the Williams exercises more than 60 years ago, the classic physical therapy approach to low back pain has included the pelvic tilt. This maneuver flattens the lumbar lordosis by rotating the pelvis in an anterosuperior direction. It is a technique best mastered lying supine and is a useful starting point for developing abdominal strengthening exercises. In pattern 4, walking with a pelvic tilt can substantially increase the distance before the onset of leg pain. For an older population possessing little trunk muscle strength or endurance, beginning an abdominal exercise routine may be the most appropriate initial management. In contrast to the other three patterns, these patients require continued or repeated professional supervision thus blurring the boundaries between acute care and chronic rehabilitation.

The goal is sustained posture correction. Repetitive

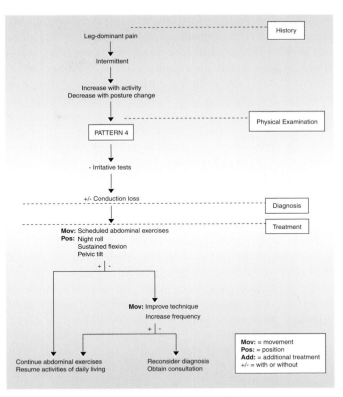

Figure 4 Low back pain treatment algorithm—pattern 4.

movement has little to offer beyond the temporary elimination of the exercise-induced leg pain with flexion. Because pain at rest is not a frequent component of this pattern, back supports or other aids seldom are required.

Medication

Most acute nontraumatic, nonmalignant spinal pain has a mechanical origin. Because education, physical modalities, and selected movements or positions can generally accomplish rapid pain control, medication plays a distinctly secondary role. Providing a prescription as the initial, perhaps as the only response to a patient's complaint serves to strengthen the widely held perception that physicians lack the technical skills exhibited by many practitioners of alternative medicine to deal with the pain.

Conversely, adding a suitable medication when mechanical recovery falters or is incomplete offers an optimal therapeutic routine. The role of medication in acute back pain is not curative; it is just another means of hastening remission. Because the effects are short term and address only the symptoms, the medications should be selected not only for their effectiveness but also, perhaps more importantly, for their lack of side effects.

Acetaminophen and aspirin are the most commonly prescribed analgesic medications. Acetaminophen does not possess the same degree of anti-inflammatory activity as aspirin but is an equally effective pain reliever. For short-term use in therapeutic doses, acetaminophen is relatively nontoxic. The sustained high dose levels associated with hepatic toxicity are not appropriate in the management of short-term low back pain. The anti-inflammatory doses of aspirin may require up to 6 grams daily in divided doses. The analgesic effect, more appropriate in the management of acute spinal pain, is produced at a substantially lower intake. As with most nonsteroidal anti-inflammatory drugs (NSAIDs), gastrointestinal toxicity may occur.

NSAIDs are prescribed commonly in spite of the fact that their beneficial effects are unpredictable. Acetic acid derivatives such as indomethacin, oxicams such as piroxicam, and propionic acid derivatives such as ibuprofen or naproxen all share the same problem of adverse reactions involving the gastrointestinal tract. Symptoms of nausea, epigastric pain, heartburn, diarrhea, and generalized abdominal distress have all been reported. In light of the self-limiting, benign nature of most nontraumatic spinal pain, this class of drugs should be used judiciously in all cases and probably is contraindicated in high-risk patients with a history of gastrointestinal problems. NSAIDs should not be prescribed for the management of back pain during pregnancy or in patients with renal insufficiency.

The cyclooxygenase-2 (COX-2) inhibitors are currently the most frequently prescribed anti-inflammatory medications in North America. Celecoxib and rofecoxib possess the same analgesic and anti-inflammatory properties as the older NSAIDs, but their selective COX-2 inhibition reduces the potential for serious gastrointestinal irritation. It is a widely held misconception that this class of NSAIDs is a more potent anti-inflammatory agent than the previous generations. In fact, the therapeutic response is approximately the same. Their great advantage is the apparent significant decrease in potentially dangerous side effects. This fact alone is enough to recommend them for the symptomatic treatment of a transiently painful, non-life-threatening condition.

The short-term use of opiate analgesics should rarely be necessary. Their frequent or indiscriminate use may have less to do with the severity of the patient's pain than with the clinician's inability to deal more directly with the underlying mechanical problem. Pertinent education, physical modalities, and appropriate pain control activities can often eliminate the need for narcotic drugs.

Muscle relaxants occasionally are considered as an option in the treatment of acute nontraumatic spinal pain. They should not be used on a routine basis. This class of drugs includes central nervous system anxiolytics, hypnotics, and sedatives whose effects are more central than peripheral. Drugs such as diazepam, cyclobenzaprine, and orphenadrine have the potential for major side effects including drowsiness and depression. Although they appear more effective than placebo they have not been shown to be more effective than NSAIDs. Combining muscle relaxants and NSAIDs produces no additional benefit.

Antidepressant medications such as monoamine oxidase inhibitors or serotonin re-uptake inhibitors are not recommended for the treatment of acute low back pain. The short-term benefit is negligible and the potential for long-term dependency is significant.

Although oral corticosteroids can be used in the treatment of radicular pattern 3 symptoms, presumably to reduce acute nerve root inflammation, their routine use is not recommended. They have significant side effects, and pain control can generally be accomplished without exposing the patient to these unnecessary risks. There is no place for oral corticosteroids in the treatment of mechanical back-dominant pattern 1 or pattern 2 pain.

Follow-Up

The primary management of acute nontraumatic spinal pain not only lies outside the usual medical paradigm, it also confounds conventional expectations. The usual course of mechanical back pain is both rapid and predictable. In most cases, pain control or at least pain reduction can be accomplished within the first 24 hours. For a pattern 1 fast responder or a patient with pattern 2 symptoms, the pain may be eliminated during the consultation. For this reason, early follow-up is strongly recommended. Waiting the customary week before the first review visit interposes confounding factors that may obscure the patient's initial response.

Because each of the mechanical patterns suggests a specific course of action, a positive response to the treatment validates the initial presumptive categorization. A patient with pattern 1 pain not only has typical back-dominant pain aggravated by forward bending but also responds to the specific mechanical measures designed to reduce pattern 1 symptoms. The patient with a clearly defined history and physical examination whose clinical course follows the anticipated path to complete pain abolition requires no further investigation or intrusive medical management. The feedback reinforces the original premise. It is the patient with the vague history, conflicting physical assessment, and unsatisfactory clinical course who requires immediate attention. Unnecessary delay in these patients can result in potentially serious complications.

The optimal reassessment should take place 24 to 48

hours after the original consultation. An overview of the patient's situation is helpful. Ask, "Generally speaking during the past 24 hours with reference to your typical pain, are you better, worse, or the same?" This general inquiry sets the tone of the interview and is followed by a more detailed analysis of the changes in the clinical picture. Four distinct questions represented by the acronym LIFE focus on the separate elements of the situation.

What is the Location of the pain compared to where it was felt initially? Movement of the pain toward the midline, centralization, is an indicator of improvement. Conversely, movement of the pain into the periphery suggests that the selected strategy is not working.

The Intensity of the pain can be a measure of success. Recording the pain on a 0 to 10 scale at the initial visit then asking the patient for a new rating at the first review is helpful. The pain scale has no validity between patients but is a useful measure of progress for a given individual. Patients may not be aware that centralization can be accompanied by a transient increase in pain. In this instance, what the patient sees as failure may, in fact, may be a sign of success.

The Frequency of the pain may be gauged either as the amount of time spent in pain or, more optimistically, as the amount of time spent pain free. A pain described as constant in the initial history that becomes intermittent during the treatment period strongly supports the chosen approach. Each treatment program has a number of distinct components.

The Effect of each element should be assessed separately. Distinguishing between the benefits of a counterirritant, a posture-correcting device, or a pain-control exercise will direct the next stage of treatment.

Before attributing a lack of improvement to improper pattern selection or serious underlying nonmechanical pathology, consider the more common reasons for failure: Is the patient actually doing the pain control activities, using the recommended physical modalities, or taking the prescribed medication? Noncompliance with the therapeutic regimen is a frequent cause of failure. Is the patient using the correct techniques, and if so are they being used frequently enough? In addition to hearing the patient's account, the first follow-up of a nonresponsive patient should include direct observation of the pain-control maneuvers. Even compliant patients can misunderstand the original instructions. Have there been additional pain-producing episodes? Although avoidance of painful activities is not mandatory, reducing their frequency is often helpful. When this is not possible or when following the initial evaluation the patient is required to undertake additional pain-producing pursuits, the anticipated positive response may not occur.

There is a significant distinction between controlling a single acute episode of nontraumatic spinal pain and permanently solving the problem. Within the first year, more than half the patients will have a recurrence. Patients whose symptoms always return at the resumption of normal activity require a more detailed evaluation and definitive treatment. Those for whom simple, short-term mechanical back pain has been superseded by the development of pain-focused behavior require intensive and prolonged therapy. For both groups as well as for those whose pain has led to a significant loss of conditioning, the recognition of a clinical back pain syndrome offers, at best, a transient goal. For everyone else, dealing with the acute episode in an active intelligent fashion offers the best chance of lasting control.

The patient has two options. One is to accept an unintelligible medical diagnosis, endure needless apprehension, passively observe nonparticipatory therapy, and face the prospect of prolonged disability. The other is to gain a rudimentary but sufficient understanding of the problem, actively pursue self-directed treatment with limited medical assistance, and increase the probability of rapid recovery. The choice is between medical domination and medical support, between dependency and self-sufficiency. The necessary transfer of responsibility is not easy for either the practitioner or the patient. Relinquishing professional control requires the confidence of both parties that this apparently simple approach to diagnosis and pain management is both safe and effective. For the physician, given the method's wide digression from the traditional medical model, this is not an easy determination. For the patient, controlling the pain demands knowledge and physical skill, and accepting responsibility means accepting the blame for failure. The change in roles may not be comfortable but given the medical establishment's conspicuous failure to deal successfully with acute nontraumatic spinal pain, the status quo is not acceptable.

Distinguishing patterns of pain based on the same categories used in the low back is equally effective for the cervical spine. The identification of the two neck-dominant patterns is complicated only by the fact that neck dominant can apply to pain felt along the trapezius ridge or medial scapular border, over the occiput, and as far forward as the retro-orbital area, to the jaw or anterior chest and descending down the upper arm. All of these locations reflect referred mechanical pain. Only when the most intense pain occurs in the arm below the deltoid insertion should the clinician entertain a diagnosis of pattern 3, radicular pain from direct cervical root irritation. The mechanical patterns may be intermittent but neurogenic arm pain must be constant.

In the neck, the condition most analogous to the low-back pattern 4, neurogenic claudication from stenosis, is cervical myelopathy. It usually results from narrowing of the cervical canal by osteophytic ridges or ligament calcification. The symptoms are a mix of upper and lower motor neuron involvement affecting both the arms and legs. Cervical myelopathy has a different and more ominous prognosis than compression of the cauda equina. In advanced cases, treatment, if possible, is frequently surgical. Except for measures of protection and activity modification, there is no effective early conservative care.

The physical examination focuses on the same findings as for the lumbar spine. Pain produced by flexion and intensified with a head-forward posture is pattern 1. It may be constant or intermittent. This pattern alone encompasses nearly all the patients who present with acute neck-dominant pain. Pain designated as pattern 2 occurs only during cervical extension. It is always intermittent and highly unusual. Physical confirmation of pattern 3 is hindered by the lack of a specific test for nerve root irritation comparable to straight leg raising. The occasional finding of a motor or reflex loss, most commonly at C6 or C7, clarifies the picture but many patients with neurogenic pain are initially recognized only on the basis of a history of constant, arm-dominant pain.

The principals of treatment are also the same. Most mechanical and neurogenic pain will improve with time. Educating the patient about what to expect, adding professionally administered or self-directed pain-relieving measures, and providing positive modifications to the patient's daily activities may be all that is necessary.

Specific pain-modifying movements reverse the generation of the pain. For pattern 1, correcting a head-forward posture is helpful and ironically often is achieved by using a lumbar support. When recumbent, a rolled towel along the lower edge of the pillow supports the cervical spine and reduces pain. Regular practice of cervical retractions adds a dynamic component. The rare patient with pattern 2 pain need only gently flex the chin to the chest, but finding a relatively pain-free rest position for pattern 3 can be a challenge. Patients with C7 irritation, for example, are sometimes more comfortable resting the affected forearm on top of their head. Whatever brings a measure of relief is appropriate.

The one exception is the use of a soft cervical collar. Although its support may provide a brief period of pain reduction, the presence of the collar promotes a head-forward posture and interferes with more effective active means of control. Physical and psychological dependence develop rapidly and delay recovery. The collar is a tempting substitute for the arduous and time-consuming task of engaging the patient in the process of recovery. But apparent early progress may come at the expense of timely complete recuperation.

Once again medication holds a secondary role. Early structured follow-up is advantageous. The prognosis is generally far better than either the patient or the practitioner believes.

The treatment of dorsal pain is unique. Most thoracic symptoms are, in reality, referred from the cervical area. The diagnosis of true dorsal pain should be made only after ruling out all possibility of a pain source in the neck. There has been considerable speculation about the clinical significance of thoracic disc protrusions. During the acute phase and in the absence of long tract signs, the conjecture has no relevance to the treatment. Acute mechanical thoracic pain often responds optimally to direct manual therapy rather than training, physical modalities, or medication. The best chance for rapid pain control may be the nonspecific manipulation of an undetermined physical problem, the antithesis of conventional medical care.

Annotated Bibliography

Borenstein DG: A clinician's approach to acute low back pain. *Am J Med* 1997;102:16S-22S.
  Treatment should return patients to regular activity as quickly as possible in a cost-effective manner. Conditions are identified that require urgent or emergent care. All other patients start conservative therapy without radiographic or laboratory tests regardless of the presumed diagnosis.

Burton AK, Waddell G, Tillotson KM, Summerton N: Information and advice to patients with back pain can have a positive effect: A randomized controlled trial of a novel educational booklet in primary care. *Spine* 1999;24:2484-2491.
  A double-blind randomized controlled trial demonstrates that a booklet stressing fear avoidance, positive attitudes, and rapid return was more effective than a conventional brochure. Effectiveness was measured by a reduction in self-reported disability. The intervention did not affect the pain.

Carter JT, Birrell LN: *Occupational Health Guidelines for the Management of Low Back Pain at Work: Principle Recommendations.* London, England, Faculty of Occupational Medicine of the Royal College of Physicians, 2000.
  These guidelines take an evidence-based approach. Everyone involved should be aware that delayed return to activity quickly leads to chronic pain and disability. They recommend against the use of speculative diagnostic labels that may have a detrimental effect on outcome.

Deyo RA, Phillips WR: Low back pain: A primary care challenge. *Spine* 1996;21:2826-2832.

Most patients come to the physician with uncomplicated low back pain. Identifying the rare patient with significant pathology is like looking for a needle in a haystack. Assessment must be rapid with limited extensive investigation, a rational for a simple, pragmatic approach.

Fritz JM, George S: The use of a classification approach to identify subgroups of patients with acute low back pain: Interrater reliability and short-term treatment outcomes. *Spine* 2000; 25:106-114.

This classification defines four groups using information gathered from the physical examination and patient self-reports. The classification guides treatment. It emphasizes the importance of the appropriate reliability coefficient. The study demonstrated differences in initial patient characteristics and treatment outcomes.

Keen S, Dowell AC, Hurst K, Klaber Moffett JA, Tovey P, Williams R: Individuals with low back pain: How do they view physical activity? *Fam Pract* 1999;16: 39-45.

Although an early return to activity is advocated by the current guidelines, it may be hindered by the patient's fear of pain. This study examines the relationship between levels of physical activity and the patient's perception of his or her pain-induced limitations.

Laslett M, van Wijmen P: Low back and referred pain: Diagnosis and a proposed new system of classification. *NZ J Phys* 1999;27:5-14.

Low back pain is categorized into 12 groups. The article describes the Quebec Task Force and McKenzie classifications. An appendix defines terms such as centralization and peripheralization used by physical therapists in the early treatment of acute low back pain.

Marshall KW: Practical implications of cyclooxygenase-2-specific inhibitors in orthopaedics. *Am J Orthop* 1999;28(suppl 3):19-21.

The study indicates a higher than anticipated risk of significant side effects with conventional NSAIDs. The odds ratio of serious gastrointestinal complications is approximately 2.5. The unpredictability of side effects in this group makes the COX-2 inhibitors an excellent alternative.

McKenna F: COX-2: Separating myth from reality. *Scand J Rheumatol Suppl* 1999;109:19-29.

Rankings of the COX-2/COX-1 inhibition ratios of various NSAIDs related to the agents' toxicities have been used to support COX-2 selectivity as an important factor in upper gastrointestinal safety. None of these claims has been supported by endoscopy studies.

Rainville J, Sobel JB, Banco RJ, Levine HL, Childs L: Low back and cervical spine disorders. *Orthop Clin North Am* 1996;27:729-746.

Management of neck and back pain maximizes the natural history and minimizes the resulting disability. When no medical or reversible causes are found, intervention is aimed at improving tolerance for physical activities and a rapid return to a normal lifestyle.

van den Hoogen HJ, Koes BW, van Eijk JT, Bouter LM, Deville W: On the course of low back pain in general practice: A one year follow-up study. *Ann Rheum Dis* 1998;57:13-19.

This is a 1-year follow-up on 443 consecutive cases of low back pain in general practice. The majority experienced at least one relapse within the first year. The pain and disability diminished more rapidly after a recurrence than after the initial episode.

Vroomen PC, de Krom MC, Knottnerus JA: Consistency of history taking and physical examination in patients with suspected lumbar nerve root involvement. *Spine* 2000;25:91-97.

This is a cross-sectional study of interobserver variability. All patients had significant referred leg pain. Limited straight leg raising occurred in two thirds and one third had abnormal neurology. The consistency of data improved when history and physical examination were combined and concordant.

Wilson L, Hall H, McIntosh G, Melles T: Intertester reliability of a low back pain classification system. *Spine* 1999;24:248-254.

The classifications in this article were subjected to a prospective intertester reliability study. Using pairs of physical therapists and a cohort of 204 patients, intertester reliability was 80.2%. A kappa coefficient of 0.614 indicated a low probability of chance agreement.

Classic Bibliography

Agency for Health Care Policy and Research, Bigos SJ (ed): *Acute Low Back Problems in Adults*. Rockville, MD, US Department of Health and Human Services, AHCPR Publication 95-0642, Clinical Practice Guideline #14, 1994.

Bush T, Cherkin D, Barlow W: The impact of physician attitudes on patient satisfaction with care for low back pain. *Arch Fam Med* 1993;2:301-305.

Donelson R, Silva G, Murphy K: Centralization phenomenon: Its usefulness in evaluating and treating referred pain. *Spine* 1990;15:211-213.

Hall H, Hadler NM: Controversy: Low back school. Education or exercise? *Spine* 1995;20:1097-1098.

McKenzie RA: *The Lumbar Spine: Mechanical Diagnosis and Therapy*. Waikanae, New Zealand, Spinal Publications, 1989.

Malmivaara A, Hakkinen U, Aro T, et al: The treatment of acute low back pain: Bed rest, exercises or ordinary activity? *N Engl J Med* 1995;332:351-355.

Report of the Quebec Task Force on Spinal Disorders: Scientific approach to the assessment and management of activity-related spinal disorders: A monograph for clinicians. *Spine* 1987;12(suppl 7):S1-S59.

Chapter 19

Nonsurgical Management of Acute Injuries to the Spine

James Kimbro Maguire, Jr, MD

Most acute injuries to the spine, whether to the skeleton or the soft tissues, are often managed nonsurgically. However, the term nonsurgical is not synonymous with the term conservative. In certain instances, surgical treatment might be considered more conservative than nonsurgical treatment.

Fractures of the Cervical Spine

Most fractures of the cervical spine do not require surgery. Nonsurgical management is usually appropriate in injuries without neurologic deficit and in stable injuries. Most bony injuries have the potential to heal with simple immobilization in an orthosis; ligamentous injuries heal less predictably and are more likely to require surgery.

The choice of orthosis should be based on the degree of instability of the injury and a knowledge of the ability of an orthosis to limit a particular motion. The halo vest is the most effective orthosis in controlling motion, particularly rotation and motion in the upper cervical spine. Most unstable injuries, when managed nonsurgically, are best immobilized in a halo vest. The halo vest is the only device that controls rotation to a significant degree. A comparison of different commercial halo vests did not demonstrate significant differences in their abilities to immobilize the spine.

Choices for the management of more stable injuries include soft collars, hard collars, cervicothoracic braces, or the sterno-occipital mandibular immobilizer. It is widely accepted that soft collars provide little immobilization. More restrictive devices provide greater immobilization, but a recent study demonstrated that none of these devices restricted motion to less than 19° of flexion-extension, 46° of axial rotation, or 45° of lateral bending. The Miami J collar (Jerome Medical, Moorestown, NJ) is more restrictive than either a Philadelphia collar (Philadelphia Collar, Philadelphia, PA) or the Aspen cervical thoracic orthosis (International Healthcare Devices, Long Beach, CA).

If an injury is unstable, the neck usually is immobilized for 8 to 12 weeks. At the conclusion of immobilization, flexion-extension lateral radiographs are essential to rule out instability.

Atlas Fractures

Fractures of the atlas vary in severity from simple fractures of the transverse process, to fractures involving the anterior or posterior arch, to lateral mass fractures and burst fractures. It is notable that 50% of atlas fractures are associated with other spinal fractures. Although they occasionally are associated with injuries to the greater occipital nerve or cranial nerves VI, X, XI, or XII, isolated fractures of the atlas expand the space available for the spinal cord and rarely are associated with major cord injury. Therefore, the presence of a neurologic deficit should prompt a search for an unrecognized fracture elsewhere in the spine.

Most atlas fractures can be treated nonsurgically. Isolated posterior arch fractures can be treated in a soft collar; most lateral mass and Jefferson fractures can be treated using a halo vest, usually for 3 months. Atlas fractures with a combined lateral mass displacement greater than 6.9 mm are considered less stable because of disruption of the transverse ligament. In spite of a greater degree of instability in fractures with transverse ligament disruption, nonsurgical treatment usually results in a stable spine. An initial period of traction has been advocated, but there is little support in the literature for such an approach. As with all fractures of the cervical spine that are managed nonsurgically, flexion-extension lateral radiographs are necessary at the completion of the period of immobilization, and surgical treatment should be considered when there is more than 5 mm of C1-C2 instability.

Odontoid Fractures

The classification system for odontoid fractures that was proposed by Anderson and D'Alonzo in 1974 is still most useful. There is little controversy that type I and III fractures can be managed best nonsurgically. However, the type I fracture, although appearing innocuous, can accompany occipitoatlantal instability, and the type III fracture that extends into the body, although appearing more stable, results in nonunion in 10% to 15% of cases and in malunion at a similar rate when treated in a halo.

Treatment of type II fractures is less straightforward. Patient factors to consider in choosing treatment methods for type II fractures include age and neurologic status. Fracture characteristics associated with nonunion and late instability include displacement greater than 5 mm, angulation greater than 10°, comminution, and association of other injuries, such as other fractures or ligamentous injuries. In a recent case-controlled study, age older than 50 years was found to be the most significant factor associated with failure of treatment in a halo.

There has been some support for primary surgical treatment of odontoid fractures that remain displaced more than 6 mm after an attempt at reduction or in patients older than 50 years. (Surgical indications and techniques are discussed in chapter 28, "Cervical Fractures and Dislocations.") Regarding nonsurgical treatment, one study demonstrated no significant difference in the clinical outcomes of patients treated with a halo vest versus those treated with a Philadelphia collar or similar orthosis. For those treated nonsurgically, the halo vest is the most common form of immobilization used to treat type II and III odontoid fractures. Immobilization for 12 weeks, followed by flexion-extension lateral radiographs, is recommended. Most type I fractures can be treated with a collar for 3 months, followed by flexion-extension lateral radiographs.

Traumatic Spondylolisthesis of the Axis

Fracture through the pars interarticularis of the axis, often accompanied by spondylolisthesis, is popularly referred to as a hangman's fracture. A hangman's fracture usually is not associated with neurologic injury when it occurs as an isolated injury. As many as one third of patients with this injury have another spine injury, however, so the presence of a neurologic deficit should prompt a search for additional occult injuries. The classification proposed by Levine and Edwards is the most widely used (Fig. 1). All except type III injuries (that is, those associated with a unilateral or bilateral facet joint dislocation at C2-C3) can be managed without surgery.

Type I injuries characterized by up to 3 mm of displacement and no angulation are the most stable and can be managed in a cervical collar for 8 to 12 weeks.

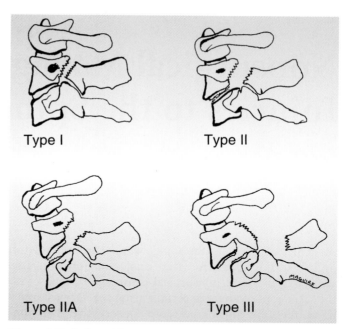

Figure 1 The Levine and Edwards classification of traumatic spondylolisthesis of the axis. Type I fractures are displaced less than 3 mm. Type II fractures are displaced with minimal angulation. The type IIA fracture subtype is identified by severe angulation; the application of traction might result in overdistraction of this injury. Type III injuries are characterized by a unilateral or bilateral facet dislocation at C2-3. (Adapted with permission from Levine AM, Edwards CC: The management of traumatic spondylolisthesis of the axis. *J Bone Joint Surg Am* 1985;67:217-226.)

Type II fractures are characterized by C2-C3 displacement and angulation. An initial period of traction has been advocated in certain type II fractures, but whether traction significantly improves outcome in these injuries is not known. When traction is being considered, it is important to rule out the type IIA fracture pattern, characterized by minimal displacement but significant angulation. These fractures are very unstable because of disruption of the disc and posterior longitudinal ligament. Traction for the patient with a type IIA fracture is contraindicated because overdistraction and iatrogenic neurologic injury can occur. With an expected union rate of 94.5%, halo immobilization is recommended for type II injuries. Gentle compression should be used when applying the halo to a patient with a type IIA fracture.

Fractures and Dislocations of the Lower Cervical Spine

Most unilateral facet dislocations, all bilateral facet dislocations, and all burst fractures associated with neurologic deficit should be treated surgically (see chapter 28). A compression fracture in the absence of posterior ligamentous injury usually will heal after 8 to 12 weeks in a rigid cervical orthosis. A wedge compression fracture should be suspected when the posterior vertebral body height exceeds the anterior height by 3 mm or more. One should suspect a posterior ligamentous injury when more than 25% of the anterior vertebral height is lost or when more than 11° of angulation exists between adjacent vertebral bodies. In such instances, the risk of developing late posttraumatic kyphosis is significant, and surgery should be considered.

Other fractures of the lower cervical spine that generally do not require surgery include isolated undisplaced fractures of the posterior elements or lateral mass fractures and low-velocity gunshot wounds. Most do well with 8 to 12 weeks of rigid cervical immobilization. The more severe variants of these injuries require surgical management (see chapter 28). Common injuries such as avulsion of the tips of spinous processes are benign but can sometimes lead to diagnostic confusion and excessive care when they are unrecognized because attention is focused on anterior elements. Careful radiographic follow-up is imperative during and after the period of immobilization to rule out instability.

Fractures of the Thoracolumbar Spine

A detailed description of all of the classification systems for fractures of the thoracolumbar spine is beyond the scope of this chapter. The classification system proposed by Denis is probably the most commonly used and is useful in making treatment decisions (Fig. 2). It is an anatomic system based on a three-column concept of the spine. The anterior column consists of the anterior longitudinal ligament, the anterior half of the vertebral body, and the associated disc and anulus. The middle column consists of the posterior half of the vertebral body, the posterior longitudinal ligament, and the associated disc and anulus. The posterior column is made up of the structures of the neural arch, the facet joints, and the associated ligamentous structures. According to this system, most fractures fall into one of four categories. Compression fractures involve failure of the middle column under compression. Burst fractures occur from failure of the anterior and middle columns under compression. Flexion-distraction injuries result because of failure of the posterior and middle columns under distraction. Fracture dislocations occur when all three columns fail and are the result of a variety of mechanisms.

Most compression fractures do not require surgery. Because many of these fractures occur in the osteoporotic spine, a clinical investigation and medical treatment for metabolic bone disease might be indicated. It is important to differentiate between benign and malignant causes of vertebral compression fractures; MRI is the most useful test for this, following a careful history and a physical examination. Benign osteoporotic com-

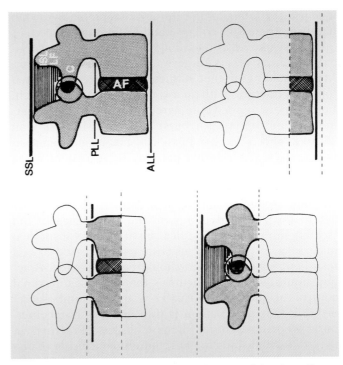

Figure 2 The Denis classification of thoracolumbar trauma is based on a three-column model of the spine. The anterior column consists of the anterior longitudinal ligament (ALL) and the anterior half of the body, disk, and anulus fibrosus (AF). The middle column is made up of the posterior longitudinal ligament (PLL) and the posterior half of the vertebral body, disk, and anulus fibrosus. The bony neural arch and associated soft-tissue suporting structures, including the supraspinous ligament (SSL), make up the posterior column. (Reproduced with permission from Denis F: The three-column spine and its significance in the classification of acute thoracolumbar spinal injuries. *Spine* 1983;8:817-831.)

pression fractures occur most commonly at the apex of the dorsal kyphus and at the thoracolumbar junction, calling for additional circumspection in evaluation of those occurring at other sites. Homogeneous alteration of the entire marrow signal of the vertebral body or the presence of a soft-tissue mass on MRI should alert the clinician to the possibility of a malignant process. Most benign compression fractures can be managed symptomatically. Activity modification and bracing might help with pain control but probably will not affect the ultimate outcome. Rigid bracing often is not well tolerated in elderly patients, but soft binders or corsets might provide some support and symptom relief. Vertebroplasty and kyphoplasty are two new techniques that offer promise in treating painful compression fractures that do not respond to noninvasive methods.

Isolated anterior column injuries in younger patients require a more cautious approach. The trauma to produce the injury is greater, and younger patients are more tolerant of bracing. A rigid brace of the Jewett or Knight-Taylor design is adequate for these fractures at the thoracolumbar junction and upper lumbar spine. It is important to maintain careful radiographic follow-up because progressive collapse and instability can occur.

Controversy exists regarding indications for nonsurgical treatment versus surgery for some burst fractures. Most would agree that surgical treatment is indicated for burst fractures with an associated neurologic deficit. Furthermore, most would agree that nonsurgical treatment is appropriate for burst fractures with less than 25° of kyphosis and less than 50% canal compromise in the neurologically intact patient. Treatment of more severe fractures in the neurologically intact patient is controversial, and there are proponents of both surgical and nonsurgical management of these injuries. To some extent the choice depends on the experience of the treating surgeon and medical institution. Nonsurgical management usually begins with a short period of bed rest. Ileus is common and should be anticipated. Bracing should be with an orthosis that provides maximal control of the spine, usually a thoracolumbosacral orthosis. Once the patient is fitted with a thoracolumbosacral orthosis, he or she is mobilized. Fractures in the low lumbar spine might require the inclusion of one thigh in the brace to limit pelvic motion. Bracing is maintained for 12 weeks, and fracture healing is monitored radiographically. An active rehabilitation program is initiated after the brace is removed.

The classic Chance fracture is a flexion-distraction injury involving transverse fracture through the bony elements of all three columns. In these cases, the anterior longitudinal ligament is intact and the injury often is stable enough to be managed nonsurgically. In less stable variants of the flexion-distraction injury, the fulcrum is within the middle column. Loss of anterior body height is the hallmark of this variant. Flexion-distraction injuries in which the plane of disruption is through ligamentous rather than bony elements heal less predictably, so surgical stabilization of this variant should be considered.

Most fracture-dislocations of the thoracolumbar spine should be managed surgically. These injuries represent disruptions of all three columns of the spine and are very unstable. Any rotational or translational displacement between the injured segments should alert the clinician to a three-column injury.

Isolated fractures of the spinous or transverse process are stable and do not require surgery. The clinician should search for such injuries when the etiology of pain following trauma is not apparent (Fig. 3).

Like all musculotendinous and ligamentous structures, those of the thoracolumbar spine are subject to sprains, strains, and traction injuries. Pain from such occurences is usually brief and responsive to simple standard measures, such as rest and ice. Permanent sequelae are infrequent and hard to document. Most

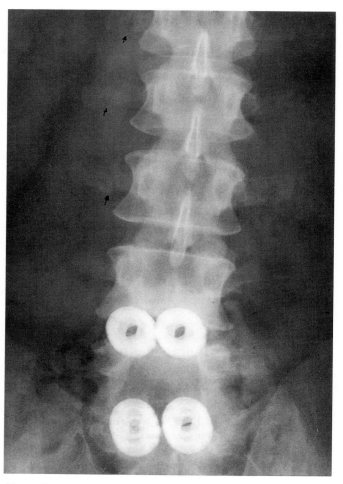

Figure 3 This 40-year-old man with a complex history of prior back trouble complained of pain in his upper lumbar spine and right flank following a motor vehicle accident. His pain was explained on the basis of multiple transverse process fractures.

often, the specific anatomic structure that is injured cannot be documented with confidence, but there are a few exceptions.

Traction or direct trauma can injure the long thoracic or, more frequently, the suprascapular nerve, causing well-defined syndromes of dorsal pain and weakness that can be documented clinically and electromyographically. The anulus fibrosus of a previously normal disc can be disrupted by violent injury, as evidence by convincing history and physical findings suggesting violent injury to a segment observed on MRI to contain a high-intensity zone in the outer anulus of a disc with normal signals in the nucleus. The presence of a high-intensity zone in the outer anulus of a disc containing other imaging signs of degeneration, such as decreased signal in the nucleus on T2, does not suggest acute injury.

If symptoms presumed to be caused by acute musculotendinous or ligamentous injuries of specific thora-

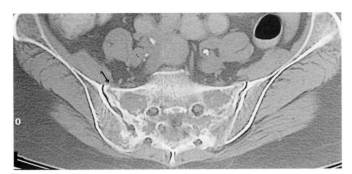

Figure 4 CT scan of patient with a fracture of the sacrum. Note the subtle disruption of the ventral cortex of the ala.

columbar tissues do not not respond quickly to rest and simple measures, they should be treated according to the principles of treatment of nonspecific back pain.

Fractures of the Sacrum

Sacral fractures are unique in that the sacrum is the junction between the spine and the pelvis. Ninety-five percent of sacral fractures occur in association with pelvic fractures, and principles common to pelvic fractures can apply in certain sacral fractures. Vertical or oblique fractures are the most common and account for 90% of sacral injuries. These injuries can be missed on plain film radiographs; careful attention to the cortices of the foramina might reveal subtle fractures. CT is the best radiographic method for defining sacral fractures (Fig. 4). Interpretation is aided by tilting the gantry to accommodate the angle of the sacrum. Sagittal reconstructions might be required to demonstrate transverse fractures. A thorough neurologic examination is essential to identify bowel or bladder dysfunction; deficits can be missed, especially in catheterized patients. A rectal examination to test sphincter tone and perineal sensation and measurement of postvoiding residual urine volume can help identify injuries to caudal nerve roots. Urodynamics and sphincter electromyography can supplement the clinical examination.

The classification proposed by Denis is the most commonly used system for vertical fractures of the sacrum (Fig. 5). In this system, the sacrum is divided into three zones. Zone 1 injuries are through the ala and have the lowest incidence of associated neurologic deficit. Zone 2 injuries are through the foramina. Zone 3 injuries involve the central canal and have the highest incidence of associated neurologic deficits.

The stability of the pelvic ring and the neurologic status usually determine treatment. The likelihood that surgery will be required is least for fractures in zone 1 and greatest in zone 3. When the pelvic ring is stable and the patient is neurologically intact, nonsurgical

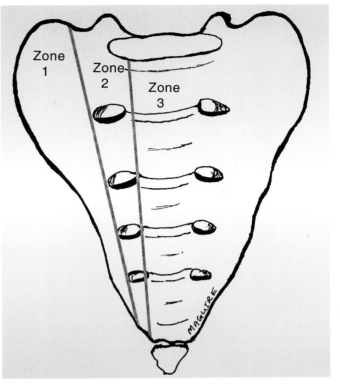

Figure 5 This classification of vertical sacral fractures is based on the work of Denis. Fractures are classified according to one of three zones of injury. The most medial extension of the fracture determines the classification. (Adapted with permission from Denis F, Davis S, Comfort T: Sacral fractures: An important problem. Retrospective analysis of 236 cases. *Clin Orthop* 1988;227:67-81.)

treatment is indicated. Early ambulation with protected weight bearing is appropriate but should be initiated with caution; also, careful follow-up is indicated because of the possibility of occult instability.

Transverse fractures of the sacrum are less common but also can be diagnostically challenging because they occur often in multiply injured patients. These fractures might not be readily seen on standard radiographic views. Frequently, they are accompanied by avulsion of lumbar transverse processes, which might be a clue to their presence. Some transverse fractures involve neurologic injury. Most can be managed nonsurgically. Flexion stress should be avoided, and weight bearing approached cautiously.

Sacral insufficiency fractures represent a different clinical entity. These are stress fractures that might occur in the absence of significant trauma. They frequently occur in patients who have undergone radiation therapy for a pelvic malignancy or in association with osteoporosis. The primary problem with these injuries is that of recognition; they should be considered in the differential diagnosis of caudal spine or posterior pelvic pain in the osteoporotic patient. A bone scan is usually diagnostic, displaying a classic H-shaped pattern of

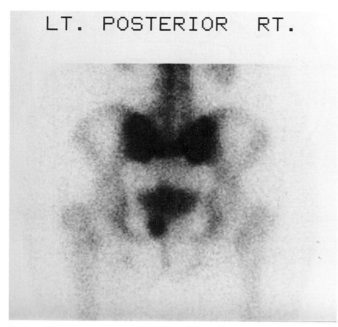

LT. POSTERIOR RT.

Figure 6 Technetium Tc 99m-medronate methylene diphosphonate scan of an elderly female who developed the spontaneous onset of low back and pelvic pain. The H-shaped pattern of tracer uptake is characteristic of sacral insufficiency fractures.

increased tracer uptake (Fig. 6). With a history of malignancy, metastatic disease must be considered, and the patient should be evaluated by MRI. Treatment is with activity modification, use of a walker, and symptomatic management. Resolution of symptoms can be expected within 3 months.

Whiplash-Associated Disorders

Considerable controversy surrounds whiplash-associated disorders of the cervical spine. The terminology surrounding this entity is not uniform. Other terms are used synonymously with whiplash, including acceleration injury to the neck, cervical sprain, and cervical hyperextension injury. It is likely that the term whiplash actually is applied to many different injuries of varying severity. This injury to the cervical spine is frequently linked to a specific injury mechanism: rear-end motor vehicle collisions. Often implicit in this mechanism are the issues of fault and associated legal ramifications; all of these factors can affect treatment and influence ultimate patient outcome.

There are very few well-done studies related to whiplash. As part of the investigation conducted by the Quebec Task Force, more than 10,000 publications related to whiplash-type injuries were reviewed. Of these, only 294 were considered eligible for consideration after the application of a standardized review process, and very few of these were considered to be of sufficient quality to allow firm recommendations to be

made. The report ended with a plea for better research.

Whiplash is a diagnosis of exclusion of other identifiable injury. The best diagnostic approach is to obtain plain radiographs, including flexion-extension lateral views of the cervical spine, after a thorough history and physical examination. Additional testing, including MRI and a bone scan, is indicated in patients who fail to respond to treatment.

Most treatments for patients with whiplash-associated disorders have not been evaluated scientifically; nevertheless, the general consensus is that prolonged immobilization is to be avoided. A short period in a collar is acceptable, but mobilization therapy should be initiated early. Nonsteroidal anti-inflammatory drugs and analgesics are commonly prescribed. It is believed that early, active intervention is crucial to limit the duration of symptoms. Educating the patient is an important component of treatment. Statistics related to the prognosis vary among studies, but it is clear that, for the majority of patients, this is a benign condition with complete recovery. A small percentage of patients will not recover as expected. The patient with chronic symptoms is best managed with a multidisciplinary approach, as any patient with chronic pain would be.

Soft-Tissue Injuries of the Neck

Injuries to the ligamentous structures supporting the cervical spine can occur by mechanisms other than vehicular trauma. Cervical sprains are graded based on the severity of the injury. Grade I sprains are partial tears with no defect or instability. Grade II sprains are characterized by a palpable defect but no instability. Grade III sprains are diagnosed by subluxation of the facet joint without dislocation, and grade IV sprains are complete ligamentous disruptions with dislocation. Grade I and II sprains are stable and can be managed nonsurgically.

The hallmarks of treatment of these stable injuries include the control of pain, the maintenance of motion, the prevention of muscle atrophy, and the avoidance of chronicity. Temporary immobilization with a cervical collar can be useful in reducing the pain acutely, but prolonged use of a collar is to be avoided. An early exercise program that includes isometric and isotonic exercises can help maintain muscle tone and flexibility, thus reducing the chances for chronic pain. In addition to an active rehabilitation program, potential treatment modalities for the patient with acute neck strain include pharmacologic agents, education, manipulation, and injection therapy. A few points bear emphasis. The scientific basis for any of these modalities is limited. Drugs commonly used include nonsteroidal anti-inflammatory drugs, analgesics, and muscle relaxers. None of the various anti-inflammatory drugs has proved to be more effective than the others. Two new drugs with more specificity for the cyclooxygenase-2 enzyme hold promise, but their increased efficacy is unproven. Narcotic analgesics are appropriate for acute pain, but their use must be monitored closely. The benefit of muscle relaxers is questionable. However, whether a formal neck school program could make a significant difference in these patients is debatable. Spinal manipulation is becoming more accepted but remains controversial. Injection of tender "trigger points" might provide some relief, but the mechanism of pain reduction is not understood.

Although many disc herniations occur in the absence of demonstrable trauma, the disc can herniate as a result of an acute injury. Most cervical disc herniations respond favorably to a nonsurgical management program. Recommended management includes traction, specific therapeutic exercises, oral anti-inflammatory medication, and patient education. Cervical epidural corticosteroids can be useful, but their risk-benefit ratio has not been established. High patient satisfaction with nonsurgical care has been demonstrated; therefore, surgery should be considered only after nonsurgical management has failed.

Annotated Bibliography

Fractures of the Cervical Spine

An HS: Cervical spine trauma. *Spine* 1998;23:2713-2729.

This is an excellent, comprehensive review of this subject with an extensive bibliography.

Askins V, Eismont FJ: Efficacy of five cervical orthoses in restricting cervical motion: A comparison study. *Spine* 1997;22:1193-1198.

This radiographic study of 20 normal volunteers investigated the effectiveness of several commercially available cervical orthoses. The NecLoc orthosis (Jerome Medical) was the most effective in restricting motion, followed by the Miami J collar.

Glaser JA, Jaworski BA, Cuddy BG, et al: Variations in surgical opinion regarding management of selected cervical spine injuries: A preliminary study. *Spine* 1998;23:975-983.

Thirty-one orthopaedic surgeons and neurosurgeons who deal with cervical trauma were given clinical information and radiographic studies for five selected cervical injuries. A large variety of opinion regarding treatment choices was noted, implying a wide variation in accepted standard management for many of these injuries.

Greene KA, Dickman CA, Marciano FF, Drabier JB, Hadley MN, Sonntag VK: Acute axis fractures: Analysis of management and outcome in 340 consecutive cases. *Spine* 1997;22:1843-1852.

Nonsurgical treatment was recommended for most type II odontoid fractures. Indications for surgery included instability in spite of external immobilization, transverse ligament disruption, displacement of at least 6 mm, and association with a hangman's fracture.

Hart R, Saterbak A, Rapp T, Clark C: Nonoperative management of dens fracture nonunion in elderly patients without myelopathy. *Spine* 2000;25:1339-1343.

This retrospective study of a group of elderly patients with mobile nonunions of the odontoid process treated nonsurgically demonstrated good results. No patient developed myelopathy and none of the fractures developed increased instability. A nonsurgical treatment protocol might be appropriate in patients who are poor candidates for surgical fusion.

Lennarson PJ, Mostafavi H, Traynelis VC, Walters BC: Management of type II dens fractures: A case-control study. *Spine* 2000;25:1234-1237.

The risk of failure of halo immobilization was found to be 21 times higher in patients older than 50 years of age. The authors advised surgical intervention for type II odontoid fractures in older patients.

Mirza SK, Moquin RR, Anderson PA, Tencer AF, Steinmann J, Varnau D: Stabilizing properties of the halo apparatus. *Spine* 1997;22:727-733.

This cadaveric study demonstrated that vest fit and tightness were important to maximize the effectiveness of the halo apparatus. There was no significant difference in effectiveness among various commercially available halo vests.

Polin RS, Szabo T, Bogaev CA, Replogle RE, Jane JA: Nonoperative management of types II and III odontoid fractures: The Philadelphia collar versus the halo vest. *Neurosurgery* 1996;38:450-457.

This retrospective study compared union rates and late instability in patients with odontoid fractures treated with either a halo or a rigid cervical orthosis. There was no significant difference among results for the two treatment methods, even in type II fractures. A case is made for the use of a rigid orthosis rather than a halo for the nonsurgical management of these fractures.

Sandler AJ, Dvorak J, Humke T, Grob D, Daniels W: The effectiveness of various cervical orthoses: An in vivo comparison of the mechanical stability provided by several widely used models. *Spine* 1996;21:1624-1629.

This study demonstrated that cervical orthoses do not provide a high level of mechanical restriction of motion. The sterno-occipital mandibular immobilizer was the most restrictive device tested, but the difference was not great and might not be enough to justify one of the more expensive or less comfortable orthoses. A criticism of this study is that segmental spinal motion was not evaluated.

Thoracolumbar and Sacral Fractures

Chow GH, Nelson BJ, Gebhard JS, Brugman JL, Brown CW, Donaldson DH: Functional outcome of thoracolumbar burst fractures managed with hyperextension casting or bracing and early mobilization. *Spine* 1996;21:2170-2175.

This is a retrospective review of 26 patients with unstable burst fractures treated nonsurgically. Good clinical results were noted in spite of the fact that the patients had ligamentous injury to the posterior column.

Seybold EA, Sweeney CA, Fredrickson BE, Warhold LG, Bernini PM: Functional outcome of low lumbar burst fractures: A multicenter review of operative and nonoperative treatment of L3-L5. *Spine* 1999;24:2154-2161.

This retrospective study of 42 patients advocates nonsurgical treatment of these less common fractures. The results of nonsurgical treatment were comparable with those of surgical treatment.

Shen WJ, Shen YS: Nonsurgical treatment of three-column thoracolumbar junction burst fractures without neurologic deficit. *Spine* 1999;24:412-415.

Thirty-eight patients with single-level burst fractures associated with posterior-element fractures were studied retrospectively. The patients in this study were rapidly mobilized, and only minimal bracing was used. Results were similar to those of patients treated with more restricted protocols.

Whiplash-Associated Disorders

Borchgrevink GE, Kaasa A, McDonagh D, Stiles TC, Haraldseth O, Lereim I: Acute treatment of whiplash neck sprain injuries: A randomized trial of treatment during the first 14 days after a car accident. *Spine* 1998;23:25-31.

Immobilization and sick leave for patients were associated with a poorer outcome than were mobilization and continuation of normal activities.

Lord SM, Barnsley L, Wallis BJ, Bogduk N: Chronic cervical zygapophysial joint pain after whiplash: A placebo-controlled prevalence study. *Spine* 1996;21:1737-1745.

This well-done, placebo-controlled study indicates that the cervical zygapophyseal joint is a common pain generator in patients who have developed chronic pain after whiplash injury. The C2-C3 joint was usually responsible in patients with upper neck pain and headache. The C5-C6 joint was the usual source in patients with lower cervical axial pain and referred arm pain.

Pettersson K, Hildingsson C, Toolanen G, Fagerlund M, Bjornebrink J: Disc pathology after whiplash injury: A prospective magnetic resonance imaging and clinical investigation. *Spine* 1997;22:283-288.

The authors conclude that it is not advisable to use MRI in patients with whiplash injuries during the acute phase because of the high proportion of false-positive findings.

Pettersson K, Toolanen G: High-dose methylprednisolone prevents extensive sick leave after whiplash injury: A prospective, randomized, double-blind study. *Spine* 1998; 23:984-989.

This small study suggests that treatment with methylprednisolone within 8 hours after injury shortens the duration of symptoms in patients with whiplash injury. This treatment is not benign and more studies, including an assessment of the risks versus benefits of this approach, are needed before this treatment can be recommended.

Soft-Tissue Injuries to the Neck

Cummins CA, Messer TM, Nuber GW: Suprascapular nerve entrapment. *J Bone Joint Surg Am* 2000;82:415-425.

The authors review more than 100 articles published since the syndrome of suprascapular nerve injury and dysfunction was reported in 1959. Direct trauma, traction injury, or entrapment of the suprascapular nerve can cause dorsal pain with weakness and atrophy of the infraspinatus and/or supraspinatous muscles—a syndrome easily overlooked or confused with other cervical or dorsal syndromes.

Hodges SD, Castleberg RL, Miller T, Ward R, Thomburg C: Cervical epidural steroid injection with intrinsic spinal cord damage: Two case reports. *Spine* 1998;23:2137-2142.

Two patients who sustained spinal cord injury at the time of epidural corticosteroid injection are reported. The injuries occurred in spite of the fact that fluoroscopy was used. The authors speculate that intravenous sedation prevented the patient from reporting the usual symptoms associated with spinal cord irritation. It is recommended that the patient be fully awake at the time of injection.

Saal JS, Saal JA, Yurth EF: Nonoperative management of herniated cervical intervertebral disc with radiculopathy. *Spine* 1996;21:1877-1883.

    In this longitudinal cohort study, 24 of 26 patients with cervical disc herniation were successfully managed with an aggressive nonsurgical treatment plan.

Classic Bibliography

Anderson LD, D'Alonzo RT: Fractures of the odontoid process of the axis. *J Bone Joint Surg Am* 1974;56: 1663-1674.

Denis F: The three-column spine and its significance in the classification of acute thoracolumbar spinal injuries. *Spine* 1983;8:817-831.

Denis F, Davis S, Comfort T: Sacral fractures: An important problem. Retrospective analysis of 236 cases. *Clin Orthop* 1988;227:67-81.

Francis WR, Fielding JW, Hawkins RJ, Pepin J, Hensinger R: Traumatic spondylolisthesis of the axis. *J Bone Joint Surg Br* 1981;63:313-318.

Levine AM, Edwards CC: The management of traumatic spondylolisthesis of the axis. *J Bone Joint Surg Am* 1985;67:217-226.

Newhouse KE, el-Khoury GY, Buckwalter JA: Occult sacral fractures in osteopenic patients. *J Bone Joint Surg Am* 1992;74:1472-1477.

Spitzer WO, Skovron ML, Salmi LR, et al: Scientific monograph of the Quebec Task Force on Whiplash-Associated Disorders: Redefining "whiplash" and its management. *Spine* 1995;20(suppl 8):1S-73S.

Wolf JW Jr, Johnson RM: Cervical orthoses, in Cervical Spine Research Society Editorial Committee (eds): *The Cervical Spine*, ed 2. Philadelphia, PA, JB Lippincott, 1989, pp 97-105.

Chapter 20

Pharmacologic Care of Arthritic and Metabolic Disorders of the Spine

David Borenstein, MD

A variety of illnesses can affect the structures of the spine. Mechanical disorders can cause degenerative changes in the lumbar spine associated with pain and local inflammation that manifest as vertebral osteoarthritis (OA). Spondyloarthropathies (SPAs) are a group of inflammatory disorders that cause calcification of paraspinous structures, resulting in limitation of motion and eventual fusion of the axial skeleton. In contrast with SPAs, which affect the entire spine, rheumatoid arthritis (RA) primarily damages the cervical spine. In addition, the muscles that support the axial skeleton can be damaged by mechanical and inflammatory processes. Disorders that affect paraspinous muscles include muscle strain and polymyalgia rheumatica. Osteoporosis (OSP) is a disorder of bone associated with loss of bone mass per unit volume. In the axial skeleton, the reduction of bone mass is most noticeable in the thoracic spine and lumbar spine.

No single therapy is effective for all of the illnesses that cause spinal disease. Different categories of drugs are effective for the control of symptoms and signs associated with specific illnesses. The nonsurgical therapy of spinal disease involves a process of choosing the appropriate combination of agents to maximize function for patients with spinal pain and inflammation. In a majority of individuals with mechanical disorders, a single agent is adequate to decrease pain. However, the more inflammatory the disorder, the greater is the need for a combination of multiple drug categories to obtain symptomatic control of spinal disease.

Nonsteroidal Anti-Inflammatory Drugs

Nonsteroidal anti-inflammatory drugs (NSAIDs) are the most frequently prescribed class of agents. NSAIDs are indicated for a variety of musculoskeletal diseases, including muscle injuries, OA, SPAs, and RA. NSAIDs possess antipyretic, analgesic, anti-inflammatory, and antithrombotic characteristics. NSAIDs have analgesic properties when given in single doses and are anti-inflammatory and analgesic when given long-term in larger doses. The limiting factor in the utility of NSAIDs is their toxicities, which include gastrointestinal dysfunction (dyspepsia, bowel perforations, obstruction) and renal dysfunction (proteinuria, renal failure).

Both the therapeutic effects and potential toxicities of NSAIDs are related to the inhibition of the synthesis of prostaglandins (PGs) by the cyclooxygenase (COX) enzyme. A single COX enzyme was thought to regulate the production of PGs for the maintenance of organ function (gastric mucosal integrity) and the promotion of an inflammatory response. However, understanding of the mechanism of action of the NSAIDs has been advanced by the identification of two forms of the COX enzyme.

COX-1 is a constitutive form that produces PGs that maintain organ function. COX-1 is inhibited by most of the available NSAIDs (for example, ibuprofen, naproxen, and indomethacin). Inhibition of COX-1 activity induced by the NSAIDs is associated with increased risk of gastrointestinal toxicity, potential renal dysfunction in at-risk patients, and decreased aggregation of platelets associated with increased risk of bleeding. COX-2 is an inducible enzyme that develops at inflammatory sites with the stimulation of inflammatory cytokines, growth factors, and endotoxin. COX-2 is also inhibited by the same number of NSAIDs.

The two isoforms of the COX enzymes differ in the shape of their active sites. The active site of COX-1 has a linear configuration, whereas the COX-2 active site is located in a side pocket off the main channel of the enzyme. The original NSAIDs had chemical forms that easily fit into both active sites. Since 1998, though, spe-

The author or the department with which he is affiliated has received something of value from a commercial or other party related directly or indirectly to the subject of this chapter.

cific COX-2 inhibitors that have been approved by the Food and Drug Administration for use in pain, OA, and RA, have side chains that fit into the COX-2 active site, inhibiting the production of inflammatory PGs. The same side chain physically excludes COX-2 drugs from entering the COX-1 active site. The clinical result of COX-2 inhibition is the control of inflammation and pain to a degree similar to that measured with COX-1/COX-2 inhibitors, with a significant decrease in associated toxicity in the gastrointestinal tract, kidney, and platelets. For example, in distinction from patients taking COX-1/COX-2 inhibitors, individuals taking COX-2 inhibitors have a normal bleeding time. Also, COX-2 patients are able to take their medication up to the time of their invasive procedures without the exacerbation of disease associated with the discontinuation of their NSAID.

Studies demonstrating the efficacy of COX-2 inhibitors in the treatment of acute pain, OA, and RA have been completed, although no studies are available documenting the efficacy of COX-2 inhibitors in SPAs. In general, however, doses effective for RA are also useful for the control of spinal inflammation associated with SPAs.

The NSAIDs and COX-2 inhibitors currently available for the treatment of spinal disorders are listed in Table 1. The choice and dosage of NSAIDs depend on factors related to the medical condition and to the individual patient. Acute mechanical conditions occurring in young individuals require NSAIDs with rapid onset of action and analgesic properties. The duration of NSAID therapy in these acute mechanical disorders is 2 to 4 weeks. Concerns regarding toxicity are less significant in these acute disorders with rapid resolution in young individuals without concomitant medical disorders (eg, heart disease) compared with older patients.

OA of the lumbar spine is a chronic condition that occurs in elderly individuals. OA is a painful, locally inflammatory arthritis. Elderly patients with OA of the lumbar spine have a great likelihood of suffering from concomitant medical disorders, such as diabetes, hypertension, or congestive heart failure. The presence of OA in elderly patients necessitates the use of NSAIDs at the lowest effective dose for extended periods of time, measured in months to years. In the past, these patients would have been at risk for NSAID-associated toxicity. Today, OA patients with prior gastrointestinal ulcerations are appropriate recipients of COX-2 inhibitors.

Patients with a SPA or RA have a systemic inflammatory disorder. NSAIDs are an essential component of therapy used for the control of these disorders and must be used at maximum dosages for extended periods of time, measured in years. NSAIDs with prolonged half-lives require less-frequent dosing for persistent anti-inflammatory effect. NSAIDs with shorter half-lives but in sustained-release formulations offer similar characteristics. Of course, NSAIDs should be taken with food to decrease gastrointestinal toxicities.

The clinician should take into account the characteristics of both the patient and the drug in deciding on the best agent for a particular individual. Of greatest importance is efficacy. A drug should be used until it reaches a steady-state level (five half-lives) before determining efficacy. If an agent helps for a portion of the day but then loses effect, an additional dose at the end of a day might be appropriate. Also, an effective drug might cause toxicity. Alterations in certain social habits (alcohol and coffee consumption, smoking) or adding proton-pump inhibitors or misoprostol are useful to limit toxicity. Individuals who have failed other NSAIDs, who have a history of gastrointestinal ulceration, or who are taking corticosteroids are appropriate candidates for COX-2 inhibitors.

Disease-Modifying Antirheumatic Drugs

RA is a destructive, inflammatory arthropathy. The disease process causes joint destruction early in the course of the illness. RA usually affects the cervical spine at a time when the appendicular joints have developed destructive synovitis. Therefore, RA patients with cervical spine involvement have a stage of disease that requires more aggressive therapy. The traditional RA therapeutic pyramid included the prolonged use of NSAIDs before the initiation of disease-modifying antirheumatic drugs (DMARDs). DMARDs were added when NSAIDs were determined to be ineffective. However, this protocol resulted in needless joint destruction and increased morbidity and mortality. Currently, a consensus has been reached that the use of DMARDs is indicated in the early stages of RA. A combination of NSAIDs and DMARDs, with or without corticosteroids, is necessary for adequate control of joint synovitis. Currently available DMARDs are listed in Table 2.

A number of DMARDs with modes of action different from those of currently available DMARDs have been approved by the FDA for the treatment of RA. These DMARDs are as effective as methotrexate (MTX) for the treatment of RA. MTX, a purine inhibitor, is the DMARD against which the other DMARDs are measured. The usual dose of MTX ranges from 7.5 to 25 mg orally over 24 hours once a week. MTX decreases inflammation within 4 to 6 weeks. The dose should be raised in increments of 2.5 mg until control of joint inflammation is achieved. Sustained improvement for more than 10 years has been documented in patients with RA who have taken continuous

TABLE 1 | Nonsteroidal Anti-Inflammatory Drugs

Drug (Chemical Class)	Trade Name	Size (mg)	Max Dose (mg/day)	Frequency (x/day)	Onset (h)	Half-life (h)
Salicylates						
Aspirin	Bayer	325	5,200	4-6	1-2	4
Enteric coated	Ecotrin	325	5,200	4-6	1-2	4
Enteric coated	Easprin	975	3,900	4	1-2	4
time-release	Zorprin	800	3,200	2	2	4
Substituted Salicylates						
Diflunisal	Dolobid	250/500	1,500	2-3	1 (with loading)	11
Salsalate	Disalcid	500/750	3,000	2	2	4
Choline magnesium trisalicylate	Trilisate	500/750	3,000	2	2	4
Aspirin/antacid	Ascriptin	325	5,200	4-6	2	4
Propionic acid						
Ibuprofen	Motrin	400, 600, 800	4,800	4-6	1-2	1-3
Naproxen	Naprelan	375, 500	1,500	2-3	2	13
	Anaprox	275, 550	1,100	2	1-2	13
Fenoprofen	Nalfon	200, 300, 600	3,000	3-4	2	2-3
Ketoprofen	Orudis	25, 50, 75	300	3-4	2	3-4
Extended release	Oruvail	100, 150, 200				
Flurbiprofen	Ansaid	50, 100	300	2-3	1-2	6
Oxaprozin	Daypro	600	1,800	1-2	3-5	25
Pyrole acetic acid						
Sulindac	Clinoril	150, 200	450	2-3	2	18
Indomethacin	Indocin	25, 50, 75 SR, suppositories	225	1-3	2	4
Tolmetin	Tolectin	200, 400	1,600	4	1	4
Benzeneacetic acid						
Diclofenac sodium	Voltaren	25, 50, 75, 100 SR	225	2-3	2-3	2
Diclofenac potassium	Cataflam	25, 50	150	2-3	1	2
Diclofenac/Misoprostol	Arthrotec	50/75	225	2-3	1	2
Oxicam						
Piroxicam	Feldene	10, 20	20	1	5	38-45
Pyranocarboxylic Acid						
Etodolac	Lodine	200, 300, 400 XL, 500 XL	1,600	2-4	2	6
Fenemate						
Meclofenemate	Meclomen	50, 100	400	4	1	4
Pyrrolopyrrole						
Ketorolac	Toradol	10	40	4	1	4-6
Naphthylalkanone						
Nabumetone	Relafen	500, 750	2,000	2	4	26
COX-2 inhibitors						
Celecoxib	Celebrex	100, 200	400	2	3	11
Refecoxib	Vioxx	12.5, 25, 50	50	1	1	18
Meloxicam	Mobic	7.5	7.5	1	5	15

(Adapted with permission from Borenstein DG, Wiesel SW, Boden SD: Medical therapy, in Low Back Pain: Medical Diagnosis and Comprehensive Management, *ed 2. Philadelphia, PA, WB Saunders, 1995, pp 626-627.)*

TABLE 2 | Disease-Modifying Antirheumatic Drugs

Drug	Size (mg)	Dosage (mg)	Toxicities	Comment
Hydroxychloroquine	200	200-400	Retinopathy	Requires 6 mo to work
Sulfasalazine	500	1,000-2,000	GI, anemia	Sulfa allergy
Gold (PO)	3	3-9	GI, anemia	Requires 3-6 mo to work
Gold (IM)	5 mg/mL	10-50	Thrombocytopenia, proteinuria	Requires 2 mo to work
Penicillamine	125, 250	125-750	Thrombocytopenia, proteinuria	Requires 2 mo to work
Methotrexate	2.5	5-25	Hepatitis, pneumonitis	Requires 6 wk to work
Azathioprine	50	50-300	Hepatitis, leukopenia	Requires 3 mo to work
Cyclosporine	25, 50, 100	Up to 5 mg/kg	Hypertension	Limited by toxicity
Leflunomide	10, 20, 100	20	Diarrhea, alopecia	100 × 3 day initially, onset at 4 wk
Etanercept (IM)	25	25 twice a week	Injection site pain, URI	Requires 3 mo to work
Infliximab (IV)	100	3 mg/kg	Nausea, URI	Best with MTX

IM = intramuscularly; IV = intravenously; PO = per os (orally); URI = upper respiratory infection; GI=gastrointestinal

MTX therapy. Monitoring potential MTX toxicities requires complete blood count and liver function tests every 6 to 8 weeks. Alopecia and oropharyngeal ulcerations are mitigated through the use of folic acid 1 mg every day except the day of MTX ingestion.

Leflunomide (LEF), a pyrimidine inhibitor, is a new immunomodulator that inhibits cell proliferation in activated lymphocytes in patients with active RA. The onset of action, at 4 weeks, is earlier than that of MTX. Functional improvement is greater with LEF than with sulfasalazine or MTX. Like other DMARDs, LEF delays the rate of progression of radiologically measured RA. The half-life of LEF is 2 weeks. With such a prolonged half-life, the initial dose of drug is 100 mg for 3 days, then 20 mg/day. The most common adverse reactions include diarrhea, elevated liver enzyme (ALT or AST > 49 mL), and alopecia. The dose can be decreased to 10 mg if toxicity appears. LEF is contraindicated in pregnancy, and women contemplating pregnancy must undergo a drug-elimination program with cholestyramine to remove LEF from enterohepatic circulation. LEF and MTX taken together have a synergistic effect in diminishing joint inflammation without a significant increase in drug toxicity.

Tumor necrosis factor-alpha (TNF-α) is a proinflammatory cytokine produced primarily by activated macrophages and monocytes. TNF-α induces vasodilation and vascular permeability; activates platelets; increases production of collagenase and superoxide radicals; and mediates fever, anemia, and cachexia. In patients with active RA, TNF-α levels are elevated in serum and synovial fluid. The biologic activity of TNF-α is mediated by specific transmembrane receptors on inflammatory cells. A TNF-α molecule cross-links with two receptors to initiate a response. The extracellular portions of the TNF-α receptors are shed by cells and act as functional antagonists of TNF-α. The degree of TNF-α–mediated inflammation depends on the balance between TNF-α and its soluble receptor.

Etanercept is a dimeric fusion protein consisting of two copies of the extracellular receptor ligand for TNF-α linked by the constant portion of human immunoglobulin G (IgG). Infliximab is a chimeric monoclonal antibody directed against TNF-α. This antibody consists of an Fc human constant portion of IgG combined with a Fab murine variable region with binding properties for TNF-α. Both of these antibody therapies are effective in decreasing synovitis associated with RA. Etanercept is administered as a 25-mg intramuscular injection twice a week. It can be given individually or in combination with other DMARDs. Onset of effect is within 4 weeks. Toxicities include injection site pain and increased risk of upper respiratory infections. Infliximab is administered intravenously at a dose of 3 mg/kg at 0, 2, and 6 weeks initially and then at 8-week intervals. Improvement can occur after the second infusion. Toxicities include infusion-related fever and chills, upper respiratory infections, and autoantibody production.

Another consideration regarding TNF-α inhibitors, however, is their expense. Both etanercept and infliximab are appreciably more expensive than other DMARDs.

Corticosteroids

Corticosteroids, primarily in the form of oral prednisone, play a role in the therapy of RA and polymyalgia rheumatica (PMR). Prednisone at low doses is indicated in the therapy of RA. Unless acute, life-threatening complications such as RA vasculitis are present, doses of prednisone greater than 7.5 mg are rarely indicated. Doses of 7.5 mg or less can be used for extended periods of time without the development of diabetes, hypertension, weight gain, or even OSP.

Prednisone therapy should be decreased gradually as RA patients improve. One-milligram prednisone tablets are used to taper corticosteroid therapy slowly in single-milligram decrements. The dose can be decreased even more slowly by taking a 1-mg lower dose every other day until a steady state has been achieved. Once symptoms are stable, the lower dose can be used on a daily basis. The rate of decrease depends on continued control of joint inflammation. The time frame for successful tapering of prednisone is measured in weeks to months.

Prednisone is also used for therapy of PMR. Doses of 15 to 25 mg are required to improve clinical symptoms of morning stiffness and pain in the proximal muscles over the buttocks, thighs, and shoulders. The clinical activity of PMR is associated with an elevated erythrocyte sedimentation rate (ESR; > 20 mm/h). The dose of prednisone necessary to control PMR is predicated upon the amount needed to decrease the ESR to a normal level. Once the ESR has returned to normal, prednisone can be slowly tapered. Patients with an initially lower ESR are more likely to resolve their disorder within a year. At least a third of individuals, however, never resolve their disorder and require continual low-dose corticosteroids.

Treatment of Osteoporosis

The treatment of OSP starts with prevention at an early age through maximizing bone mass. Prevention strategies include maximizing peak bone mass during adolescence, maintaining bone mass during adulthood, and minimizing postmenopausal bone loss. Physical exercise increases stress on the skeleton and enhances bone growth. Weight-bearing exercise augments bone mineral density (BMD). Exercise is helpful for all age groups, including the elderly, to prevent bone loss from disuse. Adequate calcium intake is essential for the development and maintenance of a normal skeleton. Bone mass is increased in children and adolescents who consume higher levels of calcium supplements. However, high calcium intake during the postmenopausal period has no effect or only a minimal protective effect against bone loss. In Caucasian women, the recommended calcium intake is 800 mg/day until age 10 years, 1,500 mg/day during adolescence and pregnancy, and 1,200 mg/day during adulthood. Vitamin D, 400 to 800 IU, is a valuable supplement used in conjunction with calcium supplements. Vitamin D is particularly helpful for elderly individuals who have limited exposure to sunlight or who have nutritional deficiency. The combination of these supplements decreases the risk of hip fractures in the elderly. However, vitamin D and calcium are unable to increase BMD.

Estrogen Replacement Therapy

Estrogen deficiency after menopause leads to bone loss and OSP. The greatest rate of bone loss occurs in the first years after cessation of ovarian function. Estrogen replacement therapy (ERT) should be instituted soon after the onset of menopause in women without contraindications for estrogen therapy. Contraindications for ERT include a history of breast or uterine cancer or thromboembolic disorders. Conjugated estrogens, at a dose of 0.625 mg/day, are necessary to prevent bone loss. Progesterone is recommended for women with an intact uterus to decrease uterine cancer. Controversy remains concerning the relationship between ERT and breast cancer. Recent epidemiologic studies suggest a small association. However, the use of ERT is a personal choice.

Raloxifene is a selective estrogen-receptor modulator that has estrogen-like effects on bone resorption without stimulating the breast tissue or uterine endometrium in postmenopausal women. Raloxifene at 60 mg/day modestly increases BMD and decreases the risk of vertebral or femoral neck fracture. Toxicities associated with raloxifene include hot flashes, leg cramps, and rare episodes of venous thrombosis.

Bisphosphonates

Bisphosphonates are analogs of pyrophosphates but are impervious to enzymatic hydrolysis. Bisphosphonates are avidly adsorbed onto the surface of hydroxyapatite crystals in bone, the sites of active bone remodeling. Bisphosphonates alter bone remodeling by reducing bone resorption.

Etidronate is a bisphosphonate that is approved for the treatment of Paget's disease. This drug also has been used to prevent osteoporotic fractures. However, etidronate decreases bone mineralization and is associated with osteomalacia when used daily for extended periods. Therefore, the OSP regimen is limited to 400 mg/day for 14 days every 3 months. Etidronate is not approved for treatment of OSP by the FDA and might not be as effective after 2 years of continuous therapy.

Alendronate, a second-generation bisphosphonate, is effective for the prevention and treatment of OSP. Alendronate is a potent inhibitor of bone turnover but does not affect bone mineralization. Studies of women with established OSP found that alendronate 10 mg/day prevented postmenopausal bone loss and increased BMD in the spine by approximately 4% to 6% during a 3-year period. Alendronate also has a beneficial effect on increasing BMD of the femoral neck. Alendronate 5 mg/day is comparable to estrogen in preventing bone loss. Also, the effect on bone is prolonged because the half-life of alendronate is 10 years. Younger women of childbearing age are not candidates for this agent, however.

Risedronate is a third-generation bisphosphonate that has been effective for Paget's disease at a dose of 40 mg/day. At a dose of 5 mg/day, risedronate decreases the risk of vertebral and femoral neck fractures as well as increasing BMD in these locations. This drug has been recently approved by the FDA for the treatment of postmenopausal OSP.

A common characteristic of the bisphosphonates is poor intestinal absorption. These drugs must be taken on an empty stomach. For example, alendronate should be taken in the morning with a large glass of water after an overnight fast. The patient also should remain upright for 30 minutes to ensure that the medication remains out of the esophagus. The primary toxicity of the bisphosphonates is gastrointestinal. Esophagitis is a common complaint. Ongoing studies are investigating the efficacy of alendronate 70 mg once a week for the treatment of OSP. This weekly regimen would decrease the frequency of exposure of the gastrointestinal tract to irritation.

For individuals who are unable to tolerate oral bisphosphonates, an intravenous form of the drug is available. Pamidronate is a bisphosphonate approved for the treatment of hypercalcemia of malignancy and Paget's disease. Intravenous pamidronate, 30 mg every 3 months, has been associated with increases in spinal BMD in postmenopausal patients.

Calcitonin

Calcitonin is a peptide hormone that reduces osteoclastic bone resorption. Calcitonin derived from salmon is more effective than human calcitonin for OSP. Calcitonin is effective when given by injection (50 or 100 IU/day) or intranasally (200 IU/day). Bioavailability of nasal calcitonin is 10% of that achieved by injection but is better tolerated. Calcitonin treatment results in slight gains in spinal BMD—somewhat less than the gains achieved with ERT or bisphosphonates. Nasal calcitonin decreases the risk of spinal fractures but might not significantly alter the risk of hip fractures. However, one of the added benefits of calcitonin is its analgesic effect, particularly on bone fractures. Nasal calcitonin should be considered as an adjunctive pain therapy for individuals who have sustained osteoporotic fractures.

The therapy of OSP is imperfect. The interventions given currently need to be sustained for long periods to have a beneficial effect. The only therapy available to increase osteoblast function is fluoride, which increases not only BMD but also bone fragility. Fluoride also is irritating to the stomach and can cause musculoskeletal pain, associated with rapid bone remodeling, in the appendages. Its therapeutic window is too narrow to be an effective therapy for most OSP patients. In the future, the use of parathyroid hormone peptides or other growth factors will likely become available to stimulate bone growth to complement the antiresorptive agents for more effective prevention and treatment of OSP.

Annotated Bibliography

Nonsteroidal Anti-Inflammatory Drugs/ Cyclooxygenase-2 Inhibitors

Bensen WG, Fiechtner JJ, McMillen JI, et al: Treatment of osteoarthritis with celecoxib, a cyclooxygenase-2 inhibitor: A randomized, controlled trial. *Mayo Clin Proc* 1999;74:1095-1105.

In a double-blind, placebo-controlled, 12-week trial of celecoxib, naproxen, and placebo in 1,003 patients with OA of the knee, celecoxib was similar to naproxen in efficacy compared with placebo.

Crofford LJ, Lipsky PE, Brooks P, Abramson SB, Simon LS, van de Putte LB: Basic biology and clinical application of specific cyclooxygenase-2 inhibitors. *Arthritis Rheum* 2000;43:4-13.

This is a review of the mechanism of action and clinical ability of cyclooxygenase-2 inhibitors.

Langman MJ, Jensen DM, Watson DJ, et al: Adverse upper gastrointestinal effects of rofecoxib compared with NSAIDs. *JAMA* 1999;282:1929-1933.

Rofecoxib is associated with a significantly lower incidence of perforations, ulcerations, and bleeding compared to treatment with NSAIDs in patients with OA.

Schnitzer TJ, Truitt K, Fleischmann R, et al: The safety profile, tolerability, and effective dose range of rofecoxib in the treatment of rheumatoid arthritis: Phase II rofecoxib rheumatoid arthritis study group. *Clin Ther* 1999;21:1688-1702.

In a double-blind, placebo-controlled, 8-week trial of rofecoxib versus placebo in 658 patients with RA, 25 mg/day and 50 mg/day were significantly better than 5 mg/day and placebo for the control of inflammation and pain.

Simon LS, Weaver AL, Graham DY, et al: Anti-inflammatory and upper gastrointestinal effects of celecoxib in rheumatoid arthritis: A randomized, controlled trial. *JAMA* 1999;282:1921-1928.

Celecoxib is effective for the treatment of RA and is associated with fewer endoscopic gastrointestinal ulcerations compared with naproxen.

Wolfe MM, Lichtenstein DR, Singh G: Gastrointestinal toxicity of nonsteroidal antiinflammatory drugs. *N Engl J Med* 1999;340:1888-1899.

NSAIDs cause increased morbidity and mortality associated with damage to the upper gastrointestinal tract.

Rheumatoid Arthritis

Maini RN, Breedveld FC, Kalden JR, et al: Therapeutic efficacy of multiple intravenous infusions of anti-tumor necrosis factor alpha monoclonal antibody combined with low-dose weekly methotrexate in rheumatoid arthritis. *Arthritis Rheum* 1998;41:1552-1563.

This was a double-blind, placebo-controlled, 26-week infusion study of 101 patients with RA who received infliximab at 1, 3, or 10 mg/kg, with or without MTX. Infliximab at 10 mg/kg with MTX had a sustained effect of decreasing inflammation at 26 weeks.

Moreland LW, Schiff MH, Baumgartner SW, et al: Etanercept therapy in rheumatoid arthritis: A randomized, controlled trial. *Ann Intern Med* 1999;130:478-486.

In a double-blind, placebo-controlled, 6-month trial of etanercept versus placebo in 234 patients with RA, etanercept reduced disease activity by 59% versus 11% for placebo as measured by the American College of Rheumatology (ACR) 20% response.

Pincus T, O'Dell JR, Kremer JM: Combination therapy with multiple disease-modifying antirheumatic drugs in rheumatoid arthritis: A preventive strategy. *Ann Intern Med* 1999;131:768-774.

This report is an evidence-based review of studies supporting the efficacy of combination therapy with DMARDs for RA.

Strand V, Cohen S, Schiff M, et al: Treatment of active rheumatoid arthritis with leflunomide compared with placebo and methotrexate: Leflunomide rheumatoid arthritis investigators group. *Arch Intern Med* 1999;159: 2542-2550.

A double-blind, placebo, and active-controlled 1-year study of 482 patients with RA reported that LEF reduced disease activity by 52% versus MTX (46%) versus placebo (26%) as measured by the ACR 20% response. Initial response was more rapid with LEF, and LEF delayed radiographically documented disease progression.

Weinblatt ME, Maier AL, Fraser PA, Coblyn JS: Longterm prospective study of methotrexate in rheumatoid arthritis: Conclusion after 132 months of therapy. *J Rheumatol* 1998;25:238-242.

MTX remains an effective treatment for the control of RA inflammation for periods of time over a decade.

Corticosteroids

Weyand CM, Fulbright JW, Evans JM, Hunder GG, Goronzy JJ: Corticosteroid requirements in polymyalgia rheumatica. *Arch Intern Med* 1999;159:577-584.

This study differentiates 27 PMR patients into three distinct groups with variable responses to corticosteroid therapy. PMR patients with low initial ESR had the best opportunity to resolve their illness within 1 year.

Osteoporosis

Cummings SR, Black DM, Thompson DE, et al: Effect of alendronate on risk of fracture in women with low bone density but without vertebral fractures: Results from the Fracture Intervention Trial. *JAMA* 1998;280: 2077-2082.

Alendronate decreases the risk of first vertebral fractures in women with low BMD of the spine in the osteopenic range.

Eastell R: Treatment of postmenopausal osteoporosis. *N Engl J Med* 1998;338:736-746.

This is a review of all the forms of therapy for postmenopausal OSP.

Ettinger B, Black DM, Mitlak BH, et al: Reduction of vertebral fracture risk in postmenopausal women with osteoporosis treated with raloxifene: Results from a 3-year randomized clinical trial: Multiple outcomes of raloxifene evaluation (MORE) investigators. *JAMA* 1999;282:637-645.

This study reported on the fracture rate of 7,705 postmenopausal women who took raloxifene 60 mg/day or 120 mg/day versus placebo over a 36-month period. Raloxifene at

120 mg/day reduced new vertebral fractures by 50% compared with placebo. BMD was increased in the spine (2.7%) and femoral neck (2.4%) compared with placebo. Raloxifene is associated with an increased risk of venous thromboembolic events.

Harris ST, Watts NB, Genant HK, et al: Effects of risedronate treatment on vertebral and nonvertebral fractures in women with postmenopausal osteoporosis: A randomized, controlled trial: Vertebral efficacy with risedronate therapy (VERT) study group. *JAMA* 1999;282:1344-1352.

This is a report of a double-blind, placebo-controlled trial of 2,458 postmenopausal women with at least one vertebral fracture followed for a 3-year period. Risedronate at 5 mg/day reduced new vertebral fractures by 41% over 3 years. Bone mass was increased by 5.4% over a similar period.

Watts NB: Treatment of osteoporosis with bisphosphonates. *Endocrinol Metab Clin North Am* 1998;27: 419-439.

This article is a review of the mechanism of action of bisphosphonates. The clinical parameters for using the drugs are discussed.

Classic Bibliography

Chrousos GP: The hypothalamic-pituitary-adrenal axis and immune-mediated inflammation. *N Engl J Med* 1985;312:818-822.

Gabriel SE, Jaakkimainen L, Bombardier C: Risk for serious gastrointestinal complications related to use of nonsteroidal anti-inflammatory drugs. A meta-analysis. *Ann Intern Med* 1991;115:787-796.

Harris ST, Watts NB, Jackson RD, et al: Four-year study of intermittent cyclic etidronate treatment of postmenopausal osteoporosis: Three years of blinded therapy followed by one year of open therapy. *Am J Med* 1993;95:557-567.

Hench PS, Kendall EC, Polley HF: Effects of cortisone acetate and pituitary ACTH on rheumatoid arthritis, rheumatic fever and certain other conditions. *Arch Intern Med* 1950;85:545-666.

Liberman UA, Weiss SR, Broll J, et al: Effect of oral alendronate on bone mineral density and the incidence of fractures in postmenopausal osteoporosis. The Alendronate Phase III Osteoporosis Treatment Study Group. *N Engl J Med* 1995;333:1437-1443.

Mitchell JA, Akarasereenont P, Thiemermann C, Flower RJ, Vane JR: Selectivity of nonsteroidal antiinflammatory drugs as inhibitors of constitutive and inducible cyclooxygenase. *Proc Natl Acad Sci USA* 1993;90:11693-11697.

Overgaard K, Hansen MA, Jensen SB, Christiansen C: Effect of calcitonin given intranasally on bone mass and fracture rates in established osteoporosis: A dose-response study. *Br Med J* 1992;305:556-561.

Weinblatt ME, Coblyn JS, Fox DA, et al: Efficacy of low-dose methotrexate in rheumatoid arthritis. *N Engl J Med* 1985;312:818-822.

Chapter 21

Manipulative Therapy

Eric L. Hurwitz, DC, PhD

Scott Haldeman, MD, PhD

Introduction

In 1992, Shekelle and associates concluded from the results of a meta-analysis that spinal manipulation confers short-term benefit for acute pain patients but that long-term efficacy could not be determined and that data at that time were insufficient to permit firm conclusions to be made regarding the efficacy of spinal manipulation for chronic low back pain, sciatica, and other lumbar spine disorders. In 1994, guidelines for the treatment of acute low back pain published by the Agency for Health Care Policy and Research (renamed the Agency for Healthcare Research and Quality in 1999) included the use of acetaminophen and non-steroidal anti-inflammatory drugs (NSAIDs) for pain, certain aerobic activities and conditioning exercises, and spinal manipulation (in patients without radiculopathy). Although few data were available on adverse events, the risk of serious complications resulting from lumbar spinal manipulation was estimated to be very small. Complications following cervical spine manipulation were considered to be more serious but still rare. Spinal manipulation in the mid 1990s was regarded as being of some benefit for patients with acute, uncomplicated low back pain, with small likelihood of serious adverse reactions. The value of spinal manipulation in the treatment of other low back conditions, sciatica, and other neuromusculoskeletal disorders, and its role in pain prevention, had not been clearly established in randomized trials or in systematic reviews of the literature.

This chapter summarizes findings from recent clinical trials, well-designed observational studies, and systematic reviews of manipulation and mobilization to describe how understanding of this topic is changing and to establish the basis for current indications and contraindications of this treatment approach. Because practitioners of chiropractic and osteopathy provide the great majority of spinal manipulation delivered in the United States, relevant studies from these fields also are included.

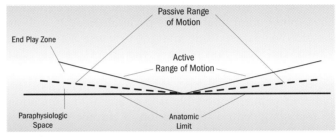

Figure 1 Joint motion comprises active range of motion and passive range of motion. Passive range of motion consists of end play where mobilization is performed and the paraphysiologic space where manipulation is performed. *(Reproduced with permission from Haldeman S, Hooper PD, Phillips RB, Scaringe JG, Traina AD: Spinal manipulative therapy, in Frymoyer JW (ed): The Adult Spine: Principles and Practice, ed 2. Philadelphia, PA, Lippincott-Raven, 1997, pp 1837-1861.)*

Manipulative Therapy

Although manipulative therapy encompasses a large array of manual articular and nonarticular manipulative and adjustive procedures performed by chiropractors, osteopaths, physical therapists, medical physicians, and other manual therapists, this chapter focuses solely on spinal manipulation and mobilization.

Spinal manipulation is defined as a controlled, judiciously applied, passive dynamic thrust of high or low velocity and low-amplitude force directed to one or more spinal joint segments within patient tolerance. These procedures might take joints into the "paraphysiologic" space, resulting in possible joint cavitation. The paraphysiologic space is between the joint's passive end range and its anatomic end range (Fig. 1). Joint cavitation is heralded by the sound commonly heard during manipulation.

Spinal mobilization is defined as a controlled, judiciously applied, passive force of low velocity and variable amplitude directed to one or more spinal joint segments. Mobilization procedures usually take place within the joint's physiologic space—that is, they do not take joints beyond the passive range of motion and do not typically result in joint cavitation.

Mechanism of Action

In general, manipulation and mobilization are used to reduce pain and facilitate joint motion in restricted spinal segments. Manipulation has been shown to result in relatively greater joint motion than does mobilization alone. Explanations for the physiologic effects of manipulation include the release of entrapped synovial or disc tissue, stretching and breaking of adhesions, release of endorphins, somatosomatic and viscerosomatic reflex responses, and muscle relaxation. These explanations have not been subjected to adequate experimental study, although isolated effects, such as muscle relaxation, changes in skin pain threshold, reflex responses in muscles, and increased range of motion, have been reported. It is possible and even probable that spinal manipulation has psychological as well as physiologic effects that interact to cause a favorable clinical outcome. Furthermore, the effect can vary, and different mechanisms might come into play, depending on the source, chronicity, and other properties of the patient's pain. The possible role of spinal manipulation in inhibiting central sensitization in chronic pain states and in autonomic dysfunction through effects at the spinal level and via descending inhibitory pathways has been postulated and is being studied. Despite increased, recent documentation of the specific biomechanical forces imposed by manipulation and a greater understanding of the effects of compression on neural function and the rate of somatosomatic and somatovisceral reflexes, the steps required to understand the relationship between the physiologic effects of mechanical forces on spinal tissues and the reported clinical outcomes have yet to be elucidated.

Low Back Pain and Sciatica

Chiropractors deliver the majority of manipulative care in the United States. Their caseload of patients with low back pain exceeds that of family physicians and orthopaedic surgeons. The authors of a 1998 utilization study of chiropractic services in the United States and Canada found that two thirds of chiropractic patients sought the services of a chiropractor because of low back pain. Spinal manipulative therapy was noted in more than 80% of the almost 2,000 abstracted records from chiropractic offices. Patients with low back pain had an average of 14 visits (median, 7) per episode of care.

Efficacy/Effectiveness

Low Back Pain

Episodes of low back pain of 3 months' duration or less are defined as acute or subacute, whereas episodes of more than 3 months' durations are considered to be chronic. Findings from three randomized clinical trials (RCTs) that compared chiropractic with physical therapy for low back pain have been published recently. In a 1995 update of their trial of chiropractic versus hospital outpatient management of low back pain in England, Meade and associates found no clinically significant differences in pain and disability outcomes. However, chiropractic patients were significantly more satisfied at 2 and 3 years, with a greater benefit observed in patients with more severe baseline pain and disability and in those who had had previous chiropractic care. The investigators of an RCT conducted in Sweden that compared back and neck pain treatment by chiropractors with treatment by physical therapists reported no differences between groups at 6 months or 1 year in terms of pain, function, cost, or sick leave, although chiropractic was slightly more favorable for patients with episodes of less than a week's duration and physical therapy more favorable for patients with episodes of more than a month's duration. Chiropractic patients were more likely to report that their expectations had been fulfilled. In a 1998 RCT, chiropractic and McKenzie physical therapy yielded similar rates of patient satisfaction and similar improvements in pain and disability after 2 years of follow-up, but these groups had only slightly better outcomes than did patients randomized to a minimal (provision of an educational booklet) intervention group.

A 1995 RCT that compared chiropractic spinal manipulation with sham manipulation and back education for chronic low back pain patients showed a small benefit in favor of chiropractic spinal manipulation versus sham at 2 and 4 weeks in terms of pain and disability. The authors of a 1999 clinical trial comparing osteopathic care with standard medical care in a managed care setting found equivalent pain and disability outcomes and satisfaction among patients with subacute (3 weeks to 6 months) low back pain after 12 weeks of care but greater prescription medication and physical therapy use in the medical care group. A well-designed observational study in North Carolina published in 1995 showed that among patients with low back pain of less than 10 weeks' duration who were seen by primary care physicians, chiropractors, and orthopaedic surgeons, pain and functional status outcomes were similar at 6 months, but patient satisfaction was highest among chiropractic patients.

The authors of a 1996 review of eight chiropractic RCTs, four of which included chronic patients only, concluded that insufficient evidence was available to show chiropractic as more (or less) beneficial than the comparison treatments (such as physical therapy, mobilization, traction, exercises, massage, corset, transcutaneous electrical nerve stimulator, bed rest, drugs, and back school) for patients with acute or chronic low back pain. One year later, authors from the same institution identified and performed a systematic review of 16 RCTs of manipulation for acute low back pain and of nine RCTs for chronic low back pain. They concluded that manipulation might be more effective than placebo for acute low back pain, but because of inconsistent results and poor study quality, the authors found that spinal manipulation had not been established to have an advantage over massage, shortwave diathermy, exercises, or analgesics. However, they found good evidence in favor of manipulation over placebo, general practitioner care, bed rest, analgesics, and massage for patients with chronic low back pain.

Sciatica
Findings from RCTs before 1995 and recent case series demonstrate that spinal manipulation might be a safe and effective alternative to surgery for patients with lumbar radiculopathy. However, no well-designed clinical trials or other comparative studies have been published recently addressing the efficacy of spinal manipulation for sciatica or radiculopathy. Coupled with the lack of convincing evidence before 1995, the efficacy of manipulative therapy for patients with these conditions, although promising, cannot be determined at this time.

Although numerous case reports and case series describe the successful use of manipulation under anesthesia (MUA) on patients with a variety of low back-related conditions, including chronic lumbosacral and sacroiliac strain and sciatica, MUA has not been subjected to well-designed observational or randomized clinical studies. Its value relative to manipulation without anesthesia or to other noninvasive or surgical treatments is therefore unknown.

Complications
A 1996 literature review of case reports, surveys, and review articles reporting complications from spinal manipulative therapy showed that complications resulting from spinal manipulation for low back pain are extremely rare. Almost half of the lumbar spine complications, predominantly cauda equina syndrome (CES), reported in the literature occurred following MUA. Given the much lower frequency of MUA compared with manipulation without anesthesia, the risk of CES with manipulation under anesthesia is most likely much greater than without anesthesia. Overall, the rate of occurrence of CES has been estimated to be about one case per 100 million low back manipulations performed without anesthesia.

Findings from 1996 and 1997 surveys of Swedish and Norwegian chiropractic practices showed that minor side effects from spinal manipulation, such as local discomfort, are common but benign and short lived, and that women are somewhat more likely to be affected than men. The temporal association between the treatments and the reactions suggests a causal relationship; however, coincidental effects cannot be discounted. These surveys did not detect any cases of CES or other serious adverse reactions following chiropractic spinal manipulation, and none of the clinical trials of spinal manipulation for low back pain have reported any serious complications.

Appropriateness
In a retrospective study, Shekelle and associates developed appropriateness criteria according to the RAND Corporation consensus method and used these criteria to judge the appropriateness of chiropractic spinal manipulation initiated for low back pain among chiropractic patients whose records were randomly selected from a cluster sample of six sites in the United States and Canada. "Appropriate" was defined as an indication for which the expected health benefits exceed the expected health risks by a sufficiently wide margin that spinal manipulation was considered reasonable. Initiation of spinal manipulation was judged to be appropriate for almost half (46%) of patients and inappropriate for a little more than a quarter (29%). These figures are similar to the proportions of medical procedures that have been judged to be appropriate for other conditions using the same criteria. Indications involving patients with acute low back pain with no neurologic findings and no sciatic nerve irritation were the most frequently judged as appropriate. Many of the inappropriate and uncertain indications were for patients with subacute or chronic low back pain for which little or inconsistent data were available at the time the consensus document was formulated.

Neck Pain
Neck and headache pain is second only to back pain as the most common reason for providing manipulative therapy. Data from the utilization of chiropractic services indicated that chiropractors provide between 18 and 38 million cervical manipulations per year for neck pain and headaches, although the overall use of cervical manipulation is much higher.

Efficacy/Effectiveness
A 1996 systematic literature review of manipulation and mobilization of the cervical spine identified nine RCTs that assessed the effectiveness of cervical spine manipulation or mobilization for neck pain. The manipulation

RCTs focused primarily on subacute and chronic pain, whereas three of the mobilization RCTs addressed acute pain.

Acute Neck Pain

One RCT compared neck collar, collar and transcutaneous electrical nerve stimulator, or collar and mobilization among patients with neck pain of less than 3 days' duration. After 1 week, the mobilization group had higher mean improvements in cervical mobility and pain reduction. No differences between groups were detected at 6 weeks and 3 months.

Two trials compared Maitland mobilization with other treatments for patients with acute flexion-extension sprains. One study compared rest and analgesics, Maitland mobilization and McKenzie exercises, and neck collar and advice on posture and exercises; the other study compared Maitland mobilization to cervical collar. In the first study, the groups receiving Maitland mobilization and neck collar plus advice about mobilization had decreases in pain intensity and increases in lateral flexion movement after 1 and 2 months; these were different from the decreases in pain intensity and increases in movement in the group that received rest and analgesics but were not different from each other. The group receiving Maitland mobilization in the second study had less pain after 4 and 8 weeks and a greater increase in cervical range of motion at 8 weeks than did the cervical collar group.

Subacute and Chronic Neck Pain

Two RCTs assessed the immediate effect of manipulation compared with mobilization for patients with predominantly subacute and chronic neck pain. One study showed equivalent decreases in pain in both groups after the data were adjusted for pretreatment differences between groups. The group receiving manipulation in the second study showed an improvement in the pressure pain threshold (the amount of pressure required to produce pain) in the neck. Neither study reported long-term outcomes.

Two additional RCTs assessed the effect of a muscle relaxant and rotational cervical spine manipulation versus the muscle relaxant alone. A greater proportion of the manipulated groups reported subjective improvement in pain or felt treatment was helpful 3 weeks after one to three treatments, compared with patients in the muscle relaxant groups. Another trial included patients with both chronic neck and chronic back complaints and compared manual therapy (including manipulation and mobilization), physical therapy, placebo, and usual general practitioner care. The study measured functional outcomes and reported long-term results (12 months) that showed a modest benefit favoring the group treated with manual therapy. Among the 64 patients with chronic neck complaints, no appreciable differences in severity of neck pain were detected between the manual therapy and the other groups at three and 12 weeks.

Another RCT compared salicylate and mobilization with salicylate and massage, traction, and electrical stimulation, and with a third group that received salicylate alone as treatment for patients with subacute and chronic neck pain. One week after concluding 3 weeks of treatment, the patients who received mobilization had a greater improvement in self-reported pain. A 1998 RCT in Denmark that compared intensive training of the cervical musculature, active and passive physiotherapy, and chiropractic manipulation for patients with neck pain of 3 months' duration or longer showed improvements in all groups at 4 and 12 months but no differences between groups with respect to pain, disability, and medication use.

Manipulation, mobilization, or physiotherapy are all probably more effective than muscle relaxants or usual medical care in producing short-term pain relief among some patients with subacute or chronic neck pain, and manipulation is probably slightly more effective than mobilization or physical therapy. Only one study so far has reported long-term results, so the long-term effects of manipulation are poorly understood.

The Quebec Task Force on Whiplash-Associated Disorders concluded that the value of manipulation has not been established for patients with postwhiplash head and neck symptoms. The task force also concluded that mobilization might be effective for some patients in the short term, but long-term effectiveness is unknown. (The Quebec Task Force also concluded that cervical pillows, postural alignment training, acupuncture, spray and stretch, transcutaneous electrical nerve stimulation, ultrasound, laser, short-wave diathermy, heat, ice, massage, epidural or intrathecal injections, muscle relaxants, and psychosocial interventions have no proven value for patients with postwhiplash neck pain, headache, and other related symptoms.)

Complications

Two comprehensive reviews of complications from cervical spine manipulation have been published recently. One review of English language articles documented more than 110 cases of complications allegedly arising from cervical spine manipulation. A few additional cases also have been published recently. Although no systematic data are available, the risk of complications from cervical spine mobilization is probably very small. The vast majority of complications from manipulation involved vertebrobasilar artery (VBA) dissections with consequences such as brainstem and/or cerebellar infarction. Recent prospective studies have shown manipulation to be associated with minor side effects, such as local discomfort and headache and, much less commonly, nausea and dizziness.

It is difficult to estimate the frequency of VBA dissections and other complications among patients undergoing cervical spine manipulation because of the uncertainty of both the number of complications and the number of cervical manipulations that patients receive over time. Separating causal from coincidental associations also is problematic. Estimates of VBA or stroke rates associated with cervical manipulation have ranged from 1 per 400,000 to 1 per 10 million manipulations. Using data from a community-based study of the use of chiropractic services and published case reports, the rate of VBA or other serious complication as a result of cervical spine manipulation was recently estimated to be 1 per 1 million manipulations. The death rate from cervical spine manipulation was estimated to be 2.68 per 10 million manipulations. Complication rates from other cervical spine treatments, such as surgery and drugs used to relieve cervical symptoms, are estimated to be much higher. A 1995 risk assessment of cervical manipulation versus NSAIDs for the treatment of neck pain showed NSAIDs to carry an appreciably greater relative risk of serious complications and death. A recent systematic review of reported cases of VBA dissections from manipulation and other forms of neck trauma, as well as spontaneous dissections, was not able to identify any risk factors for these incidents, including history of neck trauma; risk factors for vascular disease such as diabetes, hypertension, or smoking; or type or frequency of manipulation. The only potential risk factor was the acute onset of new and unusual neck pain and headache, which might reflect a dissection in progress.

Appropriateness

Appropriateness criteria have recently been developed for manipulation and mobilization of the cervical spine for neck pain in the same manner as criteria were developed for low back pain by Shekelle and associates. The level of consensus, however, was less than that for low back pain. Because these criteria have yet to be applied to cervical spine patients, the rate of appropriate and inappropriate manipulative therapy is not known. The clinical factors for neck pain rated as appropriate (that is, expected benefit exceeds expected risk) for manipulation tended to include pain anatomically consistent with musculotendinous distribution, no evidence of radiculopathy, and no contraindication for manipulation (this latter factor being poorly defined). Manipulation was judged as inappropriate in the presence of substantial trauma with no radiographs to rule out fractures, radiographic contraindications suggesting destructive pathology, and disc herniation or spinal canal stenosis

with radiculopathy. For the latter two conditions, mobilization was thought to be reasonable.

Other Neuromusculoskeletal Conditions

Although manipulative therapy is routinely used as a primary or adjunctive treatment for neuromusculoskeletal disorders other than low back and neck pain, scientific evidence establishing the efficacy or effectiveness of manipulative therapy for these conditions is lacking. With the possible exceptions of treatment for muscle-tension, cervicogenic, and migraine headaches, there are currently insufficient data to support or refute the use of manipulation for shoulder, arm, or hand pain, thoracic outlet syndrome, carpal tunnel syndrome, and temporomandibular joint disorders. There are, however, encouraging findings from recent case series and observational studies. A single RCT that compared chiropractic treatment with ibuprofen in patients with carpal tunnel syndrome showed improvement in both treatment groups but without significant differences between the groups. The ibuprofen group, however, had a much higher rate of intolerance (22%) and complication rate than did the chiropractic group.

Relative Cost of Manipulative Therapy

The costs of chiropractic care and medical care for workers' compensation back-injury claimants and other back or neck-pain patient populations have been compared in six retrospective studies and three prospective studies (including two RCTs) since 1995. Lack of comparability of chiropractic and medical patients and insufficient clinical data preclude determining valid estimates of cost differences in the retrospective studies. Chiropractic and physical therapy for back or neck pain resulted in comparable costs and outcomes in one RCT. A second RCT showed chiropractic and McKenzie physical therapy to have similar costs but to be more expensive than a booklet for low back pain patients. In a prospective cohort study, patients with low back pain who received care from primary care providers had lower average treatment costs than did patients of chiropractors and orthopaedic surgeons. With the exception of satisfaction, which was highest among chiropractic patients, long-term clinical outcomes were similar between groups. RCTs of chiropractic (or manipulative therapy) and other therapeutic strategies with the inclusion of formal cost-effectiveness analyses have not been published to date.

Research in Progress

Two major ongoing RCTs should offer findings regarding the relative effectiveness of spinal manipulation for low back pain with and without leg pain and of spinal manipulation versus mobilization for patients with neck pain. These two studies, being conducted in a managed care setting, include cost and utilization data and will incorporate formal cost-effectiveness analyses. The neck pain study also includes the systematic collection of data on adverse reactions associated with treatment, which should contribute to the limited knowledge of the relative frequency of side effects from manipulation versus mobilization. A well-designed cohort study addressing the effectiveness of manipulation under joint anesthesia for low back pain with radiculopathy also is under way. A proposal for assessing the frequency of appropriate use of cervical spine manipulation and mobilization in the United States is currently under review. Other studies in progress are looking at the relative complication rates of manipulation and NSAIDs and the cost of chiropractic and medical treatment in the workers' compensation system. Further animal experimental studies on the biomechanical and neurophysiologic theories of manipulation also are under way.

Summary

The efficacy, effectiveness, safety, and appropriateness of manipulative therapy and chiropractic care for low back pain, neck pain, and other spinal disorders remain topics of ongoing and future studies. It tentatively can be concluded that spinal manipulation is probably more beneficial than placebo therapy for low back pain; is at least as beneficial as other routine treatments for acute low back pain; and might be more effective than other common management strategies such as general medical care, bed rest, analgesia, and massage for patients with chronic low back pain. Spinal mobilization is probably of at least short-term benefit for patients with acute neck pain; spinal manipulation is probably slightly more effective than mobilization for patients with subacute or chronic neck pain; and both are probably superior to usual medical care.

Insufficient evidence exists to establish the long-term effectiveness of spinal manipulation for any condition or for the short-term or long-term effectiveness of manipulation for patients with sciatic nerve irritation, radiculopathy, or other neuromusculoskeletal disorders. Minor adverse reactions following spinal manipulation are common but transient. The frequency of serious complications from lumbar spine manipulation is negligible, whereas cervical spine manipulations are associated with more severe, albeit very rare, complications. The rate of severe adverse reactions from medications and surgery prescribed for back and neck pain appears to be much greater than the complication rates from manipulative therapy. Almost half of initial chiropractic

spinal manipulative treatments for low back pain have been judged as appropriate.

Priorities for future research include anatomic, biomechanical, and biochemical studies to address the mechanisms of manipulative therapy; more well-designed RCTs comparing manipulative therapies in combination with other manual methods and with other treatments (and self-care) for low back pain, neck pain, and sciatic nerve root irritation; and the identification of subgroups of patients for whom manipulative therapy is most beneficial. Costs, utilization of services (for example, the frequency of visits or manipulations), and clinical outcomes are under study to measure and compare the effectiveness of alternative management strategies.

Annotated Bibliography

Andersson GB, Lucente T, Davis AM, Kappler RE, Lipton JA, Leurgans S: A comparison of osteopathic spinal manipulation with standard care for patients with low back pain. *N Engl J Med* 1999;341:1426-1431.

Patients with subacute episodes of low back pain randomized to osteopathic manual therapy or standard medical care had similar pain and disability outcomes after 12 weeks. Medication use was greater in the medical group. Ninety percent of all patients were satisfied.

Assendelft WJ, Koes BW, vander Heijden GJ, Bouter LM: The effectiveness of chiropractic for treatment of low back pain: An update and attempt at statistical pooling. *J Manipulative Physiol Ther* 1996;19:499-507.

Eight RCTs of chiropractic care for low back pain were identified. Poor study quality and heterogenous outcome measures precluded a meta-analysis. However, a narrative review yielded little evidence for the effectiveness of chiropractic for acute or chronic low back pain.

Carey TS, Garrett J, Jackman A, McLaughlin C, Fryer J, Smucker DR: The outcomes and costs of care for acute low back pain among patients seen by primary care practitioners, chiropractors, and orthopedic surgeons: The North Carolina Back Pain Project. *N Engl J Med* 1995;333:913-917.

Patients with acute low back pain who sought care from primary care providers, orthopaedic surgeons, or chiropractors had similar clinical outcomes. Outpatient costs were greatest among patients of orthopaedic surgeons and chiropractors; satisfaction was highest among chiropractic patients.

Cherkin DC, Deyo RA, Battie M, Street J, Barlow W: A comparison of physical therapy, chiropractic manipulation, and provision of an educational booklet for the treatment of patients with low back pain. *N Engl J Med* 1998;339:1021-1029.

In this RCT, chiropractic and McKenzie physical therapy resulted in better 1-year and 2-year pain and disability outcomes compared with receiving a booklet. Costs and satisfaction were less in the booklet group.

Coulter ID, Hurwitz EL, Adams AH, et al: The appropriateness of manipulation and mobilization of the cervical spine. RAND Corporation Publication MR-781-CCR, 1996.

Criteria were developed for manipulation and mobilization for neck pain and other cervical spine disorders. Manipulation was judged as appropriate for musculotendinous neck pain without radiculopathy, and inappropriate for trauma-associated pain without radiographs, radiographic contraindications, and disc herniation and spinal stenosis with radioculpathy.

Dabbs V, Lauretti WJ: A risk assessment of cervical manipulation vs NSAIDs for the treatment of neck pain. *J Manipulative Physiol Ther* 1995;18:530-536.

Studies addressing the risks and benefits of cervical manipulation and NSAIDs were identified and reviewed. No RCTs of NSAIDs specifically for neck pain were identified. The authors concluded that cervical manipulation for neck pain is safer and no less effective than NSAID use.

Davis PT, Hulbert JR, Kassak K, Meyer JJ: Comparative efficacy of conservative medical and chiropractic treatments for carpal tunnel syndrome: A randomized clinical trial. *J Manipulative Physiol Ther* 1998;21:317-326.

The efficacy of ibuprofen and manipulation were compared. Outcome measures were self-reported physical and mental distress, nerve conduction studies, and vibrometry. Improvements in perceived comfort and function, nerve conduction, and finger sensation were similar in both groups.

Haldeman S, Kohlbeck FJ, McGregor M: Risk factors and precipitating neck movements causing vertebrobasilar artery dissection after cervical trauma and spinal manipulation. *Spine* 1999;24:785-794.

This systematic review of the literature looked at VBA dissections following cervical manipulation and minor and major trauma as well as dissections reported as spontaneous. The literature at this time does not provide evidence that allows for the identification of the patient at risk or the type of neck movement likely to cause a VBA dissection.

Hurwitz EL, Aker PD, Adams AH, Meeker WC, Shekelle PG: Manipulation and mobilization of the cervical spine: A systematic review of the literature. *Spine* 1996;21:1746-1760.

Articles describing the efficacy/effectiveness of cervical spine manipulation and mobilization, and related complications, were identified. The authors concluded that manipulation and mobilization might be of short-term benefit for some patients with neck pain and headache, and the complication rate is small.

Hurwitz EL, Coulter ID, Adams AH, Genovese BJ, Shekelle PG: Use of chiropractic services from 1985 through 1991 in the United States and Canada. *Am J Public Health* 1998;88:771-776.

Sixty-eight percent of randomly selected chiropractic charts from five US and one Canadian site showed that care was sought for low back pain. Spinal manipulation therapy was recorded in 83% of all charts. The chiropractic use rate in these sites is twice that of estimates made 15 years ago.

Jordan A, Bendix T, Nielsen H, Hansen FR, Host D, Winkel A: Intensive training, physiotherapy, or manipulation for patients with chronic neck pain: A prospective, single-blinded, randomized clinical trial. *Spine* 1998;23:311-319.

Pain, disability, and medication use after 4 and 12 months were similar among patients with neck pain of at least 3 months' duration who were randomized to intensive training of cervical musculature, active and passive physiotherapy, and chiropractic spinal manipulation.

Lebouf-Yde C, Hennius B, Rudberg E, Leufvenmark P, Thunman M: Side effects of chiropractic treatment: A prospective study. *J Manipulative Physiol Ther* 1997;20:511-515.

Six hundred twenty-five patients of 66 chiropractors (1,858 visits) recorded self-reported unpleasant reactions after spinal manipulation. Two thirds of the reactions involved local discomfort in the treatment area; 10% involved pain in other areas; and most symptoms disappeared within 24 hours. Women were more likely than men to report reactions.

Senstad O, Leboeuf-Yde C, Borchgrevink CF: Side-effects of chiropractic spinal manipulation: Types frequency, discomfort and course. *Scand J Prim Health Care* 1996;14:50-53.

Ten chiropractors collected data on reactions reported by 10 consecutive patients per chiropractor. Although side effects were reported in one third of the 368 treatments among 95 patients, 90% of the reactions were rated as moderate or slight, and 83% had disappeared within 24 hours.

Shekelle PG, Coulter I, Hurwitz EL, et al: Congruence between decisions to initiate chiropractic spinal manipulation for low back pain and appropriateness criteria in North America. *Ann Intern Med* 1998;129:9-17.

Criteria developed for the appropriate use of spinal manipulation for low back pain were applied to patients randomly selected from chiropractic practices in the United States and Canada. Spinal manipulation was appropriately initiated in 46% of the cases.

Skargren EI, Carlsson PG, Oberg BE: One-year follow-up comparison of the cost and effectiveness of chiropractic and physiotherapy as primary management for back pain: Subgroup analysis, recurrence, and additional health care utilization. *Spine* 1998;23:1875-1884.

The group of patients with back and neck pain randomized to chiropractic providers had similar improvement, costs, and recurrences as those randomized to physiotherapy after 6 and 12 months. Chiropractic patients were more likely to report that their expectations had been fulfilled.

van Tulder MW, Koes BW, Bouter LM: Conservative treatment of acute and chronic nonspecific low back pain: A systematic review of randomized controlled trials of the most common interventions. *Spine* 1997;22:2128-2156.

RCTs of low back pain treatments were identified and scored. Manipulation was found to be better than placebo; more effective than general practitioner care, bed rest, analgesics, and massage for chronic pain; and not better than modalities, exercises, or drugs for acute pain.

Classic Bibliography

Bigos SJ (ed): Acute Low Back Problem in Adults. Rockville, MD, US Department of Health and Human Services (Clinical Practice Guideline #14: AHCPR Publication No. 95-0642), 1994.

Brodin H: Cervical pain and mobilization. *Int J Rehabil Res* 1984;7:190-191.

Cassidy JD, Lopes AA, Yong-Hing K: The immediate effect of manipulation versus mobilization on pain and range of motion in the cervical spine: A randomized controlled trial. *J Manipulative Physiol Ther* 1992;15:570-575.

Hadler NM, Curtis P, Gillings DB, Stinnett S: A benefit of spinal manipulation as adjunctive therapy for acute low-back pain: A stratified controlled trial. *Spine* 1987;12:702-706.

Howe DH, Newcombe RG, Wade MT: Manipulation of the cervical spine: A pilot study. *J R Coll Gen Pract* 1983;33:574-579.

Koes BW, Assendelft WJ, van der Heijden GJ, Bouter LM, Knipschild PG: Spinal manipulation and mobilisation for back and neck pain: A blinded review. *BMJ* 1991;303:1298-1303.

Koes BW, Bouter LM, van Mameren H, et al: Randomised clinical trial of manipulative therapy and physiotherapy for persistent back and neck complaints: Results of one year follow up. *BMJ* 1992;304:601-605.

MacDonald RS, Bell CM: An open controlled assessment of osteopathic manipulation in nonspecific low-back pain. *Spine* 1990;15:364-370.

McKinney LA: Early mobilisation and outcome in acute sprains of the neck. *BMJ* 1989;299:1006-1008.

McKinney LA, Dornan JO, Ryan M: The role of physiotherapy in the management of acute neck sprains following road-traffic accidents. *Arch Emerg Med* 1989;6:27-33.

Meade TW, Dyer S, Browne W, Frank AO: Randomised comparison of chiropractic and hospital outpatient management for low back pain: Results from extended follow up. *BMJ* 1995;311:349-351.

Meade TW, Dyer S, Browne W, Townsend J, Frank AO: Low back pain of mechanical origin: Randomised comparison of chiropractic and outpatient hospital treatment. *BMJ* 1990;300:1431-1437.

Mealy K, Brennen H, Fenelon GC: Early mobilization of acute whiplash injuries. *Br Med J* 1986;292:656-657.

Nordemar R, Thorner C: Treatment of acute cervical pain: A comparative group study. *Pain* 1981;10:93-101.

Report of the Quebec Task Force on Spinal Disorders: Scientific approach to the assessment and management of activity-related spinal disorders. A monograph for clinicians. *Spine* 1987;12(suppl 7):S1-S59.

Shekelle PG, Adams AH, Chassin MR, Hurwitz EL, Brook RH: Spinal manipulation for low-back pain. *Ann Intern Med* 1992;117:590-598.

Sloop PR, Smith DS, Goldenberg E, Dore C: Manipulation for chronic neck pain: A double-blind controlled study. *Spine* 1982;7:532-535.

Spitzer WO, Skovron ML, Salmi LR, et al: Scientific monograph of the Quebec Task Force on Whiplash-Associated Disorders: Redefining "whiplash" and its management. *Spine* 1995;20(suppl 8):1S-73S.

Triano JJ, McGregor M, Hondras MA, Brennen PC: Manipulative therapy versus education programs in chronic low back pain. *Spine* 1995;20:948-955.

Vernon HT, Aker P, Burns S, Viljakaanen S, Short L: Pressure pain threshold evaluation of the effect of spinal manipulation in the treatment of chronic neck pain: A pilot study. *J Manipulative Physiol Ther* 1990;13:13-16.

Chapter 22

Spinal Injections for Diagnosis and Treatment

Christopher J. Rogers, MD

Paul Dreyfuss, MD

General Considerations

Interventional diagnostic and therapeutic spinal injections represent significant additions to the management of painful spine conditions. Awareness of the efficacy and relative safety of spinal injections, and knowing when their use is indicated or contraindicated, allows physicians to provide safe and effective clinical care.

Contraindications and Potential Complications

Diagnostic and therapeutic spinal injections should be performed by an experienced injectionist to minimize the risk of complications. Most adverse events are minor and self-limiting and include regional muscle spasm or postinjection pain. Inappropriate needle placement can cause injury to tissues other than those targeted for injection; these include the vertebral artery and spinal cord at the cervical levels, pleura and lungs at the thoracic levels, and spinal nerves and dura at all levels.

Absolute contraindications to injections include bleeding diathesis, use of anticoagulant or antiplatelet agents, local or systemic infection, spinal malignancy, or significant allergy to any of the injected solutions (contrast, local anesthetic, and corticosteroid). Patients receiving anticoagulation therapy can undergo spinal injections when the medication is withheld for a period sufficient to normalize coagulation. Risk of allergy can be determined by assessing the response to a low-volume (0.5 mL) subcutaneous injection of the suspected agent before spinal injection.

The risk of an inadvertent dural puncture is estimated at 0.1% to 5% during a cervical or lumbar epidural steroid injection (ESI) and 0.6% with a caudal epidural injection. The incidence of dural puncture during a transforaminal ESI has not been studied but is thought to be a rare occurrence when the needle is not advanced more than halfway into the neuroforamen. Dural puncture is associated with postdural puncture headache, a condition that is usually self-limiting. When dural puncture is not recognized, injection of local anesthetic into the subarachnoid space can result in spinal anesthesia, sympathetic block, hypotension, and, at the cervical level, respiratory compromise. The use of contrast-enhanced fluoroscopic guidance allows the injectionist to identify a potential subarachnoid or subdural injection before injecting such agents.

The overall incidence of inadvertent intravascular needle placement during contrast-enhanced, fluoroscopically guided lumbar spinal injections varies according to the type of injection employed. Caudal and transforaminal ESIs have the highest rates—6.4% to 10.9% and 8.8% to 12.7%, respectively—followed by lumbar zygapophysial joint (6.1%), sacroiliac joint (5.3%), and lumbar interlaminar (1.9%) injections. In up to 74% of cases, preinjection aspiration fails to produce a flash at the needle hub when intravascular placement has occurred. Inadvertent intravascular injections can cause anesthetic toxicity, including seizures and cardiac dysrhythmias. The risk of intravascular injection is eliminated with the use of contrast-enhanced fluoroscopic guidance.

Lumbar epidural hematoma, infection, and nerve root injury are extremely rare but have been reported. The most common effects after injection are related to the use of corticosteroids. Reactions include facial flushing, insomnia, agitation, anxiety, and low-grade fever. These effects are transient and rarely last longer than 5 to 7 days. The administration of three weekly epidural injections of 80 mg triamcinolone acetate has been shown to suppress plasma cortisol levels for a median duration of 1 month, with levels normalizing by 3 months. These effects should be considered in patients who will undergo surgery shortly after injection of corticosteroids. However, no documented complications exist related to hypothalamic suppression after ESIs.

Selective Nerve-Root Block

Selective nerve-root blocks (SNRBs) are used to establish the presence of radicular pain when the clinical presentation is not straightforward. The procedure is optimally performed with fluoroscopic guidance to allow precise injection of local anesthetic into the epiradicular sheath. To maximize SNRB specificity, total volumes usually are maintained at less than 1 mL in the cervical spine and less than 2 mL in the lumbar spine. Although commonly used clinically, scientific assessment of the predictive value of cervical and thoracic SNRBs is lacking; however, studies exist on lumbar SNRBs.

Derby and associates retrospectively assessed the value of SNRB (lidocaine with corticosteroid) for predicting surgical outcome in 78 consecutive patients with leg pain greater than low back pain. They selected patients who achieved more than 80% immediate anesthetic relief after a SNRB performed within 1 month before surgery. In addition, because corticosteroid was used with the anesthetic, a positive steroid response was described as pain relief greater than 50% for at least 1 week. A positive surgical response was described as leg pain relief greater than 50% for at least 6 months. In patients with leg pain of more than 1 year, a positive steroid response predicted a positive surgical outcome with a positive predictive value of 85%. A negative steroid response predicted a negative surgical outcome with a negative predictive value of 95%. An important limitation of the study was the retrospective manner in which patients were asked to recall information 8 months after the intervention.

Surgical outcomes were not assessed by Stanley and associates, who prospectively studied SNRBs. However, 95% of those who received complete symptom relief with SNRBs were noted to have surgical confirmation of nerve root pathology. Similar results were described by Haueisen and associates, who found surgical confirmation in 93%. Dooley and associates, studied patients who received complete relief from SNRBs who underwent subsequent decompression of the involved nerve root. Of the patients with a herniated lumbar disc, 100% obtained complete leg pain relief and 78% obtained complete back pain relief. Of the patients with lumbar stenosis, 82% obtained complete leg pain relief. Seventy-one percent of the patients with epidural fibrosis and 8% with arachnoiditis obtained complete relief. Similar results have been described by van Akkerveeken, who correlated the immediate anesthetic relief aspect of the SNRB result with surgical outcomes and found a positive predictive value of 95%. Although initial results are promising, randomized trials are needed to evaluate the true prognostic value of SNRBs in the evaluation of radicular pain.

Epidural Steroid Injection

The first published report of ESI for the treatment of sciatic pain was that done by Robecchi and Capra in 1952. Multiple studies have since been reported on the use of ESIs for the treatment of radicular pain.

The primary indication for the implementation of an ESI rests on the presence of radicular pain that cannot be managed by other means. Radicular pain is characteristic in that it is referred into the affected extremity in a dermatomal pattern and often is associated with paresthesia, dysesthesia, or hypesthesia. The patient might exhibit loss of motor function or muscle stretch reflexes in a myotomal distribution. Dural tension signs also might be present. CT or MRI can show disc pathology capable of producing inflammation of the involved neural tissues. Electrodiagnostic studies can demonstrate findings consistent with spinal nerve pathology. Radicular pain should be differentiated from somatic referred pain, which is usually described as deep or aching without physical examination findings that would suggest neural involvement. Somatic referred pain is not expected to improve with ESI treatment. Patient characteristics that predict an unfavorable response include longer duration of symptoms, absence of radicular pain, unemployment because of pain, a greater use of medications, a greater number of previous treatments, nicotine habituation, and pain that does not increase with activity or is not relieved with medications. The best responses to ESIs are reported within 3 months from the onset of radicular pain.

The therapeutic effects of ESIs are believed to be mediated through the anti-inflammatory action of corticosteroids. Commonly used corticosteroids include betamethasone, methylprednisolone, and triamcinolone. Histologic and biochemical evidence of nerve root inflammation has been identified in patients with radicular pain. Acute disc injuries release phospholipase A_2 (PLA_2), a proinflammatory enzyme that stimulates the release of arachidonic acid, a precursor to prostaglandins and leukotrienes. Demyelination of nerve roots and ectopic discharges have been demonstrated with epidurally injected PLA_2 and a significant reduction in PLA_2 concentration has been shown with epidurally administered steroids in animal models. Steroids also inhibit leukocyte aggregation and granulocyte degranulation and promote lysosomal membrane stabilization. Finally, steroids have been shown to block nociceptive C-fiber transmission.

ESIs have become an integral part of the nonsurgical management of lumbar disc herniations and radiculopathy and are endorsed by the North American Spine Society and the Agency for Health Care Policy and Research. The most commonly quoted beneficial response rates are that 60% to 75% of patients receive at least some radicular pain relief. Controlled, prospective, randomized, double-blind studies on the efficacy of lumbar ESIs have provided mixed results. Unfortunately, these studies contain significant design flaws, including a lack of fluoroscopic guidance during injection or the use of advanced imaging to assist in locating potential neural tissue inflammation. When fluoroscopy is not used, 20% to 40% of attempted lumbosacral ESIs can miss the epidural space.

A recent randomized control trial by Carette and associates showed the greatest benefit of nonfluoroscopically guided interlaminar corticosteroid ESIs to occur in the first 6 weeks following treatment; however, this same study found no long-term difference between the active and placebo groups at 3 months postinjection. Because of this fact, most clinicians use this window of pain reduction in the first 1 to 2 months following an ESI to facilitate an active rehabilitation plan.

Uncontrolled, prospective studies of transforaminal ESIs that use fluoroscopic guidance to accurately inject at the site of pathology offer promising results. Weiner and Fraser prospectively studied 30 patients who had CT evidence of a lumbar disc herniation and radicular pain of an average duration of 3 months. Patients were treated with a single fluoroscopically guided transforaminal ESI. At 3 weeks, 90% had at least moderate relief, and at an average follow-up of 3.4 years, 78% continued to have at least moderate relief.

Lutz and associates prospectively studied 69 patients who had MRI confirmation of a lumbar disc herniation and radicular pain of a mean duration of 22 weeks. Patients received an average of 1.8 fluoroscopically guided transforaminal injections, followed by up to 12 weeks of physical therapy. At an average follow-up of 80 weeks, 75% obtained more than 50% relief of preinjection pain.

Bush and Hillier studied 165 patients with CT evidence of a lumbar disc herniation and radicular pain of more than 4 months' duration. An initial caudal ESI without fluoroscopy was followed by one or two fluoroscopically guided transforaminal ESIs as needed over the course of 1 year. At 1-year follow-up, 86% of the patients were treated successfully without surgery, with a mean decrease in visual analog scale of 94%.

Riew and associates have conducted the only prospective, randomized, controlled, double-blind study of fluoroscopically guided transforaminal ESI. Fifty-five patients with radiographic confirmation of nerve root compression who had requested surgical intervention were randomized to receive a transforaminal selective nerve root injection with bupivacaine or bupivacaine with betamethasone. Each patient received up to three injections on request. At follow-ups of 13 to 26 months,

33.3% of the control group versus 71.4% of the group receiving the corticosteroid elected not to undergo surgery because of substantial pain reduction. Further studies of this caliber will be required to validate the efficacy of ESIs.

Clinicians have reported good to excellent pain relief or neurologic improvement in 41% to 76% of patients after cervical ESI (CESI). However, no prospective, randomized, controlled studies of CESI exist. The best results are reported with the use of fluoroscopically confirmed injection techniques in patients with radicular symptoms of less than 6 months caused by a herniated disc.

Bush and Hillier described the response to CESIs for radicular pain in a prospective, noncontrolled fashion. They studied 68 subjects with neurologic deficits of 2 months' average duration and abnormal MRI studies that correlated with the side and level of radicular symptoms. A nonfluoroscopically guided lateral approach was first performed at the seventh cervical segment. If symptoms were not "significantly improved," then a second fluoroscopically guided, contrast-enhanced transforaminal approach was performed no more than 1 month after the first injection. A third CESI was performed using fluoroscopy when the first two injections were not completely successful. An average of 2.5 injections per patient was required for adequate pain control. At 7 months' follow-up, 47% of the patients had partial and 46% had full neurologic recovery. Ninety-four percent reported pain relief, with none requiring surgery. Despite the lack of a placebo control for natural history, this study suggests that CESIs might provide a nonsurgical treatment alternative for painful cervical radiculopathy.

Thoracic ESIs have not been studied to any extent, probably because thoracic disc herniations account for less than 1% of all symptomatic disc herniations. However, radicular pain caused by herpes zoster, trauma, degenerative scoliosis, and diabetes also have been reported to improve with thoracic ESIs.

ESIs can be repeated but no more than two ESIs should be given without regard to response. Most practitioners limit the number to three or four injections per year based on a desire to limit the corticosteroid dose. Patients who obtain a good initial sustained response might benefit from an additional injection if symptoms recur. Patients who experience transient but not sustained relief are not candidates for further injections.

Zygapophysial Joint Injection

The posterior paired joints of the spine are commonly called facet joints or, more formally, zygapophysial joints (z-joints). The lumbar z-joints were first recognized as a potential source of low back pain in 1911.

Injection of hypertonic saline into the joints with fluoroscopic guidance has been shown to produce low back and lower extremity pain. In 1976, relief of low back pain and lower extremity pain after injection of local anesthetic into the lumbar z-joints was first described.

The z-joints are true synovial joints with a joint space, hyaline cartilage, synovial membrane, and a fibrous capsule. Lumbar z-joints are innervated with nociceptive fibers that travel through the medial branches of the dorsal rami. Autonomic nerve fibers and mechanoreceptors have been demonstrated in lumbar z-joint capsules.

The cause of most lumbar z-joint pain is unknown. Pain can occur with systemic inflammatory arthritides, such as rheumatoid arthritis and ankylosing spondylitis. Fractures, capsular tears, articular cartilage splits, and hemorrhage have been documented in postmortem studies of trauma victims with normal radiographs. Osteoarthritis is another potential source of lumbar z-joint pain. Villonodular synovitis, synovial cysts, and infection can rarely cause z-joint pain. Multiple other causes of z-joint pain have been proposed, including synovial impingement, joint subluxation, chondromalacia facetae, capsular and synovial inflammation, and joint capsule injury caused by restriction of normal articular motion.

To date, no pathognomonic, noninvasive radiographic, historic, or physical examination findings allow definitive identification of z-joints as sources of spine pain. The diagnosis of z-joint–mediated pain is based on controlled diagnostic blocks of the joint or its nerve supply. Based on responses to comparative blocks of the lumbar z-joint, the prevalence of z-joint–mediated chronic low back pain in younger patients was determined to be 15%. In patients with a median age of 59 years, the prevalence of chronic z-joint–mediated low back pain was 40%, using placebo-controlled joint blocks. The L4-5 and L5-S1 z-joints are the most commonly symptomatic z-joints in the lumbar spine. In a group of 68 patients with whiplash injuries, a randomized, placebo-controlled, double-blind study using triple blocks demonstrated a worst-case prevalence of chronic cervical z-joint pain to be 46%. The most commonly symptomatic z-joints in the cervical spine are C2-3 and C5-6. The prevalence of z-joint pain in patients with acute spine pain is unknown.

The thoracic z-joints have been shown to be capable of mediating local and referred pain, and their innervation from the medial branch division of the dorsal ramus has been described. However, the prevalence of thoracic z-joint pain is unknown.

The lateral atlantoaxial (LAA) and atlanto-occipital (AO) joints have the capacity to cause cervical and cranial pain. Referral patterns into the head and neck have been described. Unusual complaints, such as visual disturbances, dizziness, nausea, tongue numbness, and ear pain, also have been attributed to LAA and AO joint-mediated pain. Injection methods for the LAA and AO joints have been described, but the efficacy of intra-articular corticosteroids has not yet been validated.

Diagnostic and potentially therapeutic blocks of the z-joint or its innervation (the medial branch of the dorsal ramus) are used when noninvasive conservative treatment has failed. Z-joint injections should not be commonly used in patients with new neurologic impairment as determined by dermatomal sensory loss, muscle weakness, or neural tension signs. Normal imaging of the lumbar z-joints is not a contraindication to injection when the clinical presentation suggests the possibility of z-joint pain.

No scientific studies advocate z-joint injection procedures that do not use fluoroscopic guidance. Fluoroscopy is used to visualize a joint arthrogram after a minimal amount of contrast medium has been injected. Injectant volume should be approximately 1 to 2 mL in the lumbar spine and less than 1 mL in the cervical and thoracic spine to minimize the risk of capsular disruption and extravasation.

Block of the z-joint innervation by medial branch blocks is confirmed with anatomically appropriate contrast spread without venous uptake. The target specificity of cervical and lumbar medial branch blocks has been established, and the physiologic ability of lumbar medial branch blocks to anesthetize the z-joint occurs at a rate of 89% provided venous uptake does not occur. Venous uptake is noted to occur at a rate of 6.1% with lumbar z-joint injections and 8% with medial branch blocks. The false-negative rate is 50% when venous uptake occurs during medial branch blocks in spite of needle repositioning. When joint entry cannot be obtained, medial branch blocks provide an equally valuable diagnostic option for z-joint pain. No evidence exists that the concomitant use of corticosteroids with medial branch blocks provides a long-term beneficial effect.

Five open, uncontrolled trials on cervical z-joint injection of corticosteroid have shown it to be beneficial in reducing neck pain. There is also one randomized, double-blind, controlled trial on intra-articular corticosteroids for 42 patients with chronic z-joint–mediated pain following whiplash injury. The subjects were randomized to receive intra-articular corticosteroid or bupivacaine in symptomatic joints, established through comparative medial branch blocks. There were no other cointerventions such as physical or manual therapy. Less than 50% of subjects had pain relief for more than 1 week, and more than 20% had relief for more than 1 month, irrespective of the agent used. The median time to a 50% return of baseline pain level was 3 days in the corticosteroid group and 3.5 days in the anesthetic group. This difference was not significant. There are only case reports on the positive effect of intra-articular thoracic z-joint corticosteroid injections and no controlled trials.

Low back and leg pain relief lasting more than 6 months after intra-articular injection of lumbar z-joint corticosteroids has ranged from 18% to 63% in open, uncontrolled clinical studies. Five placebo-controlled studies of intra-articular corticosteroid lumbar z-joint injections have been performed, with conflicting results. The study with the strongest methodology regarding lumbar intra-articular z-joint injections evaluated 101 patients with low back pain of more than 6 months' duration. Patients who received more than 50% relief with a single z-joint block were randomized to intra-articular saline or intra-articular methylprednisolone. At 1 month postinjection, a significant difference was not found, with 42% of the treatment group and 33% of the control group having gained significant pain relief. At 6 months postinjection, 46% of the treatment group and 15% of the control group continued to experience marked relief. The difference was statistically significant but limited because of cointerventions (physical therapy) in the treatment group. The greatest flaw in the study was the failure to exclude placebo responders who had a more strict criterion for inclusion (only used greater than 50% relief with a single block). However, the results imply that intra-articular steroid injections combined with physical therapy might be an effective treatment option for patients who have failed other means of conservative treatment.

Predictors of an anesthetic response to intra-articular lumbar z-joint blocks have been studied and include absence of exacerbation with coughing, forward flexion, hyperextension, or extension with rotation, or with arising from a flexed position; older age; and relief when recumbent. In another study, although the clinical features traditionally believed to predict the presence of z-joint pain were no more common in patients who gained relief after z-joint injection, the intensity of pain after activities and motions thought to stress the z-joints (lumbar extension, hip hyperextension, standing, and walking) were diminished after the block.

A study of 58 patients with low back pain found that those with facetal uptake on single-photon emission computed tomography (SPECT) scan had a 95% response rate at 1 month and a 79% response rate at 3 months to z-joint injections with steroid and anesthetic. In contrast, those with negative SPECT scans were unchanged after injection of corticosteroid into the facet joints. Relatively long-term relief has been reported in 45% of patients with presumed symptomatic spondylolysis. In recent retrospective audit of 30 patients with lumbosacral radicular pain from sympto-

matic synovial cysts who underwent intra-articular corticosteroid injections, one third at a mean follow-up of 26 months had long-lasting acceptable benefit from z-joint injections for their radicular pain.

The therapeutic benefit of z-joint injections remains controversial. Current therapeutic z-joint injection studies are limited by a lack of precise knowledge regarding the therapeutic mechanism of intra-articular corticosteroid injections. The effect of the steroids on intracapsular inflammation is presumptive and based on the known anti-inflammatory action of steroids. No formal studies have addressed the mechanism of steroid action within the z-joint or have documented the presence of intra-capsular inflammation.

No long-term side effects from intra-articular corticosteroid injections have been reported, and the appropriate dose remains empiric. There is no role for repeated injections of the z-joint when pain relief lasting longer than several months does not occur after the first injection. Patients who, after an intra-articular injection, receive significant relief that is limited in duration might subsequently be evaluated with a medial branch block. Medial branch blocks are used in this context to determine the possible value of medial branch nerve neurotomy.

Dual blocks of the z-joint or the medial branches are recommended to obtain a secure diagnosis of this condition because of the false-positive rates of 38% and 27% with single z-joint injections in the lumbar and cervical spine, respectively. In a double-blind, controlled study of chronic neck pain, the false-negative rate of time-contingent relief (longer relief with bupivacaine than with lidocaine) with dual medial branch blocks was high (46%) compared with placebo, but the false-negative rate of non–time-contingent relief (relief not necessarily longer with bupivacaine) was 0. Eighty-eight percent of those with and 65% of those without time-contingent relief after dual medial branch blocks failed to have relief after a placebo challenge. Dual medial branch blocks substantially reduce the likelihood of a false-positive response; however, only a placebo injection can absolutely exclude a true placebo response. Non–time-contingent relief following dual medial branch blocks is a reasonable diagnostic compromise between single medial branch blocks and placebo blocks, which incur additional time and expense. With this approach, the sensitivity remains high (near 100%) and specificity is greatly improved compared with a single diagnostic block.

Medial Branch Radiofrequency Neurotomy

Radiofrequency (RF) lesioning of nerves that supply painful tissues can provide an effective treatment once the pain source is identified. Neurotomy of the medial branch nerves was devised based on the premise that pain from a z-joint could be relieved by coagulation of its afferent nerve supply. The greatest volume of literature regarding z-joint denervation considers RF lesioning, although methods using cryoneurolysis and phenol injection have been described.

RF lesioning involves the placement of a percutaneous needle electrode with a 5- to 10-mm noninsulated active tip parallel to the medial branch nerve. An adhesive surface-dispersive electrode on the skin surface completes the circuit. When a high-frequency alternating current is applied, ionic currents are created in the tissue adjacent to the active electrode tip. Heat is generated as a result of friction. Denervation of tissues occurs when the application of heat energy exceeds the early cytotoxic range for nervous tissue (45°C to 50°C). Clinically, temperatures of at least 85°C to 90°C for 60 to 90 s are recommended for irreversible lesions.

The innervation of the z-joints has been well described. The AO and LAA joints are not z-joints because of their anterior location and are innervated by the ventral rami of C1 and C2, respectively. Thus, RF neurotomy is not an option for these joints because of safety concerns. RF neurotomy is an option for recalcitrant C2-3 to L5-S1 z-joint pain. The C2-3 joint is innervated mostly by the third occipital nerve (TON) and superficial medial branch of C3 dorsal ramus, with some innervation from a communicating loop that joins the TON and C2 dorsal ramus.

Each cervical z-joint from C3-4 to C7-T1 is innervated from the medial branches of the dorsal rami, with each joint supplied from the branch above and below that joint. Therefore, the C5-6 z-joint is innervated by the C5 and C6 medial branches, which cross over the "waist" of the same numbered articular pillar. The T1-2 to T11-12 z-joints are innervated by two medial branch nerves that cross over the superolateral aspect of the same numbered transverse processes. The T12-L1 to L4-5 joints are innervated by two medial branch nerves that travel over the transverse process just lateral to the superior articular process. Therefore, the L4-5 z-joint is innervated by the L3 and L4 medial branch nerves that cross the L4 and L5 transverse processes. Similarly, the T4-5 z-joint is innervated by the T3 and T4 medial branch nerves that cross the T4 and T5 transverse processes. The L5 dorsal ramus crosses the sacral ala and divides into a medial and intermediate branch, with the medial branch nerve and L4 medial branch nerve providing innervation for the L5-S1 z-joint.

Patients most likely to benefit from RF lesioning of the medial branches have been diagnosed with z-joint pain based on two non–time-contingent z-joint or medial branch blocks that have offered more than 80% relief.

Outcomes are inferior when single medial branch blocks with less strict criteria are used. Studies that have selected patients on clinical grounds alone or with single intra-articular blocks have generally reported poor results.

Only one prospective, double-blind, controlled study on the treatment of chronic cervical z-joint pain with RF lesioning exists. The diagnosis was confirmed after three double-blind, placebo-controlled medial branch blocks yielded complete pain relief with anesthetic and not after placebo injection. The median time that elapsed before pain returned to 50% of the pretreatment level was significantly longer in the group treated with RF lesioning (263 days) than in the group treated with sham RF lesioning (8 days). McDonald and associates found that the median duration of relief following a successful cervical medial branch neurotomy was 422 days and that pain relief can be reinstated with repeat neurotomy. No peer-reviewed reports using current anatomic considerations exist on thoracic medial branch neurotomy.

The first prospective, randomized, double-blind study on the effects of lumbar medial branch RF lesioning demonstrated only modest results. Subjects who received more than 50% relief after a single z-joint block were treated with RF lesioning. The control group was treated with sham lesioning. Significantly more successes (at least 50% pain relief) were found in the RF group at 3-, 6-, and 12-month follow-ups. However, only a minority of subjects received more than 90% relief.

A more recent prospective audit studied patients with very strict inclusion criteria. Patients with low back pain for at least 1 year with more than 80% relief after two separate sets of medial branch blocks were treated with RF lesioning at the involved levels. More than 90% of the nerves were lesioned, as determined by normal presegmental specific multifidus electromyographic versus posttreatment electromyographic evidence of denervation in the same segmental multifidus related to the lesioned medial branch nerve. Sixty percent of the subjects had more than 90% relief at a 1-year follow-up, and an additional 27% had at least 60% pain relief. Statistically significant improvements in visual analog scale, Roland-Morris disability scale, McGill Pain questionnaire, and Medical Outcomes Study 36-Item Short Form Health Survey measures were found at 6 weeks and 3, 6, and 12 months postneurotomy compared with baseline. These studies show that proper patient selection and accurate surgical technique are critical to the successful management of low back pain with RF neurotomy.

Sacroiliac Joint Injection

The sacroiliac (SI) joint is a link between the spine and the lower extremities and as such is subjected to significant mechanical stresses. It is a diarthrodial joint with hyaline cartilage on the sacral side and pseudofibrous cartilage on the iliac side. The joint is contained by a fibrous joint capsule. A strong posterior interosseous and SI ligamentous complex stabilizes the joint by enmeshing with fibers from the gluteus maximus, gluteus medius, and thoracodorsal fascia. The weak anterior ligament is a thickening of the joint capsule and is in close proximity to the lumbosacral plexus. Additional support is provided from the sacrotuberous, sacrospinous, and long dorsal SI ligaments.

Innervation of the upper dorsal SI joint is provided from the L5 ventral ramus; the lower dorsal SI joint is innervated by the lateral branches of the S1 to S4 dorsal rami. The upper ventral aspect of the SI joint is supplied by the L5 ventral ramus, and the lower ventral aspect of the SI joint is innervated by the ventral ramus of S2 or branches from the sacral plexus. These free nerve endings convey pain, thermal sensation, pressure, and position sense. Therefore, the joint and its capsule and ligamentous complex can be a source of extraspinal pain. The differential diagnosis of SI joint-mediated pain includes joint capsule tears, ligamentous sprains, stress fracture, infection, ankylosing spondylitis, psoriatic arthritis, Reiter syndrome, osteoarthritis, calcium pyrophosphate crystal deposition disease, gout, synovial villoadenomas, iatrogenic instability from iliac bone graft harvest, and osteitis condensans ilii.

The intra-articular administration of approximately 2 mL of local anesthetic is believed to specifically block the SI joint and has been used as the gold standard to diagnose this clinical entity. Using diagnostic SI joint blocks, the incidence of SI joint mediated pain was studied in a group of 43 chronic low back pain patients with pain below the L5 level. Using controlled blocks as the diagnostic criteria for SI joint mediated pain, the prevalence of SI joint pain in this group was at least 13% and as high as 30%. Using dual intra-articular blocks of the SI joint as the gold standard for diagnosis, the prevalence of SI joint pain in 54 patients with maximal pain below L5 was 19%.

Under fluoroscopic guidance, a spinal needle can be introduced into the inferior aspect of the joint from a posterior approach. The administration of contrast will outline the auricular shape of the joint on an oblique view. Diverticula, ventral capsular tears, and attenuated areas can be visualized. In addition, routes of communication between the SI joint and neural tissues can be identified. These include a posterior subligamentous extension into the dorsal sacral foramina, superior recess extravasation into the L5 epiradicular sheath, or leakage from a ventral tear to the lumbosacral plexus. These findings have not yet been correlated with any pattern of clinical presentation.

Cannulation of the SI joint is rarely possible without fluoroscopic or CT guidance. A prospective study evaluated the ability to inject the SI joint with a mixture of bupivacaine, methylprednisolone, and iohexol without radiographic guidance. CT was performed immediately after the injection. Intra-articular injection was accomplished in only 22% of the patients. Epidural injection was observed in 24% of the patients. This study underscores the necessity of fluoroscopic visualization for accurate joint injection.

To date, no specific or pathognomonic historic features have been validated scientifically that accurately identify a painful SI joint. Variable pain referral patterns might occur because of the complex innervation of the joint, multiple sites of potential joint injury, and irritation of adjacent neural structures. Referred pain has been described as occurring in the region of the posterior superior iliac spine, lower lumbar spine, lateral buttock, groin, and distal lower extremity.

In addition, physical examination has been unable to predict which patients will obtain relief after an SI joint block. Dreyfuss and associates studied accepted diagnostic historic and physical examination findings of 45 patients who obtained more than 90% relief from a fluoroscopically guided SI joint block against a cohort of subjects without SI joint-mediated pain. None of the commonly accepted historic or physical examination tests that are purported to diagnose SI joint pain correctly predicted the response to injection. Maigne and associates prospectively studied 54 patients with normal CT and more than 75% relief of low back pain following double SI joint blocks. Physical examination maneuvers such as the compression test, distraction test, Gaenslen's test, Patrick test, and others failed to predict the response to SI joint block. Similar results attesting to the limitation of physical examination in the diagnosis of SI joint-mediated pain have been found by Slipman and associates and Schwarzer and associates.

Corticosteroid injection has been shown to be efficacious in the treatment of sacroiliitis caused by spondyloarthropathy. A prospective, double-blind, randomized, controlled study in a small group of subjects found at 1-month follow-up that intra-articular corticosteroids provided 85.7% good or very good results (more than 70% relief) in the group that received 1.5 mL cortivazol compared with 0 in the group that received saline injection. At 3- and 6-month follow-ups, 62% and 58%, respectively, continued to demonstrate significant improvement. A prospective case series on the effects of CT-guided intra-articular corticosteroid injection in spondyloarthropathy-induced sacroiliitis evaluated subjects with low back pain for at least 2 months. At 10 months' follow-up, 92.5% of patients had obtained more than 30% pain relief. The pretreatment and posttreatment mean visual analog scales were 8.8 and 3.3, respectively. In addition, a significant reduction in the enhancement factor on dynamic contrast-enhanced MRI was noted. These studies imply a therapeutic role for intra-articular SI joint corticosteroid injection when the diagnosis of true sacroiliitis has been established. The long-term efficacy of SI joint injection for other possible causes of SI joint-mediated pain has not yet been studied.

Conclusion

Diagnostic injections of the spinal nerve, facet joint, medial branch nerves, and SI joint provide additional tools for establishing the source of spinal pain. ESIs, z-joint and SI joint injections, and medial branch RF neurotomy provide nonsurgical options in the management of painful spinal conditions. These procedures can allow the patient to avoid potentially unnecessary treatments or continuing pain. Their diagnostic and potentially therapeutic role has now become well accepted, and their use continues to increase.

Annotated Bibliography

Contraindications and Potential Complications

Sullivan W, Willick S, Chira-Adisai W, et al: Incidence of intravascular uptake in lumbar spinal injection procedures. *Spine* 2000;25:481-486.

The authors report an incidence of intravascular uptake during lumbar spinal injection procedures of 8.5%. Absence of flashback of blood upon preinjection aspiration did not predict extravascular needle placement. Contrast-enhanced, fluoroscopic guidance was recommended when doing lumbar spinal injection procedures to prevent inadvertent intravascular uptake of injectate.

Windsor R, Pinzon E, Gore H: Complications of common selective spinal injections: Prevention and management, in Lennard T (ed): *Pain Procedures in Clinical Practice*, ed 2. Philadelphia, PA, Hanley & Belfus, 2000, pp 10-24.

This chapter on the complications of spinal injections covers patient preparation, monitoring, management and a review of the available literature.

Epidural Steroid Injections

Bush K, Hillier S: Outcome of cervical radiculopathy treated with periradicular/epidural corticosteroid injections: A prospective study with independent clinical review. *Euro Spine J* 1996;5:319-325.

The authors of this prospective study of patients undergoing serial periradicular/epidural corticosteroid injection in managing cervical radiculopathy over a 10-year period found a satisfactory recovery without the need for surgical intervention with an average of 2.5 injections per patient.

Canon D, Aprill C: Lumbosacral epidural steroid injections. *Arch Phys Med Rehabil* 2000;81:S87-S98.

This is a general review of the use of lumbosacral epidural steroid injections for the treatment of lumbar radicular pain.

Carette S, Leclaire R, Marcoux S, et al: Epidural corticosteroid injections for sciatica due to herniated nucleus pulposus. *N Engl J Med* 1997;336:1634-1640.

The authors of this randomized, double-blind trial administered up to three epidural injections of methylprednisolone acetate to patients with sciatica due to a herniated nucleus pulposus. After 6 weeks, the only significant difference was the improvement in leg pain. After 3 months, there were no significant differences between the groups. At 12 months, the cumulative probability of back surgery was 25.8% in the placebo group.

Koes B, Scholten R, Mens J, et al: Epidural steroid injections for low back pain and sciatica: An updated systematic review of randomized clinical trials. *Pain Digest* 1999;9:241-247.

This meta-analysis scored the results of clinical trials. Of the four best studies, two reported positive outcomes and two reported negative results. Overall, six studies indicated that the epidural steroid injection was more effective than the reference treatment and six reported it to be no better or worse than the reference treatment.

Lee H, Weinstein J, Meller S, et al: The role of steroids and their effects on phospholipase A2: An animal model of radiculopathy. *Spine* 1998;23:1191-1196.

Behavioral pattern changes observed in the irritated nerve root model in the rat are caused in part by a high level of phospholipase A_2 activity initiated by inflammation. The mechanism of action of epidural steroid injection is inhibition of phospholipase A_2 activity.

Lutz G, Vad V, Wisneski R: Fluoroscopic transforaminal lumbar epidural steroids: An outcome study. *Arch Phys Med Rehabil* 1998;79:1362-1366.

The authors of this prospective case series investigated the outcome of patients with lumbar herniated nucleus pulposus and radiculopathy who received fluoroscopic guided transforaminal epidural steroid injections. Seventy-five percent of patients had a successful long-term outcome, reporting at least a greater than 50% reduction between preinjection and postinjection pain scores, as well as an ability to return to or near their previous levels of functioning after only 1.8 injections per patient.

Lutze M, Stendel M, Vesper J, Brock M: Periradicular therapy in lumbar radicular syndromes: Methodology and results. *Acta Neurochir* 1997;139:719-724.

The study evaluated the therapeutic success of CT- versus fluoroscope-guided periradicular injections of local anesthetics and corticoids. CT-guided injection demonstrated superior results when compared with fluoroscope-assisted treatment.

Riew KD, Yin Y, Gilula L, et al: The effect of nerve-root injections on the need for operative treatment of lumbar radicular pain: A prospective, randomized, controlled, double-blind study. *J Bone Joint Surg Am* 2000; 82:1589-1593.

The data indicate that selective nerve-root injections of corticosteroids are significantly more effective than those of bupivacaine alone in obviating the need for surgery for up to 13 to 28 months after injections in candidates for surgery.

Rozenberg S, Dubourg G, Khalifa P, et al: Efficacy of epidural steroids in low back pain and sciatica. *Rev Rhum* 1999;66:79-85.

A critical appraisal by a French Task Force of randomized clinical trials found that five trials demonstrated greater pain relief within the first month in the steroid group as compared to the control group. In eight trials no measurable benefits were found.

Weiner B, Fraser R: Foraminal injection for lateral lumbar disc herniation. *J Bone Joint Surg Br* 1997;79: 804-807.

The authors prospectively studied the effects of transforaminal steroid injection for the management of foraminal and extraforaminal disc herniation. Seventy-nine percent of the patients available for long-term follow-up had considerable and sustained relief from their symptoms.

Zygapophysial Joint Injections

Dolan AL, Ryan, PJ, Arden, NK, et al: The value of SPECT scans in identifying back pain likely to benefit from facet joint injection. *Br J Rheum* 1996;35: 1269-1273.

The authors studied the response to intra-articular corticosteroid zygapophyseal joint injection after SPECT imaging. The percentage of scan-positive patients who reported improvement was 95% at 1 month and 79% at 3 months, significantly greater than the control group. Within 6 months, pain improvement in the SPECT-positive group was no longer statistically significant.

Dreyer S, Dreyfuss P, Cole A: Posterior elements (facet and sacroiliac joints) and low back pain. *Phys Med Rehabil State Art Rev* 1999;13:443-471.

A concise review of the literature regarding zygapophyseal and SI joint injection is presented.

Dreyfuss P, Schwarzer AC, Lau P, Bogduk N: The target specificity of lumbar medial branch and L5 dorsal ramus blocks: A computed tomography study. *Spine* 1997;22: 895-902.

A cross-sectional study to determine the validity of lumbar medial branch blocks demonstrated that when the appropriate technique is used, medial branch blocks are target specific.

Fukui S, Ohseto K, Shiotani M, et al: Referred pain distribution of the cervical zygapophysial joints and cervical dorsal rami. *Pain* 1996;68:79-83.

The distribution of referred pain from the cervical zygapophyseal joints and the cervical dorsal rami (C3 to C7) was studied by injection of contrast medium into the joints or by electrical stimulation of the dorsal rami. Each joint and dorsal ramus produced referred pain with a characteristic distribution.

Fukui S, Ohseto K, Shiotani M: Patterns of pain induced by distending the thoracic zygapophysial joints. *Reg Anesth* 1997;22:332-336.

The study was designed to investigate the patterns of referral pain associated with the thoracic zygapophyseal joints (C7-T1 to T2-3, and T11-12). The referred pain distribution for the joints C7-T1 to T2-3 showed significant overlap and the T11-12 joint referred to the iliac crest.

Fukui S, Ohseto K, Shiotani M, et al: Distribution of referred pain from the lumbar zygapophysial joints and dorsal rami. *Clin J Pain* 1997;13:303-307.

Under fluoroscopic control the joints from L1-2 to L5-S1 were stimulated by injection of contrast medium and the lumbar medial branches of the dorsal rami from T12 to L5 underwent electrical stimulation. The distribution of referred pain from the L1-2 to L5-S1 zygapophyseal joints, and the medial branches of the dorsal rami from L1 to L5 were similar for each level stimulated, and the overlap of referred pain between each level was considerable.

Kaplan M, Dreyfuss P, Halbrook B, Bogduk N: The ability of lumbar medial branch blocks to anesthetize the zygapophysial joint: A physiologic challenge. *Spine* 1998;23:1847-1852.

The authors of this randomized, controlled, single-blinded study demonstrated the physiologic effectiveness of lumbar medial branch blocks. When properly performed, lumbar medial branch blocks successfully inhibit pain associated with capsular distention of the lumbar zygapophysial joints at a rate of 89%.

Lord S, Barnsley L, Wallis B, et al: Chronic cervical zygapophysial joint pain after whiplash: A placebo-controlled prevalence study. *Spine* 1996;22:1737-1744.

The reliability of comparative blocks of the medial branches of the cervical dorsal rami in the diagnosis of cervical zygapophysial joint pain were studied. Comparative blocks were found to have a specificity of 88%, but only marginal sensitivity (54%). Expanding the comparative blocks diagnostic criteria to include all patients with reproducible relief, irrespective of duration, increases sensitivity to 100% but lowers specificity to 65%.

Parlier-Cuau C, Wybier M, Nizard R, Champsaur P, Le Hir P, Laredo JD: Symptomatic lumbar facet joint synovial cysts: Clinical assessment of facet joint steroid injection after 1 and 6 months using long-term follow-up in 30 patients. *Radiology* 1999;210:509-513.

Facet joint intraarticular steroid injection in patients with symptomatic lumbar facet joint synovial cysts were studied. After 1 month, the nerve root pain outcome was excellent or good in 67% of these patients. After 6 months, only 50% of these patients still had excellent or good results.

Revel M, Poiraudeau S, Auleley G, et al: Capacity of the clinical picture to characterize low back pain relieved by facet joint anesthesia: Proposed criteria to identify patients with painful facet joints. *Spine* 1998;23:1972-1976.

The presence of five among seven variables (age greater than 65 years and pain that was not exacerbated by coughing, not worsened by hyperextension, not worsened by forward flexion, not worsened when rising from flexion, not worsened by extension-rotation, and well-relieved by recumbency), distinguished 92% of patients responding to zygapophyseal joint injection of lidocaine and 80% of those not responding in the lidocaine group.

Radiofrequency Neurotomy

Dreyfuss P, Halbrook B, Pauza K, et al: Efficacy and validity of radiofrequency neurotomy for chronic lumbar zygapophysial joint pain. *Spine* 2000;25:1270-1277.

In this prospective audit, 60% of the patients undergoing lumbar radiofrequency neurotomy obtained at least 90% relief of pain at 12 months, and 87% obtained at least 60% relief.

Lord S, Barnsley L, Wallis B, et al: Percutaneous radiofrequency neurotomy for chronic cervical zygapophysial joint pain. *N Engl J Med* 1996;335:1721-1726.

The median time that elapsed before the pain returned to at least 50% of the pretreatment level was 263 days in the active-treatment group and 8 days in the control group of subjects with chronic cervical zygapophysial joint pain after whiplash injury.

McDonald GJ, Lord SM, Bogduk N: Long-term follow-up of patients treated with cervical radiofrequency neurotomy for chronic neck pain. *Neurosurgery* 1999;45:61-67.

Complete relief of pain was obtained in 71% of patients after an initial procedure with a median duration of relief of 422 days when only successful cases are considered.

Van Kleef M, Barendse G, Kessels A, et al: Randomized trial of radiofrequency lumbar facet denervation for chronic low back pain. *Spine* 1999;24:1937-1942.

This prospective double-blind randomized trial of 31 patients found RF lumbar zygapophysial joint denervation results in a significant alleviation of pain and functional disability in a select group of patients with chronic low back pain.

Sacroiliac Joint Injections

Bollow M, Braun J, Taupitz M, et al: CT-guided intraarticular corticosteroid injection into the sacroiliac joints in patients with spondyloarthropathy: Indication and follow-up with contrast enhanced MRI. *J Comp Assist Tom* 1996;20:512-521.

This prospective randomized trial showed a statistically significant abatement of subjective complaints for at least 5 months after treatment. The severity of inflammation and the response to therapy can be determined quantitatively by dynamic MRI.

Dreyfuss P, Michaelsen M, Pauza K, et al: The value of history and physical examination in diagnosing sacroiliac joint pain. *Spine* 1996;21:2594-2602.

This prospective study evaluated the diagnostic utility of historically accepted SI joint tests. No historic feature, none of the 12 SI joint tests, and no ensemble of these 12 tests demonstrated worthwhile diagnostic value.

Fortin J, Kissling R, O'Connor B, Vilensky JA: Sacroiliac joint innervation and pain. *Am J Orthop* 1999;28:687-690.

This article reviews current knowledge on the innervation of the human SI joint.

Maigne JY, Aivaliklis A, Pfefer F: Results of sacroiliac joint double block and value of sacroiliac pain provocation tests in 54 patients with low back pain. *Spine* 1996;21:1889-1892.

This prospective study evaluating the double SI block in patients with low back pain suggests the SI joint is an uncommon but real source of low back pain.

Maigne JY, Boulahdour H, Chatellier G: Value of quantitative radionuclide bone scanning in the diagnosis of sacroiliac joint syndrome in 32 patients with low back pain. *Eur Spine J* 1998;7:328-331.

This prospective study compared the results of radionuclide bone scanning with those of an SI joint anesthetic block in patients with unilateral low back pain. The sensitivity, specificity, and positive and negative predictive values of the quantitative bone scanning in the unilateral mechanical SI joint syndrome were 46.1%, 89.5%, 85.7%, and 72%, respectively.

Maugars Y, Mathis C, Berthelot J: Assessment of the efficacy of sacroiliac corticosteroid injections in spondylarthropathies: A double-blind study. *Br J Rheum* 1996; 35:767-770.

The authors demonstrated at 1 month, 80% of SI joints injected with corticosteroid described a relief of greater than 70%, in comparison to 0 of the placebo group. Results were still significant at 3 months (62%) and 6 months (58%).

Rosenberg J, Quint T, de Rosayro A: Computerized tomographic localization of clinically-guided sacroiliac joint injections. *Clin J Pain* 2000;16:18-21.

Intra-articular injection was accomplished in only 22% of patients when CT guidance was not utilized during injection. Epidural injected material was seen 24% of the time.

Slipman C, Jackson H, Lipetz J, et al: Sacroiliac joint pain referral zones. *Arch Phys Med Rehabil* 2000;81: 334-338.

Positive diagnostic responses to fluoroscopically guided SI joint injection were studied. Pain referral from the SI joint does not appear to be limited to the lumbar region and buttock.

Slipman C, Sterenfeld E, Chou L, et al: The predictive value of provocative sacroiliac joint stress maneuvers in the diagnosis of sacroiliac joint syndrome. *Arch Phys Med Rehabil* 1998;79:288-292.

To determine the clinical validity of provocative SI joint maneuvers in making the diagnosis of SI joint syndrome, patients' responses to a fluoroscopically guided SI joint block were studied. Results did not support the use of provocative SI joint maneuvers to confirm a diagnosis.

Classic Bibliography

Barnsley L, Bogduk N. Medial branch blocks are specific for the diagnosis of cervical zygapophysial joint pain. *Reg Anesth* 1993;18:343-350.

Barnsley L, Lord S, Wallis B, Bogduk N: Lack of effect of intra-articular corticosteroids for chronic pain in the cervical zygapophysial joints. *N Engl J Med* 1994;330: 1047-1050.

Barnsley L, Lord S, Wallis B, Bogduk N: False-positive rates of cervical zygapophysial joint blocks. *Clin J Pain* 1993;9:124-130.

Bush K, Hillier S: A controlled study of caudal epidural injections of triamcinolone plus procaine for the management of intractable sciatica. *Spine* 1991;16:572-575.

Carette S, Marcoux S, Truchon R, et al: A controlled trial of corticosteroid injections into the facet joints for chronic low back pain. *N Eng J Med* 1991;325: 1002-1007.

Chua W, Bogduk N: The surgical anatomy of thoracic facet denervation. *Acta Neurochirurgica* 1995;136: 140-144.

Derby R, Kine G, Saal J, et al: Response to steroid and duration of radicular pain as predictors of surgical outcome. *Spine* 1992;6:S176-S183.

Dooley J, McBroom R, Taguchi T: Nerve root infiltration in the diagnosis of radicular pain. *Spine* 1988;13: 79-83.

Dreyfuss P, Michaelsen M, Fletcher D: Atlanto-occipital and lateral atlanto-axial joint pain patterns. *Spine* 1994;19:1125-1131.

Dwyer A, Aprill C, Bogduk N: Cervical zygapophysial joint pain patterns: I. A study of normal volunteers. *Spine* 1990;15:453-457.

Grob K, Neuhuber W, Kissling R: Die innervation des sacroiliacalgelenkes beim Menschen. *Zeitschr Rheumatol* 1995;27:117-122.

Haueisen D, Smith B, Myers S, et al: The diagnostic accuracy of spinal nerve injection studies. *Clin Orthop* 1985;198:179-183.

Ikeda R: Innervation of the sacroiliac joint: Macroscopic and histological studies. *J Nippon Med School* 1991;58: 587-596.

Jamison R, VadeBoncouer T, Ferrante F: Low back pain patients unresponsive to an epidural steroid injection: Identifying predictive factors. *Clin J Pain* 1991;7: 311-317.

Lilius G, Laasonen E, Mylynen P, et al: Lumbar facet joint syndrome: A randomized clinical trial. *J Bone Joint Surg Br* 1989;71:681-684.

Lord S, Barnsley L, Bogduk N: The utility of comparative local anesthetic blocks versus placebo-controlled blocks for the diagnosis of cervical zygapophysial joint pain. *Clin J Pain* 1995;11:208-213.

Mooney V, Robertson J: The facet syndrome. *Clin Orthop* 1976;115:149-156.

Robecchi A, Capra R: Lidrocortisone (composto F): Prime esperienze cliniche in campo reumatologico. *Minerva Med* 1952;98:1259-1263.

Schwarzer A, Aprill C, Derby R, et al: The false positive rate of uncontrolled diagnostic blocks of the lumbar zygapophysial joints. *Pain* 1994;58:195-200.

Schwarzer AC, Aprill CN, Derby R, et al: Clinical features of patients with pain stemming from the lumbar zygapophysial joints: Is the lumbar facet syndrome a clinical entity? *Spine* 1994;19:1132-1137.

Schwarzer A, Wang S, Bogduk N, et al: Prevalence and clinical features of lumbar zygapophysial joint pain: A study in an Australian population with chronic low back pain. *Ann Rheum Dis* 1995;54:100-106.

Schwarzer AC, Wang SC, O'Driscoll D, et al: The ability of computed tomography to identify a painful zygapophysial joint in patients with chronic low back pain. *Spine* 1995;20:907-912.

Schwarzer AC, Scott AM, Wang S, et al: Abstract: The role of bone scintigraphy in chronic low back pain: Comparison of SPECT and planar images and zygapophysial joint injection. *Aust NZ J Med* 1992;22:185.

Schwarzer A, Aprill C, Bogduk N: The sacroiliac joint in chronic low back pain. *Spine* 1995;20:31-37.

Slipman C: Diagnostic nerve root blocks, in Gonzalez E, Materson R (eds): *The Nonsurgical Management of Acute Low Back Pain*. New York, NY, Demos Vermande, 1997, pp 115-121.

Stanley D, McLaren M, Euinton H, Getty C: A prospective study of nerve root infiltration in the diagnosis of sciatica: A comparison with radiculography, computed tomography, and operative findings. *Spine* 1990;6:540-543.

van Akkerveeken P: The diagnostic value of nerve root sheath infiltration. *Acta Orthop Scand* 1993;64:61-63.

Chapter 23

Chronic Pain Management: The Pain Clinic

T. Samuel Shomaker, MD, JD

Michael A. Ashburn, MD, MPH

Introduction

Given the propensity with which human beings seem to injure their backs and the relatively long life span that individuals in western societies currently enjoy, it is inevitable that many physicians, among them orthopaedic surgeons, neurosurgeons, and other spine care physicians, will see a large number of patients with chronic back pain. Although some of these patients can be cured by surgery, many cannot, and thus it is important for physicians to know the rudiments of care for the patient with chronic back pain.

Chronic pain, as distinguished from acute pain and cancer-related pain, is commonly defined as pain that lasts longer than would be expected for healing of the original injury to take place or as pain associated with progressive, nonmalignant disease. Statistics show that about 10% of patients with back pain do not get better in 4 to 6 weeks and that more than half of patients who recover from an initial episode of acute low back pain will have another episode within a few years. Some of these patients are destined to develop chronic back pain.

Chronic back pain is a complex medical condition that includes both physical and psychosocial factors. In fact, up to 85% of patients with low back pain cannot be given a definitive diagnosis because of poor association among symptoms, physical findings, and imaging results. In many cases, chronic back pain persists long after the tissue damage that initially triggered the onset of pain has resolved. Indeed, in some patients, chronic back pain is present without any antecedent injury or tissue damage.

Chronic back pain frequently results from changes in the peripheral or central nervous system in response to tissue injury. Some of these changes, especially in the peripheral nervous system, persist even after tissue damage has resolved. Changes in the processing of stimuli from nociceptive receptors within the central nervous system also can result in persistent pain. If these nervous system changes are the source of the patient's pain complaint, then surgical intervention at the site of the original tissue damage is not likely to treat the pain successfully.

The Effect of Chronic Pain

Chronic pain has a more pervasive effect on a patient's life than does acute pain. Patients with chronic pain frequently experience depression, sleep deprivation, decreased overall physical capability, and enhanced fatigue. Their pain complaint comes to affect their lives profoundly, influencing mood, personality, and social relationships. Patients frequently experience diminished satisfaction with life and a loss of self-esteem. They are often subjected to a seemingly endless continuum of workups that fail to reveal a specific cause of the pain problem, or they are put through expensive tests that do not reveal why the pain is occurring. They are frequently exposed to health professionals who are skeptical that a real medical problem is at the root of their discomfort. Gradually, many patients withdraw from their normal activities and fail to participate in recreational or social events that once were important to them. In short, their pain complaint becomes the central focus of their life.

Given the complex interaction of physical, psychological, and social issues in chronic pain syndromes, physical pain is only one of the many issues that must be addressed in the management of patients with chronic pain. In reality, chronic pain syndromes are chronic diseases and, in most cases, it is unrealistic to expect that patients will be cured and their pain removed. Thus, the goal of therapy is to assist patients in controlling pain and to rehabilitate them so that they can achieve the highest level of functioning of which they are capable.

Evaluation of Chronic Back Pain

Back pain has many potential causes and, when it becomes chronic, is often a complex, multifactorial problem. Whereas treating the patient with acute back pain can be a relatively straightforward matter, treating the patient with chronic back pain is frequently highly challenging and, indeed, often frustrating. Given that these are complicated, demanding patients with essentially an incurable disease, it often makes sense for the spine care physician who does not specialize in chronic pain care to refer these individuals to specialists in pain management.

Pain Treatment Facilities

Many types of facilities and health care professionals offer pain treatment services, but the literature suggests that patients with chronic pain are most effectively treated in an interdisciplinary clinic format. This approach brings together pain physicians, psychologists or psychiatrists, physical therapists, occupational therapists, vocational counselors, nurse specialists, and pharmacists in a setting in which each contributes a particular strength to the treatment of the pain problem. The gold standard for interdisciplinary pain programs is provided by accreditation by the Commission on Accreditation of Rehabilitation Facilities (CARF), which evaluates pain programs on structural, process, and outcomes measures. It is advisable to refer patients with complex chronic back pain to CARF-accredited interdisciplinary pain programs. (A guide to pain facilities published by the American Pain Society gives a self-reported list of services provided by each facility.) The coordinated, multifaceted approach provided by a multidisciplinary pain program is capable of dealing with the multiple and complex factors that contribute to chronic back pain and, therefore, carries the greatest chance of preserving and enhancing patient functionality.

Multidisciplinary pain centers (MPCs) date from the 1950s. The first comprehensive MPC was founded at the University of Washington in 1961 by John Bonica, an anesthesiologist, who believed that chronic pain could best be managed by a well-coordinated team of specialized individuals working together. By 1990, an estimated 1,000 pain clinics existed in the United States alone.

The MPC is the most comprehensive type of pain treatment facility. It includes a wide variety of health care professionals, provides multiple therapeutic modalities, is affiliated with a major health science institution, and offers both evaluation and treatment services in inpatient and outpatient settings. Other levels of pain treatment facilities provide less comprehensive facilities and treatment and evaluation options. They are also staffed in a more limited fashion.

The complexity of patients with pain seen in MPCs is illustrated by a recent meta-analysis that reviewed 65 treatment outcome studies containing a total of 3,089 patients. These patients were a heterogeneous group but had an average pain duration of 7.1 years; more than 50% had had at least one pain-related surgery, and more than 50% were taking opioid medications at the time of the study. The prevalence of depression among the patients in the studies was estimated at 50%. A number of other distinguishing characteristics make MPC patients more complex than patients treated in more conventional medical facilities. These include higher levels of emotional distress, a higher prevalence of work-related injuries, greater health care utilization, more negative attitudes about the future, more constant pain, and greater functional impairment.

A number of outcome studies have found MPCs to be effective in dealing with the complex pain problems their patients present with. Outcome measures that have been used to assess the effectiveness of MPCs include pain reduction, a reduction or elimination of opioid use, an increase in activity levels, return to work, decreased utilization of health care resources, and closure of disability claims. In the area of pain reduction, MPCs have been marginally successful (in the range of 20% to 30%), but results are similar to those of other types of therapy, such as conventional medical and surgical treatment. In general, treatment offered by MPCs appears to be effective in reducing or eliminating opioid intake in patients with chronic pain; up to 73% of patients have decreased opioid use at the time of treatment termination. Substantially greater increases in activity level were observed in MPC patients (65%) versus those treated in a more conventional fashion (35%). MPC treatment also appears to help patients return to work, reduce utilization of health care resources, and close claims for disability.

In addition to their medical effectiveness, MPCs appear to be cost effective compared with other forms of treatment. One study reported a significant reduction in medical costs following MPC treatment, from $13,000 spent in the year before treatment to $5,500 in the year after treatment. Savings also are incurred in the amount of disability payments disbursed to patients in MPCs. Thus, although only a relatively small number of patients are treated annually in MPCs (currently around 8,000, versus nearly 300,000 patients who undergo surgery for back pain), MPCs appear to be cost effective and clinically successful in terms of restoring patients to greater degrees of functionality.

The Pain Treatment Plan

In the interdisciplinary clinic setting, many types of health professionals are involved in caring for the patient, but it is the pain physician who oversees and organizes the team's efforts. The first step is screening of the patient by a member of the core team, who determines which members of the team will be needed to develop and implement a comprehensive treatment plan. Communication among team members and with the patient is a key step in the development of this care plan, which is tailored to the individual needs of the patient and should include measurable treatment goals agreed upon by the team and the patient. Treatment possibilities can range anywhere from simple education and pharmacologic therapy to intensive inpatient rehabilitation lasting 3 to 4 weeks.

In designing the treatment plan, it is imperative that the treating team address the patient's expectations. Many patients have unrealistic expectations that their pain will be eliminated and they will be able to return to a preinjury state of full functionality. This is often not achievable, and a realistic goal is the reduction, rather than elimination, of pain and the improvement of current levels of physical functioning, mood, and associated symptoms. Another important goal is helping patients develop active coping skills. The ultimate objective is to rehabilitate the patient to the extent that he or she can return to as many normal daily activities, such as work, recreation, and hobbies, as possible.

Once the treatment plan has been established and treatment begins, continual communication among team members is essential so that the patient's progress can be optimized. Ongoing monitoring of achieved treatment goals allows the course of therapy to be adapted and adjusted as necessary, based on the patient's response. In addition to intrateam communication, ongoing communication with the patient provides insight into how the patient is dealing with the pain problem and any surrounding issues. Many patients with chronic back pain require intensive initial therapy and ongoing long-term therapy. Follow-up might be provided by pain clinic personnel but often is handled by the referring physician, based on consultation with MPC staff.

Treatment Methods

The many potential approaches to the treatment of chronic back pain include nerve block therapy, pharmacologic management, behavioral modification, neural stimulation, and physical therapy. In chronic back pain, single-treatment modalities are rarely effective; therefore, a combination of techniques is often the preferred approach.

Interventional Therapy

Nerve block therapy is frequently used in the management of chronic pain. Nerve blocks are procedures that involve the administration of local anesthetics, corticosteroids, or neurodestructive agents centrally, to visceral plexi, or to peripheral nerves and muscles. Despite the fact that they are used frequently, nerve blocks have a limited role in the treatment of chronic pain. The use of nerve blocks alone seldom results in the cure of a chronic pain condition. Nerve blocks are, in fact, more useful to facilitate the patient's participation in physical therapy than as a stand-alone treatment modality. The goal of enhanced participation in physical therapy is to improve range of motion and strength, thereby decreasing disability. Thus, although nerve blocks are rarely curative, they do have a role, albeit a limited one, in the management of chronic back pain.

A trigger point is a discrete, well-defined area of hyperirritability within a muscle or fascia. Trigger points take the form of a palpable and tender nodule or a band of tissue within a muscle that prevents the full range of motion of that muscle. Patients with back pain frequently develop trigger points, most often in response to pain-induced changes in their posture that persist for weeks or months. Trigger points also can develop after acute injury to musculoskeletal structures. Trigger points can be treated with injections of local anesthetic directly into the site of maximal tenderness. However, to be most effective, the injections must be used in conjunction with physical therapy and guided exercise.

Facet joint injections also have gained some currency in the treatment of back pain. Injections directly into the facet joint capsule or blockade of the median dorsal branch of the posterior primary division can be done using standard regional anesthesia techniques under radiographic guidance. Diagnostic blocks with local anesthetics are sometimes followed by radio frequency lesioning or cryolesioning intended to produce longer-term analgesia, allowing the patient to participate in physical therapy to enhance mobility and strength. The use of neuroablation techniques for the spinal or epidural nerve roots, although developed in the context of treatment for low back pain, is no longer advocated for this purpose unless the pain is of malignant origin and cannot be controlled by other methods. Neurolytic blockade carries a high incidence of undesirable side effects, such as motor weakness, bladder and sexual dysfunction, bowel incontinence, arachnoiditis, proprioceptive dysfunction, and dysesthesias.

A variety of stimulation techniques also has been used to blunt the perception of chronic back pain. These include both transcutaneous electrical nerve stimulation (TENS) and dorsal column stimulation. The postulated mechanism of action of both techniques is explained by the gate control theory of pain transmission. Chronic back pain carried by slow-transmitting A omega or C fibers can be drowned out by the stimulation of larger, faster-transmitting fibers of the A alpha or A beta variety. Modulation of the noxious stimulus probably takes place in the dorsal horn of the spinal cord.

TENS involves the application of an electric current

to the painful area of the back by either unipolar or bipolar electrodes placed on the skin surface overlying the area. The effectiveness of the electric stimulus depends on its intensity, wave form, and duration. When pain relief is produced, it will be noted within 10 to 15 minutes after the initiation of treatment. Efficacy is in the range of 10% to 15%. TENS is noninvasive and easy for patients to learn. It does not interfere with other forms of treatment and does not have serious side effects. In addition to its other beneficial effects, TENS also might help relieve muscle spasm associated with back injury.

Dorsal column stimulation, an invasive procedure involving the surgical implantation of electrodes into the epidural space, is becoming more popular for patients with chronic noncancer pain. Because of its invasive nature, it is rarely a first-line treatment. Before implantation therapy is considered, a specific diagnosis should be established and patients should undergo psychological evaluation to rule out drug dependency, major psychiatric disorders, or the possibility of secondary gain. Implantation for failed back syndrome is now the most common use of spinal cord stimulation in the United States. Spinal cord stimulation is more effective for radicular back pain, arachnoiditis, or epidural fibrosis than for axial or mechanical pain because the technique works best when the stimulation paresthesia overlays the anatomic distribution of pain.

Spinal cord stimulators consist of electrodes and leads, a pulse generator/receiver, and a programmer. Electric current flows from the positive anode to the negative cathode, and nerve fibers are depolarized by the accumulation of current at the cathode. Leads available today can contain up to eight electrodes, which are placed in the epidural space, allowing a wide array of anode and cathode configurations and thereby permitting precise control of the stimulating pattern. Pulse generators are either totally implantable or are radio frequency driven. The totally implantable generators contain lithium batteries that have an effective life of between 2 and 7 years, depending on patient usage. The pulse generator is controlled by means of a transcutaneous programmer. The radio frequency system involves an implanted receiver with a transmitting device that is worn outside the body. The patient is able to access and change the parameters of the system in a radio frequency device. Features that can be adjusted include amplitude, frequency, and pulse width. The device is set so as to give the patient a comfortable paresthesia that will modulate the pain sensation.

Prior to permanent implantation, all patients undergo temporary placement to evaluate the effectiveness of dorsal column stimulation in individual cases. If, after a trial period of several days to several weeks, a patient notes a consistent reduction in pain of at least 50%, along with increased functional status and stable or decreased analgesic usage, permanent implantation is then considered. Temporary placement is performed under fluoroscopic guidance with the use of local anesthesia and minimal sedation, but permanent implantation almost always is done in the operating room and is done either percutaneously or in an open fashion through a laminectomy. Side effects include technical difficulties relating to the positioning of the leads or inability to access the epidural space, inadvertent dural puncture and nerve root injury, and postoperative lead migration, the incidence of which can be as high as 25%.

A recent study found that of patients who underwent permanent implantation, 52% reported at least a 50% reduction of pain at 7-year follow-up. In general, the success rate of spinal cord stimulation for low back pain ranges from 40% to 70%.

Recently a new treatment modality, percutaneous electrical nerve stimulation (PENS), which combines the effects of TENS and acupuncture, has been evaluated in the treatment of back pain. The technique involves the use of acupuncture-like probes that are placed in the soft tissue or muscles overlying the affected area to stimulate peripheral sensory nerves at dermatomal levels corresponding to the injured site. A recent study showed promising results in comparison to the use of placebo, TENS, or exercise therapy.

Pharmacologic Management

Classes of drugs available for the treatment of chronic pain include opioids, nonsteroidal anti-inflammatory drugs (NSAIDS), antidepressants, anticonvulsants, and a number of miscellaneous drugs. Regardless of the pharmacologic therapy chosen, the initial approach should be the same. Patients should be assessed and a treatment plan developed. The patient must give informed consent and agree to the proposed plan. Once therapy has started, ongoing monitoring and assessment of patient progress is required; based on the patient's response, adjustment in the regimen might be necessary. Consultation with other specialists also is sometimes required to deal with issues that arise during the course of treatment.

Drug combination therapy frequently is employed; in these situations, special precautions must be taken. The practitioner must be aware of the potential for drug interactions posed by the use of multiple agents and also should be vigilant for the occurrence of side effects, which are sometimes cumulative with multiple drugs.

Despite the perception of the widespread perils of their misuse, opioids are a valuable treatment modality for providing analgesia in chronic pain syndromes and can be used effectively with minimal problems, as long as there is a disciplined approach to their use. Opioids should be used in a scheduled, time-contingent manner, with regular doses of any one of a number of opioid medications selected according to the circumstances of the individual patient's problem. In general, opioids work by binding to various types of opioid receptors in the central nervous system, opening potassium channels and closing calcium channels, resulting in the inhibition of ascending pain pathways and thereby altering the patient's perception of and response to pain.

Opioids have a common profile of adverse effects. About 40% of patients on morphine experience constipation; 40% experience nausea; and a slightly lesser number report dizziness. Equianalgesic doses of other opioids have a similar profile of side effects. Tolerance — the need for a higher dose to achieve the same pharmacologic effect — appears frequently in patients on long-term opioid therapy. Tolerance can be difficult to address. Sometimes it can be dealt with by changing the opioid or the route of administration.

Certain types of pain are opioid insensitive, that is, the pain does not respond to a progressive increase in opioid dose. Most commonly, opioid-insensitive pain is a result of nerve compression or nerve destruction. Thus, in patients suffering from sensory disturbance as a component of back pain, opioids might not be effective in dealing with the pain problem. Movement-related pain is also difficult to manage in patients with chronic pain. Doses of oral opioid required to control movement-related pain might be excessive when the patient is at rest and the pain stops.

Opioids are effective in many chronic pain states but are underprescribed because of societal fears about chemical dependence and substance abuse. Opioids can be used safely and responsibly in chronic pain states when prescribed on a regularly scheduled treatment regimen and when patients are adequately monitored to assess the effectiveness of the therapy. However, opioids should never be prescribed casually, and the use of these drugs requires a commitment on the part of the prescribing physician to follow patients closely and keep careful records.

NSAIDs are often prescribed for chronic and acute pain conditions. Despite their widespread use, NSAIDs have a fairly limited role in the treatment of chronic pain because they are often ineffective and carry a substantial risk of adverse side effects.

Antidepressant medications, particularly the tricyclic antidepressants, are frequently effective in the treatment of chronic pain conditions. The exact mechanism for the successful use of these medications is unclear, but it appears to be independent of their antidepressant effects. It might be that tricyclic drugs enhance endogenous pain-inhibiting mechanisms within the central nervous system by blocking the reuptake of serotonin and norepinephrine at the nerve synapse. In addition to their analgesic effects, tricyclic medications also can assist in the treatment of other common symptoms present in patients with chronic pain, such as depressed affect and sleep disorder.

Newer antidepressant medications that work through the mechanism of selective serotonin reuptake inhibition have found some use in the treatment of chronic pain. These medications are characterized by a much less significant potential side effect profile. In addition to their effect on chronic pain perception, these medications also might assist in the treatment of other manifestations of chronic pain, such as depression and sleep disorder.

Neuropathic pain resulting from injury to central or peripheral nerves is a difficult chronic pain problem. Neuropathic pain probably results from damage to afferent nociceptive axons. Damage in these neurons is believed to produce excitation caused by the loss of normal inhibition within the nerve. Neuropathic pain can be quite severe and disabling. Treatment is often initiated through the use of anticonvulsant medications such as carbamazepine or phenytoin. One hypothesized mechanism for the usefulness of anticonvulsants in neuropathic pain is the stabilization of sodium channels, which might suppress firing in the polysynaptic neurons that process nociceptive signals within the central nervous system. In severe pain states, full anticonvulsive doses are necessary to achieve some degree of effect. Carbamazepine appears to be more effective than phenytoin, but carbamazepine does have some undesirable side effects, such as the risk of blood dyscrasias, including neutropenia, leukopenia, pancytopenia, or thrombocytopenia. Thus, when indicated, the use of carbamazepine must be accompanied by the monitoring of blood counts to track the development of these potential side effects. Another anticonvulsant that has been used with some success and which has fewer side effects, gabapentin, also has shown some potential. In many cases, anticonvulsant and tricyclic antidepressant effects appear to be additive, if not synergistic, in the treatment of chronic pain.

Other drugs, such as the autonomic nervous system agents clonidine and baclofen, and ketamine, an *N*-methol-D-aspartate receptor antagonist, have been used with limited success in the treatment of chronic back pain. The use of these drugs also is associated with a number of undesirable side effects.

As previously stated, a well-planned treatment regimen for chronic back pain often includes the use of multiple modalities of therapy, including several drugs, behavioral modification, and physical therapy. When multiple drugs are used, the medications should be added one at a time, the effect should be observed, and the patient should be monitored for the development of drug interactions or adverse side effects. Potentially beneficial combinations include opioids and tricyclics; opioids and anticonvulsants; and opioids, tricyclics, and anticonvulsants. With the use of multiple drugs, patient monitoring becomes an even more significant issue, and patients should be seen relatively frequently to assess progress, adjust medication doses, and check for side effects.

Behavioral Approaches

Behavioral approaches to chronic pain therapy are designed to give patients some control over their lives and attitudes. Providing patients with tools to help them address their own issues is often a useful approach, especially when integrated into an interdisciplinary treatment program, which includes other strategies such as pharmacotherapy and exercise. A number of behavioral methods are available to assist in the treatment of chronic pain, including relaxation techniques, hypnosis, biofeedback, and cognitive behavioral therapy.

Cognitive behavioral therapy is widely used in interdisciplinary pain centers. It is a psychological method that seeks to change the patient's approach to his or her life by altering patterns of negative thoughts and dysfunctional attitudes to foster a healthier, more adaptive approach in day-to-day life. Cognitive behavioral therapy starts with patient education and skills acquisition. The patient is then called on to rehearse the new approach, to generalize it to day-to-day living, and finally to use this new thought process in a consistent fashion.

Relaxation techniques are often effective in the treatment of chronic back pain, as well. These include meditation, progressive muscle relation, deep breathing, and other forms of controlled respiration.

Biofeedback techniques provide patients with physiologic information intended to help them achieve a state of relaxation. Electromyographic, galvanometric, and electroencephalographic readings, as well as body temperature, are examples of physiologic data that can be used in the biofeedback process. Hypnosis is another technique to help patients achieve a state of directed relaxation. It uses the suggestion of a specific goal as a central principle.

Physical Therapy

Physical therapy is a cornerstone of treatment for all chronic pain syndromes, including chronic back pain. Patients with chronic back pain are often reluctant to use their bodies for fear that movement will initiate a vicious pain response. However, additional pain and disability are created through the disuse of muscles and joints. In addition, the perceived inability to exercise can also create further psychological problems and a growing sense of disability and hopelessness. Therefore, physical therapy is a key component of an interdisciplinary approach to chronic pain management. Physical therapists design specific exercise protocols to improve patient functionality and teach patients how to exercise safely with a minimum of pain. Patients who exercise have an enhanced sense of well being and an improved attitude, leading to greater life satisfaction and an improved ability to deal with stress.

A significant consideration in physical therapy is that movement-related pain is difficult to control in patients with chronic pain problems. At times, it is appropriate to use nerve blocks with local anesthetics to enable patients to begin the process of exercising and to break the cycle of growing disability. Movement-related pain is difficult to treat with oral opioids because doses sufficient to cover pain on exertion are often excessive for the resting state. Therefore, behavioral modification techniques are often used as adjuncts to physical therapy.

Summary

Chronic low back pain is frequently a disabling and debilitating medical problem. The development of chronic back pain is often associated with the onset of other social, psychological, and behavioral problems, and these can be as difficult and intractable to treat as the underlying pain. Perhaps the most important aspect to keep in mind in treating patients with chronic back pain is that they might well have a chronic disease for which there is no quick fix. These patients frequently require long-term and sometimes life-long therapy. Treatment in an MPC often is appropriate and desirable. A multifaceted approach to the patient's multiple problems is usually necessary to make any progress toward returning the patient to increased functional status. Thus, careful evaluation of the patient and the construction of a well-planned treatment regimen that includes consultation with the patient is of critical importance. Treatment plans commonly include pharmacologic, behavior-modifying, and exercise therapies. The physician responsible for the patient's long-term progress should periodically review the course of treatment and compare the patient's progress against predetermined treatment objectives. In the end, the goal of both physician and patient should be for the patient with chronic back pain to improve functionality and gain a sense of physical and mental well-being. In most cases, achieving these goals requires a patient to accept some limitation on previous levels of activity. A patient with realistic expectations is happier in the long run.

Annotated Bibliography

American Pain Society: Pain facilities. Accessed at http://www.ampainsoc.org/facility/finding.htm on July 25, 2000.

This site lists nationwide pain treatment centers and their services.

Ashburn M, Rubingh C: The role of nonopioid analgesics for the management of postoperative pain. *Acute Pain Control* 1999;6:10-13.

The authors provide a description and assessment of nonopioid pain medication options for use in acute pain settings.

Ashburn MA, Staats PS: Management of chronic pain. *Lancet* 1999;353:1865-1869.

This article provides a broad overview of the current approach to the management of chronic pain problems.

Collins SL, Faura CC, Moore RA, McQuay HJ: Peak plasma concentrations after oral morphine: A systematic review. *J Pain Symptom Manage* 1998;16:388-402.

The authors present a review of 69 studies on the pharmacokinetics and pharmacodynamics of oral morphine. No accumulation of morphine was seen in the use of multiple versus single doses.

Federation of State Medical Boards of the United States: *Model guidelines for the use of controlled substances for the treatment of pain*. Euless, TX, Federation of State Medical Boards of the United States, 1998.

These are authoritative and well-researched guidelines for the use of opioids to provide analgesia in pain conditions.

Feine JS, Lund JP: An assessment of the efficacy of physical therapy and physical modalities for the control of chronic musculoskeletal pain. *Pain* 1997;71:5-23.

The authors present an analysis of review articles showing that patients are helped by most forms of therapy during the period they are being treated.

Ghoname EA, Craig WF, White PF, et al: Percutaneous electrical nerve stimulation for low back pain: A randomized crossover study. *JAMA* 1999;281:818-823.

The authors describe PENS and compare it with TENS and placebo.

Hubbard JE, Tracy J, Morgan SF, McKinney RE: Outcome measures of a chronic pain program: A prospective statistical study. *Clin J Pain* 1996;12:330-337.

This study shows the effectiveness of the interdisciplinary approach to pain management. Patients with chronic pain within the program had improved functional status.

Loeser JD: *Desirable Characteristics for Pain Treatment Facilities*. Seattle, WA, International Association for the Study of Pain, 1998.

The author describes the characteristics of various types of pain treatment facilties.

McQuay H: Opioids in pain management. *Lancet* 1999; 353:2229-2232.

This article is a guide to the use of opioid analgesics in the treatment of acute and chronic pain conditions.

Moulin DE, Iezzi A, Amireh R, Sharpe WK, Boyd D, Merskey H: Randomised trial of oral morphine for chronic non-cancer pain. *Lancet* 1996;347:143-147.

This study concludes that oral morphine is an effective analgesic with a low risk of addiction in the treatment of chronic noncancer pain. Little improvement was seen in functional status.

NIH Technology Assessment Panel on Integration of Behavioral and Relaxation Approaches into the Treatment of Chronic Pain and Insomnia: Integration of behavioral and relaxation approaches into the treatment of chronic pain and insomnia. *JAMA* 1996;276: 313-318.

The study presents an assessment of the use of behavioral and relaxation techniques as a part of the management strategy for chronic pain conditions. Relaxation, hypnosis, cognitive behavioral therapy, and biofeedback were all shown to be strongly or moderately effective.

North RB, Roark GL: Spinal cord stimulation for chronic pain. *Neuro Surg Clin N Am* 1995;6:145-155.

Dorsal column stimulation is discussed.

Turk DC: Efficacy of multidisciplinary pain in the treatment of chronic pain. In Campbell JN, Cohen MJ (eds): *Pain Treatment Centers at Crossroads: A Practical Concept Reappraisal*. Seattle, WA, International Association for the Study of Pain Process, 1996, p 257.

The author reviews the effectiveness of MPCs.

Turk DC, Stacey BR: Multidisciplinary pain centers in the treatment of chronic back pain, in Frymoyer JW, Ducker TB, Hadler NM, Kostuick JP, Weinstein JN, Whitecloud TS III (eds): *The Adult Spine: Principles and Practice*, ed 2. Philadelphia, PA, Lippincott-Raven 1997, vol 1, pp 253-274.

This chapter describes the organization role and approach of interdisciplinary pain clinics in the treatment of chronic back pain.

Classic Bibliography

Allison MC, Howatson AG, Torrance CJ, Lee FD, Russell RI: Gastrointestinal damage associated with the use of nonsteroidal antiinflammatory drugs. *N Engl J Med* 1992;327:749-754.

Bonica JJ: Pain management: Past and current status, including the role of the anesthesiologist, in Stanley TH, Ashburn MA, Fine PG (eds): *Anesthesiology and Pain Management.* Dordrecht, The Netherlands, Kluwer Academic, 1991, pp 1-30.

Bogduk N, Long DM: Percutaneous lumbar medial branch neurotomy: A modification of facet denervation. *Spine* 1980;5:193-200.

Clive DM, Stoff JS: Renal syndromes associated with nonsteroidal anti-inflammatory drugs. *N Engl J Med* 1984;310:563-572.

Coles PG, Thompson GE: The role of neurolytic blocks in the treatment of cancer pain. *Int Anesthesiol Clin* 1991;29:93-104.

Flor H, Fydrich T, Turk DC: Efficacy of multidisciplinary pain treatment of centers: A meta-analytic review. *Pain* 1992;49:221-230.

Fordyce WE, Fowler RS Jr, Lehmann JF, Delateur BJ, Sand PL, Treischmann RB: Operant conditioning in the treatment of chronic pain. *Arch Phys Med Rehabil* 1973;54:399-408.

Frank A: Low back pain. *BMJ* 1993;306:901-909.

Goldenberg D: Fibromyalgia syndrome: An emerging but controversial condition. *JAMA* 1987;257:2782-2787.

Melzack R, Wall P: Pain mechanisms: A new theory. *Science* 1965;150:971-979.

North RB, Kidd DH, Zahurak M, James CS, Long DM: Spinal cord stimulation for chronic, intractable pain: Experience over two decades. *Neurosurgery* 1993;32:384-394.

North RB, Han PR, Zahurak M, Kidd DH: Radiofrequency lumbar facet denervation: Analysis of prognostic factors. *Pain* 1994;57:77-83.

Onghena P, Van Houdenhove B: Antidepressant-induced analgesia in chronic non-malignant pain: A meta-analysis of 39 placebo-controlled studies. *Pain* 1992;49:205-219.

Schuster GD, Infante MC: Pain relief after low back pain surgery: The efficacy of transcutaneous electrical nerve stimulation. *Pain* 1980;8:299-302.

Swerdlow M: Anticonvulsant drugs and chronic pain. *Clin Neuropharmacol* 1984;7:51-82.

Chapter 24

Pharmacologic Management of Chronic Pain

Jerome Schofferman, MD

Introduction

The treatment of spinal pain can include muscle strengthening, body mechanics training, spinal injections, and surgery. Although most patients improve, some continue to have severe pain and marked reduction in function. For some well-chosen patients, palliative pharmacologic pain management can result in marked improvements in quality of life.

To help their patients with refractory pain, impairment, and disability, spine specialists should know the basic concepts of pharmacologic pain management and be familiar with at least a few drugs from each category. This chapter will familiarize the reader with the classifications of drugs and particular medications that are the most helpful and have favorable risk-to-benefit ratios.

The classes of drugs most useful for chronic pain are the opioid analgesics, tricyclic antidepressants, and anticonvulsants, although other medications can be helpful for selected patients (Table 1).

Classifications of Pain Disorders

Acute Pain Versus Chronic Pain

Most physicians are trained to treat acute pain but not chronic pain. Acute pain has a recent onset, usually is treatable by specific means, can be associated with overactivity of the sympathetic nervous system, and is expected to follow a familiar natural history. Chronic pain is quite different. It is not just acute pain that does not resolve; it is pain that persists well beyond its expected duration, although formerly, some physicians defined chronic pain as any pain that lasted more than 6 months. Specific treatment in the patient with chronic pain will have been tried and will have failed. Signs of sympathetic overactivity seen in the patient with acute pain have been replaced by vegetative symptoms such as sleep disturbance and changes in appetite and weight. In addition, the patient often has a depressed mood. These symptoms are usually results of the pain, not the causes of the pain.

TABLE 1	Categories of Medications Useful for Chronic Spinal Pain	
Very Useful	**Occasionally Useful**
Analgesics	Sedative-hypnotics (sleep)
Peripherally acting	Glucocorticosteroids (flares)
Centrally acting	Muscle relaxants
Tricyclic antidepressants	Antihistamines (nausea)
Anticonvulsants (neuropathic pain)	Stimulants (side effects of opioids)
	Anti-arrhythmics (neuropathic pain)
	Alpha adrenergic blockers (for CRPS)

CRPS = complex regional pain syndrome (formerly called reflex sympathetic dystrophy)

Nociceptive Versus Neuropathic Pain

It is useful to divide chronic refractory spinal pain into nociceptive and neuropathic pains. The distinction is clinically important because some medications are more effective for one type than for the other. Nociceptive pain is caused by a structural disorder that stimulates small nerve endings (nociceptors)—for example, one or more painful, degenerated discs. Nociceptive pain is most responsive to opioids and nonsteroidal anti-inflammatory drugs (NSAIDs), although tricyclic antidepressants (TCAs) also can help.

Neuropathic pain is caused by nerve damage or injury. A damaged nerve is the source of the pain even though the nerve is no longer being stimulated. In addition, because the nerve is sensitized, pain may increase with only minimal stimulation. Examples include a "battered root," arachnoiditis, and complex regional pain syndrome (formerly called reflex sympathetic dystrophy). The drugs of choice for neuropathic pain are the TCAs and anticonvulsants. Some patients will respond to opioids, but higher doses might be needed. Some patients can have both nociceptive and neuropathic pain, a mixed-pain syndrome.

Analgesics

Analgesics can be divided into those that act in the periphery and those that act in the central nervous system. Each can have a role in the treatment of chronic spinal pain.

Peripherally Acting Analgesics

The peripherally acting analgesics are acetaminophen, aspirin, and the NSAIDs. They are useful for mild to moderate pain and also act synergistically with centrally acting analgesics. In addition to their anti-inflammatory effects, NSAIDs appear to produce analgesia by other mechanisms. Empiric support for this includes the facts that analgesia can begin in less than an hour, long before any anti-inflammatory activity could occur, and that NSAIDs can relieve pain even when no inflammation is present.

One way to select an NSAID is by the speed of onset and duration of analgesia. If the NSAID is to be used by the patient as needed for pain, then a drug with a rapid onset is preferable, although the duration of analgesia will be shorter. If the NSAID is to be used chronically, then a drug with a longer duration of analgesia would be preferable, even though it could take days for benefits to occur. Because of the variability in patient responses, several NSAIDs might have to be tried.

Centrally Acting Analgesics

The most important centrally acting analgesics are the opioids. Opioids produce analgesia primarily by binding with opiate receptors in the central nervous system. They work best for nociceptive pain but can be effective for neuropathic pain. Controversy still exists regarding the long-term use of opioids for chronic pain, although far less than was the case 10 years ago. Recent surveys have shown that many physicians use opioids for chronic low back pain, osteoarthritis, and other painful musculoskeletal disorders.

Concerns About the Use of Opioids

The major considerations that have discouraged some physicians from using opioids for long-term treatment are: (1) concerns about producing addiction and dependence, (2) fear of causing organ toxicity, (3) apprehension about possible disciplinary action by medical licensing boards, (4) concerns about tolerance, and (5) drug efficacy.

The most important concern should be efficacy. Do opioids produce pain relief without significant risk of harm? For years, physicians believed that these drugs were ineffective for long-term treatment and the risks too great, but these opinions were not based on medical evidence. The evidence published over the past decade is quite convincing that long-term opioid therapy can be safe and effective for many well-selected patients with low back pain and osteoarthritis. Most studies were longitudinal cohort studies, but a few have been randomized and placebo controlled. No recent studies show lack of efficacy. Efficacy has been well maintained in the long-term studies, although none has followed patients for more than a year. No evidence of serious organ toxicity or of a high incidence of addictive behavior or abuse has been reported.

No single opioid has proven to be superior to others. About 15% of patients are not able to tolerate long-term opioid use because of side effects. Of the patients who can tolerate long-term use of opioids, about 75% experience meaningful pain relief and most, but not all, also experience an increase in function. About 10% of patients disabled because of low back pain are able to return to work.

Addiction is a disease that is both psychological and biologic. It is defined as the compulsive use of a psychoactive substance resulting in biologic, psychological, or social harm. There is loss of control. The prevalence of addiction in patients treated with opioids for pain is low, and although opioids can activate an underlying addictive disease, they do not cause it. However, chronic opioid use will usually cause dependence, a physiologic state induced by chronic use of a psychoactive substance (for example, alcohol or opioids) characterized by an abstinence syndrome on the abrupt discontinuation of that substance. Dependence is rarely a clinical problem.

Opioids are not toxic to the liver, kidneys, brain, or other organs. Respiratory depression is very rare with oral opioids except in persons with significant pulmonary disease, sleep apnea syndrome, or other serious medical conditions. Side effects are common but usually can be managed with adjunctive medications.

Tolerance is not a limiting factor. Tolerance is the need for progressively higher doses of an analgesic to produce the same effect. True tolerance is a biologic process. In painful spinal disorders, the need for higher opioid doses is usually the result of progression of the structural disorder or an increase in activity level rather than of tolerance. Therefore, it is necessary to adjust the opioid doses to a point of optimal balance between analgesia, activity level, and side effects. Experience with opioid analgesics in cancer patients who survive for years has shown that tolerance is not a clinical problem.

Fear of disciplinary action by medical societies or government agencies should not be a reason to withhold opioids. It is appropriate medical practice to prescribe long-term opioids for chronic pain, and physicians who prescribe opioids for appropriate clinical indications are acting well within the scope of good medical practice.

Guidelines for Safe and Effective Use of Opioids

The decision to treat a patient with long-term opioids for chronic pain is a serious one, partly because it could be a life-long treatment. To maximize the chances for success and minimize the risks to the patient and doctor, the Federation of State Medical Boards of the United States issued guidelines for the use of controlled substances for pain, patterned on guidelines published by the Medical Board of California in 1996. The guidelines include a careful evaluation of the patient; a written treatment plan that states the goals of therapy; informed consent (verbal or written); periodic review to assess and document efficacy, side effects, and problems; consultation, when necessary; and the maintenance of good medical records.

Opioids should not be used to treat nonspecific pain. There must be a well-defined stimulus that cannot be definitively treated, and the pain level should be consistent with the structural disorder. Aggressive conservative care must have failed; there should be no significant psychological illness or history of addiction or drug abuse; and the opioids should be prescribed and refilled in person, not by telephone.

The patient must use the drugs as directed, not receive drugs from other doctors, and faithfully keep follow-up appointments. Also, it might be best for the prescribing physician to obtain a second opinion from a psychiatrist or pain management specialist who is familiar with the use of opioids for pain. Then, once opioids are started, the patient should be seen on a regular basis, and the improvements in pain and/or function should be documented to justify continuing use.

Despite the best screening, some patients will abuse or misuse opioid analgesics. If abuse or misuse is suspected, the patient should be referred for consultation to a specialist in addiction medicine. Certain actions have been identified as being highly suggestive of addictive behavior. These include selling prescription drugs; forging prescriptions; repeatedly borrowing drugs from friends or family; the concurrent use of large amounts of alcohol; the use of any illicit street drugs; the "loss" of prescriptions or pills; seeking prescriptions from other doctors, including emergency room personnel; and frequent missed appointments. Other signs that should raise the suspicion of drug abuse include frequent complaints that the dose is too low, requests for specific drugs, unsanctioned dose escalations, or use of the drug to treat other symptoms. However, some of these behaviors might be the result of inadequate pain control, sometimes called pseudoaddiction.

Dosing Intervals

Analgesics can be prescribed in two ways: as pain-contingent or as time-contingent dosing. Pain contingent means taking the analgesic when pain occurs. Time contingent means taking the analgesic on a regular schedule based on the analgesic half-life of the drug. Time-contingent dosing, which avoids large swings in blood or brain levels, usually provides better analgesia and fewer side effects. More analgesic is needed to reduce severe pain than to maintain mild to moderate pain. Time-contingent dosing is almost always preferable for chronic pain, with rescue doses available for breakthrough pain.

Short-Acting Versus Long-Acting Opioids

It is best to use a continuous-release or long-acting opioid for long-term opioid analgesic therapy, although short-acting opioids should be available for breakthrough pain. The short-acting opioids such as codeine, hydrocodone, or immediate release oxycodone are not usually used for long-term therapy because of the wide swings in the blood levels, which in turn lead to poor pain control and more side effects. For those rare patients who do better with a short-acting opioid, the drug should be prescribed in a time-contingent manner.

Choice of Opioid Analgesic

Currently five opioids suitable for long-term use are available (Table 2). No one drug is best for every patient. In fact, some patients respond preferentially to some opioids but not to others, which might make it necessary to try several different ones in a patient. Continuous-release morphine is available generically and therefore is less expensive than continuous-release oxycodone, but both are effective and reasonably easy to use. The opioid is released continuously from the tablet and slowly absorbed from the gut with little accumulation in body tissues. Analgesia is effective for 8 to 12 hours, and the dosing interval is adjusted accordingly. The continuous-release opioids are available in many dose sizes, which makes dose titration convenient. The dose can be titrated upward once or twice weekly until good pain control is achieved or significant side effects occur.

Methadone is a long-acting opioid. It is inexpensive and somewhat more difficult to titrate to the optimal dose than morphine or oxycodone, but provides excellent analgesia. This lipophilic drug is well absorbed from the gut and is then distributed in body fat, taking about 5 to 7 days to reach a steady state. Therefore, the dose should be adjusted only once per week. Once a steady state is reached, however, 8 to 12 hours of pain relief can be achieved. Some patients initially might hesitate to try methadone because of its association with the treatment of addicts, but they usually will accept it after the difference in uses is explained. Transdermal fentanyl also is effective, but it provides less dosing flexibility, and some people have difficulty keeping the patches

TABLE 2 | Opioid Analgesics (Narcotics) Most Useful for Chronic Pain

Chemical Name	Brand Names	Duration of Analgesia	Comments
Morphine	MS Contin	8 to 12 h	Multiple dose sizes; convenient
	Oramorph	8 h	
Oxycodone	Oxycontin	8 to 12 h	Multiple dose sizes; convenient; expensive
Methadone	Dolophine	8 to 12 h	Very inexpensive
Fentanyl	Duramorph	48 to 72 h	Transdermal
Levorphanol	Levo-dromoran	6 to 8 h	Only 2-mg dose size; inconvenient

on. Levorphanol is a long-acting opioid that is also quite effective.

Meperidine should not be used long term because it is poorly absorbed, provides unreliable analgesia, and is associated with an unacceptably high level of toxic neurologic side effects. Buprenorphine is a mixed agonist/antagonist opioid that has been tried for low back pain. However, it is not a good choice because many patients cannot tolerate its side effects. Also, it is short acting, and if it is inadvertently given to a patient who is already opioid dependent, buprenorphine might precipitate an abstinence syndrome.

Routes of Administration and Doses
In chronic pain, continuous-release or long-acting opioids are administered by oral or transdermal routes in a time-contingent manner at intervals based on the duration of analgesia of the particular drug (Table 2). There should be rescue doses of an immediate-release opioid available for breakthrough pain or flares. The dose and dosing interval are adjusted based on the degree and duration of pain relief and side effects until there are good control of baseline pain and minimal side effects. There is no best or correct dose.

Side Effects
Most patients taking opioids have side effects, but the types and intensity vary greatly. The most worrisome are somnolence and changes in mental status. Interestingly, chronic severe pain can result in an alteration of cognitive abilities, and when opioids relieve pain effectively, cognitive abilities actually improve. Sedation is common, particularly at the initiation of treatment or when doses are raised, but this usually improves over time despite continued treatment. When the opioid is effective but the patient experiences excessive sedation, methylphenidate (Ritalin) can be of value.

Nausea is common, especially when the opioid is first begun. The nauseated patient usually responds to expec-

tant treatment with prochlorperazine or transdermal scopolamine. Constipation occurs in most patients, and prophylaxis is important; stool softeners, 2 to 4 tablets at night, can be used. Other side effects include itching, sweating, dry mouth, and dizziness. Occasionally sexual dysfunction caused by opioid-induced lowered testosterone might occur; this is treated with a testosterone patch.

Intrathecal Opioids (ITOs)
No discussion of long-term opioids is complete without a mention of ITOs. Limited data are available about the efficacy of ITOs for chronic nonmalignant pain. Before patients are considered for ITOs, they must be candidates for long-term opioid analgesic therapy in general, have good pain relief with oral or transdermal therapy, but also have intolerable side effects. Only then should ITOs be considered.

Antidepressants

Antidepressants have many uses in the management of chronic spinal problems, including the treatment of neuropathic pain, low back pain, sleep disturbance, and depression. The TCAs work better than other types of antidepressants for pain. They are most effective for neuropathic pain but also can provide meaningful relief of low back pain. They are effective in patients with no evidence of depression; and the analgesic effect occurs at far lower doses than does the antidepressant effect. The view that antidepressants improve pain through the treatment of a "masked" depression is no longer held. However, many patients with chronic pain do develop depression that requires specific treatment. To treat depression, the selective serotonin reuptake inhibitors (SSRIs) are usually more effective than TCAs, although several other types of antidepressants can be effective as well (Table 3).

TABLE 3	Some Antidepressant Considerations for Patients With Chronic Pain			
Generic	Brand Name	Value for Pain	Value for Depression	Value for Sleep
Nortriptyline	Pamelor	High	Medium	Medium
Amitriptyline	Elavil	High	Medium	High
Desipramine	Norpramine	High	Medium	Low
Trazodone	Desyrel	Low	Low	High
Fluoxetine	Prozac	Low	High	Poor
Sertraline	Zoloft	Low	High	Poor
Paroxetine	Paxil	Low	High	Low
Citalopram	Celexa	Low	High	Low
Doxepin	Sinequan	Low	Medium	High
Bupropion	Wellbutrin	Low	Medium	Poor
Venlafaxine	Effexor	Low	High	High

Mechanism of Action

The TCAs block the presynaptic reuptake of norepinephrine; this action appears to be the most important mechanism for pain relief. The TCAs also have other effects, a fact that accounts for some of the other beneficial effects as well as the side effects (Tables 3 and 4). The SSRIs block the reuptake of serotonin, which accounts for their usefulness in the treatment of depression. Bupropion acts on dopamine as well as on norepinephrine and serotonin. It is not very effective for pain, but it is effective for depression and in helping patients stop smoking. Only the sustained-release form should be used to minimize the risk of seizures. Venlafaxine at low doses acts on serotonin but at higher doses affects norepinephrine. It is not very effective for pain, but it works well for depression.

Choice of Antidepressant

The choice of antidepressant depends on the target symptoms—pain, depression, or sleep disturbance. The TCAs nortriptyline, desipramine, and amitriptyline are the antidepressants most effective for pain. Fluoxetine, sertraline, paroxetine, and citalopram can be the most useful SSRIs for depression. Citalopram has very few drug interactions, so it might be preferable for patients who take multiple medications. When a patient does not respond to selected TCAs or SSRIs, however, referring the patient to a psychiatrist might be the best course of action.

Dosing Guidelines

The initial dose of nortriptyline, desipramine, or amitriptyline is 10 mg at night, which is then increased every 5 days or so in 10-mg increments to 50 mg. After 50 mg, the dose can be increased in 25-mg increments to a target of 75 or 100 mg. Fluoxetine is started at 20 mg each morning, sertraline at 50 mg, paroxetine at 20 mg, and citalopram at 20 mg. Higher doses are best left to specialists in psychopharmacology.

Side Effects

Side effects are common but vary in intensity according to the drug and individual patient susceptibility (Table 4). The TCAs are sedating, so they are usually given at night to help with sleep. Some patients might experience excessive daytime sedation. Other side effects include dry mouth, urinary retention, constipation, weight gain, blurry vision, and orthostatic hypotension. Usually side effects are mild and decrease with continued use. The SSRIs can cause irritability and sexual dysfunction.

Anticonvulsants

Anticonvulsants can be effective for neuropathic pain but rarely for low back pain. Gabapentin is currently used most often, although its use for pain is off label. It may be useful for neuropathic extremity pain caused by iatrogenic nerve injury, arachnoiditis, or prolonged neu-

| TABLE 4 | Relative Side Effects of Commonly Used Antidepressants |

	Sedation	Insomnia	Orthostasis	Anticholinergic*
Amitriptyline	3	0	3	3
Nortriptyline	2	0	1	2
Desipramine	1	1	1	1
Fluoxetine	0	2	0	0
Trazodone	3	0	2	0

0 = no effect, 1 = mild effect, 2 = moderate effect, 3 = major effect

*Anticholinergic side effects include blurred vision, dry mouth, sinus tachycardia, constipation, urinary retention, and memory dysfunction

ral compression and for peripheral neuropathy. Gabapentin is started at 300 mg at night, then increased to 300 mg every 8 h over the next few days. It is then gradually titrated upward over several weeks until good pain relief is achieved or significant side effects occur. Pain relief can occur at 900 mg/day, but often 1,800 to 3,600 mg/day is necessary. Side effects include dizziness, somnolence, ataxia, and headaches, but these are usually seen at the higher dose levels.

Clonazepam, a benzodiazepine, also can be useful for neuropathic pain and is very effective in reducing myoclonic jerks, a potential side effect of opioids. It is started at 0.5 mg at night and increased in 0.5-mg increments as necessary to a maximum dose of 2 to 4 mg/day in three divided doses. Carbamazepine and sodium valproate also can be helpful for neuropathic pain, but these drugs are more complicated to use because of the potential for serious side effects. Their use probably is best left to specialists in neuropharmacology.

Muscle Relaxants

Muscle relaxants often are prescribed for patients with acute, nonspecific low back pain, based on the assumption that muscle spasm, strain, or sprain can be a significant cause of pain. Although muscle spasm might be a cause of acute low back pain, in chronic low back pain, any muscle involvement usually is secondary to an underlying structural problem. Therefore, although muscle relaxants might have a temporary role in acute low back pain or flares of chronic low back pain, their use for chronic pain should be limited. There is little evidence that these drugs specifically relax tight muscles. They are sedating, and they might cause dependence. Most of their effects are central rather than peripheral.

That said, cyclobenzaprine is chemically similar to amitriptyline and can be useful for patients with a sleep disturbance who decline antidepressants. The dose is 10 mg at night. Baclofen can be effective for the relief of painful spasms and also might have a role in neuropathic pains. Its action is in the central nervous system rather than on the muscles. Baclofen is started at 10 mg at night and gradually titrated up to 10 mg every 6 hours. Occasionally, higher doses are needed. Other muscle relaxants include orphenadrine, carisoprodol, methocarbamol, metaxalone, and tizanidine. No good evidence supports choosing one over another. Diazepam is too sedating to use regularly, but lorazepam is occasionally effective for muscle spasms.

Sedative-Hypnotics

The role of sedative-hypnotics in chronic spinal pain also is limited. Chronic sleep disturbance, frequently present in chronic pain, responds better to trazodone or TCAs. However, for occasional sleep problems, especially during flares of chronic pain, a sedative-hypnotic might be useful. Zolpidem, 10 mg at bedtime, might be the safest drug because it is less likely to produce dependence, rebound insomnia, or daytime sedation. Benzodiazepines such as clonazepam or temazepam also might be prescribed for occasional use.

However, the use of sedative-hypnotics for long periods is fraught with problems. Long-acting drugs such as diazepam or flurazepam can accumulate with chronic use and produce cognitive impairment and depression. Rebound insomnia can result when the drugs are discontinued.

Miscellaneous Drugs

Antihistamines

Antihistamines can help control opioid-induced nausea, vomiting, and itching, but contrary to popular belief, they do not enhance opioid analgesia. Hydroxyzine and promethazine are effective for nausea, and both hydroxyzine and cetirizine work well for itching. Diphenhydramine also can be used but is more sedating. Antihistamines should not be used as hypnotics; far better drugs are available for this purpose.

Topical Analgesics

Capsaicin

Capsaicin is a topical analgesic cream that depletes substance P in small nociceptors and thereby can provide pain relief in patients with peripheral neuropathy, arthritis of small joints, and, occasionally, complex regional pain syndrome.

Lidocaine 5% Patch

The lidocaine 5% dermal patch is another useful topical treatment. The patch is applied over small areas of neuropathic pain. Anecdotally, some patients with very focal nociceptive pain also respond. The patches are worn for 12 h, then removed for 12 h, but the analgesia is sustained.

Annotated Bibliography

Atkinson JH, Slater MA, Williams RA, et al: A placebo-controlled randomized clinical trial of nortriptyline for chronic low back pain. *Pain* 1998;76:287-296.

In a prospective study of back pain without depression, nortriptyline reduced back pain significantly more than placebo did, with a 22% mean reduction of pain. Patients with radicular plus low back pain did better than those with only low back pain.

Model Guidelines for Use in Regulating the Prescribing of Controlled Substances for the Management of Pain. Federation of State Medical Boards of the United States, Euless, TX, 1998.

The Federation developed model guidelines for use in regulating the prescribing of controlled substances for the management of pain. Their goals were to facilitate effective pain control by educating the medical community and to protect legitimate medical use of controlled substances for the treatment of pain while preventing drug diversion and inappropriate prescribing.

Hale ME, Fleisschmann R, Salzman R, et al: Efficacy and safety of controlled-release versus immediate-release oxycodone: Randomized, double-blind evaluation in patients with chronic back pain. *Clin J Pain* 1999; 15:179-83.

In a short-term study of patients with moderate to severe low back pain, both controlled-release and immediate-release oxycodone resulted in significant improvements.

Jamison RN, Raymond SA, Slawsby EA, Nedeljkovic SS, Katz NP: Opioid therapy for chronic noncancer back pain: A randomized prospective study. *Spine* 1998;23: 2591-2600.

In a 1-year prospective study of low back pain, patients on a titrated dose of continuous-release morphine showed significantly better relief of pain and emotional distress than did those on a fixed dose of oxycodone or naproxen.

Joranson DE, Ryan KM, Gilson AM, Dahl JL: Trends in medical use and abuse of opioid analgesics. *JAMA* 2000;283:1710-1714.

The use of opioids for pain control has increased substantially, but there has not been an increase in the health consequences of opioid analgesics, such as addiction or other forms of abuse.

McQuay HJ, Tramer M, Nye BA, Carroll D, Wiffen PJ, Moore RA: A systematic review of antidepressants in neuropathic pain. *Pain* 1996;68:217-227.

In a review of published studies, antidepressants were reported to provide more than 50% reduction in neuropathic pain in 30% of patients. Analgesia occurred independently of change in mood. TCAs were better than other groups of drugs.

Rosenberg JM, Harrell C, Ristic H, Werner RA, de Rasayro AM: The effects of gabapentin on neuropathic pain. *Clin J Pain* 1997;13:251-255.

In a retrospective study, gabapentin resulted in significant reduction in neuropathic pain, particular in patients with direct nerve injuries, but there was no reduction in low back pain.

Roth SH, Fleischmann RM, Burch FX, et al: Around-the-clock, controlled-release oxycodone therapy for osteoarthritis-related pain. *Arch Int Med* 2000;160: 853-860.

In a randomized, placebo-controlled trial for osteoarthritis pain, continuous-release oxycodone produced significant improvements in pain and function compared to placebo. Analgesia was sustained long term, side effects decreased over time, and there was no evidence of tolerance.

Schofferman J: Long-term opioid analgesic therapy for severe refractory lumbar spine pain. *Clin J Pain* 1999; 15:136-140.

In a 1-year prospective study of 33 patients with refractory low back pain treated with titrated doses of opioids, 15% could not tolerate opioids and 75% of the remainder had significant improvements in pain and function.

Sindrup SH, Jensen TS: Efficacy of pharmacological treatments of neuropathic pain: An update and effect related to mechanism of action. *Pain* 1999;83:389-400.

This is an extensive review of the literature. TCAs might be the most effective class of drugs, but other drugs that work almost as well might be better tolerated.

Classic Bibliography

Action Report: Medical Board of California. *Treatment of Intractable Pain: A Guideline.* 1996;57:1-6.

Kalso E, McQuay HJ: *Opioid Sensitivity of Chronic Noncancer Pain.* Seattle, WA, IASP Press, vol 14, 1999.

Max M: Antidepressants as analgesics, In Fields HL, Liebeskind JC (eds): *Pharmacological Approaches to the Treatment of Chronic Pain: New Concepts and Critical Issues.* Seattle, WA, IASP Press, 1994.

Portenoy RK: Opiod therapy for chronic nonmalignant pain: Current status, in Fields HL, Liebeskind JC (eds): *Pharmacological Approaches to the Treatment of Chronic Pain: New Concepts and Critical Issues.* Seattle, WA, IASP Press, 1994.

Schofferman J: Medication considerations in low back pain, in Cole A, Herring S (eds): *The Low Back Pain Handbook: A Practical Guide for the Primary Care Physician.* Philadelphia, PA, Hanley & Belfus, 1997.

Turk DC, Brody MC, Okifuji A: Physicians' attitudes and practices regarding the long-term prescribing of opioids for non-cancer pain. *Pain* 1994;59:201-208.

Chapter 25

Psychosocial Care for Spinal Disorders

Peter B. Polatin, MD

Robert J. Gatchel, PhD

Introduction

Low back pain is perhaps the most problematic of musculoskeletal problems for the clinician to treat. Patients' complaints are largely subjective and are not easily correlated with objective findings, particularly as the pain becomes chronic and more refractory to both conservative and surgical treatment. When a patient with low back pain fails to improve with appropriate treatment, the clinician should reevaluate the patient using a biopsychosocial frame of reference, scrutinizing issues other than the actual physical complaint.

The biopsychosocial model, first elaborated by Turk and Rudy, incorporates cognitive, affective, psychosocial, behavioral, and physiologic factors that interact in producing and perpetuating the chronic pain experience. Disability-engendering factors and background information are elicited with a detailed patient history, a format for which is suggested in Table 1. Also, to appreciate fully any possible secondary gain issues on the part of a patient, the clinician should understand the medicolegal jurisdiction of any financial claim. A summary of different jurisdictions is presented in Table 2. In addition, the clinician should undertake an inquiry into psychosocial factors relevant to the patient to uncover possible symptoms of somatization, symptom magnification, depression, anxiety, and dysfunctional coping. Methods of performing this psychosocial screening evaluation are suggested in Table 3. If these screening tests for disability-engendering factors, secondary gain issues, and psychosocial factors are positive, then a full mental health evaluation should be performed on the patient.

Gatchel has carefully delineated how practitioners should evaluate psychosocial and personality factors to better help care for patients with chronic pain. It must not be assumed that a single instrument can serve as the best assessment method for all patients. Rather, for many patients, several assessments will be required. Psychosocial personality assessment should be viewed as a stepwise process, proceeding from global indices of emo-

TABLE 1	Interview Format for Evaluating Patient History and Possible Disability-Related Issues

Job

  Time on the job

  Job satisfaction

  Relationships at work (supervisor, coworkers)

  Previous jobs and their durations

  Plan (return to job, new job, retire)

Education

  Years of high school and college

  Vocational training

  Future vocational interests

Finances

  Current weekly or monthly benefits from all sources (temporary income, short-term disability, long-term disability, pensions, alimony, etc)

  Deferred payment protection (loans, mortgage, alimony)

Litigation/Dispute

  Settlement issues regarding impairment, indemnity, punitive damages, "buy-out" from work, etc

Social support for or against disability

  Family

  Employer, coworkers

  Insurance adjuster

  Attorney

TABLE 2 | Medicolegal Jurisdictions and Possible Secondary Gains

Type of Compensation	Jurisdiction	Secondary Gain		
		Financial Gain	**Job Manipulation**	**Vocational Retraining**
Workers' Compensation	State	X	X	X
Federal Employees Compensation Act	Federal (eg, postal workers, VA employees)		X	
Federal Employees Labor Act	Railroad workers	X	X	
Longshore Harbor Workers' Act and Maritime Jones Act	Maritime and off-shore workers	X		
Personal Injury	Negligence litigation; nonsubscriber work injury	X		
Short-term/Long-term Disability	Individual policy coverage	X		X
Social Security Disability	Federal disability retirement	X		

TABLE 3 | Psychosocial Screening

Interview/Examination

   Somatization: nonorganic (Waddell) signs

   Depression: feeling sad most of time; sustained loss of enjoyment

   Anxiety: increased nervousness, panic attacks, avoidant behavior

   Poor coping: disheveled appearance, admits when asked

   Alcohol/drugs: breath odor, pupils, vital signs, ataxia, slurred speech, mental status

Screening Tests

   Pain drawing (nonanatomic, exaggerated)

   Million Visual Pain Analog Scale, Oswestry Low Back Pain Disability Questionnaire (self-perception of disability)

   Beck Depression Inventory (BDI)

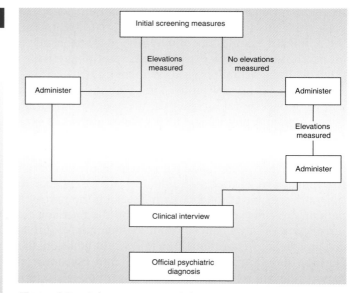

Figure 1 Stepwise assessment approach for delineating potential personality and psychosocial problems in patients with chronic pain.

tional distress and disturbance to more detailed evaluations of specific clinical diagnoses and personality disorders. A flow chart for such a stepwise assessment process is shown in Figure 1.

Psychosocial Management: An Overview

The Management of Socioeconomic Disability Factors

The clinician and the patient frequently can be at cross purposes because of a lack of understanding of disabil-

ity factors involved in the case. In some instances, the patient has unrealistic expectations of an eventual case settlement. In other situations, the physician might not be aware of the documentation required to settle a case, thereby inadvertently stimulating the possible perception by a patient that his or her needs are being ignored. For patients with demonstrated socioeconomic barriers to recovery, disability case management might be initiated to improve the patient's motivation for functional improvement and return to work. Any pertinent secondary gain issues are first identified by extended interview. The patient must then be guided to an appropriate resolution by rapport building, education, and negotiation. Other interventions might include those regarding job modification, vocational counseling, or vocational retraining. The desirable outcomes are functional recovery, return to work at the highest possible level, and case closure.

Cognitive-Behavioral Treatment

Patients with low back pain and accompanying psychological distress are most effectively treated with counseling that has a cognitive-behavioral orientation, utilizing a combination of education, training in self-modulation, and reorganization of goals. A multimodal disability management program based on a cognitive-behavioral approach to crisis intervention has been advocated. Such a program focuses on helping a patient overcome physical and psychosocial difficulties that interfere with returning to a productive and functional lifestyle.

The program includes four major components. (1) Individual and group counseling emphasizes a crisis-intervention model (for example, to cope with employment and family problems). (2) Behavioral stress-management training involves initial training in muscle relaxation, followed by exercises and guided imagery in which patients practice relaxing while imagining themselves in various stressful situations. Patients also might receive biofeedback sessions during which they refine their relaxation skills, with the understanding that these skills will help them cope more effectively with residual pain and discomfort. (3) Cognitive-behavioral skills training includes instruction in assertiveness, the identification of rational versus irrational thinking, and learning methods of stress and time management. (4) Meetings organized by family counseling professionals encourage family members to take an active role in the patient's rehabilitation process and also provide the family with information about the philosophy and specific details of a multimodal disability management program.

Careful psychosocial assessment precedes the effective administration of an individually tailored multimodal disability management program. It is of great importance that each patient be viewed as unique and be evaluated individually so that the treatment program is carefully tailored to the patient. Blindly administering the same disability management program to all patients, regardless of their unique individual needs, can lead to failure.

Medication Management

Antidepressants, anxiolytics, neuroleptics, and mood stabilizers, as well as more conventional analgesics, muscle relaxants, and adjunctive medication, are used to control the patient's pain and accompanying symptoms of emotional distress. The antidepressants can have multiple functions for the control of pain and anxiety as well as depression. Insofar as a patient's emotional distress affects compliance and the ability to treat the patient, psychopharmacologic stabilization is essential to ensure a good response to therapy. Table 4 summarizes the more commonly used psychotropic agents and their applications.

Among the antidepressants, the older tricyclic agents (amitriptyline, nortriptyline, doxepine, imipramine, desipramine) have the longest track record for the treatment of pain, at lower doses than is required for the treatment of depression and with a more rapid onset of therapeutic effect. Some of these agents, particularly amitriptyline and doxepine, also are sedatives. Unfortunately, they have side effects that could become problematic, such as causing weight gain, cardiac arrhythmia, postural hypotension, and oversedation.

The newer selective serotonin reuptake inhibitors ([SSRIs] fluoxetine, paroxetine, sertraline, and citalopram) have become the drugs of first choice for the treatment of depression but only recently have been found to have any mitigating effect on pain. Some of these agents can have a sedative effect (for example, paroxetine), and several have been found to be effective for the treatment of anxiety or obsessive compulsive symptoms (fluoxetine, paroxetine, sertraline). The SSRIs have a lower side-effect profile but can cause increased anxiety, headaches, flushing, diarrhea, and sexual dysfunction in some patients.

Some studies suggest that there is a pain-mitigating effect with other antidepressants (mirtazepine, maprotiline, venlafaxine). Trazodone, mirtazepine, and nefazodone are sedatives. Others work well on symptoms of anxiety (venlafaxine) or for obsessive-compulsive disorder (fluvoxamine). In addition, the monoamine oxidase inhibitors (MAOIs), although proven to be effective for both depression and pain, are not commonly used because of side-effect potential, the requirement for a tyramine-free diet, and the need to avoid concomitant use of common over-the-counter decongestants, stimulants, and weight-loss aids.

The benzodiazepines (alprazolam, diazepam, clonazepam, lorazepam, chlorazepate, and oxazepam) are effective as immediate-onset antianxiety agents. Therefore, they might be used as needed for acute symptoms as well as regularly for prophylaxis. Clonazepam particularly might have some mitigating effect on pain, but generally it is thought that any pain-reducing effect that others of these agents have is related to a decrease in anxiety and resulting muscle relaxation. Buspirone is an alternative agent that decreases anxiety but not panic

TABLE 4 | Psychopharmacological Agents for Problematic Low Back Pain

	P	I	D	A	O	I-2	P-2
Tricyclic antidepressant agents	+++	++	+++				
SSRIs	+	++	++++	++	++	++	
Other antidepressant agents							
Trazodone		+++	++				
Mirtazepine	+	+++	++++				
Venlafaxine	+	++++	+++				
Nefazodone	?	++	++++				
Fluvoxamine	?	++	++++	+	++		
Bupropion	?		+++				
Maprotiline	+	+	+++				
Antianxiety agents							
Benzodiazepine		+		++++		++	
Buspirone	+			++			
Antipsychotics		+		+	+	+	++++
Mood stabilizers	+++		+			+	++++
Sedatives		++++					

P = pain; I = insomnia; D = depression; A = anxiety/panic; O = obsessive/compulsive symptoms; I-2 = irritability; P-2 = psychosis mania; + = slightly indicated; ++ = mildly indicated; +++ = moderately indicated; ++++ = strongly indicated; ? = no known effect

attacks. It must be taken for a few weeks and titrated to an effective dose, much like an antidepressant. It also might have a mitigating effect on pain.

Mood-stabilizing agents for symptoms of mania include lithium (carbonate or citrate), carbamazepine, divalproex, phenytoin, and gabapentin. The anticonvulsants in this category, particularly gabapentin, also have an established mitigating effect on neuropathic pain.

Finally, the other psychotropic agents listed in Table 4 (antipsychotic agents and sedatives) have applicability for specific emotional dysfunction symptoms in patients with low back pain but have no modifying effects on pain itself.

The Context of Psychosocial Care

Psychosocial care refers to the treatment of psychosocioeconomic barriers to recovery in patients with low back pain. These patients' physical illnesses are placed within the frame of reference of other factors in their lives, including their jobs, financial status, family and relationship dynamics, exposure to stress, and psychological and psychopathologic diagnoses. Psychosocial therapies are made use of at a secondary or tertiary level of care. In secondary level care (therapeutic exercise, reconditioning, work conditioning, work hardening), such interventions are introduced as adjuncts to the progression of physical and occupational therapy on an as-needed basis and outside the therapy milieu. In tertiary care (pain management, functional restoration), rehabilitation incorporates the psychosocial therapies into the core curriculum of the program, with interdisciplinary communication and feedback for the patient.

Psychosocial Intervention at a Secondary Care Level

A patient with low back pain in work conditioning or work hardening might fail to progress or might verbalize an unwillingness to engage in therapy because of severe pain. Alternatively, he or she might exhibit aberrant behavior in the treatment milieu, which stymies progress. Such a patient should be referred for an evaluation of socioeconomic and psychosocial barriers to recovery. After such a reassessment, a decision might be made about whether to continue secondary level care.

When the patient does not exhibit a severe level of emotional distress but socioeconomic issues need to be discussed and clarified, the patient might continue in the previous program but in addition be assigned a disability case manager to clarify and negotiate closure of secondary gain issues. Without the involvement of a case manager, the therapists inadvertently might take an overly directive approach because of a poor understanding of the issues of the case, possibly alienating the patient and potentially leading to treatment failure and prolongation of disability.

When the patient has some degree of emotional distress, then psychotropic medication and/or psychotherapy, obtained through outside consultation while the patient remains in the secondary level program, might be warranted. For a patient who is motivated to recover, even assuming a mild degree of depression or anxiety, such an extended program might lead to success. However, sometimes the outside psychotherapist or psychopharmacologist is placed at odds with the secondary level of care program because of lack of communication with the physical or occupational therapists or because of conscious or unconscious manipulation by the patient to "split" the various therapists. If this occurs, then tertiary level care should be considered.

Psychosocial Care in Tertiary Level Programs

Pain management and functional restoration are both interdisciplinary programs in which all necessary rehabilitation services (physical therapy, occupational therapy, disability case management, psychological counseling, medication management, and adjunctive therapies) are represented by a team that works with the patient, meets in regularly scheduled staffings to review progress, and is under the supervision of a managing physician who also attends the staffings and meets with the patient on a regular basis. Gatchel and Turk have delineated the essential ingredients of interdisciplinary pain management.

The involvement of the psychologist and the case manager complements this team orientation because they are able to assist the other therapists in devising strategies to overcome pain behaviors that interfere with patient progress. At the same time, the psychologist and case manager are able to follow the actual progress of the patient in the various therapies and dis-

TABLE 5	Risk Factors Associated With Chronic, Disabling Low Back Pain

Elevation of Minnesota Multiphasic Personality Inventory scale 3 (hysteria)

Depression

Low activity/high pain behavior

Negative beliefs/fear of pain

Job dissatisfaction

Blue collar/heavy physical work

Older age

Severe psychological stress or abuse

High subjective pain intensity

Substance abuse

Receiving compensation and unemployment benefits

cern important but subtle differences between the patient's behavior and overt communication. A patient claiming improvement but not progressing in physical therapy, for example, can be gently confronted by his or her counselor or case manager to directly explore unresolved psychosocioeconomic issues still interfering with treatment. A patient who has been placed on psychotropic medication but who still exhibits symptoms that interfere with progress should be referred for a readjustment of the medication.

Finally, it must be emphasized that communication is a key ingredient in successful interdisciplinary care. A communicating interdisciplinary team is unified in its treatment philosophy, and the message given to the patient is consistent. Sabotage of treatment goals by "splitting" behaviors and by miscommunication is minimized. When interdisciplinary tertiary care services are denied, even though all the elements might have been provided separately, outcomes are adversely affected. The clinical efficacy and cost effectiveness of a comprehensive interdisciplinary treatment program have been well defined in recent studies.

Conclusion

When a patient with low back pain fails to progress as expected with appropriate treatment, a biopsychosocial reevaluation is indicated, including scrutiny of financial, social, family, vocational, and psychological factors. When financial or vocational secondary gain issues are believed to be affecting treatment response, disability case management can improve the prospects for a successful therapeutic outcome. If emotional distress or dysfunction is identified, it must be treated. Therapies can include psychological counseling and medication management with various psychotropic agents. Secondary level programs will be successful with complicated patients when these programs can provide such services to deal with psychosocioeconomic barriers to recovery. However, the more distressed and refractory patients will require a tertiary level of care in which these services are integrated into an interdisciplinary program with full communication among the treatment team members.

Finally, as further evidence of the often complex psychosocial issues that need to be addressed with chronic pain patients, Sanders has recently provided a brief overview of risk factors that appear to predict the occurrence of low back pain as well as the development of chronic disability (that is, pain disability lasting 3 months or more). Table 5 presents these 11 factors, the majority of which are psychosocial, behavioral, or environmental in nature. Identifying and modifying these psychosocioeconomic risk factors allows the clinician to prevent the development of disabling, chronic low back pain to manage these patients more effectively.

Annotated Bibliography

Atkinson JH, Slater MA, Wahlgren DR, et al: Effects of noradrenergic and serotonergic antidepressants on chronic low back pain intensity. *Pain* 1999;83:137-145.

This is a thorough discussion of the applicability of the newer antidepressants for the treatment of low back pain.

Deschner M, Polatin PB: Interdisciplinary programs: Chronic pain management, in Mayer TG, Gatchel RJ, Polatin PB (eds): *Occupational Musculoskeletal Disorders: Function, Outcomes and Evidence*. Philadelphia, PA, Lippincott-Williams & Wilkins, 2000, pp 629-637.

This is a comprehensive review of the interdisciplinary treatment approach to chronic pain management. The key components of this approach are detailed.

Drugs for depression and anxiety. *Med Lett Drugs Ther* 1999;41:30-38.

This is a quick summary, in easily understood format, of currently available drugs for the treatment of depression and anxiety.

Gatchel RJ: How practitioners should evaluate personality to help manage patients with chronic pain, in Gatchel RJ, Weisberg JN (eds): *Personality Characteristics of Patients With Pain*. Washington, DC, American Psychological Association, 2000, pp 241-257.

A stepwise approach to psychosocial assessment is presented. This approach is advocated to determine the sequence in which assessment testing should be undertaken to best understand potential personality and psychosocial problems that might be encountered in treating patients with chronic pain.

Gatchel RJ: Psychosocial assessment and disability management in the rehabilitation of painful spinal disorders, in Mayer TG, Mooney V, Gatchel RJ (eds): *Contemporary Conservative Care for Painful Spinal Disorders*. Philadelphia, PA, Lea & Febiger, 1991, pp 441-454

The key elements of a multimodal disability management program for the treatment of chronic painful spinal disorders are reviewed and discussed.

Gatchel R, Noe C, Gajraj N, Vakharian A, Polatin P, Deschner M, Pulliam C: The negative therapeutic impact on an interdisciplinary pain management program of insurance "treatment carve out" practices. *J Workers Comp*, in press.

This recent research study clearly documents the detrimental impact of managed care on the efficacy of the interdisciplinary treatment of chronic pain. In the future, outcome studies such as this one will have the potential to affect managed care policies.

Gatchel RJ, Turk DC: Interdisciplinary treatment of chronic pain patients, in Gatchel RJ, Turk DC (eds): *Psychosocial Factors in Pain: Critical Perspectives*. New York, NY, Guilford Press, 1999, pp 435-444.

The authors comprehensively discuss the major components required for a successful interdisciplinary pain-management program. The cost effectiveness of such a program also is reviewed.

Judd LL: A decade of antidepressant development: The SSRIs and beyond. *J Affect Disord* 1998;51:211-213.

This is an academic discussion of the newer agents for the treatment of depression.

Leeman G, Polatin P, Gatchel R, Kishino N: Managing secondary gain in patients with pain-associated disability: A clinical perspective. *J Workers Comp* 2000;9:25-44.

This article outlines a useful clinical methodology for the evaluation and treatment of secondary gain factors, with the emphasis on financial secondary gain. The role of the disability case manager is discussed in detail, as are the various jurisdictions governing such cases.

Matheson LN: Job analysis, job matching, and vocational intervention, in Mayer TG, Gatchel RJ, Polatin PB (eds): *Occupational Musculoskeletal Disorders: Function, Outcomes and Evidence.* Philadelphia, PA, Lippincott-Williams & Wilkins, 2000, pp 609-627.

This chapter provides an overview of three approaches to job analysis and focuses on aspects of the job analysis process that are particularly important in the treatment of occupational musculoskeletal disorders.

Mayer TG, Polatin PB: Tertiary nonoperative interdisciplinary programs: The functional restoration variant of the outpatient chronic pain management program, in Mayer TG, Gatchel RJ, Polatin PB (eds): *Occupational Musculoskeletal Disorders: Function, Outcomes and Evidence.* Philadelphia, PA, Lippincott-Williams & Wilkins, 2000, pp 639-649.

This chapter presents a detailed review of how functional restoration has been successfully applied for the effective treatment of chronic musculoskeletal disorders.

Polatin PB, Gatchel RJ: Psychosocial factors in spinal disorders, in Garfin SR, Vaccaro AR (eds): *Orthopaedic Knowledge Update: Spine.* Rosemont, IL, American Academy of Orthopaedic Surgeons, 1997, pp 149-152.

This chapter discusses the various psychosocial and socioeconomic factors that might affect the management of spinal disorders. Methods of screening for such factors, as well as the content of such a screening or assessment process, are reviewed.

Rush J, Polatin P, Gatchel R: Depression and chronic low back pain: Establishing priorities in treatment. *Spine* 2000;25:2566-2571.

This is a comprehensive discussion of the evaluation and treatment of depression in patients with chronic low back pain, including diagnosis, treatment, and comorbidity factors.

Rosenberg JM, Harrell C, Ristic H, Werner RA, de Rosayro AM: The effect of gabapentin on neuropathic pain. *Clin J Pain* 1997;13:251-255.

This is a review of the efficacy of a new anticonvulsant for the treatment of neuropathic pain.

Sanders SH: Risk factors for chronic disability low-back pain: An update for 2000. *American Pain Society Bull* 2000;10:4-5.

In this brief article, the author provides an overview of 11 major risk factors that have been shown in the research literature to predict the initial occurrence of low back pain as well as the subsequent development of chronic disability.

Turk DC, Gatchel RJ: Psychosocial assessment of chronic occupational musculoskeletal disorders, in Mayer TG, Gatchel RJ, Polatin PB (eds): *Occupational Musculoskeletal Disorders: Function, Outcomes and Evidence.* Philadelphia, PA, Lippincott-Williams & Wilkins, 2000, pp 587-608.

The major focus of this chapter is providing an introduction to the concepts and process of the psychosocial evaluation of patients with persistent chronic pain. A method for conducting such a comprehensive assessment is provided.

Turk DC, Rudy TE: Towards a comprehensive assessment of chronic pain patients. *Behav Res Ther* 1987;25: 237-249.

This article presents the heuristic value of employing a biopsychosocial model to the assessment and treatment of pain. This model incorporates affective, behavioral, cognitive, physiological, and psychologic factors that interact in initially producing and then perpetuating the chronic pain experience.

Wesley AL, Polatin PB, Gatchel RJ: Psychosocial, psychiatric, and socioeconomic factors in chronic occupational musculoskeletal disorders, in Mayer TG, Gatchel RJ, Polatin PB (eds): *Occupational Musculoskeletal Disorders: Function, Outcomes and Evidence.* Philadelphia, PA, Lippincott-Williams & Wilkins, 2000, pp 577-586.

This chapter provides a comprehensive review of the role of psychosocial, psychiatric, and socioeconomic factors in the development and maintenance of chronic occupational musculoskeletal disorders.

Chapter 26

Functional Restoration of Patients With Chronic Spinal Pain

Tom G. Mayer, MD

Introduction

Spine surgeons have a vital interest in the outcomes of treatment for spinal disorders. Unlike many other surgical specialties, spine surgery evolved to its present eminence, in part through the fact that the orthopaedic surgeon was a complete musculoskeletal physician, rather than simply a surgeon whose nonsurgical care was provided by others. As such, knowledge of trends in rehabilitation for postoperative or chronically disabled patients is vital.

Functional restoration is a type of tertiary nonsurgical care for patients with chronic, disabling spinal disorders. Functional restoration of the patient with spinal pain involves special problems related to the chronic disability. To address these problems, assessment and care must be defined to provide a broad context of nonsurgical assessment, treatment, and prevention.

Severity of Injury

The first major issue regarding functional restoration of patients with chronic spinal pain is the severity of injury. Particularly in the industrial setting of workers' compensation, the severity of a musculoskeletal injury depends much more on the patient's disability and its chronicity than on the event that caused the injury. The situation is in contrast to that of severe orthopaedic trauma. Fractures and dislocations to a musculoskeletal area usually predict not only the type of treatment but also the duration of a patient's incapacity and ultimate outcome. Most spinal disorders are soft-tissue injuries with "sprains and strains" of musculoligamentous tissues that, in most cases, have a relatively brief healing period.

Incomplete or imperfect healing can cause permanent impairment of important supporting musculoskeletal elements. The socioeconomic impact can be great because of lost productivity, medical costs, and disability-related indemnity benefits. Most studies show that the mean cost of low back pain care is more than 10 times greater than the median cost, implying that the relatively small number of chronic cases encompasses the major share of social and financial costs. The patient with chronic low back and neck pain accounts for 80% of the cost of degenerative spine problems through the combined costs of medical treatment, lost productivity, indemnity costs, and government support.

Chronic spinal pain can develop in many contexts. Because low back pain is an almost universal phenomenon and recurrences follow in 50% of back pain episodes, episodic spinal disorders are commonplace. The etiology is controversial, despite the fact that most clinicians attempt to satisfy patients' desire for a cause of their pain by providing explanations. Degenerative changes, strength deficits, instability, neural compression, and psychological factors all have been cited as potential causes of back and neck pain. In most cases, patients themselves might be uncertain about the event that triggered the back pain episode.

However, a small but important group of patients must report injury as the origin of their spinal pain: individuals with compensable injuries (that is, workers' compensation claims, personal injury and other third-party claims, and claims for various forms of long-term disability payments). Although before the 1930s spinal pain was not considered a compensable event, during the past 70 years the criteria for causation have been extensively liberalized, so that virtually any claim of injury today, no matter how tenuous, is ultimately accepted as compensable. The acceptance by an insurance carrier of such a claim can result in the patient's receiving both medical benefits and financial wage supplementation for any disability created by the injury. In addition, the acceptance within the past 15 years of repetitive or cumulative trauma as an injury has further expanded the definition of compensable spinal disorders. Part of the issue of severity is related to socioeconomic (that is, compensation-related) and psychosocial factors. This chapter considers a treatment approach applicable to all patients with chronic spinal pain while stressing the special relationship to patients claiming disability and efforts to help them overcome that disability.

Three Levels of Nonsurgical Care

The taxonomy of nonsurgical care in the context of disabling compensable injuries must be related to the chronologic severity of an injury (ie, the increasing severity of the injury sequelae with the passing of time and persistence of disability). Because the outcome of legal and administrative indemnity issues hinges on the rehabilitation process, the identification of three distinct levels of nonsurgical care is useful. Primary treatment is that generally applied in acute cases and is designed for symptom control. Treatment generally involves the use of medication and some degree of rest, supplemented by use of the so-called passive modalities (such as temperature modalities, electrical stimulation, manual techniques). These might be accompanied by low-intensity, supervised exercises and education. The vast majority of patients who require medical care for spinal pain receive this treatment and nothing more.

Secondary treatment is appropriate in the postacute phase of injury. It is the first level of reactivation treatment of medium intensity. In addition to spinal injections and pharmacologic interventions, secondary treatment involves more restorative exercise and education designed to prevent deconditioning. Secondary treatment usually is provided by physical or occupational therapists, sometimes accompanied by consultative psychological, disability management, and multidisciplinary physician services.

Tertiary treatment is appropriate for the relatively small number of chronically disabled patients who can benefit from physician-directed, intensive, interdisciplinary team treatment with multiple professionals on site. Programs usually are organized along the lines of traditional pain clinics but can follow diverse patterns. Functional restoration is one of the modes of tertiary treatment with proven outcomes in workers' compensation settings in multiple venues.

Cervical and Lumbar Injuries

In providing functional restoration treatment to individuals with cervical or lumbar injuries, an initial aspect of care is recognizing the similarities and differences between the anatomy and physiology of these two spinal areas. Disability related to cervical injuries occurs less frequently than does disability related to low back pain. These two conditions together, with their associated neurologic alterations of the extremities, account for 60% to 65% of all cases of disability, thus making advisable the use of a common guide to permanent

impairment. Obvious anatomic similarities include the three-joint complex controlling joint motion and the bilateral exit of segmental nerve roots. The spinal cord, however, is not a factor in the lumbar spine region because the conus medullaris terminates near T12-L1. Significant upper motor neuron injury is a risk only in the cervicothoracic spine. Physiologic similarities involve the relative size and stabilization of the anatomic structures to accept the relative load of the head (cervical) or trunk (lumbar) and the relative freedom of mobility (compared with the thoracic spine) created by segmented conduits supported by musculotendinous soft-tissue structures. It is reasonable to conclude that the lower stability, higher mobility, and greater reliance on soft-tissue support probably accounts for the greater susceptibility of the cervical and lumbar regions to degenerative disc and facet disease and to the higher likelihood of the development of disabling symptoms associated with deconditioning.

Work-related disabilities often are related to ergonomics and job demands unique to the symptomatic area. In the cervical spine, for example, sedentary jobs that require persistent static positioning (sitting, writing, computer viewing, driving) and upper extremity activities (reaching, pushing over shoulder) are often affected. In the lumbar spine, by contrast, heavy activities requiring transmission of load from hands through the trunk (lifting, carrying), particularly with the individual in bent or rotated positions, generally are associated with symptom development. Recognizing these similarities and differences is necessary before a rehabilitation program for specific spinal disorders can be designed (Tables 1 and 2).

TABLE 1　Similarities Between the Cervical and Lumbar Regions

Three-joint complex (disc and posterolaterally oriented diarthrodial joints) positioned to maximize mobility while protecting neurologic structures

Laterally placed neuroforamina

Posterior ramus innervation of posterolateral musculoskeletal structures

Anterior ramus innervation of a single extremity

Size and orientation of structures related to biomechanical loads commonly encountered

Good resistance to compression but low resistance to bending/twisting moments

Degenerative disease and/or disc injury frequently associated with nerve root compression

---

TABLE 2 | Differences Between the Cervical and Lumbar Regions

Condition	Cervical	Lumbar
Motion	Three planes (sagittal, coronal/axial)	Mainly two planes (sagittal/coronal)
Upper motor neuron	Common (spinal cord vulnerable)	Unlikely (cauda equina)
Muscular support	Paravertebral musculature dominant	Both paravertebral and abdominal support
Biomechanical links	Linked to shoulder	Linked to hip/pelvis function, girdle function
Associated peripheral nerve entrapment and/or vascular engorgement	Common (associated "double crush" carpal tunnel, cubital tunnel, thoracic outlet syndromes)	Unusual association

Psychosocial and Socioeconomic Factors

The second major issue regarding functional restoration of patients with chronic spinal pain involves psychosocial and socioeconomic factors in disability that often accompany chronic and postoperative spinal disorders. The term disability refers to the inability to perform all of the usual functions of daily living and is frequently linked to prolonged episodes of severe spinal pain. Treatments of chronic pain derive from concepts about pain and methods of evaluation. Traditionally, clinicians have searched for causes of pain, seeking a physiologic basis for pain complaints that, once identified, could be eliminated or blocked. When no physical basis was identified, a psychological cause was assumed—hence the term psychogenic pain. The traditional view of persistent pain embraces a simple dichotomy: the pain is either physical or psychological. However, so simple a dichotomy is inadequate. Traditional medical approaches to chronic pain problems are ineffective, with long-term success rates below 30%. A range of psychosocial factors occurs secondary to an injury or disease.

Quantification of Physical and Functional Capacity

Functional restoration, because it treats only chronic disabling conditions, involves several concepts not generally considered relevant as part of acute and post-acute nonsurgical care. The first of these is the concept of deconditioning. Other concepts are psychosocial barriers to recovery and disability outcome monitoring. Disuse and immobilization can lead to many physically deleterious effects on joint mobility, muscle strength, endurance, and soft-tissue homeostasis.

The quantitative assessment of function is a vital aspect of developing an effective treatment program for disabling spinal disorders. The extremities offer good visual feedback for the examiner. Joints are easily seen, with mobility subject to goniometric measurements. Muscle bulk is easily assessed by inspection and tape measurements. Right-left comparisons between normal and abnormal sides can usually be made. By contrast, the spine offers inadequate direct visual feedback of physical capacity. This deficiency often forces clinicians to rely on a patient's subjective self-report or on physical examination findings that can be inaccurate or irrelevant. Physical examination findings are poor guides to the physical functional capacity of the low back. More accurate methods of objective testing are necessary to guide treatment recommendations.

As in the extremities, the critical physical capacity measures in the spine are mobility, strength, endurance, and the ability of the involved spinal region to mesh with adjacent body parts to perform musculoskeletal and neurologic tasks. In the spine, the most relevant tests involve cervical or lumbar regional isolated mobility, isometric or isokinetic regional strength, and the ability to perform relevant activities of daily living, such as lifting, bending, carrying, reaching, and walking. Cervicothoracic dysfunction often is accompanied by a limitation of upper extremity functional capacity and not infrequently by secondary upper extremity pathologic, vascular, or neuropathic diagnoses (carpal tunnel syndrome, cubital tunnel syndrome, thoracic outlet syndrome, tendinitis, or causalgia). Lower extremity dysfunction similarly often accompanies low back disability, often associated with a substitution of lower extremity performance for activities customarily performed, at least partially, by the low back (for example, squat lifting versus bent lifting).

At the tertiary level of nonsurgical treatment, with a goal of achieving specific socioeconomic outcomes, reliance on the observational skills of therapists to guide reconditioning is not adequate. Objective, quantitative measurement of human performance leads to specific, individualized training approaches. Objective measurement, however, is not generally part of the training curriculum of physical therapists, occupational therapists, or even most physicians. These skills therefore must be acquired. Qualitative, observational methods of guiding care to achieve outcome goals are adequate in secondary care but not in functional restoration.

Spinal range of motion does not lend itself to measurement by simple hinged goniometers because of multisegmental regional linkage. Motion above and below the region in question must be distinguished from regional motion.

Enhancing support musculature for the cervical and lumbar spinal segments is vital in restoring function. Isometric and/or isokinetic methodologies are available for assessing performance. The scientific literature reports a strong relationship between strength performance and imaging (CT, MRI) in assessing differences between the normal and pathologic states.

Lifting capacity is the most relevant functional capacity test related to both cervical and lumbar dysfunctions. Lifting is most frequently correlated with industrial injury events, and restoration of lifting capacity is of critical importance in a large number of blue-collar occupations. Other relevant daily living tasks (such as bending, reaching, repetitive motion, and vibration are difficult to measure, with few devices available to do so. As such, isometric, isokinetic, and/or isoinertial lifting techniques from floor to waist and waist to shoulder are the dominant functional capacity measures, respectively, for thoracolumbar and cervicothoracic functional capacity. Cardiovascular fitness can be measured simultaneously with lower extremity endurance through standard bicycle ergometry. Upper body ergometers are available to assess upper extremity endurance relevant to cervicothoracic dysfunctions. Additionally, a number of obstacle courses and work-simulation stations are available for observing a patient's ability to perform other functional tasks.

Psychosocial Barriers to Recovery

In a work environment, when injury is associated with compensation for disability, physical problems are rarely the only factor to be considered in organizing a tertiary treatment program for chronic disabling spinal disorders. Many psychosocial and socioeconomic problems can confront the patient recovering from a spinal disorder, particularly a patient accustomed to a productive lifestyle. Inability to see a "light at the end of the tunnel" can produce severe situational depression, often associated with anxiety and agitation about income, family responsibilities, and interactions with insurance

adjusters and lawyers. The back injury itself might be a sign of emotional factors involving, for example, authority conflicts or job dissatisfaction. Personality changes might manifest as anger, hostility, and noncompliance directed at the therapeutic team. Minor head injuries, organic brain dysfunction resulting from age or the use of alcohol or drugs, or limited intelligence can produce cognitive errors and dysfunctions that make patients difficult to manage and refractory to education. A variety of preexisting personality disorders also can complicate treatment.

Many chronic spinal disorders exist within a "disability system." That is, workers' compensation laws initially were devised to protect workers' income and provide timely medical benefits following industrial accidents. In return for providing these worker rights, employers were absolved of certain consequences of negligence, generally including cost-capped liability for any injury, no matter how severe, and set by state or federal statute. Unfortunately, certain disincentives to rational behavior can emerge within this system. For example, one possible outcome of a guaranteed paycheck during the period of temporary total disability is the lack of a clear incentive for the patient to return to work as soon as possible. Also, an aggressive approach to surgical decision-making and rehabilitation without awareness of compensation-related factors might be taken by a patient as "validation" of a spurious claim and create an incentive for further deconditioning and healthcare–seeking behaviors, making recovery more problematic. Complicating matters even further is the fact that, even though the employer has a verifiable financial incentive to have patients return as soon as possible to productive status, the employer usually is screened from the details of a claim by the insurance carrier. In other words, health professionals, attorneys, insurance companies, and vocational rehabilitation specialists all could have limited motivation or ability to combat a disabled patient's foot-dragging.

Before 1960, efforts to distinguish between functional (nonorganic) and organic low back pain did not meet with success. As mentioned earlier, the complex nature of chronic pain makes it difficult to categorize component factors as either purely physical or psychological. Chronic pain must be understood as an interactive, psychophysiologic behavior pattern wherein the physical and the psychological overlap. The focus of psychological evaluation of the patient with low back pain must shift away from functional versus organic distinctions to the identification in each patient of psychological characteristics with behavioral motivators. These characteristics affect a patient's disability and his or her response to treatment efforts. Identification of such characteristics facilitates treatment planning and assists with the prediction of treatment outcome. Psychosocial assessment should be organized in a standardized fashion and reported to an interdisciplinary team. Certain simple self-report tests (such as pain drawing, Million Visual Analog Scale, Beck Depression Inventory, Medical Outcomes Study 36-Item Short Form Health Survey) can be repeated frequently throughout the treatment process to assess patient perception of progress. Other tests also might help as part of the standard assessment.

Any efforts to assess patients are not designed simply to categorize or label patients but to assist the interdisciplinary team in dealing with patients' specific disability factors to facilitate return to function and productivity. It is a fallacy to believe that patients with noncompensable injuries fail to display many of the psychosocial and socioeconomic problems demonstrated by patients with compensable injuries. The development of chronic pain itself, particularly sustained rather than episodic pain, leads to feelings and behaviors that resonate with physical deconditioning and fear-avoidance in social and work situations. In time, this interaction between the mind and body can result in what was initially perceived as simply nontraumatic spinal pain developing into a full-blown compensable injury (leading to long-term disability payments, Social Security disability payments, or delayed reporting of a workers' compensation claim). Any clinician, whether a surgeon or not, must be aware of the complex interplay between physical and psychological factors in the progression of chronic disabling spinal disorders.

Functional Restoration Treatment

Functional restoration is a type of tertiary care that uses a patient's physical and functional capacity and psychosocial assessments to organize a physician-directed, interdisciplinary-team treatment approach whose primary goal is to restore patients to productivity. This approach varies from that of the traditional pain clinic, whose primary goal of relieving pain often encourages the use of such palliative measures as multiple injections or opiates while discouraging patient independence and participation in sports medicine–style exercise, which often induces pain associated with temporary overuse (Fig. 1). In functional restoration, return to activity is of paramount importance, with pain relief anticipated only after initial pain increases during the reconditioning process. Multiple disciplines are required on site, with all patients having access to each specialized group of health-care providers in an intensive program individualized to the initial assessments. An additional feature of functional restoration programs is the attention to outcome monitoring for all patients, with structured clinical

interviews at 1 year. These interviews focus on the specific objective factors of cost and disability.

Phase I Treatment

Following the initial assessment of a patient, a preliminary phase of treatment is initiated on a regular basis for which duration and frequency are determined by the degree of a patient's physical inhibition and the psychosocial barriers that interfere with participation in the tertiary care team approach. In this phase, the physical and occupational therapists are involved primarily in individual confidence-building to help the patient overcome fear and inhibition producing limited physical performance. Mobilization and stretching exercises are designed to prepare the patient for the intensive muscle-training portion of tertiary care. Adjunctive interventions might be used, such as providing zygapophyseal or epidural injections to facilitate overcoming segmental rigidity or nerve irritability that can impair the progression of rehabilitation.

The supervising physician should manage the patient's psychotropic medications and facilitate the patient's detoxification from opiates and tranquilizers before intensive exercise is initiated. Anti-inflammatory analgesics might be useful. Psychologists should be available to deal with a patient's psychological issues (such as depression or substance dependence) and disability managers to address the patient's social concerns (such as financial matters, transportation issues, and family responsibilities).

Intensive Treatment Phase: Reconditioning

After physical and emotional stabilization, the patient enters an intensive phase of the tertiary care program. Depending on an individual's needs, program duration, education, and individual counseling are tailored to the patient's requirements, taking advantage of the benefits offered by the site's environment of function that is critical to tertiary rehabilitation. Physical progress occurs through a quantitatively directed exercise progression program supplemented by periodic, objective, human performance testing to document a patient's progress, and by the educational and supervisory skills of the physical and occupational therapists. If necessary, a lower-intensity work-transition phase can be adopted for individuals without jobs to return to, those who require work simulation for particularly strenuous jobs, or those who might have to move directly into focused vocational rehabilitation placement or a retraining option.

For the reconditioning and work simulation aspects of the program, therapists use active treatment processes. In other words, patient participation in exer-

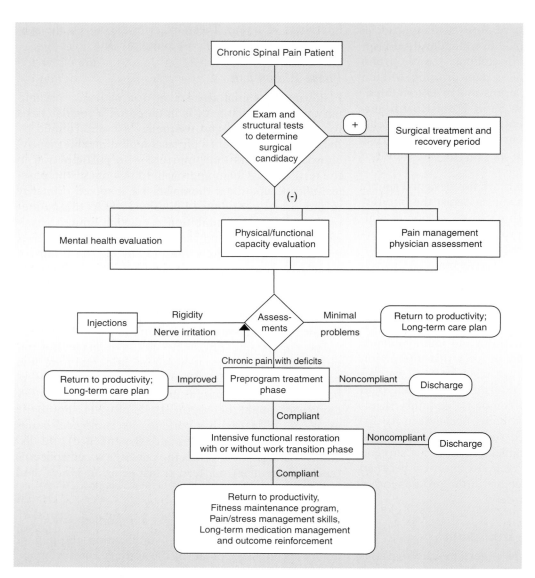

Figure 1 Functional restoration algorithm.

cise and activity stimulation, rather than passive pain-control techniques applied to the patient, is the norm. Further efforts at mobility reacquisition, begun during phase I, are intensified with encouragement and feedback from repeated motion measures. Strengthening of the injured musculoskeletal spinal region (or weak link), endurance building, and development of coordination through a variety of exercise techniques are added in this phase. Quantification is necessary for these aspects of the program. The indirect assessments confirm a patient's functional deficits and psychosocial barriers to effort and so lead to a combination of education and exercise training to resolve the deconditioning syndrome. Initial treatment is directed toward mobilizing and strengthening the "weak link" in the biomechanical chain identified through testing, while whole-body work simulation integrates the performance

of this link with other areas of the body that have been deconditioned by inactivity. A computerized expert system to standardize the exercise progression, based on age, gender, body mass, and testing performance factors, can markedly increase the efficient delivery of such a program.

In addition, when active treatment assessment has determined the diagnosis of a patient's psychosocioeconomic barriers to functional recovery, then a cognitive-behavioral multimodal disability management program should focus on specific solutions for these problems. The initial treatment might be pharmacologic, as mentioned above, requiring detoxification from habituating opiate and tranquilizer medications and the use of antidepressants, anti-inflammatory medications, and, occasionally, major tranquilizers. Remaining treatments include a cognitive, behaviorally based program of education and counseling, including stress management, that is time limited and aggressively oriented toward sequential goal-setting.

Patient Goals

Failure to pursue mutually prearranged goals could result in termination of the treatment program by the facility because failure to agree on goals makes it unlikely that expected outcomes will be achieved. However, the goals of treatment can be quite flexible. The type of patient who usually completes the program sets goals of returning to productivity that include a sustainable work plan with sufficient physical capacity to fulfill family responsibilities and enjoy recreational pursuits. The patient's acquisition of improved functional capacity also should help prevent recurrent injury and the need for significant amounts of future health-care utilization for the treated spinal disorder. In some cases, however, retirement or disability financial support might preclude returning to work as the patient's primary goal. In other cases, abbreviated programs might be considered as completed when an early discharge leads to returning to work and undertaking a home fitness maintenance program. Noncompletion of treatment, though, generally implies noncompliance with the requirements for attendance, drug detoxification, or minimum levels of program participation.

Postoperative care does not differ markedly from the care of patients who have not undergone surgery but who have also developed chronic dysfunction. Although surgery in compensable injury has been shown in multiple studies often to be associated with diminished work and pain report outcomes, recent data have shown that the combination of spine surgery and functional restoration in both the neck and back can provide superior pain relief, with socioeconomic outcomes identical to those of cohorts of chronic spinal pain patients who have not undergone surgery. Other studies have confirmed that despite repeat or extensive surgical care, recurrent injury rates and postrehabilitation surgery and health-care utilization rates after functional restoration are low. Finally, although extended periods of disability (up to 15 years) might show a trend toward poorer rehabilitation outcomes, those outcomes remain cost effective compared with the failure to provide tertiary care at all. The costs to society of continued lost productivity and poor physical and mental health, leading to persistent health-care utilization and comorbidities, cannot be overestimated.

Outcome Monitoring

Once the intensive phase of treatment is completed, the patient's ultimate socioeconomic outcome depends on maintaining treatment goals. Based on the training level a patient has achieved under supervision, a much higher level of physical and functional capacity can be reached by continuing with a fitness maintenance program for which the patient has been educated. Relevant pieces of durable medical equipment or membership in appropriately equipped fitness centers may be suggested. Repeated objective, physical quantification leads to feedback to the patient on maintenance of physical capacity, which can be correlated with job demands. In addition, follow-up interview information can be combined with the patient's preprogram demographic data to provide statistical comparisons of the ability of a comprehensive functional restoration program to deal with disability and cost problems.

Functional restoration might be appropriate for some patients even before a normal soft-tissue healing period (4 to 6 months postinjury) has concluded. Although secondary treatment is usually preferable for patients before 4 months postinjury, the availability of effective tertiary care that offers cost-limited and duration-limited programs might make these programs desirable for selected patients. In particular, with employer involvement through transitional work-return programs, with the recognition that early psychosocial stressors potentially can lead to enhancement of disability, and with the advent of treatment guidelines to inform health-care providers and administrative agencies of demonstrated ways to achieve treatment goals, tertiary treatment could be instituted in selected patients within 6 to 8 weeks of injury or disability. A variety of criteria can be used to distinguish the suitability of secondary or tertiary care in these patients, including the match between physical capacity and job demands, recent prior injury, age, the presence of other medical conditions, response to previous treatment, preexisting psychosocial barriers, and job availability.

The future of rehabilitation of chronically disabled patients with neck and back pain lies in finding solutions that promote cooperation between those with a stake in the various compensation systems (long-term disability, Social Security Disability Income, workers' compensation, third-party claims). The patient should be given an opportunity to receive appropriate medical care, to be rehired at his or her place of employment, and to be compensated for any injury that meets legal compensability criteria. When objective structural documentation cannot provide adequate means for assessing impairment, scheduled or functional assessment-based awards might be considered for the patient. Any planned surgical treatment must be carefully evaluated, not purely on the basis of a pain or structural issue but in terms of the impact surgery will have in a workers' compensation system, including any effect on the patient's socioeconomic outcomes discussed above. Partnerships between surgeons and rehabilitation specialists, based not on higher health-care utilization but on proven outcomes, could become the rule. The surgical treatment of a structural lesion alone rarely can be expected to result in a return to work in complex, chronically disabled patients. A network of occupational medicine professionals, surgeons, and providers of secondary and tertiary care is the most likely solution for achieving acceptable outcomes. Accomplishing these goals is the challenge for the next decade of spine surgeons and rehabilitation specialists.

Annotated Bibliography

Andersson G, Cocchiarella L (eds): *American Medical Association Guides to the Evaluation of Permanent Impairment*, ed 5. Chicago, IL, American Medical Association, 2000.

The methodology for making a nonmedical determination of loss of bodily function for compensation purposes must be fair, reproducible, and simple to perform. Two methodologies are used for the spine, involving a purely diagnosis-related system, complemented by a physical examination-based system involving neurologic examination and inclinometric spine mobility measurements.

Bendix AF, Bendix T, Haestrup C: Can it be predicted which patients with chronic low back pain should be offered tertiary rehabilitation in a functional restoration program? A search for demographic, socioeconomic, and physical predictors. *Spine* 1998;23:1775-1784.

The authors present a factor analysis to identify predictors of outcomes in a functional restoration program.

Flicker PL, Fleckenstein JL, Ferry K, et al: Lumbar muscle usage in chronic low back pain: Magnetic resonance image evaluation. *Spine* 1993;18:582-586.

This study evaluated the changes in MRI of the lumbar musculature associated with exercise.

Flores L, Gatchel RJ, Polatin PB: Objectification of functional improvement after nonoperative care. *Spine* 1997;22:1622-1633.

This literature review provides documentation of the various methods for objective assessment of functional improvement. The methods are discussed with respect to nonsurgical care, but they are also applicable to postsurgical assessment.

Garcy P, Mayer T, Gatchel RJ: Recurrent or new injury outcomes after return to work in chronic disabling spinal disorders: Tertiary prevention efficacy of functional restoration treatment. *Spine* 1996;21:952-959.

The occurrence of recurrent injury claims (particularly associated with lost time) is an important socioeconomic outcome that can be objectively measured as a relevant cost driver in industry. This study of a large number of chronically disabled workers undergoing functional restoration is the first to identify the prevalence of recurrent (or new) injury after tertiary rehabilitation in such a population.

Gatchel RJ, Mayer T, Dersh J, Robinson R, Polatin P: The association of the SF-36 health status survey with 1-year socioeconomic outcomes in a chronically disabled spinal disorder population. *Spine* 1999;24:2162-2170.

This study correlates objective socioeconomic outcome variables for work-related spinal disorders with the self-reported changes in the SF-36 before and after rehabilitation.

Hildebrandt J, Pfingsten M, Saur P, Jansen J: Prediction of success from a multidisciplinary treatment program for chronic low back pain. *Spine* 1997;22:990-1001.

This study demonstrates that the most important variable in predicting treatment outcome is the multidisciplinary counseling and training that leads to a reduction in the subjective feelings of disability in patients.

Jordan KD, Mayer TG, Gatchel RJ: Should extended disability be an exclusion criterion for tertiary rehabilitation? Socioeconomic outcomes of early versus late functional restoration in compensation spinal disorders. *Spine* 1998;23:2110-2117.

This study examines chronic spinal pain patients treated early (4 to 8 months) and late (more than 18 months) after a work-related injury date. Outcomes are comparable except that early-intervention patients have less spinal surgery. Late-disability patients show a trend to poorer outcomes as disability duration increases beyond 5 years.

Mayer TG, Polatin P, Smith B, et al: Spine rehabilitation. Secondary and tertiary nonoperative care. *Spine* 1995;20:2060-2066.

The authors review the principles involved in secondary and tertiary nonsurgical care, including historic background and principles incorporated in pain clinics and functional restoration.

Mayer TG, Kondraske G, Beals SB, Gatchel RJ: Spinal range of motion: Accuracy and sources of error with inclinometric measurement. *Spine* 1997;22:1976-1984.

This study demonstrates physics-based principles in assessing spinal range of motion using inclinometers. Test administrator errors in measurement are found to be the greatest source of error in providing accurate measurements, whereas device error is the least important factor.

Mayer T, McMahon MJ, Gatchel RJ, Sparks B, Wright A, Pegues P: Socioeconomic outcomes of combined spine surgery and functional restoration in workers' compensation spinal disorders with matched controls. *Spine* 1998;23:598-606.

This functional restoration study compares lumbar discectomy and fusion patients with matched control cohorts. The study demonstrates socioeconomic outcomes equivalent to findings for untreated control subjects, in marked contrast to meta-analyses of spinal surgery in workers' compensation, which demonstrated low work-return rates relative to noncompensation populations.

Mayer T, Robinson R, Pegues P, Kohles S, Gatchel R: Lumbar segmental rigidity: Can its identification with facet injections and stretching exercises be useful? *Arch Phys Med Rehabil* 2000;81:1143-1150.

This article, accompanied by a small cohort study, describes the use of facet injections in chronic lumbar disorders for dealing with observable segmental rigidity rather than a facet syndrome based on patient self-report of pain. It is suggested that injections administered for more objective physical findings, such as segmental rigidity or lower extremity neurologic disturbance, are likely to be far more effective in outcome studies than procedures based only on subjective statements.

Torstensen TA, Ljunggren AE, Meen HD, Odland E, Mowinckel P, Geijerstam S: Efficacy and costs of medical exercise therapy, conventional physiotherapy, and self-exercise in patients with chronic low back pain: A pragmatic, randomized, single-blinded, controlled trial with 1-year follow-up. *Spine* 1998;23:2616-2624.

This randomized trial shows that efficiency in dealing with chronic low back pain helps in preventing future sick leave.

Turner JA, Ersek M, Herron L, et al: Patient outcomes after lumbar spinal fusions. *JAMA* 1992;268:907-911.

This meta-analysis of spinal surgery studies demonstrates poorer outcomes in compensation injuries.

Wright A, Mayer TG, Gatchel RJ: Outcomes of disabling cervical spine disorders in compensation injuries: A prospective comparison to tertiary rehabilitation response for chronic lumbar spinal disorders. *Spine* 1999;24:178-183.

This study compares a cervical workers' compensation cohort to previously described lumbar cohorts, showing minimal differences in socioeconomic outcomes. However, delay in referral of cervical patients, particularly postoperative ones, is noted.

Classic Bibliography

Brady S, Mayer T, Gatchel RJ: Physical progress and residual impairment quantification after functional restoration: Part 2. Isokinetic trunk strength. *Spine* 1994;19:395-400.

Curtis L, Mayer TG, Gatchel RJ: Physical progress and residual impairment quantification after functional restoration: Part 3. Isokinetic and isoinertial lifting capacity. *Spine* 1994;19:401-405.

Hazard RG: Spine update: Functional restoration. *Spine* 1995;20:2345-2348.

Hazard RG, Fenwick JW, Kalisch SM, et al: Functional restoration with behavioral support: A one-year prospective study of patients with chronic low-back pain. *Spine* 1989;14:157-161.

Kishino ND, Mayer TG, Gatchel RJ, et al: Quantification of lumbar function: Part 4. Isometric and isokinetic lifting simulation in normal subjects and low-back dysfunction patients. *Spine* 1985;10:921-927.

Mayer TG, Barnes D, Nichols G, et al: Progressive isoinertial lifting evaluation: Part 2. A comparison with isokinetic lifting in a disabled chronic low-back pain industrial population. *Spine* 1988;13:998-1002.

Mayer T, Brady S, Bovasso E, Pope P, Gatchel RJ: Noninvasive measurement of cervical tri-planar motion in normal subjects. *Spine* 1993;18:2191-2195.

Mayer T, Gatchel RJ, Keeley J, Mayer H, Richling D: A male incumbent worker industrial database: Part 1. Lumbar spinal physical capacity. *Spine* 1994;19:755-761.

Mayer T, Gatchel RJ, Keeley J, Mayer H, Richling D: A male incumbent worker industrial database: Part 2. Cervical spinal physical capacity. *Spine* 1994;19:762-764.

Mayer T, Gatchel R, Keeley J, Mayer H, Richling D: A male incumbent worker industrial database: Part 3. Lumbar/cervical functional testing. *Spine* 1994;19:765-770.

Mayer TG, Gatchel RJ, Kishino N, et al: Objective assessment of spine function following industrial injury: A prospective study with comparison group and one-year follow-up. *Spine* 1985;10:482-493.

Mayer TG, Gatchel RJ, Mayer H, Kishino ND, Keeley J, Mooney V: A prospective two-year study of functional restoration in industrial low back injury: An objective assessment procedure. *JAMA* 1987;258:1763-1767.

Mayer TG, Tencer AF, Kristoferson S, Mooney V: Use of noninvasive techniques for quantification of spinal range-of-motion in normal subjects and chronic low-back dysfunction patients. *Spine* 1984;9:588-595.

Mayer TG, Vanharanta H, Gatchel RJ, et al: Comparison of CT scan muscle measurements and isokinetic trunk strength in postoperative patients. *Spine* 1989;14:33-36.

Newton M, Waddell G: Trunk strength testing with iso-machines: Part 1. Review of a decade of scientific evidence. *Spine* 1993;18:801-811.

Ward NG: Tricyclic antidepressants for chronic low-back pain: Mechanisms of action and predictors of response. *Spine* 1986;11:661-665.

Chapter 27

Spinal Cord Injury Rehabilitation

David F. Apple, Jr, MD

Spinal cord injury has an approximate incidence of 32 patients per million, or roughly 10,000 persons per year in the United States. Approximately 200,000 Americans have spinal cord injuries. Recent changes in the epidemiology of spinal cord injury have shown an increase in the percentage of paraplegic patients and thus a concomitant decrease in the percentage of quadriplegic patients. The percentage of patients with spinal cord injury caused by violence also has increased, although motor vehicle accidents still account for the largest percentage of these patients (Table 1). In the cervical spine, the most common level of injury is C5, followed by C4, then C6. In the remainder of the spine, the most common level of injury is T12. Approximately 80% of paralyzed patients are male. The percentages of plegic African-American and Hispanic males are disproportionately high compared with their relative percentages in the population as a whole.

Evaluation

Whether evaluation of the spinal cord-injured patient takes place at the time of the injury or during consultation for further management, an accurate dermatome delineation, such as that depicted in Figure 1, is necessary. The motor evaluation requires knowledge of the basic key muscles according to the root level (Table 2). Each muscle should be graded on a scale of 0 to 5 in

TABLE 1 | Etiology of Spinal Cord Injury

	1980	1990
Motor vehicle accident	47%	37%
Violence	14%	27%
Falls	15%	21%
Sports	15%	7%
Other	8%	8%

(Reproduced with permission from Maynard FM Jr: International Standards for Neurological and Functional Classification of Spinal Cord Injury. Atlanta, GA, American Spinal Injury Association, 1996.)

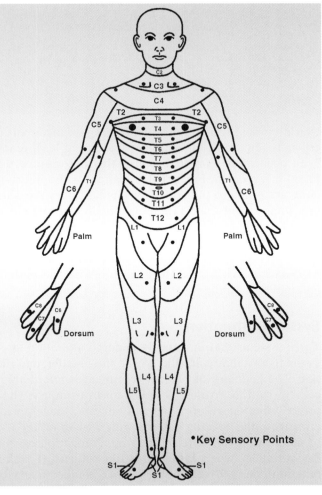

Figure 1 A competent neurologic examination should include dermatome functional evaluation, both sensory and motor. *(Reproduced with permission from Maynard FM Jr: International Standards for Neurological and Functional Classification of Spinal Cord Injury. Atlanta, GA, American Spinal Injury Association, 1996, p. 10.)*

TABLE 2	Components of a Motor Dermatone Functional Examination

Spinal Cord Level	Function
C5	Elbow flexors (biceps, brachialis)
C6	Wrist extensors (extensor carpi radialis longus and brevis)
C7	Elbow extensors (triceps)
C8	Finger flexors (flexor digitorum profundus) to the middle finger
T1	Small finger abductors (abductor digiti minimi)
L2	Hip flexors (iliopsoas)
L3	Knee extensors (quadriceps)
L4	Ankle dorsiflexors (tibialis anterior)
L5	Long toe extensors (extensor hallucis longus)
S1	Ankle plantar flexors (gastrocnemius soleus)

(Reproduced with permission from Maynard FM Jr: International Standards for Neurological and Functional Classification of Spinal Cord Injury. Atlanta, GA, American Spinal Injury Association, 1996.)

TABLE 3	American Spinal Injury Association Impairment Scale (modified from Frankel)

Degree of Impairment	Explanation
A = Complete	No sensory or motor function is preserved in the sacral segments S4-5
B = Incomplete	Sensory but not motor function is preserved below the neurologic level and includes the sacral segments S4-5
C = Incomplete	Motor function is preserved below the neurologic level, and more than half of key muscles below the neurologic level have a muscle grade less than 3
D = Incomplete	Motor function is preserved below the neurologic level, and at least half of key muscles below the neurologic level have a muscle grade greater than or equal to 3
E = Normal	Sensory and motor function is normal

(Reproduced with permission from Maynard FM Jr: International Standards for Neurological and Functional Classification of Spinal Cord Injury. Atlanta, GA, American Spinal Injury Association, 1996.)

which 0 is absent function and 5 is normal function. It is critically important that muscles that are at least grade 3 be accurately graded because this determines the function expected. Further delineation of the injury is done according to the American Spinal Injury Association impairment scale (Table 3). Finally, the patient is placed in one of the six clinical syndromes outlined in Table 4. Once this evaluation is complete, the spine care physician can discuss the injury and early rehabilitation expectations with his colleagues and with the patient and patient's family.

Systems Alteration

Three systems that universally undergo alteration after a spinal cord injury are the bowel, the bladder, and the skin. The hallmark of bladder treatment is intermittent catheterization. Around 4 to 6 weeks postinjury when reflex function returns the patient may develop an effective reflex voiding pattern, with or without the use of medication, and intermittent catheterization can be discontinued, when reflex function returns. If reflex function does not return, then other bladder management methods are available, including the construction of continent stomas.

Once reflex activity has returned, an effective bowel program performed every other day, usually in the evening, is the management of choice. However, individual variations might be more satisfactory because of the patient's lifestyle and/or work requirements. In certain clinical situations, a colostomy might be the best option.

Another potential complication is the breakdown of the skin. Prevention of decubitae, or pressure sores, is largely a nursing care function, with family and patient education providing the long-term impetus for skin integrity.

Fracture Care

In acute injury, especially motor vehicular trauma, long bone fractures frequently occur. The orthopaedic surgeon should be aggressive in managing these fractures with internal fixation if at all possible. Open reduction and internal fixation with the appropriate device, either in conjunction with internal fixation of the spinal fracture or shortly thereafter, is recommended. The use of a cast, external fixators, and splints over an insensitive limb is difficult at best and delays the rehabilitation process.

However, the management of a fracture in a patient who has had a spinal cord injury for longer than 6 months to a year is significantly different from care of acute injury. The use of rigid splints or casts is fraught with difficulty because of the insensitive skin. The architecture of the bone in the chronically paralyzed limb usually is not sufficient to provide good purchase for internal fixation devices, whether rods, screws, or plates. Therefore, a soft splint, such as a pillow splint for lower extremity fractures, is the management of choice. However, this type of management is not possible in some fractures such as those of the proximal femur. In spite of poor bone quality, internal fixation might be required in these cases. However, these fractures tend to develop callus more quickly and stabilize more quickly than do fractures in able-bodied patients. For instance, a fracture of the distal femur might show good callus and be clinically stable within 8 weeks of internal fixation, thus allowing discontinuance of external support.

Heterotopic Ossification

Another complication requiring orthopaedic attention is the development of heterotopic ossification. The most frequent areas for the deposition of this calcium are the hips, then the knees, the shoulders, and finally the elbows. Heterotopic ossification can start within a few weeks of the injury or be delayed many months. Twenty percent to 25% of patients with spinal cord injury develop heterotopic ossification; about half of these

cases are significant, and about a quarter of them lead to ankylosis.

Suspicion of a diagnosis of heterotopic ossification should be entertained when the physical therapist first notes some loss of motion in a major joint, usually the hip. Radiographs of the affected joint at this time usually do not show the calcification, but the alkaline phosphatase level will be elevated. When there is elevation of the alkaline phosphatase level, treatment should be instituted, the hallmark of which is the use of etidronate disodium, 20 mg/kg for 2 weeks, followed by 10 mg/kg for 3 months or until the alkaline phosphatase level nears normal. (Waiting until radiographs show the calcification makes it almost too late to start the etidronate disodium.) Other medications that can be considered are indomethacin and naproxen, but etidronate disodium appears to work better in spinal cord-injured patients than do these two medications. If the heterotopic ossification progresses and causes ankylosing of the joint, then surgery might be necessary. Surgery is most frequently needed in heterotopic ossification involving the hip joint because the hip will fuse in a position that will not allow effective sitting and can lead to skin breakdown.

Surgery should not be attempted until the alkaline phosphatase level is normal. The surgical procedure should be preceded by a 2-week course of etidronate

TABLE 4 | Incomplete Spinal Cord Injury Syndromes

Clinical Syndrome	Description	Prognosis
Central cord	A lesion, occurring almost exclusively in the cervical region, that produces sacral sensory sparing and greater weakness in the upper limbs than in the lower limbs	Lower extremities recover better than upper extremities
Brown-Séquard	A lesion that produces relatively greater ipsilateral proprioceptive and motor loss and contralateral loss of sensitivity to pain and temperature	Good prognosis for motor return
Anterior cord	A lesion that produces variable loss of motor function and of sensitivity to pain and temperature while preserving proprioception	Poor prognosis for motor recovery
Posterior cord	A lesion that produces loss of sensation, but motor function is maintained	Rare
Conus medullaris	Injury of the sacral cord (conus) and lumbar nerve roots within the spinal canal that usually results in areflexic bladder, bowel, and lower limbs	Bowel and bladder usually do not recover
Cauda equina	Injury to the lumbosacral nerve roots within the neural canal resulting in areflexic bladder, bowel, and lower limbs	Fair prognosis for motor return

(Reproduced with permission from Maynard FM Jr: International Standards for Neurological and Functional Classification of Spinal Cord Injury. Atlanta, GA, American Spinal Injury Association, 1996.)

TABLE 5 | General Goals for Spinal Cord Function

Spinal Cord Level/ Spinal Nerve	Possible Goals
C3 to C4	Control power wheelchair with sip-and-puff (mouth) or chin/head control Locomotion with modified independence Verbalize care Communicate through adaptive equipment
C5	Dress upper body (time consuming) Feed self with equipment Brush teeth, wash face with assistance Operate power wheelchair
C6	Dress upper body Dress lower body with assistance (time consuming) Groom self with equipment Perform bowel/bladder program with assistance Feed self with splints (hand or tenodesis splints) Transfer to/from wheelchair to bed, car, and toilet with some assistance Able to drive Propel power wheelchair May be able to push manual wheelchair if strength in shoulder permits
C7	Independent in transfer to bed, car, and toilet Independent in dressing with equipment Propel manual and/or power wheelchair Independent with feeding Independent with bathing and other self-care activities Bowel/bladder program with some assistance
C8 to T4	Independent in all transfers Push wheelchair Independent with self-care skills Homemaking activities with assistance Independent with bowel/bladder program
T5 to T12	Independent in all self-care Able to do all of above more easily than with above levels of injury T12: Walk with walker and long leg braces (difficult and time consuming)
L1 to L5	Independent in all self-care Walking with short or long leg braces and crutches more easily than with T5- to T12-level injuries Independent with bowel and bladder program
S1 to S5	Able to walk if able to push off ground (may need brace) Independent in all activities Bowel/bladder and sexual functioning might still be impaired

(Reproduced with permission from Maynard FM Jr: International Standards for Neurological and Functional Classification of Spinal Cord Injury. Atlanta, GA, American Spinal Injury Association, 1996.)

disodium, and the medication should be continued postoperatively for a year. Patients with multiple recurrences of heterotopic ossification might require adjunctive radiation therapy.

Pain

Pain is a common complaint in patients with spinal cord injury. Pain that is neurogenic in origin is experienced by almost 100% of patients whose spinal cord injury has been caused by a gunshot wound. Musculoskeletal pain is also possible, particularly in the chronic spinal cord-injured patients, who commonly complain of shoulder, elbow, wrist, and hand pain.

Patients with neurogenic pain usually describe it as intense, burning pain that is usually present in areas of the body that normally have no sensation, such as the buttocks and the lower extremities. The first lines of treatment are usually nonnarcotic analgesics and nonsteroidal anti-inflammatory agents. If the response to these oral medications is not good, gabapentin can be tried, starting with a dose of 100 mg three times a day and progressing to as much as 2,400 mg total daily dose. Other medications that can be considered are amytriptyline and carbamazepine. Some patients are refractory to all the medications mentioned and thus might require a pain management approach.

The spinal cord-injured patient also might complain of musculoskeletal spinal column pain, which can be treated with nonsteroidal anti-inflammatory agents and better posture in the wheelchair, with special supports. Orthoses occasionally are helpful but can cause skin-pressure problems or be too uncomfortable for the patient.

In the chronic spinal cord-injured patient, the development of rotator cuff syndrome is a frequent cause of shoulder pain because of the constant use of the wheelchair and the necessity of excessive shoulder pressure during transfer activities. Wheelchair use also can promote the development of carpal tunnel syndrome and, occasionally, complaints of elbow pain. These musculoskeletal joint pains ordinarily respond to the usual methods of treatment; however, the symptomatology might require the patient to use a power wheelchair rather than a manual chair.

Neurologic Decline

The most critical time for neurologic decline to occur is in the setting of the acute injury and immediately thereafter. A good baseline neurologic examination at the time of injury determines a starting point. If a loss of neurologic function occurs while the patient is being evaluated for stabilization, then immediate diagnostic

TABLE 6	Life Expectancy (Years) Postinjury by Severity of Injury and Age at Injury						
Age at Injury	No Spinal Cord Injury	Motor Functional at Any Level	Paraplegia	Low Tetraplegia (C5-8)	High Tetraplegia (C1-4)	Ventilator-Dependent at Any Level
20	57.2	51.6	45.2	39.4	33.8	16.2
40	38.4	33.5	27.8	23.0	18.7	7.2
60	21.2	17.5	13.0	9.6	6.8	1.2

(Reproduced with permission from Maynard FM Jr: International Standards for Neurological and Functional Classification of Spinal Cord Injury. Atlanta, GA, American Spinal Injury Association, 1996.)

procedures, usually MRI, must be undertaken to determine either soft-tissue cause or bleeding. Prompt surgical approach to the problem is mandatory, although occasionally nothing can be found to explain the neurologic decline. Rapid diagnostic testing, sometimes accompanied by surgery, also must be done in the immediate postoperative period when the patient recovers from anesthesia and is found to have a more profound neurologic loss. Occasionally, in the first 2 to 3 weeks following stabilization, a patient may experience loss of function. When this occurs, loss of fixation must be suspected and, if found, appropriate external support must be applied or secondary surgery performed.

Neurologic decline also might occur late, sometimes as early as 3 months after injury and stabilization but often not until months or years after the initial injury. The prevalence of the development of traumatic syringomyelia leading to neurologic decline is 3% to 5%. Symptoms indicating potential syringomyelia are increase in spasticity, increase in pain, and/or increase in symptomatology with flexion and/or extension. Signs of syrinx are ascending loss of pain and temperature sensation, ascending loss of tendon reflexes, and, in very flagrant instances, development of a Horner syndrome. MRI is the diagnostic test of choice in these situations. Myelography with delayed CT imaging usually is not required unless metallic internal fixation obscures accurate MRI diagnosis. Many cysts are small and either might not cause symptoms or cause symptoms so minor that they can be handled by fluid restriction measures. Large symptomatic cysts can be treated by shunting, usually to the peritoneum. Untethering the cord instead of shunting might help restore cerebrospinal fluid flow to the subarachnoid space. Shunting is more problematic in patients with incomplete spinal cord injuries.

Functional Expectations

Because the patient and the family will want to know how the patient will function postinjury, the physician must have a general idea of what can be expected with different levels of injury. A patient with a C4-level injury who is on a ventilator usually can be expected to get off the ventilator and be able to control his or her environment through the use of sip-and-puff controls on the wheelchair. Sip-and-puff controls are capable of doing more than just propelling and directing the wheelchair; they can be used to operate computers and different types of switches. In the patient with a C5-6–level tetraplegia, the shoulders and elbows will function at a grade 3 level or better, but as root return occurs in the sixth nerve root, the wrist extensors will become strong enough to significantly improve the patient's ability to participate in many activities of daily living that the C5-level tetraplegic will not be able to do. Table 5 outlines reasonable general goals for each functional level.

Life Expectancy

The effect of the spinal cord injury on life expectancy will be of great concern to the patient and family. The National Spinal Cord Injury Statistical Center has developed tables that are periodically updated. Table 6 presents life expectancy data based on information from more than 20,000 patients entered into the national database since 1973. Normal life expectancy for a patient 40 years of age at the time of injury is 38.4 years; by comparison, a 40-year-old paraplegic has a life expectancy of approximately 28 years, and a low tetraplegic, of 23 years. These life-expectancy numbers show continuous improvement, however, especially because better management of the bladder has removed complications of the urinary tract from among the top three causes of death. The causes of death with the greatest impact on reduced life expectancy in spinal cord-injured patients are pneumonia, pulmonary emboli, and septicemia. The national database shows that the cost of care for a high tetraplegic patient with injury onset at age 25 years is $1.7 million. The cost for care of a paraplegic of the same age is about half a million dollars.

Classic Bibliography

American Spinal Injury Association/International Medical Society of Paraplegia and American Paralysis Association: *International Standards for Neurological and Functional Classification of Spinal Cord Injury* (revised). Chicago, IL, American Spinal Injury Association, 1992.

Bayley JC, Cochran TP, Sledge CB: The weight-bearing shoulder: The impingement syndrome in paraplegics. *J Bone Joint Surg Am* 1987;69:676-678.

Edgar R, Quail P: Progressive post-traumatic cystic and non-cystic myelopathy. *Br J Neurosurg* 1994;8:7-22.

Marshall LF, Knowlton S, Garfin SR, et al: Deterioration following spinal cord injury: A multicenter study. *J Neurosurg* 1987;66:400-404.

Sie, IH, Waters RL, Adkins RH, Gellman H: Upper extremity pain in the postrehabilitation spinal cord injured patient. *Arch Phys Med Rehabil* 1992;73:44-48.

Stauffer ES: Neurologic recovery following injuries to the cervical spinal cord and nerve roots. *Spine* 1984;9: 532-534.

Stover SL, Niemann KM, Tulloss JR: Experience with surgical resection of heterotopic bone in spinal cord injury patients. *Clin Orthop* 1991;263:71-77.

Waters RL, Adkins RH, Yakura JS, Sie I: Motor and sensory recovery following incomplete paraplegia. *Arch Phys Med Rehabil* 1994;75:67-72.

Waters RL, Sie IH, Adkins RH: The musculoskeletal system, in Whiteneck GG, Charlifue SW, Gerhart KA, et al (eds): *Aging with Spinal Cord Injury*. New York, NY, Demos Publications, 1993, pp 53-71.

Section 3

Surgical Care

Section Editor:
Harry N. Herkowitz, MD

Chapter 28

Cervical Spine Fractures and Dislocations

Bobby K-B Tay, MD

Frank Eismont, MD

Introduction

In a recent survey of 165 trauma centers, evaluating a total of 111,219 patients, the incidence of cervical spine injury was 4.3% with a 1.3% incidence of spinal cord injury. Most studies report an incidence of 3.2 to 5.3 new spinal cord injuries per 100,000 persons at risk in the United States. The prevalence of spinal column injury is bimodal, with peaks occurring in people between 15 and 24 years of age and in people 50 years and older. The percentage of the population older than 50 years is constantly increasing as a result of longer life expectancies resulting from improvements in medical care and disease prevention. Because older adults are more active, the incidence of spinal cord injury in the elderly will certainly increase as this subset of the population expands. In addition, improvements in emergency medical care and trauma care have reduced the mortality and morbidity associated with these injuries. One report indicated that establishment of a regional spinal cord injury unit reduced the proportion of complete spinal cord injuries from 65% to 46%. The mortality from spinal cord injury also decreased from 20% to 9%. Clearly the cost savings to society from this improved care is significant.

Most patients with spinal column injury are young men; up to 30% are men in their 30s. The most common mechanism in this age group is motor vehicle accidents, followed by falls, gunshot injuries, and sports injuries. Motor vehicle accidents are the predominant mechanism of injury in the pediatric population, and falls are most common in the elderly. The proportion of spinal cord injuries from gunshot wounds is increasing, and controversy still exists as to the optimal management of a patient with a bullet in the spinal canal.

Internal fixation of spine fractures has allowed early mobilization and rehabilitation of the patient, resulting in improved overall outcomes. Internal fixation has also facilitated the ability to perform a more thorough decompression of the neural elements. Advances in the rehabilitation of patients with spinal cord injuries have maximized the overall functionality of these patients.

Clinical Evaluation

The treatment of a patient with a cervical spine injury is initiated at the scene of the injury. Without exception, all victims of trauma are suspected to have a cervical injury until proven otherwise. Cervical spine injury has been closely linked to the presence of severe head injury (odds ratio 8.5), a high-energy mechanism (odds ratio 11.6), or a focal neurologic deficit (odds ratio 58). The odds ratio in this case is the ratio of the odds of suffering a cervical spine injury in each of these instances to the odds of having one in their absence. Initial stabilization begins with the application of a rigid cervical collar, a spine board, and sandbags.

Once at the trauma center, the clinical assessment of the patient with a suspected cervical spine injury begins with evaluation of the airway, breathing, and circulation. Significant retropharyngeal soft-tissue swelling, especially in the upper cervical spine, may lead to upper airway obstruction. High cervical injuries causing diaphragmatic and chest-wall muscle paralysis will result in respiratory failure. Neurogenic shock can cause significant hypotension and bradycardia. The airway and breathing can be managed successfully by intubation and mechanical ventilation of the patient. Nasotracheal intubation remains the safest method of airway control in the acute setting because it causes less cervical spine motion than direct oral intubation. The diastolic pressure should be kept above 70 mm Hg to maximize blood flow in the spinal cord. In the polytrauma setting this is done initially with fluid resuscitation. However, once the diagnosis of neurogenic shock is established, the blood pressure should be managed with vasopressors to prevent fluid overload.

After the initial resuscitation, the primary survey can be performed to evaluate the patient for any life-threatening injuries. At this time, information from emergency medical technicians about the mechanism of injury and the accident scene can alert the treating physician to associated injuries. The secondary survey should include inspection and palpation of the entire spine. Ecchymosis, soft-tissue swelling, tenderness, crepitation, and gaps between the spinous processes suggest underlying spinal column injury. Noncontiguous spinal injuries can occur in 6% of patients, and these fractures can easily be missed in the presence of head injury, upper cervical injury, or cervicothoracic injury.

Other injuries should be assessed because they may influence the treatment of the spinal lesion and significantly affect the outcome of the patient. Much attention has been pointed to the evaluation of patients with cervical spine trauma for vertebral artery injury. A 24% overall incidence of vertebral artery injury was reported in 37 cases of nonpenetrating cervical spine trauma. The incidence of vertebral artery injury increases if the fracture extends into the foramen transversarum. A 19.7% incidence of vertebral artery injury was found by magnetic resonance angiography (MRA) in 61 patients. In this series, 83% of the patients with vertebral artery injuries had flexion-distraction or flexion-compression types of spinal injuries. Only 17% of these patients showed reconstitution of blood flow in the injured vertebral artery after a mean 25.8-month follow-up. Bilateral or dominant vertebral artery injury can cause fatal ischemic damage to the brain stem and cerebellum. Delayed cortical blindness and recurrent quadriparesis can also occur from occult vertebral artery injury after cervical trauma. The great majority of vertebral artery injuries are clinically silent. Thus, they are of unclear significance in a stable, neurologically intact patient.

Spinal Anatomy and ASIA Neurologic Examination

The careful evaluation and clear documentation of the patient's neurologic status will allow the treating physician to best determine the appropriate treatment plan and the expectations for functional recovery. The neurologic assessment of a patient with spinal cord injury requires an understanding of the basic anatomy of the spinal cord, its ascending and descending tracts, and the exiting nerve roots (Fig. 1, *A*; see also Table 2 in chapter 27).

The spinal cord comprises central gray matter (neuronal cell bodies) surrounded by white matter (axons). Within a cross section of the cord several important anatomic structures can be identified. These include the lateral spinothalamic tracts responsible for transmitting pain and temperature sensation; the lateral corticospinal tracts responsible for motor function at that level; and the posterior columns that transmit position sense, vibratory sensation, and deep pressure sensation. The spinothalamic tracts cross to the opposite side of the spinal cord within three levels of entering the cord. In contrast, the corticospinal tracts and the posterior

columns decussate at the craniocervical levels. The tracts carry a specific topographic organization; the most central portions represent the function of the more proximal areas of the body, and the more peripheral portions represent the function of the distal areas of the body.

The spinal roots exit the vertebral column through the intervertebral foramina. In the cervical spine, the C1 root exits above the C1 body, the C2 root exits below the C1 body, and the C8 root exits below the C7 body. In the thoracic and lumbar spine, each root exits under the pedicle of the same number.

The motor and sensory examination outlined by the American Spinal Injury Association (ASIA) is the most widely accepted and used system to assess the impact of spinal-cord injury on the patient (see Table 3 in chapter 27). It involves the use of a grading system to evaluate the remaining sensory and motor function. The system allows the patients to be assessed through scales of impairment and functional independence.

The sensory level is determined by the patient's ability to perceive a pinprick (using a disposable needle or safety pin) and light touch (using a cotton ball). Testing of a key point in each of the 28 dermatomes on the right and the left sides of the body as well as evaluation of perianal sensation is required. The variability in sensation for each individual stimulus is graded on a 3-point scale: 0, absent; 1, impaired; 2, normal; and NT, not testable.

The C3 and C4 nerve roots supply sensation to the entire upper neck and chest in a cape-like distribution from the tip of the acromion to just above the nipple line. The next adjacent sensory level is the T2 dermatome. The brachial plexus, C5-T1 supplies the upper extremities. ASIA also recommends testing of pain and deep pressure sensation in the same dermatomes and an evaluation of proprioception by testing the position sense of the index fingers and great toes on each side.

The motor level is determined by manual testing of a key muscle in the 10 paired myotomes from rostral to caudal (see Table 2 in chapter 27). The strength of each muscle is graded on a 6-point scale: 0, total paralysis; 1, palpable or visible contraction; 2, full range of motion of the joint powered by the muscle with gravity eliminated; 3, full range of motion of the joint powered by the muscle against gravity; 4, active movement with full range of motion against moderate resistance; 5, normal strength; and NT, not testable. For myotomes that are not clinically testable by manual muscle evaluation, the motor level is presumed to be the same as the sensory level (C1-C4, T2-L1, S2-S5).

ASIA also recommends evaluation of diaphragmatic function (via fluoroscopy, C4 level) and the abdominal musculature (via Beevor's sign, which is the upward

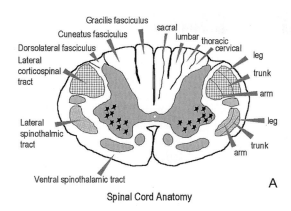

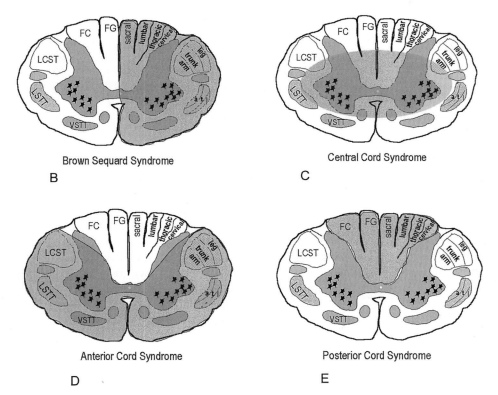

Figure 1 **A,** Cross-sectional anatomy of the cervical spinal cord showing the ascending and descending tracts and their topographic organization. **B,** Brown-Sequard syndrome with hemisection of cord. **C,** Central cord syndrome with injuries to the central portion of the spinal cord affecting the arms more than the legs. **D,** Anterior cord syndrome with sparing of only the posterior columns of the spinal cord. **E,** Posterior cord syndrome affects only the posterior columns.

migration of the umbilicus from upper abdominal contraction in the absence of lower abdominal contraction caused by paralysis at the T10 level). Evaluation of medial hamstring and hip adductor strength is also recommended but not required.

Spinal shock occurs in an initial period after spinal cord injury during which metabolic rather than structural derangements in the injured cord (depletion of adenosine triphosphate) result in spinal cord dysfunction characterized by paralysis, hypotonia, and areflexia. Once spinal shock has resolved (heralded by the return of the bulbocavernosus reflex), the motor and sensory examination allows the patient to be graded on a scale of functional impairment (see Table 3 in chapter 27).

The functionality of an individual with a spinal cord injury depends on multiple factors including age, body habitus, overall fitness, and motivation. Patients with complete spinal cord injuries often will regain one root level of function on each side over the 6 months following injury. Despite the individual variability, some generalizations can be made on the useful function that a person can attain after suffering an injury at a specific neurologic level (see Table 5 in chapter 27). In general, trauma that results in a complete spinal cord injury will also cause injury to the spinal roots exiting at the same level. These roots suffer a peripheral nerve injury because they originate from normal spinal cord just proximal to the level of damage. The function of the root is expected to return within 6 months; 66% to 80% of patients can be expected to recover at least one nerve root level of function following a complete cord injury. This must be clearly distinguished from return of cord function.

The ASIA guidelines provide an instrument, the Functional Independence Measure, to objectively evaluate and measure the impact of spinal cord injury on the patient. This instrument is widely accepted and used to evaluate the progress or lack of progress of a patient over time or after a specific treatment. It assesses six areas of functionality with two or more points of evaluation within each area. These areas include self care, sphincter control, mobility, locomotion, communication, and social cognition. The levels of functionality are graded on a 7-point scale from 1, total assistance, to 7, complete independence.

Other key components of the neurologic examination include assessment of the patient's reflexes and muscle tone, which gives clues to the possibility of cord injury, especially in comatose or seemingly uncooperative patients. The stretch reflex or deep tendon reflex is a basic mechanism to maintain tone in the muscles. The reflex is mediated by group Ia afferent neurons that monosynaptically stimulate the alpha motoneurons of the stretched muscle and postsynaptically inhibit its antagonist muscles. The reflex arc is modulated by the cerebral cortex that prevents excessive reaction with stimulation.

In addition to the evaluation of these normal reflexes, any pathologic reflexes should be sought out. The Babinski sign describes the extension of the great toe and splaying of the remaining toes when the lateral plantar surface is stroked by a sharp object. The presence of a Babinski sign is a strong indicator of a disorder of the corticospinal tract. The Oppenheim reflex is the demonstration of the Babinski sign on stroking the ipsilateral tibial crest. Hoffman's sign is demonstrated by flicking the nail of the patient's middle finger. When the sign is positive, this maneuver will lead to a prompt adduction of the thumb and flexion of the index finger, a reflex commonly associated with injury to the corticospinal tracts above C6.

Muscle tone refers to the resistance that the examiner perceives when passively manipulating the limbs of the patient. During normal circumstances, the examiner will encounter a certain amount of resistance as the muscle is brought through a range of motion. In pathologic states two abnormalities of tone may exist: hypotonia or hypertonia. Hypotonia refers to a decrease in the normal resistance encountered during passive manipulation of the limbs. Muscles will be hypotonic if their ventral roots are cut or damaged, if there is a transection of the dorsal roots that carry afferent information from the muscle, or if there are lesions in the cerebellum. Hypertonia refers to an increase in resistance to passive manipulation of the limbs and has two forms: rigidity and spasticity. Spasticity is a clasp-knife type of resistance in which there is increased resistance to passive manipulation at the initial portions of the manipulation. As the manipulation proceeds, however, the resistance suddenly decreases and disappears. Rigidity is a cogwheel type of resistance to passive manipulation.

Once the primary and secondary surveys are completed, serial neurologic examinations are necessary to detect any progression of neurologic deficit. The return of the bulbocavernosus reflex heralds the end of spinal shock. In most patients, this local reflex arc returns within 48 hours of injury. Once spinal shock ends, an accurate assessment of the patient's neurologic status can be made. If a patient has a complete neurologic deficit at the end of spinal shock, the chance for recovery of neurologic function below the level of injury is practically nonexistent.

Imaging

Plain radiographs are used as the first imaging modality for the cervical spine. The standard series includes AP, lateral, and open-mouth views. Eighty-five percent of all significant injuries to the cervical spine will be detected on the lateral view. If the standard lateral view does not adequately show the C7-T1 junction, adjunctive studies such as a swimmer's view, oblique views, or CT of this area are necessary (see chapter 7). Tan and associates retrospectively reviewed 360 trauma patients at Thomas Jefferson Hospital whose C7-T1 levels could not be adequately displayed by conventional radiography and who had no clinical evidence of lower cervical injury. Despite the lack of clinical findings, a 3.1% incidence of occult cervical fracture at the C7-T1 level was detected by CT. In this large series, the use of CT to evaluate the C7-T1 level was a cost-effective procedure. Voluntary flexion and extension views in the acute setting are not as useful as they are 1 to 2 weeks after the injury. Up to 33.5% of these views will be inadequate to assess for ligamentous injury because of voluntary guarding. In the obtunded patient or in the patient with a spinal cord injury, the entire spine must be imaged because the clinical examination may be unreliable.

Evaluation of the lateral cervical view should include assessment for prevertebral soft-tissue swelling, the sagittal alignment, and instability. The soft-tissue shadow should be less than 10 mm at C1, 4 to 5 mm at C3, and 15 to 20 mm at C6. Although this measure may be nonspecific for cervical injury, any increase in soft-tissue swelling beyond the normal values should alert the physician to rule out occult cervical trauma. The sagittal alignment of the spine should be assessed by evaluation of four imaginary lines: (1) a line formed by the anterior margins of the vertebral bodies, (2) a line formed by the posterior margins of the vertebral bodies, (3) a line formed by the anterior cortical margins of the lamina, and (4) a line formed by the tips of the spinous processes.

The presence of developmental cervical stenosis can be evaluated by calculation of the Pavlov ratio (Torg ratio), which is the ratio of the cervical spinal canal diameter to the sagittal diameter of the vertebral body. A ratio less than 0.8 indicates the presence of developmental stenosis. The space available for the spinal cord at the level of injury is also predictive of the severity of spinal cord injury. In a retrospective review of 288 patients with fractures and dislocations of the cervical spine, there were statistically significant differences in the space available for the spinal cord among patients who had complete injuries (10.5 mm), incomplete injuries (13.1 mm), isolated nerve root injuries (15.9 mm), and those with no neurologic deficit (16.7 mm).

Significant instability is commonly evaluated by using the criteria described by Panjabi and White. Although the presence of 3.5 mm of sagittal translation and angulation greater than 11° (compared with adjacent levels) are commonly used as strict criteria for instability, it is important to note that these two measurements account for only four out of five points necessary for the diagnosis of instability. Degenerative changes in the cervical spine can cause significant translation of cervical vertebrae in the absence of trauma. It has been found that 5.2% of 174 asymptomatic patients had 2 to 4 mm of anterolisthesis on lateral radiographs, especially at the C4-C5 level.

CT scanning remains the most sensitive imaging modality to evaluate fractures of the cervical spine. In a prospective study of polytrauma patients, CT used as a primary screening tool had a sensitivity of 90% and a specificity of 100% in detecting cervical injury. CT is also cost effective as a primary screening tool, especially in high and moderate risk patients. With the added benefit of sagittal, coronal, and three-dimensional reconstructed images, CT has immense power to demonstrate complex fracture patterns not easily seen on standard radiography and on the axial images.

MRI is not as good as CT or plain radiographs in the identification and evaluation of cervical fractures. It has been shown that MRI had only a 11.5% sensitivity for posterior fractures and a 36.7% sensitivity for anterior fractures. Another author reported that for acute fractures, MRI had a weighted average sensitivity of 43% compared to 48% for conventional radiography. Vaccaro and associates noted that MRI is not cost effective as a screening device in patients without a neurologic

deficit. Despite its inadequacies in evaluating bony detail, MRI is unsurpassed for the assessment of the soft-tissue elements in the cervical spine. These structures include the intervertebral disc, ligamentous structures, and the spinal cord itself. MRI is much more sensitive and specific than plain radiographs for the evaluation of prevertebral hematoma. It also is useful for the detection of spinal cord hemorrhage, which, if present, carries a poor prognosis for neurologic recovery. Acute hemorrhage has a low signal intensity on T2-weighted images (secondary to intracellular deoxyhemoglobin) and becomes hyperintense over the next several days after it becomes converted to extracellular methemoglobin.

There has been recent interest in the use of bedside fluoroscopy to clear the cervical spine in obtunded patients. A report noted that 30% of these patients could not be adequately evaluated by this technique. In addition, the risks of neurologic injury by manipulation of the cervical spine in these patients who cannot be assessed by neurologic examination may outweigh the benefits of cervical collar removal. Use of both CT and MRI may provide sufficient information to allow removal of the cervical collar without the need for manipulation of the neck.

Incomplete Spinal Cord Injury Syndromes

Greater recovery of function can be expected in patients in whom there is more initial sparing of motor and sensory function distal to the level of injury and when recovery of function is rapid. Ninety percent of incomplete injuries can be classified into either Brown Sequard syndrome (Fig. 1, *B*), central cord syndrome (Fig. 1, *C*), or anterior cord syndrome (Fig. 1, *D*).

Brown Sequard Syndrome

The pattern of neurologic deficit seen in this syndrome typically is caused by hemisection of the spinal cord from a penetrating injury such as a gunshot or a stabbing. The pattern of neurologic deficit is best understood by reviewing the local spinal anatomy at the level of injury. The corticospinal tracts (motor) and the posterior columns (proprioception, deep pressure) decussate at the craniocervical levels while the spinothalamic tracts (pain and temperature) cross to the opposite side of the cord within two to three levels of entering the spinal cord. Thus, unilateral lateral column damage results in ipsilateral muscle paralysis below the level of injury with spasticity, hyperreflexia, clonus, loss of superficial reflexes, and a positive Babinski sign. Injury to the dorsal column results in an ipsilateral loss of joint position sense, vibratory sense, and tactile discrimination below the level of injury. Damage to the lateral spinothalamic

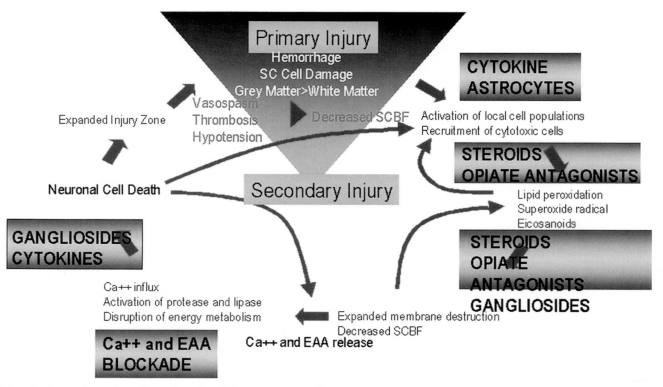

Figure 2 Primary and secondary pathways of spinal cord injury with areas amenable to pharmacotherapy.

tracts results in loss of pain and temperature sensation on the contralateral side of the body beginning one or two dermatome levels below the level of injury. Concurrent root injury may superimpose radicular symptoms over the classic Brown Sequard pattern of neurologic deficit. This type of injury carries the best prognosis for recovery of neural function, bowel and bladder function, and ambulatory capacity. In a series of 60 patients, 90% showed neurologic improvement.

Central Cord Syndrome

Central cord syndrome results from injury to the central portions of the spinal cord. This pattern most often is associated with an extension injury of the cervical spine causing a pinching of the spinal cord at the affected level. Typically, the patients are elderly and have preexisting cervical stenosis. Patients with central cord syndrome have minimal to no motor and sensory function in the upper extremities and the proximal leg muscles. Distal motor function in the lower limbs is spared. This pattern reflects the unique topographic organization of the spinal cord in which proximal motor function is represented at the more central portions of the cord while the distal musculature is represented in the more peripheral portions. Perianal sensation and rectal tone are preserved. Central cord syndrome carries the second best prognosis for recovery of ambula-

tory capacity and bowel and bladder function, with 50% of patients showing functional improvement.

Anterior Cord Syndrome

This syndrome is the result of damage to the anterior two thirds of the spinal cord, which receives its blood supply from the anterior spinal artery. The posterior columns are preserved. The classic mechanism of injury involves a flexion-compression force on the cervical spine. Patients will have minimal if any distal motor function because of damage to the lateral corticospinal tracts. Muscle groups at the level of injury will exhibit flaccid paralysis and fasciculations, and muscle groups below the level of injury will exhibit spastic paralysis. Bilateral injury to the lateral spinothalamic tracts leads to a loss of sensitivity to pain and temperature. Deep pressure and vibratory sensation is preserved. Anterior cord syndrome carries the poorest prognosis for functional recovery, with 16% of patients showing neurologic improvement.

Posterior Cord Syndrome

Posterior cord syndrome (Fig. 1, *E*) is a very rare injury isolated to the posterior columns with sparing of the anterior two thirds of the spinal cord. The patients lose their ability to discern deep pressure and vibration and joint position. Ambulation is possible only with visual feedback.

Pharmacologic Treatment of Spinal Cord Injury

Spinal cord injury occurs in multiple stages. Primary insult to the spinal cord from mechanical injury and injury to spinal blood flow is followed by a secondary injury cascade leading to increased cell death. Stabilization of the patient's medical status, reduction and restoration of spinal alignment, decompression of injured neural elements, and stabilization of fractures play key roles in minimizing and preventing progression of the primary injury.

Over the past several years, much attention has been given to pharmacotherapeutic agents that can minimize or prevent secondary injury (Fig. 2). These include but are not limited to antioxidants, free radical scavengers, excitatory amino-acid blockers, gangliosides, opiate antagonists, calcium channel blockers, potassium channel blockers, and neurotrophic factors. Basic research to identify pharmacologic agents that mitigate the secondary injury cascade in animal models of spinal cord injury are discussed in chapter 49. Methylprednisolone has been the only agent in randomized clinical trials to favorably affect neurologic recovery in spinal cord injury.

Methylprednisolone is a steroid that exerts its protective effects by decreasing lipid peroxidation, stabilizing cell membranes, enhancing spinal cord blood flow, and decreasing vascular permeability and edema. In the National Acute Spinal Cord Injury Study (NASCIS) II trials, patients with incomplete spinal cord injury treated with methylprednisolone within 8 hours of injury had a significantly better neurologic recovery than patients treated with placebo. However, patients treated after 8 hours from the time of injury had a worse outcome than those given placebo, most likely because of the relatively high rate of complications associated with the use of high-dose steroids. The results of the NASCIS III clinical trials showed improved neurologic recovery when treatment with methylprednisolone was extended to 48 hours if drug therapy was started within 3 to 8 hours from the time of injury.

The ganglioside GM-1 has also been shown in phase II clinical trials to improve motor recovery if given within 72 hours of injury. The most recent unpublished reports at the time of this writing indicate that GM-1 accelerates recovery from incomplete spinal cord injury. However, by 1 year no difference in functional outcome was noted between patients treated with GM-1 and control groups. The treatment consists of 100 mg/day for a total of 18 to 32 doses. The most promising effect of GM-1 was its ability to improve motor function in the lower extremities, suggesting that it may enhance neurite outgrowth. The mechanism of action is unclear and may include selective antagonization of excitatory amino acid overactivity, reduction of the metabolic rate in the central nervous system, and potentiation of the neuroprotective effects of nerve growth factor and fibroblast growth factor. In animal studies, GM-1 may negate the protective effects of methylprednisolone when they are given together.

Initial Stabilization of Cervical Spine Trauma

The unstable cervical spine in the acute setting usually is reduced and stabilized by skull tong traction in a rotorest bed. The use of the rotorest bed minimizes the incidence of pulmonary complications, decubitus ulcers, and deep venous thrombosis. Stainless steel tongs can be used to exert up to 140 lbs of traction and carbon fiber (MRI compatible) tongs can apply up to 65 lbs of skeletal traction safely. The pullout strength of Gardner-Wells tongs decreases with increased use. Thus skull tongs must be inspected for wear before each use (or after each use) and replaced if the internal springs are worn.

Cervical Spinal Orthosis

The two most commonly used methods of external immobilization are the cervical collar and the halo vest. Not all collars are similar in their ability to immobilize cervical fractures. Each of these forms of external immobilization is associated with its own set of complications. Cervical collars can cause pressure ulcers and increases in intracranial pressure. Polytrauma patients and comatose patients are especially at risk. Some collars also have been shown to exert pressures below closing capillary pressures and thus may decrease the risk of developing decubitus ulcers.

The halo vest provides the most secure form of external immobilization of the cervical spine. Most halo vests are MRI compatible when the study is done at 1.5 T or less. The skull pins should be tightened to 8 in-lbs in adults and 4 in-lbs in children. In the presence of osteoporosis or dysplastic bone, more pins should be used. In children, using six to eight pins will compensate for the lower torque applied to each individual pin. Increasing the tightness and improving the fit of the vest decreases the amount of motion in cadaveric specimens.

Timing of Surgery

Dislocations of the cervical spine and fractures with progressive neurologic deficit should be reduced and stabilized as soon as possible. For other injuries of the cervical spine, the optimal timing of surgical intervention is controversial. Several authors have noted either no benefit or an increased risk of neurologic deficit with early surgical intervention. However, surgical decompression and stabilization within the first 5 days allows rapid mobilization of the patient, which decreases the hospital stay, the morbidity, and the overall cost of treatment. This is especially true in the polytraumatized patient. In a retrospective review of 138 patients with cervical spine trauma in the context of polytrauma, fewer postoperative medical complications were found in patients treated within the first 72 hours. The overall recommendation is that surgery be performed as soon as the patient's medical status permits.

Specific Injuries of the Adult Spine

Atlanto-Occipital Injuries

Atlanto-occipital joint injuries are estimated to occur in between 5% and 8% of trauma victims and account for 19% to 35% of all deaths from cervical spine trauma. More than 80% of patients with occiput-C1 dislocations were reported after 1975. Improvements in on-site resuscitation and emergency transportation have increased the number of patients who survive this catastrophic injury, which typically is the result of a motor-vehicle accident. In a review of 146 traffic fatalities, there was a 5% incidence of atlanto-occipital dislocations. Children younger than 12 years of age are uniquely predisposed to this injury because they have flatter atlanto-occipital angles and a significantly greater head to body ratio than adults.

Significant retropharyngeal soft-tissue swelling at C3 will be seen on radiographs. Multiple anatomic lines mark the normal relationship of occiput to C1. A line drawn from the clivus should be tangential to the dens. Another line drawn from the opsithion to the inner aspect of the C1 lamina should be smooth in contour. The Power's ratio, the ratio of the distance from the basion to the posterior arch of the atlas divided by the distance from the opsithion to the anterior arch of the atlas, should be 1.0 or less in the absence of anterior atlanto-occipital dislocation (Fig. 3).

Because this injury is very unstable, flexion-extension views are not recommended. However, if these views are available, less than 1 mm of translation should be seen at the atlanto-occipital articulation. In children, greater than 5 mm widening of the atlanto-occipital joints should raise the suspicion of this injury.

The most commonly used classification system for occiput-C1 dislocations categorizes these injuries into three types. In type I injuries, there is anterior displacement of the occiput on the atlas. Type II injuries are the

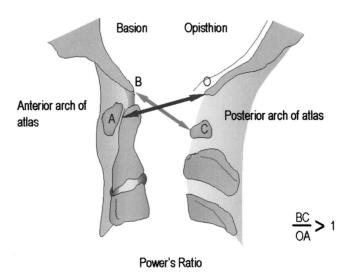

Figure 3 Calculation of the Powers ratio for anterior occipitocervical instability. A ratio greater than 1 indicates anterior occipitocervical translation.

result of longitudinal distraction. Any traction applied to a type II injury can result in progression of the existing neurologic deficit. Type III injuries involve a posterior subluxation or dislocation. Traction applied to type I and type III injuries will help reduce the dislocation and may improve the neurologic deficit.

The mortality from head on neck dislocation is extremely high, and the few survivors are likely to have deficits of the cranial nerves, brain stem, spinomedullary junction, and the upper cervical spinal cord. Vertebral artery injury may accompany the dislocation. The proposed mechanism is from an extension-rotation force. Patients with vertebral insufficiency at this level may exhibit Wallenberg's syndrome, which consists of ipsilateral defects of cranial nerves V, IX, X, and XI; ipsilateral Horner's syndrome; contralateral loss of pain and temperature sensation; cerebellar ataxia; and cruciate paralysis from injury at the level of the decussation.

All occipitocervical dislocations should be treated initially by immediate application of a halo vest. Because these injuries are unstable, stabilization of the articulation with occipitocervical fusion is the procedure of choice. This procedure can be done using a variety of techniques, including posterior wiring and structural grafting, Ransford loop fixation with wiring, and plate and screw fixation with structural grafting. The first technique will require the use of postoperative halo immobilization, whereas the latter two techniques will require only collar immobilization as external support.

Fractures of the Atlas

Atlas fractures comprise 2% to 13% of all cervical spine fractures, are seen in younger age groups (mean age 30 years), and are most commonly the result of motor vehicle accidents. These fractures are caused by axial loading and, therefore, commonly accompany head injuries in the polytrauma patient. In addition, there is an extremely high association with fractures of the C1-C2 complex and noncontiguous cervical spine fractures, including dens fractures, hangman's fractures, teardrop fractures of C2, cervical burst fractures, and lateral mass fractures.

Radiographs can differentiate between isolated posterior arch fractures, lateral mass fractures, and true Jefferson's fractures. A combined lateral mass displacement on the open mouth AP view exceeding 6.9 mm is indicative of transverse ligament insufficiency. Fine-cut CT scans in the plane of the axis will clearly delineate the fracture pattern (Fig. 4).

Treatment of fractures with a combined diastasis of less than 6.9 mm consists of immobilization in a halo vest for 3 months. After the halo vest is removed, flexion-extension radiographs are taken to test for C1-C2 instability that, if significant, can be treated by C1-C2 fusion. Treatment of fractures with greater than 6.9 mm of diastasis is controversial. Some advocate initial reduction of the fracture with skeletal traction for up to 6 to 8 weeks followed by another 6 weeks of halo vest treatment. Others have found that immediate treatment with a halo vest can result in an acceptable outcome and avoids the morbidity associated with prolonged bed rest. Both forms of treatment are acceptable, and the modality chosen will depend on the circumstances of the individual patient.

Surgical treatment is indicated if more than 5 mm of C1-C2 instability exists on flexion-extension radio-graphs once the halo vest is removed. If the posterior arch of C1 is intact, a posterior C1-C2 fusion is indicated. In the case of nonunion of the posterior arch of C1 or significant injury to the occipital condyles, occiput to C2 fusion can be performed. Isolated posterior arch fractures are caused by hyperextension of the neck. These fractures are stable injuries that can be treated in a soft collar.

Atlantoaxial Subluxation and Dislocation

Nonsurgical care of atlantoaxial rotatory subluxation, also known as Grisel's syndrome, is discussed in chapter 19. For patients who seek treatment 1 month after the subluxation occurred, an initial trial of traction can be instituted and continued for up to 3 weeks. If traction fails to reduce the deformity, open reduction and C1-C2 fusion can be performed. Many ways to achieve fusion of the C1-C2 complex have been described, including Gallie fusion, the Brooks and Jenkins technique, or C1-C2 transarticular screws supplemented with a Brooks fusion. The use of transarticular screws provides sufficient fixation to obviate the need for postoperative halo vest immobilization.

Fractures of the Odontoid

Fractures of the dens are frequently missed because of the paucity of clinical symptoms other than neck pain. In addition, if the patient suffers from head trauma or is intoxicated or obtunded, the injury can easily be missed. Both flexion and extension mechanisms can cause fractures of the dens. Hyperflexion results in anterior displacement of the dens fracture and hyperextension results in posterior displacement.

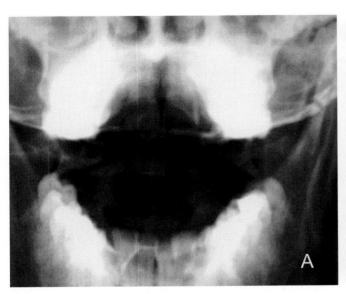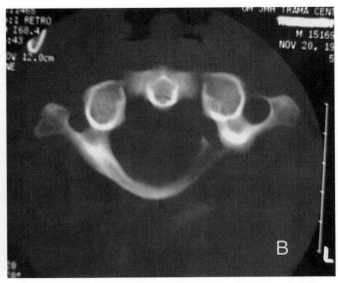

Figure 4 A, Open-mouth AP view showing widening of the lateral masses of C1 greater than 6.9 mm, denoting transverse ligament injury. **B,** CT scan though the ring of the atlas showing classic fracture pattern.

The fracture easily can be seen on open mouth and lateral radiographs of the cervical spine. Classification of these fractures is based on their location in the odontoid. The most commonly used classification scheme was

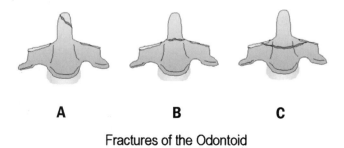

A   **B**   **C**

Fractures of the Odontoid

Figure 5 Anderson-d'Alonzo classification of odontoid fractures. **A,** Type I fractures involve the tip of the dens. **B,** Type II fractures occur at the base of the dens at the junction of the dens and the central body of the axis. **C,** Type III fractures extend into the body of the dens.

described by Anderson and d'Alonzo (Fig. 5). Type I fractures consist of injuries to the tip of the dens, type II fractures occur through the base of the dens at the junction of the dens and the central body of the axis (Fig. 6, *A* and *B*), and type III fractures extend into the body of the axis (Fig. 6, *C* and *D*).

Type I injuries can be treated nonsurgically as discussed in chapter 19. Type II odontoid fractures are more unpredictable than the other two types. The overall nonunion rate of odontoid fractures is reported to be about 32%. An increased nonunion rate was associated with fractures with greater than 5 mm of displacement, angulation greater than 10°, age over 40 years, and posterior displacement. The nonunion rate for type II fractures displaced more than 6 mm was 78%, compared to 10% when the displacement was less than 6 mm. Halo vest immobilization is the treatment of choice

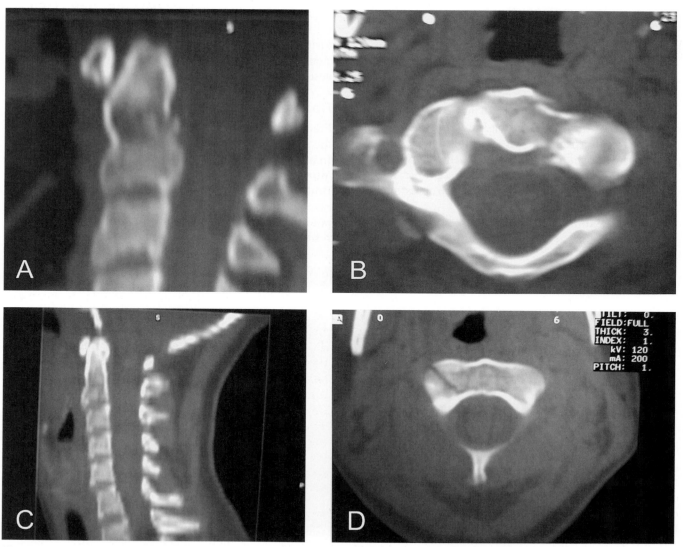

Figure 6 A, Sagittal reconstruction CT showing a type II odontoid fracture. **B,** Axial cut through the body C2 showing type II dens fracture. **C,** Sagittal reconstruction CT showing a type III odontoid fracture. **D,** Axial cut through the body of C2 showing typical extension into the body of C2.

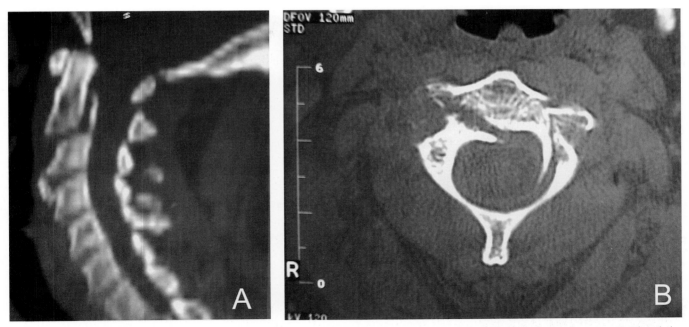

Figure 7 A, Sagittal reconstruction CT of type II variant described by Starr and Eismont. **B,** Axial cut through the body of C2 showing fracture line propagating through the posterior aspect of the vertebral body.

for undisplaced type II fractures. If the patient has two or more risk factors for nonunion, C1-C2 fusion or direct osteosynthesis with an odontoid screw is the best treatment. If primary C1-C2 fusion is selected, the patient will lose 50% of neck rotation. Primary osteosynthesis of the dens has the theoretical advantage of preserving rotation at the atlantoaxial joint; however the amount of motion preserved may not be significantly more than with C1-C2 fusion. To use osteosynthesis, the fracture needs to be transverse, noncomminuted, and reducible. The patient's chest anatomy and odontoid anatomy also must be amenable to this technique. Use of odontoid screws in the elderly is associated with a high complication rate. Treatment for type III odontoid fractures depends on the specific needs of the patient. Most authors report a 13% nonunion rate and a 15% malunion rate for type III fractures treated in a halo vest. In contrast, 96% of these fractures will heal after C1-C2 fusion.

Traumatic Spondylolisthesis of the Axis

Traumatic spondylolisthesis of the axis (hangman's fracture) can be caused by a variety of mechanisms including extension, flexion, or distraction of the cervical spine. The fracture line passes through the neural arch of the axis. These fractures are best classified using a modification of the Effendi classification. Isolated type I fractures can be treated in a rigid cervical collar for 3 months. Type II fractures demonstrate greater than 3 mm of displacement, greater than 11° of angulation, and

classically are associated with a wedge compression fracture of the inferior body of C2. Two variants of type II fractures have been described. The type IIA fracture shows significant angulation but no translation and includes significant disruption of the disc and posterior longitudinal ligament. Gross disc space distraction occurs after the application of minimal amounts of traction. In one type II variant, the fracture line propagates through the posterior aspect of the vertebral body with unilateral or bilateral continuity of the posterior cortex (Fig. 7) and is associated with a 33% incidence of neurologic deficit.

All type II fractures with the exception of type IIA are treated nonsurgically with a halo vest. Nonunions that are associated with greater than 11° of residual angulation on follow-up require posterior fusion. Type III hangman's fractures are unstable injuries, with severe displacement and angulation, associated with unilateral or bilateral facet dislocation of C2 on C3. Disruption of the anterior longitudinal ligament, the posterior longitudinal ligament, and the C2-3 intervertebral disc occur in these injuries. All type III fractures should be treated with surgical reduction and posterior C2-C3 fusion. Internal fixation can be achieved with interspinous wiring or posterior plating using pedicle screws at C2 and lateral mass screws at C3.

Injuries to the Subaxial Spine

Fractures of the subaxial spine can be grouped mechanistically using the Allen-Ferguson classification system

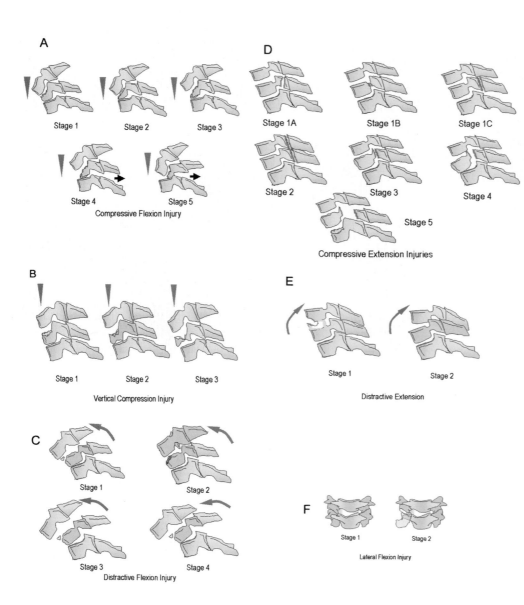

Figure 8 Allen-Ferguson classification of subaxial cervical fractures: **A,** Compressive flexion injury: Stage 1, blunting and rounding off of anterior-superior vertebral margin. Stage 2, loss of anterior height of the vertebral body and beak-like appearance anteroinferiorly. Stage 3, fracture line from the anterior surface of the vertebral body extending obliquely through the subchondral plate with fracture of the beak. Stage 4 less than 3 mm of displacement of the posteroinferior vertebral margin into the spinal canal. Stage 5, greater than 3 mm of displacement of the posterior part of the body. **B,** Vertical compression injury: Stage 1, fracture of either the superior or inferior end plate causing a central cupping of the end plate. Stage 2, fracture of both end plates. Stage 3, fragmentation and displacement of the vertebral body. **C,** Distractive flexion injury: Stage 1, facet subluxation in flexion and widening of the interspinous distance. Stage 2, unilateral facet dislocation. Stage 3, bilateral facet dislocation with less than 50% anterior vertebral body translation. Stage 4, bilateral facet dislocation with 100% anterior translation of the vertebral body. **D,** Compressive extension injury: Stage 1, unilateral vertebral arch fracture; 1A, articular process; 1B, pedicle fracture; 1C, lamina fracture. Stage 2, bilaminar fractures. Stage 3, bilateral fractures of the vertebral arches and partial anterior vertebral body displacement. Stage 4, further anterior vertebral body displacement. Stage 5, 100% translation of the anterior vertebral body. **E,** Distractive extension injury: Stage 1, failure of the anterior ligamentous complex with possible widening of the disc space and teardrop fracture. Stage 2, posterior displacement of the upper vertebral body. **F,** Lateral flexion injury: Stage 1, asymmetric compression fracture of the vertebral body with associated ipsilateral vertebral arch fracture. Stage 2, displacement of ipsilateral arch fracture.

(Fig. 8). The six major classes are based on mechanism and range from compressive flexion injuires to lateral flexion injuries. Each of these classes, in turn, is subdivided into multiple stages.

Anterior Wedge Compression Fractures

These fractures are caused by axial loading in flexion, most commonly at the C4-C5 and C5-C6 levels. Although there is minimal risk of neurologic injury, severe fractures can result in posttraumatic kyphotic deformity. Most of these injuries can be treated nonsurgically, but fusion to prevent kyphosis may be considered if angulation exceeds 11° or if there is greater than 25% loss of vertebral body height.

Cervical Burst Fractures

Cervical burst fractures are caused by a severe axial compressive load. The most common levels affected extend from C4 to C7. These types of fractures are associated with complete and incomplete spinal cord injuries from extrusion of fracture fragments into the spinal canal (Fig. 9).

Treatment of cervical burst fractures is dictated by the neurologic status. Patients with a neurologic deficit are best treated by anterior cervical corpectomy and fusion with a structural graft and internal fixation with an anterior cervical plate (Fig. 9, *D*). Although the design of anterior cervical plates has improved to the extent that they may, in many cases, be used alone in

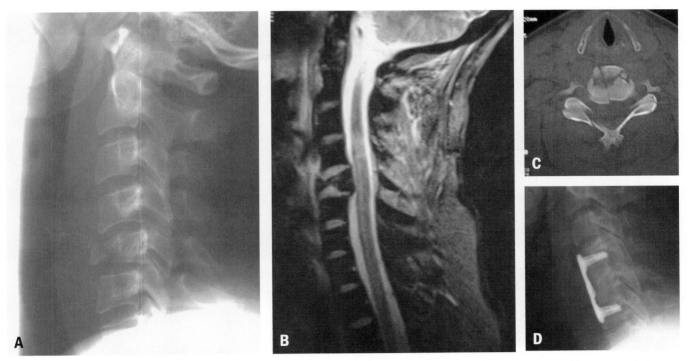

Figure 9 C5 burst fracture. **A,** lateral radiograph. **B,** T2-weighted MRI. **C,** CT image through fractured vertebra. **D,** Cervical burst fracture treated by anterior cervical corpectomy and fusion with autogenous tricortical iliac crest graft and anterior plating.

the presence of posterior injury, severe posterior element disruption may make combined anterior-posterior fusion and instrumentation necessary.

Facet Injuries

Facet injuries are among the most common injury patterns seen in cervical spine trauma. These injuries may be unilateral or bilateral and may range from pure fractures to pure dislocations.

Facet Fractures

Unilateral facet fractures can involve either the superior or the inferior facet and are caused by rotational forces with the neck in slight flexion. Superior facet fractures are the most common type of facet injury (Fig. 10), comprising about 80% of all facet fractures. Disruption of the facet capsule is accompanied by slight to moderate disruption of the interspinous ligament and partial disruption of the intervertebral disc. On lateral radiographs, the vertebral body may be slightly angulated (5° to 7°) and translated (4 to 4.5 mm). Inferior facet fractures usually begin at the base of the lamina and may have an associated lamina fracture.

Treatment of unilateral facet injuries depends on the degree of instability caused by the fracture. Nondisplaced fractures that involve only a small portion of the facet joint can be treated with a cervical orthosis. Frac-

tures with significant rotational translation are best treated with reduction and fusion over the affected level. Both anterior and posterior approaches have been described. The anterior approach has the advantage of minimizing the number of fusion levels to maintain stability. The internal fixation must be able to neutralize the rotational component of the injury.

Fracture separations of the lateral mass are extension-rotation injuries, in which fracture of the pedicle propagates through the lamina and stays parallel to the ipsilateral articular process. These predominantly unilateral fractures create two levels of instability. Patients may suffer from radiculopathy (48% incidence) and/or spinal cord injury (16% incidence). Lateral radiographs will classically show horizontalization of the lateral mass on the injured side. These injuries are very unstable and require reduction and fusion over the levels of instability. Again, both anterior and posterior approaches have been described.

Bilateral facet fractures are caused by both translational and shear forces. These fractures can be associated with significant discal disruption. The degree of translation is directly related to the severity of the injury. Bilateral facet fractures with significant translation (greater than 3.5 mm) are best treated with closed or open reduction followed by either anterior or posterior fusion with instrumentation.

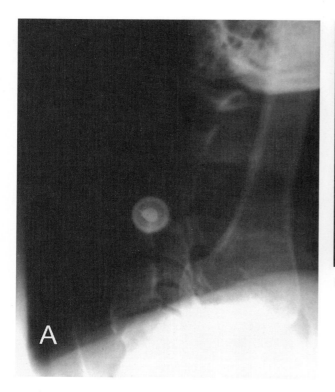

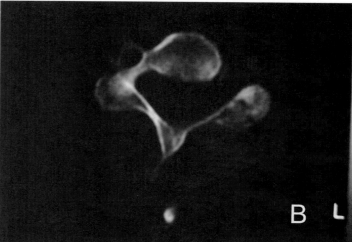

Figure 10 Unilateral facet fracture of the C5 vertebra.

Facet Subluxations and Dislocations

Unilateral and bilateral facet subluxations are flexion-distraction injuries that disrupt the posterior ligaments and facet capsules while leaving the intervertebral disc uninjured. A small amount of kyphosis (less than 10°) may be seen on lateral radiographs. These subluxations must be differentiated from more severe flexion-distraction injuries that have spontaneously reduced with neck extension.

Bilateral perched facets are more severe flexion-distraction injuries. The inferior facets slide superiorly and anteriorly over the superior facet until the tips engage on each other. Perching of the facets creates a significant kyphotic deformity of the cervical spine. Disruption of the ligamentum flavum and the posterior anulus of the disc occurs in this injury. Treatment consists of reduction and stabilization with posterior fusion and instrumentation.

Unilateral facet dislocations are caused by adding a rotational force to the flexion-distraction mechanism, resulting in attenuation of the interspinous ligament and disruption of the facet capsule and the posterolateral corner of the disc. The overall result of the injury mechanism is a rotational deformity of the spine. A 24% incidence of spinal cord symptoms and a 68% incidence of radicular symptoms were found in one series of patients with unilateral facet dislocations.

Bilateral facet dislocations are the terminal stage of the flexion-distraction injury. On lateral radiographs, there can be up to 50% anterior translation of the supe-rior vertebra. Up to 60% of bilateral facet dislocations will have associated disc disruption, and disc herniation can be present before reduction of facet dislocations in up to 55%. If the disc fragment is associated with the superior translated vertebra, reduction of the dislocation is very likely to push the herniated disc material into the spinal canal.

Controversy exists over the practicality of imaging the intervertebral disc at the level of the injury before reduction in an alert, awake, and neurologically intact patient. Despite the alarming frequency of disc herniation associated with these injuries, a large proportion of those herniations will be clinically insignificant, and most neurologic deficits have occurred during surgical reduction under general anesthesia. Thus, several studies have indicated that immediate traction and reduction of facet dislocations in alert and awake patients can be done safely without the need for preliminary MRI. These studies also indicated that immediate reduction leads to improved neurologic recovery when compared to delayed reduction. Patients in these studies were treated at either a level I trauma center or a spinal cord injury unit with staff who have developed expertise in the closed treatment of facet dislocations. Moreover, the ability to perform a detailed neurologic examination between each incremental increase in cervical traction is a critical step in the technique. Any deterioration in neurologic function can immediately be addressed.

Patients with severe spinal cord injury (Frankel

grades A and B) should undergo immediate closed reduction of the dislocation. Patients who have worsening neurologic status, those who have a spinal cord injury not explained by CT scan, and patients with dislocations that are not reducible with less than 40 to 60 lb of traction should be evaluated by MRI.

Gunshot Wounds to the Cervical Spine

As many as 500,000 gunshot wounds occur annually. Between 1973 and 1981, 13% of reported spinal cord injuries were caused by firearms, making gunshot wounds the third leading cause of spinal cord injury after motor vehicle accidents, which account for 38%, and falls, which account for 16%. Spinal cord injury from a gunshot can be caused by direct injury to the spinal cord, by concussive injury from the impact of the bullet on the vertebral column, and by chemical injury from metal toxicity (especially lead and copper bullets). The routine removal of retained bullets from the spinal canal remains controversial. In a 1991 study, removal of bullets had no significant effect on the recovery of sensation or the perception of pain. No study demonstrates that removal of bullets in the cervical spine improves motor recovery.

Sports Injuries

The incidence of cervical spine injuries in football players has been estimated to range from 10% to 15%. Linemen, defensive ends, and linebackers who perform a lot of tackling are at greater risk for these injuries. With improvements in protective equipment and tackling techniques, the overall incidence of severe cervical spine injuries as a result of contact sports has decreased. However, when cervical injuries do occur, the most likely mechanism is from flexion and axial loading of the neck. Until the injured player is brought to the emergency room, all pads and the helmet should be left on because significant alterations in cervical alignment can occur during removal of the protective equipment.

Recently, much attention has been paid to the optimal management of players who suffer transient quadriplegia during a football game. The syndrome, which is discussed in chapter 12, has an incidence of 7.3 per 10,000 athletes who play intercollegiate football.

Cervical disc herniations in athletes who are involved in tackling sports can have disastrous sequelae if ignored. Players with disc bulges without frank herniation can return to sports when radicular symptoms have resolved and after the player has achieved full and painless motion of the neck. If nonsurgical measures have failed, symptomatic cervical disc herniation can be managed effectively with anterior discectomy and fusion. The player can return to sports after a one- to two-level anterior discectomy and fusion when preoperative symptoms have fully resolved, motor strength is normal, cervical range of motion is painless, and the fusion is solid.

Unstable fractures and dislocations can be managed by either anterior, posterior, or combined approaches, depending on the nature of the injury and the direction of instability. There is no difference in surgical management between athletes who suffer these injuries and the general population. However, players who have suffered these unstable injuries should be restricted from further participation in their sport. Any fracture or unstable ligamentous injury in the upper cervical spine, especially if it requires surgery, is an absolute contraindication to continued sports participation.

Annotated Bibliography

Bracken MB, Shepard MJ, Holford TR, et al: Administration of methylprednisolone for 24 or 48 hours or tirilazad mesylate for 48 hours in the treatment of acute spinal cord injury: Results of the third national acute spinal cord injury randomized controlled trial: National acute spinal cord injury study. *JAMA* 1997;277: 1597-1604.

This multicenter study showed better improvement in neurologic recovery when methylprednisolone was continued for 48 hours if treatment was started between 3 and 8 hours of injury. Patients who received the longer steroid treatment regimen had more medical complications. When methylprednisolone was started within 3 hours of injury, there was no benefit in neurologic outcome between the 24-hour and 48-hour regimens.

Eleraky MA, Theodore N, Adams M, Rekate HL, Sonntag VK: Pediatric cervical spine injuries: Report of 102 cases and review of the literature. *J Neurosurg* 2000; 92(suppl 1):12-17.

This is a retrospective review of 102 cases of pediatric cervical spinal injury. The authors found that neurologic injury and upper cervical trauma were more frequent in children younger than age 9 years. Motor vehicle accidents were the most common mechanism of these injuries.

International Standards for Neurological and Functional Classification of Spinal Cord Injury. Chicago, IL, American Spinal Injury Association, 1996.

The handbook distributed by the ASIA describes the ASIA classification system of neurologic injury and the ASIA Functional Independence Measure.

Schlegel J, Bayley J, Yuan H, Fredricksen B: Timing of surgical decompression and fixation of acute spinal fractures. *J Orthop Trauma* 1996;10:323-330.

In this retrospective evaluation of 138 patients requiring surgical decompression, reduction, and fixation of spinal injuries between January 1986 and April 1989, the variables of timing and method of surgical intervention, level and classification of fracture, associated injuries, injury severity score, associated neurologic deficits, length of intensive care unit and hospital stays, and projected costs were analyzed for correlation with postoperative complications (pulmonary, skin, urinary, other).

Tan E, Schweitzer ME, Vaccaro L, Spetell AC: Is computed tomography of nonvisualized C7-T1 cost-effective? *J Spinal Disord* 1999;12:472-476.

Routine cervical spine radiography was performed in 360 trauma patients in whom the C7-T1 level was not adequately visualized, but there was no evidence of lower cervical spine injury. In these patients, 11 fractures of the C7-T1 level were identified by CT scanning. Based on Medicare reimbursement data the cost-effectiveness of CT for averting potential sequelae was $9,192 for each fracture identified, $16,852 for each potentially or definitely unstable fracture identified, and $50,557 for each definitely unstable fracture identified.

Torg JS, Naranja RJ Jr, Palov H, Galinat BJ, Warren R, Stine RA: The relationship of developmental narrowing of the cervical spinal canal to reversible and irreversible injury of the cervical spinal cord in football players. *J Bone Joint Surg Am* 1996;78:1308-1314.

An evaluation of 45 athletes who had had an episode of transient neurapraxia of the cervical spinal cord revealed a consistent finding of developmental narrowing of the cervical spinal canal. A Torg ratio of 0.80 or less had a high sensitivity (93%) for transient neurapraxia. The low positive predictive value of the ratio (0.2%) precludes its use as a screening mechanism for determining the suitability of an athlete for participation in contact sports.

Vaccaro AR, Daugherty RJ, Sheehan TP, et al: Neurologic outcome of early versus late surgery for cervical spinal cord injury. *Spine* 1997;22:2609-2613.

Comparison of patients who had surgery for spinal cord trauma within 72 hours of their spinal injury and patients who had surgery later than 5 days after injury showed no significant difference in length of acute postoperative intensive care stay, length of inpatient rehabilitation, or improvement in ASIA grade or motor score. Cervical spinal cord decompression after trauma less than 72 hours after injury (mean, 1.8 days) had no significant neurologic benefit compared with waiting longer than 5 days (mean, 16.8 days).

Vaccaro AR, Falatyn SP, Flanders AE, Balderston RA, Northrup BE, Cotler JM: Magnetic resonance evaluation of the intervertebral disc, spinal ligaments, and

spinal cord before and after closed traction reduction of cervical spine dislocations. *Spine* 1999;24:1210-1217.

In this prospective clinical study, awake closed traction reduction was successful in 9 of 11 patients. Two of the nine patients had disc herniations before reduction, and five had disc herniations after reduction. Despite the high incidence of disc herniations after awake reduction of cervical dislocations, no patient had neurologic worsening afterward.

Vaccaro AR, Klein GR, Flanders AE, Albert TJ, Balderston RA, Cotler JM: Long-term evaluation of vertebral artery injuries following cervical spine trauma using magnetic resonance angiography. *Spine* 1998;23:789-795.

MRA was performed at the time of injury and at a follow-up office visit in 61 consecutive patients with cervical spine injuries. Twelve of 61 patients were found to have a lack of signal flow within one of their vertebral vessels during the study period. Flow was not reconstituted in the vertebral arteries of five of six patients (83%) after an average 25.8-month follow-up period. The authors conclude that this lack of flow should be considered if future surgery is needed in this region of the cervical spine.

Classic Bibliography
Allen BL Jr, Ferguson RL, Lehmann TR, O'Brien RP: A mechanistic classification of closed, indirect fractures and dislocations of the lower cervical spine. *Spine* 1982;7:1-27.

Bohler J: Anterior stabilization for acute fractures and non-unions of the dens. *J Bone Joint Surg Am* 1982;64:18-27.

Bohler J, Gaudernak T: Anterior plate stabilization for fracture-dislocations of the lower cervical spine. *J Trauma* 1980;20:203-205.

Bohlman HH: Acute fractures and dislocations of the cervical spine: An analysis of three hundred hospitalized patients and review of the literature. *J Bone Joint Surg Am* 1979;61:1119-1142.

Clark CR, White AA III: Fractures of the dens: A multicenter study. *J Bone Joint Surg Am* 1985;67:1340-1348.

Levine AM, Edwards CC: The management of traumatic spondylolisthesis of the axis. *J Bone Joint Surg Am* 1985;67:217-226.

Panjabi M, White A III: Biomechanics of nonacute cervical spinal cord trauma. *Spine* 1988;13:838-842.

Stauffer ES, Kelly EG: Fracture-dislocations of the cervical spine: Instability and recurrent deformity following treatment by anterior interbody fusion. *J Bone Joint Surg Am* 1977;59:45-48.

Torg JS, Pavlov H, Genuraio SE, et al: Neurapraxia of the cervical spinal cord with transient quadriplegia. *J Bone Joint Surg Am* 1986;68:1354-1370.

Chapter 29

Thoracolumbar Fractures and Dislocations

Alexander R. Vaccaro, MD

Sidney M. Jacoby, BA

Introduction

Each year approximately 150,000 to 160,000 North Americans sustain a vertebral column fracture. As a result of the transition from the relatively stable thoracic spine to the flexible lumbar spine, the thoracolumbar junction is the most frequently injured portion of the spinal column. It has been estimated that nearly 15,000 major thoracolumbar injuries occur annually in the United States alone. Of those in the United States sustaining such a fracture, 4,700 to 5,000 incur significant neurologic deficits, including paraplegia.

Traumatic injuries of the thoracolumbar spine have many causes and varied clinical manifestations. For many thoracolumbar fractures, more than one treatment method has been shown to be efficacious. The choice of treatment should be tailored specifically to the individual circumstance of a particular patient thereby minimizing treatment morbidity. A variety of factors, including the patient's spinal anatomy, pathomechanics of injury, neurologic status, body habitus, and medical condition should carefully be analyzed.

For a stable thoracolumbar spinal fracture, nonsurgical care with early ambulation continues to be the management of choice. Indications for surgical intervention depend on the presence and degree of neurologic deficit and the severity of bony and ligamentous disruption. The ultimate goal is to provide the patient with a stable, painless spine, while protecting or improving neurologic function so as to improve overall functionality.

Advances in anesthesia, radiology, and surgical techniques have led to increased use of surgical treatment for selected spinal fractures. Surgical stabilization of unstable thoracolumbar injuries with or without a neurologic deficit reduces hospital stay, improves spinal alignment, shortens rehabilitation, and results in fewer medical complications compared with bed rest and nonsurgical immobilization.

Anatomic Characteristics of the Thoracolumbar Spine

Regional osteoligamentous characteristics along with the mechanism of force application contribute to the pattern of spinal injury. The thoracic spinal cord is shielded from injury by the paraspinal musculature and by the rigid thoracic rib cage. From T2 to T10, the sternum and the rib cage significantly restrict motion increasing overall stiffness. Stability of the thoracic spine is also augmented by the coronal alignment of the facet joints, which resists flexion and extension and offers minimal resistance to torsional loads. Facet orientation gradually changes to a sagittal orientation in the lumbar region, where it permits significant flexion and extension but limits rotation. The physiologic kyphosis of the thoracic spine is related to anterior wedging of the vertebral bodies, predisposing the thoracic spine to compression-flexion type injuries or progressive kyphotic deformity, particularly after surgical laminectomies or traumatic posterior element disruption.

Although the increased stability of the supporting structures in the thoracic spine provides relative protection for the spinal cord, the small diameter of the spinal canal, as compared with that in the lumbar spine, allows for minimal tolerance for canal deformities or intrusion. This difference may explain the increased incidence of catastrophic neurologic injuries associated with thoracic spine fractures.

The T11 to L1 segments represent the thoracolumbar junction and are also referred to as the transition zone. This zone is bordered superiorly by a relatively kyphotic, immobile, and stable thoracic vertebral column and inferiorly by the lumbar spine, characterized by its lordotic posture and mobile spinal units. Sixty percent of all thoracolumbar spine injuries occur at the thoracolumbar junction. It is predisposed to injury by rotational and shearing forces because the ribs are not present for stability and the facet joints have not reoriented completely from a coronal to a sagittal plane. Additionally, the thoracic vertebral bodies are not as large as the lumbar vertebral bodies and are less able to resist deformity. These factors render the thoracolumbar spine more vulnerable to injury as evidenced by its susceptibility to burst type injuries at this level.

Initial Management

Treatment of the patient with a spinal injury begins at the scene of the accident. Ultimately, the patient's outcome depends on early recognition of the injury, prompt medical resuscitation, attainment of spinal stability, prevention of additional injuries, and avoidance of complications. The initial management of a spinal trauma patient consists of (1) evaluation, (2) resuscitation, (3) immobilization, (4) extrication, and (5) transport.

With advances in the initial evaluation and management of patients with thoracolumbar trauma, the percentage of patients with partial, rather than complete, lesions is increasing. Despite these advances, however, a small percentage of all patients who have sustained a spinal cord injury deteriorate neurologically at some point during treatment. Treatment should therefore focus on restoring spinal alignment and stability while maintaining or improving neurologic function.

Patient Evaluation

Evaluation of the patient includes a primary and a secondary survey. Following the initial ABCs of trauma care (airway, breathing, circulation), a primary survey is undertaken for evidence of gross spinal deformity, tenderness, and muscle spasm. The secondary survey involves inspecting and palpating the back to look for contusions, abrasions, or lacerations that may require specific treatment.

Resuscitation and Oxygenation

Resuscitation ensures adequate oxygenation of the patient in light of a possible injury to the spinal cord. Once an airway is established, ventilation with oxygenation is begun. Maintenance of adequate circulation is also imperative to maximize perfusion of the contused spinal cord. In contrast to patients with injuries to the cervical spinal cord, patients who have neurologic deficits from an injury at the thoracolumbar level generally do not exhibit acute hemodynamic or respiratory difficulties in the absence of other injuries.

Immobilization and Extrication

Proper immobilization is essential to prevent additional spinal column and/or spinal cord injury. At the accident scene, initial in-line manual traction is recommended before moving the spine injured patient, and a hard cervical collar should be applied. After the cervical collar is in place, the patient is moved to a firm spine board for transportation. If a helmet is involved, as in football and hockey injuries, it should not be removed until arrival at the hospital. If necessary, the face mask or cage can be removed at the accident scene to perform emergency care.

Transport and Initial Treatment

The length of hospital stay and the incidence of peri-trauma-associated complications, such as pressure ulcers and mortality, are significantly reduced if the patient is admitted to a spinal-cord injury center. General guidelines for means of transportation are (1) an ambulance for distances less than 50 miles, (2) a helicopter for distances of 51 to 150 miles or heavy traffic patterns and severe injuries, and (3) a fixed-wing aircraft for distances over 150 miles.

Emergency Room Management

Following medical stabilization, a complete radiographic evaluation of the spine should be undertaken (AP and lateral). Advanced imaging modalities are then selected, depending on the nature of the thoracolumbar injury. CT is routinely performed when thoracolumbar fractures are detected because it allows more complete examination of the middle spinal column and the status of the posterior elements, especially the facet joints (Fig. 1). It is desirable to scan at least one full normal segment above and below the level of the fracture. If surgical intervention is anticipated, it is prudent to scan the entire area to be instrumented. MRI evaluates the integrity of the posterior ligamentous complex and the

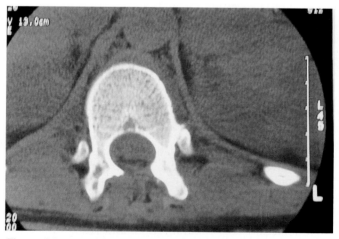

Figure 1 A transaxial CT scan revealing an empty facet sign following a bilateral facet dislocation in the thoracic spine.

presence of intracanal pathology, such as intervertebral disc displacement, spinal cord edema, or hemorrhage.

Throughout the in-hospital treatment phase, prophylaxis of deep venous thrombosis is provided by intermittent external pneumatic compression devices, static compression stockings, and, in selected cases, subcutaneous heparin (5,000 U subcutaneous every 12 h) or intravenous low-molecular-weight heparin. A proven clinical pathway in the management of spinal cord injury patients is the participation of a multidisciplinary group of medical caregivers including the spinal surgeon, rehabilitation physician, internist, and psychosocial counselors.

In an effort to standardize communication and reporting of specific neurologic injuries, the American Spinal Injury Association has developed a spinal cord injury assessment form to document both motor and sensory status. The Frankel Impairment Scale is another commonly used method for quantifying neurologic deficits. In the absence of contraindications to steroid application, it is routine today for patients who sustain spinal cord injury to receive 30 mg/kg of intravenous methylprednisolone administered for 1 h followed by 5.4 mg/kg administered over the next 23 h if administered within 3 h of injury. When methylprednisolone is initiated 3 to 8 h after injury, patients may be maintained on steroid therapy for 48 h. However, strong data documenting improvement in spinal cord, as opposed to root function, are lacking.

Spinal Stability

The concept of spinal stability is intuitive to many physicians, although its precise definition is often ellusive. Various definitions and classification systems of spinal (in)stability exist. The integrity of both the skeletal and neural structures should be considered, because both are elements in defining spinal function, treatment, and overall functional outcome.

A precise determination of spinal instability is arbitrary, due to the lack of accurate knowledge regarding the mechanism of injury and the precise understanding of compromised bony and soft-tissue anatomy and its correlation to tissue healing. Early or acute instability may result in injury to the neural structures while late instability may result in progressive deformity and chronic pain. An accurate description of stability would logically dictate appropriate therapy. Panjabi and associates defined instability as "the loss of the ability of the spine under physiological loads to maintain its pattern of displacement so that there is no initial or additional neurologic deficit, no major deformity, and no capacitating pain." In an attempt to develop an applicable clinical algorithm for the determination of spinal stability,

they proposed a clinical checklist that evaluated the degree of bony and soft-tissue disruption as well as the neurologic status of the patient after injury.

Initial attempts to recognize the spinal elements as a functional structure gave birth to the concept of the spine consisting of two load-bearing columns, anterior and posterior. The anterior column consisted of the vertebral body, disc, and anterior and posterior longitudinal ligaments, while the posterior column consisted of the pedicles, laminae, transverse and spinous processes, and all associated ligamentous structures (facet capsules, ligamentum flava, interspinous and supraspinous ligaments).

The anterior vertebral column provides most of the axial load-bearing capacity of the spine. The posterior column resists tension and shares in some of the load (approximately 20%) supported by the anterior column. With the two-column model, the integrity of the posterior ligamentous complex (PLC) is the main determinant of stability. Therefore, thoracolumbar fractures are classified as stable or unstable depending on whether the injury complex disrupts the PLC. Using this system, stable fractures are simple compression wedge fractures, burst fractures, and extension injuries. Unstable fractures consist of shear fractures and fracture-dislocations.

This led to a three-column concept, including a third, or middle column of the spine. Spinal stability was based on the number of columns disrupted (usually two) and not simply on the integrity of the PLC. In the three-column stability concept, the anterior column contains the anterior longitudinal ligament and the anterior half of the vertebral body and anulus fibrosus. The middle column contains the posterior half of the vertebral body and anulus fibrosus and the posterior longitudinal ligament. The posterior column consists of the posterior bony arch, the interspinous and supraspinous ligaments, the capsular ligaments, and the ligamentum flavum. Instability occurs after disruption of the middle column in addition to disruption of either the anterior or posterior columns; therefore, disruption of only two columns indicates instability. In addition to the mechanical model, neurologic dysfunction, especially to the spinal cord, often designates the injury as unstable.

Mechanism of Injury

Thoracolumbar injuries are usually secondary to indirect trauma. The indirect force originates either above or below the thoracolumbar region. The mechanism of injury yields insight in determining the type of fracture sustained, the stability of the traumatized vertebrae, and ultimately the treatment plan required to obtain maximum stability. Forces such as flexion, axial compression, lateral compression, flexion combined with rotation, flexion combined with distraction, and extension may all combine to result in spinal injury.

Flexion

Flexion forces result in anterior spinal compression and posterior tension. When anterior compression is < 50% of the anterior vertebral height, the middle and posterior columns usually are intact. When anterior compression is > 50% of the anterior body height, the posterior column is subjected to significant tensile force and may fail, leading to acute or delayed instability.

Axial Compression

An axial load applied to the spine may result in a variety of injury patterns. In the region of thoracic kyphosis, axial compression will usually result in an anterior flexion load to the vertebral body. Lower, at the thoracolumbar junction, a similar load results in more uniform compression of the vertebral body. As force increases, fractures of the vertebral end plates are followed by failure of the vertebral body, resulting in anterior and middle column failure. With additional flexion, there may be significant posterior element disruption.

Lateral Compression

Lateral compression creates damage similar to that caused by anterior wedge compression. The vertebral body sustains asymmetric collapse on the side of the applied load and tensile failure on the contralateral side. This combination may lead to a chronically unstable and painful deformity that develops into a focal scoliosis.

Flexion Rotation

The combination of flexion and rotation produces an injury similar to that described in pure flexion with the addition of a rotational component. This mechanism can lead to failure of all three columns and a grossly unstable injury (Fig. 2). There may be anterior column compressive failure due to the flexion force as well as posterior disruption of the facet articulations, capsules, and ligamentous structures. As the degree of rotation increases, shear occurs through the anterior, middle, and posterior columns, leading to increased displacement of the fracture fragments.

Flexion-Distraction

Flexion-distraction forces across the thoracolumbar spine often produce the typical seat-belt injury. The axis of rotation of the applied force in this type of injury is located anterior to the vertebral body, usually at the anterior abdominal wall, leading to significant tensile force through all three columns of the spine. When the

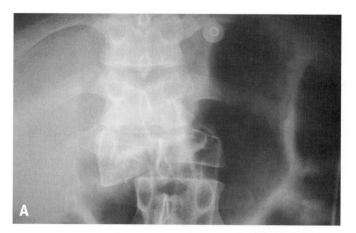

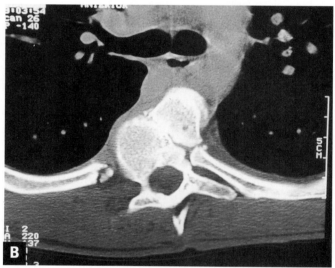

Figure 2 A, An AP plain radiograph revealing a rotatory fracture-dislocation at the L1-L2 level. **B,** A transaxial CT scan illustrates the marked rotatory displacement of the contiguous vertebral bodies at the injury level. This type of injury requires an initial posterior open reduction to accomplish adequate sagittal and coronal plane alignment, followed by consideration of an anterior decompression and/or fusion for stability.

line of force passes through bony elements alone, it is referred to as a Chance fracture. The axis of rotation may also transfer to the middle column, causing significant posterior tensile failure and anterior column compressive failure.

Extension

Posterior thrust of the head or upper trunk creates extension forces. Extension injury results in tensile failure of the anterior column involving either the anterior longitudinal ligament and disc or anterior vertebral body (Fig. 3); it frequently is manifested as an avulsion fracture of the anterior vertebral body. The posterior column is subjected to compressive forces and may sustain compression failure of the spinous process, laminae, and occasionally, the pedicles. Distraction failures

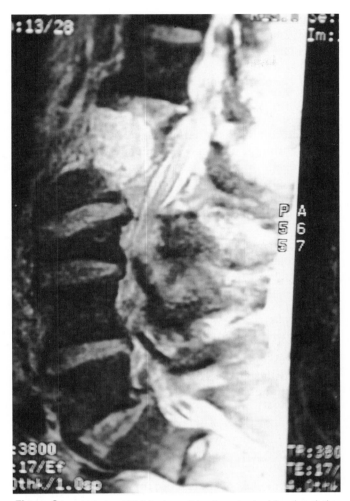

Figure 3 A sagittal plane MRI following a distraction-extension injury through the L2 vertebral body. This patient incurred a severe neurologic deficit as the result of neural element distraction.

and tensile strain through the middle and posterior columns. The posterior column may be disrupted in tension, depending on the degree of loss of anterior vertebral height (> 40% to 50%).

In burst fractures compressive failure occurs as a result of an axial load to the anterior and middle columns leading to divergent spread of the pedicles and retropulsion of bone into the neural canal. Associated radiographic findings may include a vertical lamina fracture and splaying of the posterior joints. Denis describes five types of burst fractures. Type A fractures, which involve failure of the superior and inferior end plates, are seen primarily in the low lumbar region. Type B, the most frequent, which involve failure of the superior end plate are seen primarily at the thoracolumbar junction. Type C involve failure of the inferior end plate, and type D describes a burst rotation injury usually in the mid-lumbar spine with obvious rotational misalignment as a result of an axial load associated with rotation. Type E describes a burst lateral flexion injury with asymmetric loss of vertebral height as a result of an axial load and lateral flexion.

A seat-belt injury is a flexion-distraction injury with tension failure of the middle and posterior columns and preservation or compressive failure of the anterior column depending on the location of the axis of rotation. The classic thoracolumbar flexion-distraction injury was described in 1948 as a transverse injury through the osseous structures with its fulcrum anterior to the spinal column. Severe flexion-distraction injuries that result in a disruption of the anterior hinge or anterior longitudinal ligament are referred to as fracture-dislocations. Denis also described flexion-distraction injuries as a subtype of fracture-dislocations in which there is tension failure of the anterior, middle, and posterior columns with the axis of rotation anterior to the anterior longitudinal ligament.

Fracture-dislocations involve failure of all three columns following compression, tension, rotation, or shear forces. They are associated with the highest incidence of neurologic deficit and are considered unstable. They account for approximately 20% of major thoracolumbar spine injuries and are categorized into six types by Denis. Type A is a slice fracture in which there is a rotational shear failure through the vertebral body. Type B is the result of similar torsional forces, but failure is through the disc anteriorly. Type C is a translational shear injury in which the shearing forces are directed in the posteroanterior direction, with the superior body anteriorly translated as a result of bony failure of the facet joints. The mechanism in type D is similar to that for type C, except that the neural arch is fractured and remains posteriorly as a floating lamina. Type E fractures are the result of an AP translational

entirely through discal ligamentous structures or through all three columns of the spine in certain spinal disorders, such as ankylosing spondylitis or diffuse idiopathic skeletal hyperostosis, are highly unstable shear-type injuries.

Classification of Thoracolumbar Injury

The Denis classification system divides injuries into minor and major categories on the basis of radiographic and CT imaging. Minor injuries account for 15% of all injuries and include fractures of the transverse and spinous processes, laminae, and pars interarticularis. Major injuries include compression fractures, burst fractures, flexion-distraction injuries, and fracture-dislocations.

Compression injuries are defined as fractures of the anterior column with an intact middle column. In compression-flexion injuries, loading of the flexed spine causes compressive stress through the anterior column force in which most failure is through the ligamentous structures. Type F is a three-column injury resulting from a flexion-distraction force disrupting almost all of the spinal soft-tissue and ligamentous structures with rotation and anterior translation of the superior body on the inferior vertebral body. There is usually a tethering of the functional spinal unit by the anterior longitudinal ligament.

Neurologic Injury

For adult thoracolumbar fractures, the incidence of neurologic damage to the spinal cord, or to the cauda equina, is between 10% and 38%. It can be related to the anatomic characteristics of the spine at the level of injury and to the type of deforming mechanism.

Spinal cord dysfunction following trauma may be classified as complete, incomplete, or progressive. The most critical factor determining the extent of neurologic recovery is the severity of damage sustained by the neural elements at the time of injury. Some patients recover rapidly; if no neurologic improvement is detected within 24 h, paralysis usually remains. Improvement of one nerve root may occur in 80% of patients with complete neurologic injuries, and two root levels in 20%.

In incomplete spinal cord injuries, some of the spinal cord tracts are spared. The presence of lower sacral motor or sensory function (sacral sparing) is often the only indication that a spinal cord injury is incomplete. This indicates that there is at least some structural continuity of the long spinal tracts and a possibility for functional recovery. The American Spinal Injury Association classification and the Frankel classification provide standardized methods of evaluation of motor and sensory function, which may be useful in determining functional recovery in patients with spinal cord injury.

Nonsurgical Treatment

Nonsurgical treatment may be considered when there is sufficient posttraumatic spinal stability and when the chance for progressive deformity and neurologic compromise to develop is limited. Selecting the appropriate fractures for nonsurgical treatment depends on such factors as the character of the injury, the severity of the injury mechanism, and specific host factors such as the feasibility of cast or brace wearing. Appropriate treatment selection ultimately depends on the degree of existing stability, as previously defined.

Surgical Treatment

In fractures deemed unstable, several variables must be considered in determining the suitability of surgical treatment. These include the degree and severity of spinal malalignment or deformity, the neurologic status (static versus progressive) of the patient, and the overall medical condition of the patient.

Spinal Decompression

In an effort to allow early patient mobilization and limit the consequences of prolonged bed rest, a complete spinal cord injury is often managed by spinal stabilization. Neurologic outcome of complete cord injury after spinal decompression has not been shown to significantly improve recovery as compared with stabilization alone. Although it has not been proven in acute circumstances many experienced physicians caring for patients with incomplete cord injuries believe surgery may improve functional outcome in most patients. The surgical approach is dictated by a variety of factors including the spinal level, degree and nature of canal compromise, and the experience of the surgeon.

Timing of Surgery

The optimal timing for surgical intervention, including decompression and stabilization, remains unclear in patients with spinal cord or cauda equina injury. Several clinical studies have suggested that decompression in less than 24 h may be optimal in terms of neurologic improvement. However, other centers have reported conflicting findings where surgery in less than 24 h has been associated with increased neurologic deterioration.

Animal models of spinal cord injury have consistently shown neurologic improvement with early decompression. In a canine model, early reperfusion of the spinal cord after early decompression was a critical factor in the potential for neurologic recovery. Decompression performed within 1 to 3 h of spinal injury led to recovery of electrophysiologic function. A critical window of opportunity may exist, although not yet supported by human clinical trials, in which decompression of extrinsic pressure on the spinal cord may enhance functional neurologic outcome. In the only controlled prospective randomized study to date, no significant difference in functional neural recovery was reported between patients who underwent early or late surgery.

Surgical Approaches

The surgeon may use variations of three different surgical approaches for spinal decompression, reconstruction, and stabilization: anterior, posterior, and posterolateral. The optimum approach is patient and fracture specific. Factors such as fracture type, neurologic status, degree and nature of canal compromise, spinal level, and the experience of the surgeon all contribute to the choice of surgical approach and instrumentation. Spinal instrumentation is useful in assisting in the surgical reduction of spinal alignment and rigid stabilization of the spinal elements.

Anterior Spinal Surgery

There are several indications for anterior spinal surgery in patients with acute thoracolumbar injuries. The primary indication for anterior decompression is an incomplete neurologic deficit in a compression or flexion-compression injury with marked canal compromise. Other indications include secondary decompression of residual spinal cord compression following posterior spinal realignment and stabilization or in patients with significant anterior column deficiency.

The anterior technique provides direct and therefore more predictable spinal canal decompression. At the level of the spinal cord, the anterior approach is the most reliable means of observing the compressed anterior neural elements. Minimal iatrogenic manipulation is necessary with this approach and direct observation facilitates spinal reconstruction. Following anterior decompression, Esses found that spinal canal occlusion improved from 58% preoperatively to 4% postoperatively, as compared to a posterior indirect reduction, in which canal patency improved from 44.5% preoperatively to 16.5% postoperatively.

Several anterior surgical approaches may be used depending on the fracture level. A transthoracic approach is useful for fractures of T4 to T9. Access to the upper and midthoracic spine usually requires a thoracotomy, which most often is from the right side. A thoracoabdominal approach, occasionally combined with a subphrenic extension, can be used for fractures of T10 to L1. A subpleural retroperitoneal approach is used for fractures of T12 to L5. Limited takedown of the diaphragm avoids a thoracotomy, but may not allow for adequate exposure above T12.

The upper thoracic spine is the most difficult area to approach anteriorly. Although the fracture can be observed by means of a thoracotomy, surgical manipulation of the fracture may be limited. For access to T2, T3, and T4, a lateral extrapleural parascapular approach may be useful. This approach allows for posterior spinal fixation to be applied concomitantly. If anterior access is required at the cervicothoracic junction, that is T2 or T3, an extension of the anterior cervical approach with partial manubriectomy and partial resection of the medial third of the clavicle may be performed. In some cases a sternal splitting approach may be necessary to gain exposure.

Current anterior spinal instrumentation systems are low profile and have had minimal reported device-related complications (Fig. 4). They function primarily as load-sharing devices in a neutralization mode. Sev-

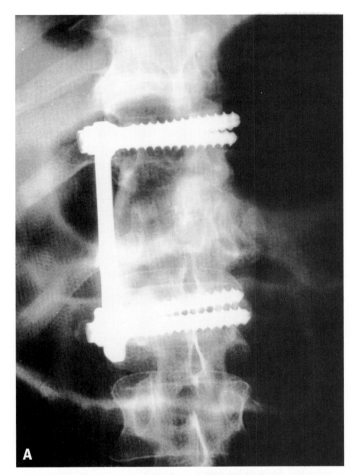

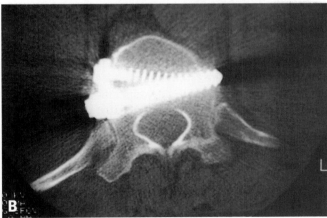

Figure 4 A, An AP plain radiograph following an L1 corpectomy and reconstruction with adjunctive anterior thoracolumbar plating. **B,** A transaxial CT scan following surgical reconstruction of this fracture. Note the orientation of the vertebral bone screws. The posterior screws are angulated anteriorly to avoid canal penetration.

eral designs allow for limited vertebral distraction and compression although care must be given to avoiding screw migration through the cancellous vertebral body. A review of 150 patients with thoracolumbar burst fractures and associated neurologic deficit treated with an anterior decompression and stabilization procedure showed good radiographic and functional results. Neurologic function improved at least one Frankel grade in 95% of patients. In nine patients, a pseudarthrosis was treated successfully with a posterolateral arthrodesis and instrumentation.

Anterior fixation devices are used more frequently in an attempt to avoid the morbidity of additional posterior surgery. Anterior surgery alone can only be used in the setting of physiologic coronal alignment. If there is extensive disruption of the posterior elements, anterior surgery alone may result in splaying of the posterior spinal elements with resultant kyphosis and instability. Although anterior instrumentation, theoretically, results in the most predictable canal clearance, several studies comparing anterior and posterior treatment methods revealed no significant difference in neurologic improvement.

A growing trend in the management of symptomatic thoracolumbar osteoporotic compression fractures without middle column compromise is the selective injection of methylmethacrylate into symptomatic levels. It is unclear at this time which patients are most suitable for this form of treatment and at what time point in their management this method of intervention is appropriate. Pain relief may be related to stability afforded to vertebrae when the cement hardens.

Posterior Spinal Surgery

Posterior spinal surgery is the most common approach used for the surgical management of thoracolumbar injuries. The mainstay of posterior surgical intervention has been distraction instrumentation. The advantages of this approach are the familiarity of the surgical anatomy and limited reliance on an assistant surgeon (often required for anterior surgery). Historically, posterior spinal instrumentation developed from efforts to stabilize and/or correct chronic spinal deformities. A natural extension of these techniques has been applied to the more acute spinal deformities related to trauma.

With posterior distraction techniques, restoration of vertebral body height, attempted correction of sagittal alignment, and partial canal clearance by ligamentotaxis or indirect manipulation through its attached soft tissues can be achieved. During ligamentotaxis, the posterior anulus fibrosus and posterior longitudinal ligament, if intact, become taut and push retropulsed fragments of bone anteriorly away from the neural elements. Canal clearance of 40% to 75% has been reported with this technique. Greater canal clearance is achieved in Denis type A burst fractures and may be related to the greater degree of bony comminution and the relative mobility of the bony fragments. In Denis type B fractures there are often one or two large intracanal bony fragments that become trapped between the two halves of the fractured vertebral body and are not easily reduced. If the retropulsed fragment is rotated, or if spinal canal occlusion is greater than 50%, ligamentotaxis is less effective. Intraoperative ultrasonagraphy or a limited laminoforaminotomy with canal exploration may be used to assess spinal canal patency following posterior indirect canal clearance through ligamentotaxis.

When choosing a posterior hook-rod distraction system, the appropriate rod length and the number of vertebral motion segments to be fused are important considerations. The primary disadvantage of posterior rodding instrumentation is the length of spinal segments that need to be spanned, usually five to six motion segments. To minimize the number of fused functional spinal units the concept of rodding long and fusing short was introduced. Ideally, only the segments above and below the fracture level are incorporated in the fusion mass, and the spinal instrumentation would be removed after approximately 1 year. Long-term problems with this technique, however, include osteoarthritis of the immobilized but unfused facets and progressive kyphosis after rod removal.

Other shortcomings of distraction hook-rod techniques include early or late hook dislodgment, with loss of sagittal and at times coronal alignment. A distraction force, although effective in restoring anterior vertebral body height, results in a kyphotic movement force over the spinal segments to which force is applied. This is especially bothersome in the mid to lower lumbar spine where distraction often leads to significant iatrogenic loss of lumbar lordosis and the development of painful flat-back deformity.

To decrease the potential of a secondary flat-back deformity, square terminal hook-rod coupling mechanisms were developed that allowed sagittal contouring of the rod with less potential for rod rotation. Alternatively, sagittal plane contouring could be maintained through three- or four-point bending forces through high-density polyethylene sleeves, termed Edwards sleeves, on the contoured rods posterior to the fractured vertebra. In the setting of an intact posterior neural arch, the sleeves are placed over the level of the pedicles of the fractured vertebra, serving as the fulcrum for a three-point bending force to reduce the kyphotic deformity and control rotation. This often allows for the instrumentation of only one spinal segment below and two spinal segments above the fracture. Using this technique, Edwards and Levine observed a reduction in kyphosis from 14° to 0°, an increase in vertebral body height from 68% to 96%, and an increase in spinal canal patency from 55% to 87%.

To help circumvent many of the complications related

to hook-rod systems in the lumbar region, pedicle screw strategies were developed to apply rigid three-column spinal fixation over a shorter fusion bed. Pedicle screw fixation allows for stabilization one level above and below the fracture of the injured spinal column without relying on the stability of the posterior neural arch for implant anchorage. This construct is especially useful in the lower lumbar region where anterior column decompression and stabilization are often technically difficult. Short-segment pedicle screw applications, however, have a high reported failure rate if used without anterior column support in the thoracolumbar junction region or without obtaining three points of fixation. If a posterior alone approach is chosen, it is usually necessary to instrument two spinal segments below, with or without an upgoing terminal infralaminar hook, and two segments above the fracture (Fig. 5). Experimental data in acute injury models have demonstrated that short-segment pedicle screw constructs provide torsional, flexural, and compressive rigidity comparable to longer hook-rod constructs. The optimum fracture patterns treated with posterior alone short-segment pedicle fixation include flexion-distraction injuries and unstable lower lumbar burst fractures. For burst fractures involving the upper lumbar or lower thoracic region, a second stage anterior reconstruction procedure often is recommended if posterior short-segment fixation fusion is used.

Posterolateral Decompression and Stabilization

Benefits of the posterolateral technique for decompressing the anterior epidural space have been documented by several authors. It is possible to decompress the neural elements (with or without grafting) and stabilize the spine posteriorly without the need for a secondary anterior procedure. The posterolateral approach allows access to the anterior thecal sac either through the pedicle (transpedicular) or lateral to the pedicle (lateral extracavitary) of the respective vertebral body. In the transpedicular approach, the fractured vertebral body is entered through its pedicle on the side of greatest canal occlusion using a high-speed drill and then a curette. Bone anterior to the retropulsed fragment can be débrided with various angled curettes and pituitaries, undermining the posteriorly displaced bone. Some mild medial retraction of the neural elements may be required, and therefore this procedure should be performed only in the lower lumbar spine below the conus. The lateral extracavitary approach is a more extensive procedure in which one or two ribs are removed to allow access to the posterolateral vertebral body. Often this technique is associated with profuse epidural bleeding, and graft placement is less than optimal due to limited visibility.

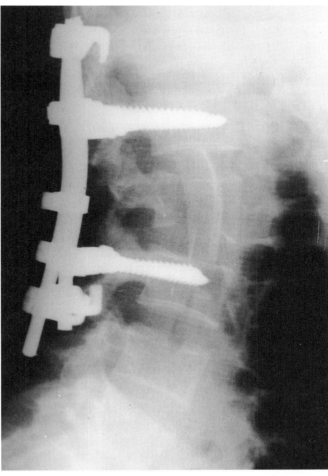

Figure 5 A lateral plain radiograph following a posterior open reduction and internal fixation of an unstable L1 burst fracture. Short-segment pedicular fixation for this unstable injury is frequently prone to instrumentation failure. A commonly used instrumentation construct involves pedicle screw fixation two vertebral levels below the injury level often with an up going infralaminar hook. A claw configuration or multilevel pedicle screw fixation anchorage points may be used cephalad to the fracture level. In this case an anterior decompression and strut fusion also were performed.

The disadvantages of posterolateral decompression include the potential for iatrogenic neural injury caused by excessive neural manipulation or inadequate neural decompression resulting from lack of direct observation. Blood loss can be excessive and graft reconstruction is often compromised due to lack of clear end plate observation. Results of clinical studies evaluating these techniques have been reported favorable with up to 77% neurologic improvement in compromised patients.

Combined Anterior and Posterior Surgical Procedures

The biomechanical stabilty and versatility of spinal instrumentation has advanced significantly over the last decade, making the need for combined anterior and posterior procedures less frequent. Currently, combined techniques are recommended in three clinical situations: (1) when the spinal canal is circumferentially compromised and requires anterior and posterior decompression, (2) when realignment or rebalancing is required to correct severe coronal or sagittal plane deformity (greater than 40°) in the setting of symptomatic anterior thecal sac compression, and (3) when anterior structural augmentation is deemed necessary following a posterior stabilization procedure.

An anterior approach followed by a posterior approach is useful in the stabilization of three-column spinal injuries or in situations of severe osteoporosis with symptomatic canal occlusion. If posterior instability is present following anterior decompression and reconstruction, a supplemental posterior stabilization is recommended. In upper thoracic or lower lumbar injuries that require an anterior decompression, adjunctive anterior instrumentation is often prominent and may impinge on the surrounding great vessels, making initial decompression and grafting followed by posterior stabilization preferable (Fig. 6).

A posterior approach followed by an anterior approach may be useful in the treatment of a displaced fracture-dislocation of the thoracolumbar spine with an incomplete neurologic deficit and spinal canal occlusion. To properly realign the spine, an initial reduction is done through the posterior approach. If, after realignment, residual symptomatic anterior neural compression is detected, an anterior decompression and reconstruction can then be done. This technique also is used less commonly in cases without significant spinal malalignment where posterior indirect reduction fails to provide adequate neural decompression and a persistent neurologic deficit exists. In about 4% of patients with an incomplete neurologic deficit and spinal canal occlusion, neural impingement persisting after a posterior reduction may warrant a posterolateral or anterior decompression.

A posterior-then-anterior surgical procedure may be necessary in patients who incur a traumatic distraction-extension spinal injury in the setting of ankylosing spondylitis or diffuse idiopathic skeletal hyperostosis. Following a posterior reduction and stabilization, an anterior column deficiency may remain. This may result in late instability if supplemental anterior reconstruction is not performed.

A simultaneous anterior and posterior spinal approach may be useful in the treatment of thoracolumbar injuries that do not involve a significant coronal plane deformity. A one-stage simultaneous procedure (anterior and posterior at the same time), results in less surgical time, less blood loss, and fewer complications, as compared with a two-stage procedure. With this approach, a second and/or third stage procedure may be avoided when performing complex revision surgery.

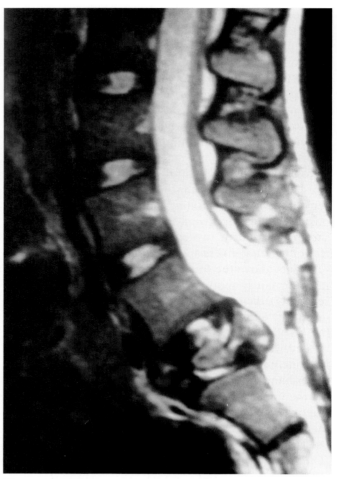

Figure 6 A sagittal plane MRI revealing evidence of an L5 burst fracture in a patient with an incomplete neurologic deficit. Due to the significant amount of canal occlusion, an anterior approach was initially attempted with reconstruction using paired autologous fibula autografts. A subsequent posterior short-segment fixation was then performed.

Comparison of Anterior Versus Posterior Spinal Surgery

The results of anterior versus posterior spinal surgery have been compared in several small studies. Esses and associates did a prospective randomized study of 40 patients with thoracolumbar injuries who underwent either a posterior approach with indirect canal clearance (AO fixateur interne) or an anterior decompression and reconstruction (using the Kostuik-Harrington device). Although the average percent canal compromise with the use of the fixateur interne changed from 44.5% preoperatively to 16.5% postoperatively, direct anterior decompression led to a decrease in canal occlusion from 58% to 4%. Kyphosis correction was 11° with the posterior approach, versus 9° with the anterior approach (not statistically significant). The authors concluded that posterior distraction can adequately decompress the canal and correct kyphosis, if performed within 72 h from the time of the injury.

In a retrospective review of 87 patients with incomplete neurologic injuries, Bradford and McBride observed that neurologic recovery was greater with anterior decompression (88%) than with posterior decompression (64%). This was more evident with regard to bladder and bowel control (65% versus 33%, respectively). Patients with inadequate posterior decompression and residual neurologic deficit improved after a subsequent anterior decompression.

In 60 consecutive patients with spinal cord injury and greater than 20% encroachment of the spinal canal, no significant change was found in neurologic improvement if posterior or anterior surgery was performed (85% and 88% respectively) and no apparent difference in the degree of canal clearance.

Management of Specific Injuries

Compression Fractures

Compression fractures involve failure of the anterior column with an intact middle column. This fracture type is prevalent among the elderly and usually is stable because of the competency of the posterior osteoligamentous complex. Most patients are successfully managed by nonsurgical or minimally invasive techniques. Surgical stabilization, although rarely necessary, may benefit those fracture subtypes with loss of anterior vertebral height greater than 50% or initial kyphosis of greater than 20° to 30° resulting from documented posterior ligamentous disruption. A four-hook, two-rod distraction system using three- or four-point fixation provides adequate stabilization. Lateral flexion-compression fractures at risk for deformity progression may also be stabilized with a distraction construct (hooks, pedicle screws-rods) on the injury side and a compression construct on the uninjured side. The potential for iatrogenic retropulsion of an intervertebral disc must be considered whenever a cantilever force is applied to reduce the spinal deformity.

Burst Fractures

Burst fractures result from axial compressive failure of the anterior and middle columns with either an intact or disrupted (compressive or tensile failure) posterior column. The management of these fractures remains controversial. Some authors believe that all patients with burst type injuries without neurologic sequelae benefit from surgical care as compared with nonsurgical management. Denis reported that surgical stabilization was better than nonsurgical treatment in all burst fractures after a retrospective study reviewing 52 patients

without evidence of a neurologic deficit. Of the 39 patients treated nonsurgically, six experienced neurologic worsening during follow-up, with 25% of patients not returning to full-time employment. Of the 13 patients treated surgically, all returned to their previous level of work unless there were unrelated disability factors. Surgical treatment, as suggested by Denis for all patients with thoracolumbar burst fractures regardless of neurologic injury, has not been supported elsewhere in the literature. Appropriate management is directed by an evaluation of kyphotic angulation at the fracture site, the degree of canal compromise from retropulsed bony fragments, and the neurologic status of the patient.

A common theme in all well-designed studies on the treatment of thoracolumbar burst fractures is the correlation of posterior ligamentous integrity and treatment approach. Burst fractures with evidence of posterior ligamentous disruption, that is, kyphosis greater than 20° to 30°, subluxation of the posterior facets, increase in the interspinous process distance, or loss of greater than 50% of anterior vertebral height, often benefit from surgical stabilization. Nonsurgical treatment in this subgroup may lead to progressive spinal instability, late pain, and the possibility of neurologic problems.

Stabilization of burst fractures may be obtained either through a posterior or anterior approach. An excessive posterior distraction force should be avoided if significant posterior ligamentous disruption is present, for fear of catastrophic tension injury to the spinal cord with worsening of the spinal deformity. A posterior hook-rod strategy may require instrument placement three levels above and two levels below the fractures at the thoracolumbar junction. If the posterior neural arch is intact, the Edwards technique may be used by instrumenting one level below and two levels above the fracture level, using a sleeve over the facet joint and pedicle of the involved vertebral body. In the setting of bony disruption of the posterior elements, a bridging sleeve construct can be used, instrumenting two to three levels above and below the fracture segment. A pedicle screw configuration in the mid and low lumbar spine may obviate immobilization of unnecessary spinal segments as well as avoid distraction resulting in flat-back deformity. Short-segment pedicle screw configurations have an early high failure rate without reconstruction of the anterior column. Consideration for pedicular instrumentation removal should be given (at around 18 months postoperatively), especially at the thoracolumbar junction if a posterior alone approach is chosen, due to the potential for instrumentation failure.

During the past two decades, anterior spinal approaches and reconstruction techniques have evolved to meet the anatomic and biomechanical challenges particular to traumatic injuries of the thoracolumbar spine.

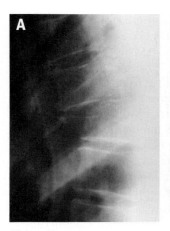
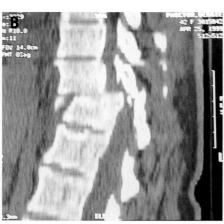
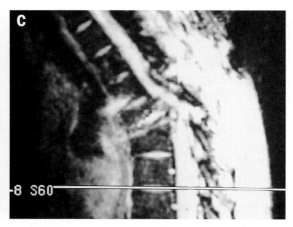

Figure 7 A, A lateral plain radiograph showing a bilateral facet dislocation at the T11-T12 level. **B,** A sagittal plane CT reconstruction of this injury demonstrates the anterior position of the inferior articular process of the cephalad vertebral body in relation to the superior articular process of the inferior vertebral body. **C,** A sagittal plane MRI of this injury demonstrates the marked posterior ligamentous disruption necessary for this injury to occur.

A stand-alone anterior decompression and fusion can be performed in the neurologically compromised patient with significant anterior thecal sac compression or when surgical intervention is delayed longer than 2 weeks, preventing adequate reduction of spinal alignment through a posterior approach. An anterior approach can also be used after failure of adequate canal decompression by posterior techniques in patients with residual neurologic dysfunction.

Flexion-Distraction Injuries

Flexion-distraction injuries can occur through bone, soft tissue, or a combination of both (Fig. 7). The management of such injuries is determined by the degree of soft-tissue or bony involvement. When these injuries extend entirely through the bony posterior elements and into the vertebral body (Chance fracture) without disc involvement, the prognosis for bony healing is good. This fracture type may be immobilized in a hyperextension cast or a total contact thoracolumbosacral orthosis for 3 months, with serial radiographic evaluation to evaluate for any fracture displacement. Caution in the use of an extension-reduction maneuver must be exercised if the middle column is comminuted for fear of bony retropulsion or if the posterior facets are incompetent preventing an adequate anatomic reduction. If the axis of rotation involves the anterior column (compression failure), a distraction hook-rod, screw construct may be utilized applying tension to the anterior longitudinal ligament with care not to overdistract the middle (that is, incompetent posterior longitudinal ligament) or posterior columns. This can be done with temporary placement of an intersegmental spinous process wire or compression hook-rod construct across the vertebral levels involving the compromised interspinous ligaments.

Fracture-Dislocations

Fracture-dislocations result from high-energy trauma involving a combination of forces. Surgical intervention is universally recommended in this fracture type. When there is no neurologic deficit, surgery is performed to realign and stabilize the spine to allow for early mobilization and to prevent deformity or neurologic injury. In the presence of a neurologic deficit, surgery is performed initially through the posterior approach to realign the spine, followed by an assessment of the spinal canal to evaluate for residual canal compromise. In patients with a complete neurologic deficit, posterior reduction and stabilization allows earlier mobilization and upright positioning, which have been shown to decrease overall morbidity and mortality from pulmonary dysfunction, skin problems, and deep venous thrombosis.

Fracture-dislocations should be treated with multisegmental posterior instrumentation at least two levels above and below the injury. Multiple points of fixation are often required to effectively immobilize the injury, prevent late construct failure, and allow mobilization without the need for prolonged external immobilization.

Distraction-Extension Injuries

Distraction-extension injuries are uncommon, highly unstable injuries that often are associated with catastrophic neurologic compromise when three-column involvement is present (Fig. 8). Supine positioning may exacerbate the deformity in patients with a preexisting kyphotic spinal posture, resulting in neurologic decline. After postural reduction, spinal stability often is obtained by posterior segmental fixation. Anterior procedures usually are not necessary in patients with this injury unless anterior column insufficiency is present

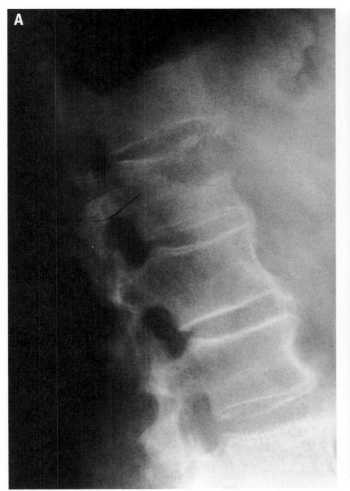 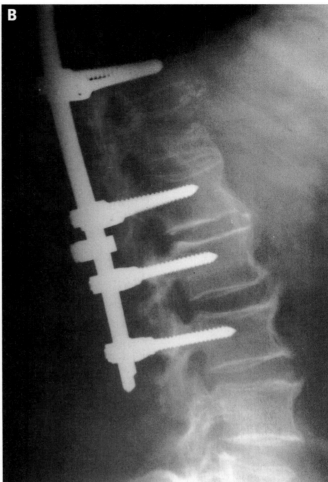

Figure 8 A, A lateral plain radiograph revealing a distraction-extension injury of the T12 vertebral body. **B,** Following a prone closed reduction, a posterior pedicle-based fixation procedure was performed.

following reduction, that is, the presence of an anterior fish-mouth type deformity.

Complications Related to Surgical Treatment of Thoracolumbar Fractures

Neurologic deterioration is one of the most serious complications following surgical treatment of thoracolumbar fractures. This occurs in approximately 1% of patients and may be the result of patient positioning with fracture fragment displacement, intraoperative iatrogenic overdistraction, overcompression, malreduction, or excessive encroachment of instrumentation within the spinal canal.

Spinal instrumentation failure may occur months after surgery and may be associated with deformity progression or lack of fracture healing. Pseudarthrosis following posterior fusion stabilization for thoracolumbar injuries has been reported to occur in approximately

2% to 8% of patients, most frequently at the thoracolumbar junction.

Occasionally, instrumentation that is less than ideally suitable for a particular fracture subtype may contribute to perioperative instability and late fracture displacement, as when Luque instrumentation is used for fractures with marked axial instability or distraction rods and hooks for shear-type injuries. Overdistraction is a potential problem with posterior hook-rod instrumentation, particularly when used in the presence of anterior or posterior longitudinal ligament disruption. A comparison of hook-rod, pedicle screws, and sublaminar Luque systems revealed no significant difference in overall complication rates. The rod-hook systems, however, had a higher rate of fixation loss and instrumentation removal.

Delayed vascular erosion can occur from metal-vessel contact and anterior instrumentation, although lower profile designs and lateral placement of these devices has decreased this risk substantially. Vertebral screw placement through the lateral vertebral body may come perilously close to the spinal canal and therefore should be started close to the posterior vertebral body border and directed slightly anteriorly during insertion. The stability of anterior dual-rod or plate instrumentation and grafting alone in the setting of significant posterior instability may lead to early implant failure with progression of spinal deformity.

Damage to the great vessels, evidenced by intimal damage and thromboembolic phenomenon or through direct vessel laceration, is an infrequent complication of anterior spinal surgery. Meticulous surgical technique and attentive assistants using well-padded retractors that are frequently released may minimize these complications. Retrograde ejaculation, due to damage to the autonomic nervous system, may occur in up to 4% of patients undergoing an anterior lumbosacral exposure. Blunt dissection with the use of peanut sponges, without use of monopolar cautery, may minimize this problem.

Fortunately, deep spinal infection is infrequent, occurring between 3% and 10% of most reported series using spinal instrumentation. At the earliest signs of infection, irrigation and débridement should be performed to remove all devitalized and necrotic tissue. Repeat débridements are then performed at 48- to 72-h intervals with the wound packed with saline-soaked vaginal tapes between débridements until the wound appears clean. Stable spinal instrumentation is not removed in the perifusion period because of its value in optimizing maturation of the fusion. Autologous bone graft, unless grossly infected, is not removed. Final closure is performed over multiple drains, usually after the second or third débridement. Antibiotics are continued intravenously for 6 weeks, followed by oral medication anywhere from 6 weeks to lifetime.

Rehabilitation

In the care of the spinal injury patient treated surgically or nonsurgically, early patient mobilization is paramount. In patients with evidence of a spinal cord injury, early passive motion exercises prevent joint contractures and facilitate a patient's participation in activities of daily living, including personal hygiene, transfer, and feeding. Early bowel and bladder training is important to decrease the level of dependency and, therefore, the financial burden on external resources.

Discussion

In recent years, advances in surgical techniques have allowed physicians to greatly improve care of patients with thoracolumbar fractures. Appropriate treatment of thoracolumbar spinal injuries requires consideration of the type of fracture, the degree of neural compromise if any, the level of the spinal fracture, the medical condition of the patient, and the surgeon's experience.

Both surgical and nonsurgical treatment can yield satisfactory results in appropriately selected patients. Although the timing of intervention for spinal injury is debated, early medical management and early surgical decompression may prove beneficial in preserving and improving neurologic function. Nonsurgical treatment is appropriate for stable spine injuries. For unstable spinal fractures, with or without neurologic deficit, rigid surgical stabilization allows for early and aggressive patient mobilization. Spine surgeons must remain attentive to the myriad of surgical approaches and the potential complications that may arise with the use of the various instrumentation systems available. Only through well-designed and controlled prospective studies will the optimum treatment regimen be better elucidated.

Annotated Bibliography

Bracken MB, Shepard MJ, Holford TR, et al: Administration of methylprednisolone for 24 or 48 hours or tirilazad mesylate for 48 hours in the treatment of acute spinal cord injury: Results of the Third National Acute Spinal Cord Injury Randomized Controlled Trial. National Acute Spinal Cord Injury Study. *JAMA* 1997; 277:1597-1604.

This double-blind randomized clinical trial compared the efficacy of methylprednisolone administered for 24 h with methylprednisolone administered for 48 h or tirilazad mesylate administered for 48 h in patients with acute spinal cord injury.

Carlson GD, Minato Y, Okada A, et al: Early time-dependent decompression for spinal cord injury: Vascular mechanisms of recovery. *J Neurotrauma* 1997;14: 951-962.

The authors investigated the importance of early spinal cord decompression on recovery of evoked potential conduction under precision loading. Results indicate that after precise dynamic spinal cord loading to a point of functional conduction deficit (50% decline in evoked potential amplitude), a critical time period exists in which intervention in the form of early spinal cord decompression can lead to effective recovery of electrophysiologic function in the 1- to 3-h postdecompression period.

Criscitiello AA, Fredrickson BE: Thoracolumbar spine injuries. *Orthopedics* 1998;20:939-944.

This article reviews some of the anatomic and mechanical aspects of thoracolumbar injuries as they relate to classification systems and stability. In addition, an overview of the initial management including surgical and conservative treatment options is provided.

Ghanayem AJ, Zdeblick TA: Anterior instrumentation in the management of thoracolumbar burst fractures. *Clin Orthop* 1997;335:89-100.

The authors describe the evolution of anterior instrumentation devices and the indication and surgical techniques for their safe and effective use.

Kaneda K, Taneichi H, Abumi K, Hashimoto T, Satoh S, Fujiya M: Anterior decompression and stabilization with the Kaneda device for thoracolumbar burst fractures associated with neurological deficits. *J Bone Joint Surg Am* 1997;79:69-83.

The authors report on 150 patients with single-stage anterior decompression and fusion. Ninety-five percent had at least one Frankel grade improvement in neurologic function, and 72% recovered complete bladder function. The fusion rate was 93%, and 86% of patients returned to their previous occupations.

McCullen G, Vaccaro AR, Garfin SR: Thoracic and lumbar trauma: Rationale for selecting the appropriate fusion technique. *Orthop Clin North Am* 1998;29:813-828.

The authors describe the treatment options and considerations involved in choosing appropriate techniques for thoracic and lumbar trauma. Emphasis is placed on the ability to define accurately the extent of the injury to both the structural and the neurologic elements of the spine as well as an understanding of the historic rationale of individual treatment methods.

Shaffrey CI, Shaffrey ME, Whitehill R, Nockels RP: Surgical treatment of thoracolumbar fractures. *Neurosurg Clin North Am* 1997;8:519-540.

This article is an overview of indications for surgery, surgical approaches, types of instrumentation, and treatment options for specific thoracolumbar injuries.

Stambough JL: Posterior instrumentation for thoracolumbar trauma. *Clin Orthop* 1997;335:73-88.

The author describes the advantages of posterior instrumentation, availability of devices, surgical techniques, and outcomes in the management of unstable thoracolumbar injuries.

Vollmer DG, Gegg C: Classification and acute management of thoracolumbar fractures. *Neurosurg Clin North Am* 1997;8:499-507.

This article focuses on Denis' three-column theory of spinal stability and its utility in categorizing five injury patterns and the forces involved: specifically, wedge compression fractures, burst fractures, flexion-distraction injuries, fracture-dislocations, and miscellaneous injuries. The authors also highlight the acute management and evaluation of patients suspected to have these types of injuries.

Classic Bibliography

Argenson C, Boileau P: Specific injuries and management, in Floman Y, Farcy JPC, Argenson C (eds): *Thoracolumbar Spine Fractures*. New York, NY, Raven Press, 1993, pp 195-214.

Bedbrook GM: Treatment of thoracolumbar dislocation and fractures with paraplegia. *Clin Orthop* 1975;112:27-43.

Bradford DS, McBride GG: Surgical management of thoracolumbar spine fractures with incomplete neurologic deficits. *Clin Orthop* 1987;218:201-216.

Crutcher JP Jr, Anderson PA, King HA, Montesano PX: Indirect spinal canal decompression in patients with thoracolumbar burst fractures treated by posterior distraction rods. *J Spinal Disord* 1991;4:39-48.

Denis F: Spinal instability as defined by the three-column spine concept in acute spinal trauma. *Clin Orthop* 1984;189:65-76.

Dickman CA, Yahiro MA, Lu HT, Melkerson MN: Surgical treatment alternatives for fixation of unstable fractures of the thoracic and lumbar spine: A meta-analysis. *Spine* 1994;19(suppl 20):S2266-S2273.

Edwards CC, Levine AM: Early rod-sleeve stabilization of the injured thoracic and lumbar spine. *Orthop Clin North Am* 1986;17:121-145.

Eismont FJ, Garfin SR, Abitbol JJ: Thoracic and upper lumbar spine injuries, in Browner BD, Jupiter JB, Levine AM, Trafton PG (eds): *Skeletal Trauma: Fractures, Dislocations, Ligamentous Injuries*. Philadelphia, PA, WB Saunders, 1992, pp 729-803.

Esses SI, Botsford DJ, Kostvik JP: Evaluation of surgical treatment for burst fractures. *Spine* 1990;15:667-673.

Garfin SR, Mowery CA, Guerra J Jr, Marshall LF: Confirmation of the posterolateral technique to decompress and fuse thoracolumbar spine burst fractures. *Spine* 1985;10:218-223.

Gurr KR, McAfee PC, Shih CM: Biomechanical analysis of anterior and posterior instrumentation systems after corpectomy: A calf-spine model. *J Bone Joint Surg Am* 1988;70:1182-1191.

Holdsworth F: Fractures, dislocations, and fracture-dislocations of the spine. *J Bone Joint Surg Am* 1970;52:1534-1551.

Jacobs RR, Asher MA, Snider RK: Thoracolumbar spinal injuries: A comparative study of recumbent and operative treatment in 100 patients. *Spine* 1980;5:463-477.

Kostuik JP, Huler RJ, Esses SI, Stauffer ES: Thoracolumbar spine fracture, in Frymoyer JW, Ducker TB, Hadler NM, Kostuik JP, Weinstein JN, Whitecloud TS III (eds): *The Adult Spine: Principles and Practice.* New York, NY, Raven Press, 1991, 1269-1329.

Levi L, Wolf A, Rigamonti D, Ragheb J, Mirvis S, Robinson WL: Anterior decompression in cervical spine trauma: Does the timing of surgery affect the outcome? *Neurosurgery* 1991;29:216-222.

Levine AM, McAfee PC, Anderson PA: Evaluation and emergent treatment of patients with thoracolumbar trauma. *Instr Course Lect* 1995;44:33-45.

Panjabi MM, Thibodeau LC, Crisco JJ, White AA: What constitutes spinal instability? *Clin Neurosurg* 1988;34: 313-339.

Saboe LA, Reid DC, Davis LA, Warren SA, Grace MG: Spine trauma and associated injuries. *J Trauma* 1991;31: 43-48.

Shiba K, Katsuki M, Ueta T, et al: Transpedicular fixation with Zielke instrumentation in the treatment of thoracolumbar and lumbar injuries. *Spine* 1994;19: 1940-1949.

Chapter 30

Sacral Fractures

Jens R. Chapman, MD

Sohail K. Mirza, MD

Introduction

As implied by its derivation from the Latin word "sacrum," meaning sacred object, the sacrum is a cross-shaped bone that lies at the intersection of the spine and the pelvis. The sacrum forms the foundation of the lumbar spine and provides the key segment to the posterior pelvic ring. As the functional anatomy of the sacrum intersects two skeletal regions, it also involves the interests of two different subspecialties, spinal surgery and pelvic trauma surgery. Optimal treatment for sacral fractures ideally combines the experience of both surgical specialties, the spine surgeon's perspective of neurologic physiology and spinal alignment and stability as well as the traumatologist's insight into patient resuscitation and pelvic ring stability. Knowledge of the treatment of sacral fractures is evolving and is based currently on a few key studies and a plethora of anecdotal reports.

Anatomic Overview

The sacrum usually consists of five fused segments that are aligned kyphotically with decreasing vertebral body and spinal canal size from rostral to caudal. The sacral kyphosis, described by the ventral surface of the sacrum, can vary from 10° to more than 90°, with the most common angulation ranging from 45° to 60°. This sacral kyphosis defines the sacral inclination angle, which in turn is the basis for lumbar lordosis. Similar to the variability of mobile lumbar segments, the actual number of sacral segments varies in the presence of transitional lumbosacral vertebrae. The transverse processes of the sacral elements are coalesced in the sacral ala, which laterally articulates with the ilium through the sacroiliac joint. The sacral ala can be a contiguous broad bony shoulder or a rather narrow and partially segmented structure. The four ventral and dorsal sacral neuroforamina lie between the junction of the sacral vertebral bodies and the ala. Areas of greatest bony density are found within the superior half of the S1 vertebral seg-

ment, the ventral first and second sacral foraminal cortices, and the sacral lamina. The sacral ala itself is composed of relatively hypodense cancellous bone, which is prone to substantially decrease in density with progressing age. The structural integrity of the sacrum relies heavily on its surrounding ligaments. These broad and well-developed ligaments anchor the sacrum to the sacroiliac joints on either side and similarly connect the most caudal lumbar vertebra to the pelvis.

Neural elements potentially directly affected by sacral trauma are the lumbosacral plexus (L4 to S1) and the sacral plexus (S2 to S4). The L5 root shoulders the sacral ala and courses distally to the lateral aspect of the sacral ala. The passage space afforded to the sacral nerve roots within the ventral foramina is proportionally narrowest at S1 and relatively most capacious at S4. Based on cadaver dissections, the S1 and S2 roots occupy one third to one fourth of the ventral sacral foraminal space as compared with the lower sacral roots of S3 and S4, which occupy one sixth of the ventral foraminal space. The caudal end of the dural sac usually is located at the S2 segment. The posterior sacral foramina contribute cutaneous rami to the cluneal nerves. Sacral root function, or chances for neural recovery may be affected adversely by angulation, translation, and direct compression of the sacral spinal canal or the ventral foramina. Maintenance of physiologic sacral alignment can have important implications for neurologic and other functions, pain, and even survival.

Evaluation

Sacral fractures can be overlooked relatively easily, both clinically and radiographically. In the presence of severe metabolic or neoplastic disease the sacrum can be subject to insufficiency fractures from low-energy injury mechanisms, which can easily be missed on plain radiographs due to indistinct radiographic landmarks and osteoporosis. These fractures are discussed in another chapter. Posterior pelvic ring fractures in metabolically healthy individuals usually result from high-energy injury mechanisms. Sacral fractures are caused most commonly by motor vehicle or motorcycle crashes or falls from heights greater than 10 feet. Survivors of such high-energy injury mechanisms commonly are affected by multiple system injuries. Concurrent injuries, such as to the cranium and the spine, can make comprehensive evaluation of patients with sacral fractures challenging. Delays of diagnosis or missed sacral fractures are believed to occur in 31% or more. A high index of suspicion and a streamlined diagnostic pathway can help reduce the frequency of these occurrences.

Initial concerns in management of patients with pelvic trauma are directed toward meeting their resuscitation needs. As suggested by the advanced trauma life support protocol, the primary radiographic evaluation includes an AP pelvic view, which should be carefully evaluated for the presence of pelvic ring disruption. If intravenous resuscitation efforts in a patient with an open book type of pelvic ring disruption are not succeeding, emergent closed pelvic ring reduction with an external fixator, pelvic clamp, or circumferential pelvic sheet can be helpful in diminishing bleeding by reducing pelvic volume.

In any patient with suspected pelvic trauma, the bony landmarks of the torso are inspected and palpated circumferentially as soon as resuscitation circumstances permit. Findings such as bruising and closed lumbosacral fascial deglovement (Morel–Lavelle lesion) over the buttocks and the posterior pelvic region are important findings of severe soft-tissue contusion. Patients with suspected pelvic or sacral trauma require rectal and, in the case of female patients, vaginal examination to rule out an occult open pelvic ring fracture. Assessment of anal sphincter function also offers the chance to examine sacral root function. Such an examination should address presence of spontaneous sphincter tone; reflex function; perianal, buttock, and posterior thigh sensation; and assessment of best-effort voluntary anal sphincter contraction. Although some of these examination components are limited or unobtainable in cognitively impaired patients, examination of sacral root function is important for sacral fractures and spinal cord injury. Lumbar and lumbosacral plexus evaluation with emphasis on L5 and S1 function are important components of the decision-making process. Presence of an L5 or S1 radicular sensitivity, as elicited by a straight leg raise test, may be caused by upper sacral foraminal root compromise.

Formal radiographic evaluation of the sacrum on a pelvis AP view is difficult because of the sacral inclination. In suspected pelvic ring injury, pelvic inlet and outlet views add important insight. The pelvic inlet view allows for assessment of the integrity of the posterior pelvic ring. The pelvic outlet view offers a frontal view of the sacrum by compensating for the sacral inclination. The Ferguson view, which is obtained at a 30° cranially inclined angle similar to the pelvic outlet view, offers a more specific coned-down view of the sacrum in AP projection. A sacrum lateral radiograph remains the most simple, yet effective radiographic tool for screening and assessment of sacral injuries.

On plain AP pelvis radiographs a variety of clues should raise the suspicion of a sacral fracture. These include presence of a fractured L5 transverse process (61% association with sacral fracture), paradoxical pelvic inlet view on a supine AP radiographic projection (92% association), and presence of a stepladder-sign along the ventral sacral foramina.

CT of the pelvic ring allows for further clarification of the injury pattern but can be limited in its demonstration of transverse sacral fractures. In the presence of a more complex appearing sacral fracture, a sacral CT with cut thickness ≤ 5 mm and sagittally and coronally reformatted views can provide meaningful insight into the injury type and can aid in selecting definitive management. The addition of three-dimensionally reformatted CT-scan images, however, usually offers little further help. Myelography and postmyelography CT scans are rarely, if ever, helpful in the management of acute sacral fractures. Although MRI can portray the contents of the sacral spinal canal, its clinical value in the treatment of acute sacral fractures remains doubtful. Indications for sacral MRI in a trauma setting exist in the presence of unexplained sacral neurologic deficits and assessment of soft-tissue lesions around the sacrum. In the postacute injury phase, MRI scans can be used to assess the lumboscaral plexus for injuries, especially when combined with an MRI neurography imaging technique.

Electrodiagnostic evaluation of patients with sacral fractures can provide better understanding of injury severity and prognosis. Sacral root function can be difficult to evaluate in polytraumatized patients with sacral fractures. In such circumstances perineal somatosensory evoked potentials and anal sphincter electromyography can be used as preoperative evaluation tools or for intraoperative monitoring. Cystomyography and post-void residual measurements have been recommended as follow-up tests for patients with neurogenic bladder dysfunction.

Classification

Fractures of the sacrum can be of confounding complexity and involve issues surrounding pelvic ring and spinal stability to varying degrees. A basic classification principle is that of differentiating any given injury into a stable or unstable category. None of the sacral fracture classification systems necessarily infer stability status with the injury type described. Factors important in assessing stability of any given pelvic trauma include the systemic injury load, adjuvant soft-tissue injury, presence and evolution of neurologic injury, fracture displacement, and ligamentous versus bony disruption. A commonly held threshold for differentiation of stable versus unstable pelvic injuries has been the 1-cm tidemark of radiographically evident fracture displacement. This measurement, however, underrepresents the actual displacement that occurs during injury and never has been validated biomechanically.

To date, there is no comprehensive classification system that succeeds in integrating the various fractures and dislocations that can occur about the pelvic ring. There are three basic categories of pelvic region fractures (Table 1). Injuries with primary focus placed on the structural integrity of the pelvic ring have been classified by Tile, Letournel, the AO/ASIF group, and others. Disruption of the integrity of the lumbosacral junction and resulting issues of stability have been classified by Isler (Fig. 1, *D*). Fractures that involve the sacrum itself can be classified usefully with the system suggested by Denis and associates (Fig. 1, *A*). Roy-Camille and associates have added a helpful subclassification system (Fig. 1, *B*) for transverse sacral fractures involving the spinal canal (Denis zone III injuries). The latter two classification systems can be seen as complementary to one another and not exclusionary. Other systems, such as introduced by Sabiston and Wing or Kaehr and Anderson are variations of the above systems, but lack comprehensiveness.

Pelvic ring fracture classification principles are described elsewhere. Physicians who treat sacral injuries should be knowledgeable of pelvic ring injury assessment and basic management needs.

Lumbosacral junction trauma has been recognized as a specific entity. These injuries may present as pure facet dislocations or complex lumbosacral fractures. Because of the strong lumbosacral junction ligaments, considerable forces are required for these injuries to occur. Numerous case reports have described various stages of lumbosacral injuries ranging from facet fractures to lumbopelvic dissociation. Such injuries may involve unilateral and bilateral L5-S1 facet dislocations and displacements in anterior, posterior, and lateral directions. Isler has proposed a systematic injury classification and inferences on necessary treatment based on location of a pelvic ring fracture relative to the L5-S1 facet joints (Fig. 1, *D*). A vertical sacral fracture lateral to the L5-S1 facet joint was found to have no relevance to lumbosacral stability. Injuries crossing through the L5-S1

TABLE 1	Overview of Pelvic Ring Fracture Classifications		
Category	**A**	**B**	**C**
Prevalent injury zone	Pelvic ring	Lumbosacral junction	Sacrum
Classification system	Tile Letournel AO/ASIF	Isler	Denis Roy-Camille (Subclassification of Denis zone III) Descriptive alphabet pattern

facet joint were differentiated into extra-articular fractures of the lumbosacral junction and articular dislocations with various stages of displacement of the L5 and S1 articular processes. Fractures crossing into the neural arch medial to the L5-S1 joint usually were found to be complex and inherently unstable.

Sacral fracture patterns also can be described using letters, which resemble the main fracture lines somewhat (Fig. 1, *C*). While not suitable for a systematic classification system, descriptive terms such as a sacral H, U, T, L or lambda fracture pattern can be used to communicate effectively some of the more common complex sacral fracture patterns.

The most helpful classification for sacral fractures remains the three-zone system proposed by Denis and associates in 1988 (Fig. 1, *A*). It was based on a retrospective review of 236 patients and differentiates sacral fractures based on the most medial excursion of the fracture lines. Alar fractures (zone I injuries) remain lateral to the sacral neuroforamina; transforaminal fractures, which usually follow a vertical pattern, do not propagate into the spinal canal and are labeled as zone II injuries; any sacral fracture extending into the spinal canal is referred to as a zone III injury. This anatomically based system has important implications in regards to the incidence and type of accompanying neurologic injuries.

The basic three injury types are also reflective of the injury incidence in general, as well as the injury mechanism. Zone I extraforaminal alar fractures were encountered in 50% of patients, with a neurologic injury rate of 5.9% affecting the sciatic nerve, most commonly its L4 and L5 roots. Zone II transforaminal injuries were found in 34% of patients, with 28% having neurologic injury to L5, S1, or S2 roots. Zone III injuries involving the spinal canal were identified in 16% of patients in this retrospective study, of which 57% were affected by neurologic injury involving the sacral roots. With injury

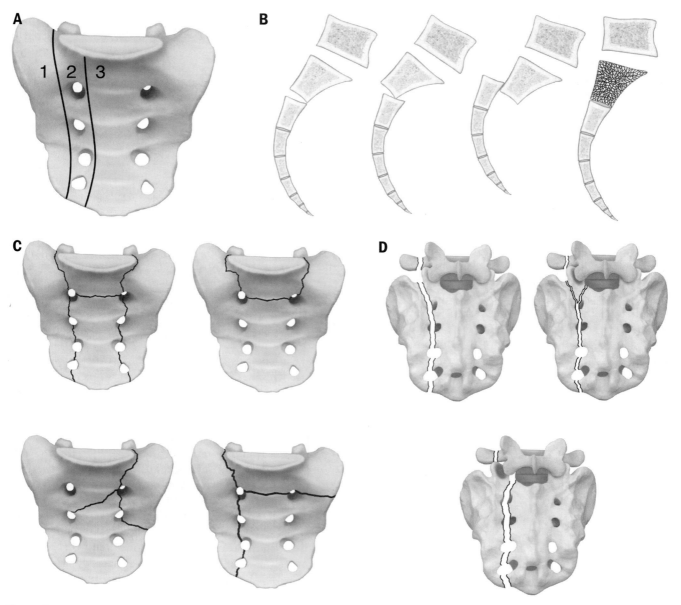

Figure 1 Sacral fracture classification systems. **A,** Three-zone system of Denis and associates (1988): zone I injuries are entirely lateral to the neuroforamina; zone II fractures involve the neuroforamina, but do not involve the spinal canal; zone III injuries extend into the spinal canal with primary or associated fracture lines. **B,** Subclassification of Denis zone III fractures as suggested by Roy-Camille and associates and modified by Strange-Vognsen and Lebech. Type 1 injuries are angulated but not translated; type 2 are angulated and translated; type 3 show complete translational displacement of upper and lower sacrum; and type 4 are segmentally comminuted due to axial impaction. **C,** Examples of complex sacral Denis zone III fractures. The fracture on top left is frequently referred to as H type, the one on top right as sacral U type. The fracture on the bottom left is a sacral lambda and the one on the bottom right a sacral T fracture. **D,** Classification of lumbosacral junction injuries as suggested by Isler. Type A injuries are lateral to the L5-S1 facet joints and may affect pelvic ring stability, but not lumbosacral stability. Type B injuries extend through the L5-S1 facet joint and are associated with a variety of displacements and neurologic injuries. Type C injuries violate the spinal canal, are invariably unstable, and usually are of complex nature.

to the lower sacral plexus, impaired bowel or bladder control or sexual function affected 76% of patients. The level of sacral canal disruption has important implications on bladder function. Patients with higher transverse sacral fractures involving the S1 through S3 segments tend to have a higher incidence of bladder dysfunction than lower sacral fractures affecting the S4 or S5 segments.

The fracture classification system of Denis and associates inherently does not address the issue of fracture displacement and injury-induced instability. Zone I and II fractures usually have a vertical orientation and are the posterior components of a pelvic ring disruption. Commonly, they are the result of lateral compression or external rotation displacement of the pelvic ring. Vertical displacement of the hemipelvis is a less common injury type and inherently very unstable. Bilateral zone I or II injuries are uncommon and may in fact represent an unrecognized zone III injury with a more obscure transverse fracture line. Denis and associates described both zone I and zone II fractures to occur as either minimally displaced, with potential for some stability, or as displaced, resulting in a loss of pelvic stability.

Sacral fractures involving the central spinal canal (Denis zone III) can be further subclassified using the system introduced by Roy-Camille and associates and modified by Strange-Vognsen and Lebech. These fractures originally were described for transverse fractures of the upper sacrum occurring in suicidal jumpers but are applicable to a wider variety of zone III injuries and trauma mechanisms. Injury severity and likelihood of neurologic injury can be inferred from progressively higher subtypes of the Roy-Camille and associates system. Type 1 injuries consist of a simple flexion deformity of the sacrum; type 2 injuries consist of a flexion and translational deformity; and type 3 injuries demonstrate complete translation of the upper to the lower sacral elements. A type 4 injury was added later by Strange-Vognsen and Lebech. It consists of a segmentally comminuted S1 vertebral body caused by axial implosion of the lumbar spine into the upper sacrum. These four subclassifications correlate with trauma severity and neurologic injury and have implications on the treatment needs of the patient.

Gibbons and associates introduced a sacral neurologic injury classification system, which addresses injury severity. They differentiated patients into having (1) no injury; (2) paresthesias only; (3) motor loss present, but bowel and bladder control intact; and (4) impaired bowel and/or bladder control. This simple and effective system has received only infrequent use to date.

Treatment

Treatment of sacral fractures is directed at optimizing chances for patient survival, assuring stability of the pelvic ring and the lumbosacral junction while maintaining them in physiologic alignment, and protecting neural structures or optimizing their recovery potential in the presence of deficits. Issues surrounding treatment choices can be divided into aspects of nonsurgical versus surgical treatment, timing of intervention, decompressive surgery, and reconstructive, stabilizing procedures.

Nonsurgical Management

The options for this treatment paradigm consist of variable time frames of activity modifications, confinement to bed rest, brace or cast immobilization using a lumbosacral construct with unilateral or bilateral hip spica extensions, or lower extremity skeletal traction (Fig. 2).

Nonsurgical management of sacral fractures has been the treatment of necessity and not choice before the advent of recently evolved surgical treatment options. To date, there are no studies comparing surgical and nonsurgical treatment paradigms and their respective outcomes. Patients with a single-system minimally displaced sacral fracture without neurologic injury may be considered for nonsurgical treatment. Posterior lumbopelvic ligamentous disruption with significant displacement generally is associated with an unfavorable outcome if treated nonsurgically. Clinical signs of a pelvic ring injury being stable are absence of significant patient discomfort with mobilization maneuvers, such as ability to tolerate turning, sitting in a wheelchair, or ambulating with assistive devices. Patients designated for nonsurgical management of more displaced fractures may require bed rest in traction for 8 to 12 weeks with a subsequent period of bracing. This form of treatment for a displaced posterior pelvic injury commonly results in a fracture malunion and is subject to morbidity typically associated with prolonged recumbence.

Timing of Intervention

Most patients with nonpathologic fractures of the sacrum will have sustained this injury as a result of high-energy trauma. The primary concern of the treating physician should therefore be directed toward adequate and timely resuscitation efforts. Patients with an open book-type pelvic ring disruption and refractory hypovolemic shock may benefit from closing down the pelvic volume. This can be achieved with a variety of techniques, such as an anterior external fixator, a pelvic clamp, or a sheet tightly draped around the pelvic ring. Timing of further treatment needs should factor in the possibility of ongoing hemorrhage and the success of restoring a stable hemodynamic status, neurologic injury, and adjuvant soft-tissue injuries. Angiographic embolization can effectively reduce active perisacral arterial bleeding. Most blood lost from displaced pelvic ring fractures involving the sacrum, however, is of venous origin and, therefore, less amenable to successful intravascular hemostasis. Presence of an open sacral fracture, such as associated with rectal perforation or soft-tissue perforation dorsally or in the perineum should be addressed by formal surgical débridement as soon as the patient's general status permits. Patients with progressive neurologic deficits referable to a sacral fracture or posterior pelvic ring disruption similarly should be considered for early surgical decompression and possible internal fixation. The timing of decompressive surgery for patients with established neurologic deficits secondary to sacral fractures remains controversial due to an unclear risk:benefit ratio. Emergent open

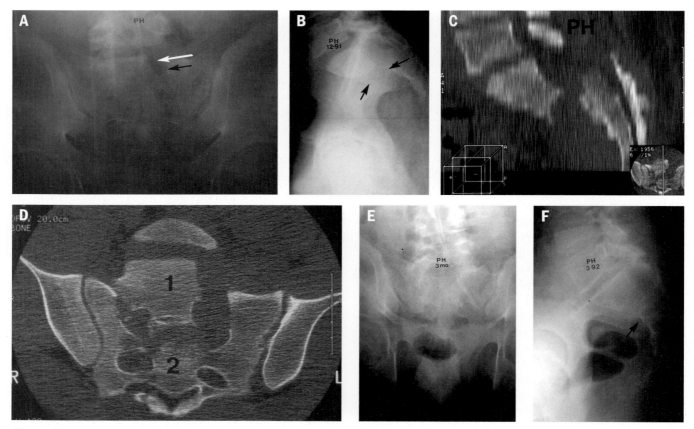

Figure 2 Nonsurgical treatment of sacral fracture. **A,** AP pelvis radiograph of a very obese 20-year-old man taken after he fell down a 30-ft embankment. Clinically the patient was neurologically normal. The arrows depict slight vertical displacement of the left hemipelvis. **B,** The lateral sacral radiograph shows significant translational sacral displacement. **C,** The axial CT and **D,** sagittally reformatted views delineate the fracture anatomy better. The patient refused any surgical intervention or blood transfusions. He was treated with 6 weeks of skeletal traction on his left followed by immobilization with a bilateral pantaloon spica. **E,** The AP and **F,** sacral lateral radiographs demonstrate the closed indirect reduction and early healing at 3 months postoperatively. The patient experienced uneventful fracture healing and an uneventful outcome.

surgical procedures performed on patients with displaced sacral fractures are likely to be associated with significant blood loss and a potentially increased wound infection risk. The thin dorsal postsacral soft-tissue layers, consisting mainly of the multifidus musculature, fascia, and skin are frequently subject to significant injury such as contusion or deglovement.

The postoperative wound infection rate following posterior open reduction and internal fixation of pelvic ring fractures has been reported to be as high as 25%. The potential for cerebrospinal fluid leakage resulting from traumatic dural laceration may add to this infection risk. Early sacral decompression surgery may be futile if primary sacral root transection occurred during trauma. In a postmortem study, 35% of transverse sacral fractures were associated with such traumatic transsections. Protracted compression of nerve roots may, however, lead to decreased chances for neurologic recovery. Unlike the timing of surgery for lumbar cauda equina decompression, the timing of sacral root decompression

has not been studied specifically. Delay of more than 2 or 3 weeks for decompression surgery in patients with traumatic lumbosacral root compression has been associated with more pronounced residual symptoms, such as pain and dysesthesia. Results of late decompressions of posttraumatic sacral root compressions have been described as disappointing. Delay of open reduction and internal fixation of a displaced pelvic or sacral fracture beyond 2 weeks renders fracture reduction eminently more difficult, as well.

Emergent surgical intervention with open reduction of a sacral fracture in a neurologically intact patient, however, is rarely indicated. Posterior sacral soft-tissue breakdown may occur with patients who have displaced and angulated transverse sacral fractures, such as a Denis zone III fracture with Roy-Camille type 3 displacement. Early surgical intervention with the goal of reposition of the fracture angulation may reduce the risk of complex soft-tissue breakdown. Aside from emergent indications, such as mentioned above, most patients with sacral fractures can be safely and effectively treated surgically, if needed, within a 48-hour to 2-week time window.

Decompression Techniques

Indications for decompression surgery for patients with neurologic injuries associated with sacral fractures remain poorly defined. As reflected in numerous studies, over 80% of patients with neurologic trauma in the presence of a sacral fracture may expect some form of improvement, regardless of surgical or nonsurgical management. Removal of a neural canal or foraminal obstruction can, however, reasonably be expected to improve chances for neurologic improvement in the face of a posttraumatic deficit.

Of the two types of sacral approaches (anterior and posterior), the posterior is by far the more clinically relevant for decompression. Anterior decompression surgery using an ilioinguinal or low transperitoneal exposure may be considered for patients with Denis zone I injuries on rare occasion to perform a neurolysis of an L5 root entrapped or tented by a ventrally displaced alar fragment or hypertrophic new bone formation. There are, however, no published reports on the success rate of such surgery.

Traumatic sacral foraminal compression mainly affects the two upper sacral foramina and can be encountered with patients who have Denis zone II fractures. Foraminal root encroachment may be present from comminution of the foramina or may occur after reduction of a pelvic ring fracture. Reduction of the size of the first or second sacral foramen by 50% or more in conjunction with sciatica-type symptoms may be considered for sacral decompression. Unilateral or bilateral parasagittal longitudinal approaches centered over the dorsal sacral foramina have been described for isolated sacral foraminotomies or open reduction and internal fixation of sacroiliac fracture-dislocations. A midline exposure with hemilaminotomy emanating from the L5-S1 laminar interspace, however, remains preferable to parasagittal approaches for a variety of reasons. Midline exposure allows for effective access to the ventral sacral foramina and improved surgical orientation, even in the presence of traumatically distorted anatomy. Comprehensive lumbopelvic stabilization can similarly be carried out from a midline exposure. In contrast, parasagittal approaches cannot sensibly be extended to the lumbar spine. For stabilization purposes, a bilateral parasagittal exposure is usually necessary. This dual surgical approach threatens to devitalize an already traumatically compromised dorsal soft-tissue envelope and has been associated with a high rate of wound-healing complications.

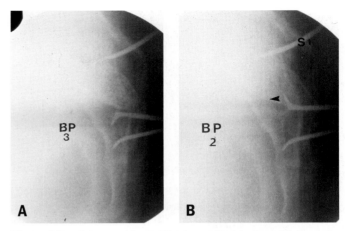

Figure 3 Sacral decompression. **A,** This intraoperative lateral sacral fluoroscopy view demonstrates a Roy-Camille type 2 injury with obvious spinal canal intrusion seen just cranial to the surgical impactor tool. **B,** Ventral spinal canal clearance was accomplished by ventral disimpaction with the impactor tool as shown.

Decompression of the central sacral spinal canal may be performed with straightforward removal of the dorsal neural arch in the sections of the affected areas of the sacrum. The sacral roots are then followed laterally until a large blunt probe can be passed around the nerve into the respective ventral sacral foramen. Should a displaced ventral sacral vertebral body tent or compress the sacral roots, decompression of the anterior canal can be achieved either with fracture reduction or kyphectomy (Fig. 3). Sacral kyphectomy can be done by isolating the sacral roots following sacral laminectomy. After controlling the dense epidural venous plexus surrounding the sacral roots, the roots and veins are laterally reflected from the area of deformity until the ventral spinal canal and its offending structures are fully exposed. The prominent fracture end can then be flattened with a high-speed burr or osteotome. Intraoperative fluoroscopy can be used to minimize the area of surgical dissection and provide helpful orientation.

Surgical Stabilization Techniques

The ability of surgeons to reduce and stabilize posterior pelvic ring elements including the sacrum has changed dramatically with the advent of segmental spinal fixation devices and the evolution of minimally invasive sacroiliac fixation techniques. Before embarking on posterior pelvic ring reduction and fixation attempts, the stabilization needs of the anterior pelvic ring should be contemplated. In pelvic ring fractures, the anterior injury component frequently is more amenable to anatomic reduction and stabilization than the usually more comminuted posterior pelvic injury. Although any anterior instrumentation technique by itself is unable to provide meaningful lasting posterior ring stabilization,

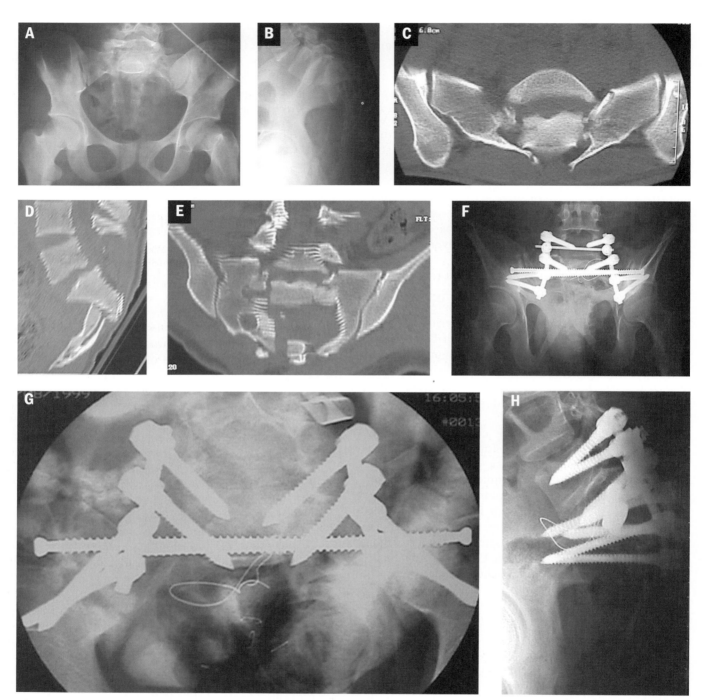

Figure 4 Open reduction and internal fixation of Denis zone III Roy-Camille fracture. This 19-year-old boy crashed with an all-terrain vehicle. He presented with complete L5 level spinal cord injury. **A,** AP trauma pelvis radiograph shows a pseudoinlet view of the S1 vertebral body typically seen with sacral zone III H and U fractures. The patient had an S1 level cauda equina type neurologic injury. **B,** The lateral sacral view confirms presence of a Roy-Camille type 3 fracture (kyphosis and translation). Axial CT **(C)** and sagittal **(D)** as well as coronal **(E)** reformatted views allow for clear delineation of this complex fracture. Following laminectomy and open reduction of the transverse sacral fracture, a pelvic trauma surgeon placed bilateral percutaneous sacroiliac screws. Definitive lumbosacral fixation was then achieved with placement of bilateral L5 and S1 pedicle screws and dual iliac screws attached to the caudal end of the lumbosacral rods. Postoperative radiographs in pelvic outlet **(F)**, inlet **(G)**, and sacral lateral **(H)** projections demonstrate stable anatomic realignment of the sacrum and iliac wings. Postoperatively the patient was mobilized without brace or other restrictions. The patient had a remarkable neurologic recovery, which included sexual function and bowel and bladder control.

it can provide a helpful realignment guide during the posterior procedure. Anterior instrumentation options include external fixation, anterior plating, and retrograde pubic screws. These techniques are described in pertinent chapters of *Orthopaedic Knowledge Update: Trauma 2*.

Posterior pelvic ring stabilization techniques have evolved from posterior transiliac threaded compression rods and posterior tension-band plates applied from open approaches to include percutaneous sacroiliac screw fixation techniques. Advantages of the latter techniques include reduced soft-tissue trauma and the ability to provide rigid stabilization to a trauma patient in supine position. Indications for such percutaneous internal fixation techniques include zone I and II sacral injuries, provided satisfactory closed reduction can be achieved and adequate C-arm visualization is present. Recently, the insertion of sacroiliac screws has been described using a CT scan. This more time-consuming variation reduces the ability to use external reduction maneuvers and is superfluous for surgeons trained in the fluoroscopically guided technique. Risks of this surgical technique consist primarily of loss of reduction and fixation in malreduction. Injuries to neural, vascular, or intestinal structures as a result of drill or screw penetration have been described as rare occurrences. In the presence of a foraminal comminution in a patient with a Denis zone II fracture, overcompression of the fracture during screw placement may lead to secondary foraminal entrapment. Anatomic limitations of percutaneous sacroiliac screw fixation include anomalous transitional lumbosacral anatomy and inability to achieve a closed fracture reduction. There are biomechanical challenges to sacroiliac screw fixation for patients with a vertically displaced Denis zone I or II sacral fracture. Segmental lumbopelvic instrumentation options may limit the likelihood of secondary loss of fracture reduction.

Sacroiliac screw fixation has also been used to stabilize Denis zone III fractures. Thirteen neurologically intact patients with Denis zone III fractures of Roy-Camille subtypes 1 and 2 displacement were successfully treated with indirect fracture reduction and percutaneous sacroiliac screw fixation. All fractures healed clinically and radiographically. One patient treated with unilateral screw placement required hardware revision as a result of disengagement of the sacroiliac screw. The insertion of bilateral sacroiliac screws, each crossing the midline, was recommended for such H and U fracture configurations. This technique was, however, not recommended for patients with displaced and unreducible Roy-Camille type 2 or 3 injuries, or if decompression of neural structures was necessary.

Internal fixation of sacral fractures, such as zone III injuries with a transverse fracture component, historically has been limited to attempts at bilateral sacral alar plating such as suggested by Roy-Camille and associates. This form of internal fixation, however, is unable to provide a meaningful stabilizing effect because of the common occurrence of fracture-site comminution and poor bicortical screw purchase in the hypodense bony composition of the ala. Conventional spinal hardware using hook or screw purchase in the dorsal sacrum is generally unsuitable because of unacceptable posterior hardware prominence and common posterior element comminution. Galveston-type lumboiliac fixation techniques used in deformity surgery lack the biomechanical stiffness and adaptability necessary for routine use in trauma. Recently, the usefulness of iliac screws connected to lumbar and sacral pedicle screw fixation systems has been demonstrated in two clinical series. Using a screw trajectory similar to the insertion technique described for the iliac component of a Luque-type rod, up to 130-mm screws of 9-mm thickness were connected to rods that were cranially attached to L5 and S1 pedicle screws. This form of fixation appears to have superior stiffness to sacroiliac screw fixation and is of low profile.

Thirty-four patients with vertically unstable zone I and II fractures were treated with unilateral segmental lumbopelvic instrumentation and early weight bearing. Successful fracture healing without displacement was found in 91% of patients (Fig. 4). A 9% incidence of wound healing complications and a 3% incidence of iatrogenic radiculopathy were some of the complications encountered. In a variation of the same concept, seven patients with vertically and rotationally displaced zone I and II pelvic ring injuries were treated with bilateral S1 screw fixation and transverse rod connection with Galveston-type rod extension into the ilium on the injured side. Satisfactory healing was reported in six patients. Complications included one deep wound infection and one patient with unresolved neurologic deficits.

For displaced Denis zone III fractures, such as encountered with the Roy-Camille subtypes 3 and 4, the most stable lumbosacral internal fixation construct following neural canal decompression and open fracture reduction can be achieved with L5 and, if possible, S1 pedicle screw fixation, bilateral iliac screw fixation, and connecting rod placement. Supplemental sacroiliac screws can be placed after the fracture reduction and prior to definitive lumbosacral posterior fixation.

Segmental lumbosacral instrumentation using pedicle screws is also the treatment of choice for patients with a lumbosacral fracture-dislocation. In one of the typically small series on this subject, five patients with Isler type 2 and 3 injuries were treated with open reduction and internal fixation using pedicle screws and plate stabilization. Anatomic reduction and brace-free ambulation with uneventful healing outcome was reported for all patients.

Annotated Bibliography

Abumi K, Saita M, Iida T, Kaneda K: Reduction and fixation of sacroiliac joint dislocation by the combined use of S1 pedicle screws and the Galveston technique. *Spine* 2000;25:1977-1983.

Seven patients with iliosacral dislocation were treated using a modification of the Galveston technique. An open reduction was carried out using an iliac bolt inserted via the Galveston technique. Stabilization was accomplished by connecting the medial rod end transversely to S1 pedicle screws. Complete fracture reduction was maintained in four patients.

Nork S, Jones CB, Harding SP, Mirza SK, Routt MLC Jr: Percutaneous stabilization of U-shaped sacral fractures using iliosacral screws: Technique and early results. *J Orthop Trauma* 2001;15:1236-tbd.

Thirteen patients with a U-shaped zone 3 Roy-Camille type 1 or 2 sacral fracture pattern were treated with early closed reduction and percutaneous fixation using sacroiliac screws. Radiographic characteristics and the diagnostic importance of the sacral lateral view for detection of U fractures are described. Seven patients experienced neurologic improvement. There were no infections; fractures in all patients healed. At final radiographic follow-up the sacral kyphosis angle remained unchanged from the initial radiograph.

Routt ML Jr, Nork SE, Mills WJ: Percutaneous fixation of pelvic ring disruptions. *Clin Orthop* 2000;375:15-29.

In this comprehensive review of percutaneous fixation options, the authors identify percutaneous sacroiliac screw fixation as helpful and safe for the treatment of sacral fractures that can be anatomically reduced.

Schildhauer TA, Josten C, Muhr G: Triangular osteosynthesis of vertically unstable sacrum fractures: A new concept allowing early weight-bearing. *J Orthop Trauma* 1998;12:307-314.

Thirty-four patients with vertically displaced zone 2 sacral fractures were treated with lumbopelvic fixation using pedicle screw fixation and long iliac screws based on a concept previously tested in cadaver specimens. The patients were mobilized without brace and progressive weight bearing. Complications included hardware loosening or loss of reduction and wound healing complications (9% of patients).

Simonian PT, Routt ML Jr: Biomechanics of pelvic fixation. *Orthop Clin North Am* 1997;28:351-367.

Biomechanical testing of cadaveric specimens with vertically displaced transforaminal sacral (zone 2) osteotomies was performed to compare different posterior pelvic ring stabilization techniques. Techniques compared included single or double sacroiliac screws, added posterior tension plates, and posterior iliac compression bars. None of these techniques provided significant biomechanical advantages over the other, and none were able to significantly decrease motion at the osteotomy site.

Classic Bibliography

Browner BD, Cole JD, Graham JM, Bondurant FJ, Nunchuck-Burns SK, Colter HB: Delayed posterior internal fixation of unstable pelvic fractures. *J Trauma* 1987;27:998-1006.

Denis F, Davis S, Comfort T: Sacral fractures: An important problem: Retrospective analysis of 236 cases. *Clin Orthop* 1988;227:67-81.

Fisher RG: Sacral fracture with compression of cauda equina: Surgical treatment. *J Trauma* 1988;28:1678-1680.

Fountain SS, Hamilton RD, Jameson RM: Transverse fractures of the sacrum: A report of six cases. *J Bone Joint Surg Am* 1977;59:486-489.

Gibbons KJ, Soloniuk DS, Razack N: Neurological injury and patterns of sacral fractures. *J Neurosurg* 1990;72:889-893.

Gunterberg B: Effects of major resection of the sacrum: Clinical studies on urogenital and anorectal function and a biomechanical study on pelvic strength. *Acta Orthop Scand* 1976;162(suppl):1-38.

Huittinen VM: Lumbosacral nerve injury in fracture of the pelvis: A postmortem radiographic and pathoanatomical study. *Acta Chir Scand* 1972;429(suppl):3-43.

Isler B: Lumbosacral lesions associated with pelvic ring injuries. *J Orthop Trauma* 1990;4:1-6.

Kaehr DM, Anderson PA, Mayo KA, Benca PJ, Benirschke SK: Classification of sacral fractures based on CT imaging. *J Orthop Trauma* 1989;3:163-164.

Kellam JF, McMurtry RY, Paley D, Tile M: The unstable pelvic fracture: Operative treatment. *Orthop Clin North Am* 1987;18:25-41.

Latenser BA, Gentilello LM, Tarver AA, Thalgott JS, Batdorf JW: Improved outcome with early fixation of skeletally unstable pelvic fractures. *J Trauma* 1991;31:28-31.

Letournel E: Traitment chirurgical des traumatisms du basin en dehors des fractures insoles du cotyl. *Rev Chir Orthop Reparatrice Appar Mot* 1981;67:771-782.

Mueller ME, Allgower M, Schneider R, Willeneger H: *Manual of Internal Fixation*, ed 3. New York, NY, Springer Verlag, 1990.

Pohlemann T, Angst M, Schneider E, Ganz R, Tscherne H: Fixation of transforaminal sacrum fractures: A biomechanical study. *J Orthop Trauma* 1993;7:107-117.

Rommens PM, Vanderschot PM, Broos PL: Conventional radiography and CT examination of pelvic ring fractures: A comparative study of 90 patients. *Unfallchirurg* 1992;95:387-392.

Routt MLC Jr, Simonian PT, Swiontkowski MF: Stabilization of pelvic ring disruptions. *Orthop Clin N Am* 1997;28:369-388.

Roy-Camille R, Saillant G, Gagna G, Mazel C: Transverse fracture of the upper sacrum: Suicidal jumper's fracture. *Spine* 1985;10:838-845.

Sabiston CP, Wing PC: Sacral fractures: Classification and neurologic implications. *J Trauma* 1986;26: 1113-1115.

Schnaid E, Eisenstein SM, Drummond-Webb J: Delayed post-traumatic cauda equina compression syndrome. *J Trauma* 1985;25:1099-1101.

Strange-Vognsen HH, Lebech A: An unusual type of fracture in the upper sacrum. *J Orthop Trauma* 1991;5:200-203.

Tile M: Pelvic ring fractures: Should they be fixed? *J Bone Joint Surg Br* 1988;70:1-22.

Wagner TA, Hanscomb D: Abstract: Pedicle screw instrumentation for reduction of acute L5/S1 fracture dislocations. *J Orthop Trauma* 1990;4:215.

Chapter 31

Pediatric Spinal Trauma

Randall T. Loder, MD

Pediatric Spine Imaging

The cervical spine should be evaluated in patients suspected of spinal trauma. Children who are at high risk for cervical spinal cord trauma are those with a history of a traumatic delivery and postpartum findings consistent with spinal shock (hypotonia, areflexia, and apnea). Plain radiographs are taken first, but are often normal. In neonates, the spine is primarily ligamentous and cartilaginous, with a much smaller percentage of ossified tissue; therefore it is amenable to ultrasound evaluation. A recent study documented the usefulness of ultrasound in the cervical spine to diagnose a cervical vertebral diastasis and concomitant spinal cord injury (noted by altered echogenicity of the cord). The ultrasound examination is preferred in the neonate because it can be performed at the bedside in the neonatal intensive care unit (ICU) without sedation or patient transport. CT or MRI evaluation is much more difficult because of problems involved with transportation of an acutely ill neonate as well as technical difficulties with ventilatory and ICU equipment in the scanning suite. The magnets in MRI scanners may interfere with ventilatory equipment.

Although these difficulties are acknowledged, MRI is still the mainstay for evaluation of the spinal cord. Children with an acute hemorrhagic pattern in the spinal cord, as manifested by a central hypointensity on T2-weighted images, have a poor prognosis for return of spinal cord function. MRI is also useful to detect abnormalities such as occult fractures, disc herniations, or epidural hematomas. These non–spinal-cord findings may alter surgical plans and should be known prior to surgery. MRI is recommended for all children with an acute or subacute spinal cord injury or children with incomplete neurologic deficits.

MRI is also useful to evaluate the soft-tissue supportive structures of the pediatric cervical spine. The most common positive MRI finding in children with cervical spine trauma is ligamentous injury. The ligamentous injury often involves more levels than initially indicated on plain radiographs; this is important information for the surgeon because the proposed fusion levels become extended. Those children with cervical spine trauma and a negative MRI study or those with flexion-extension stable cervical spines but a positive MRI study do not develop delayed instability, either clinically or radiographically.

Spinal Cord Injury Without Radiographic Abnormality

Spinal cord injury without radiographic abnormality (SCIWORA) is characterized by severe spinal cord injury without radiographic vertebral fracture or subluxation; flexion-extension lateral radiographs do not demonstrate ligamentous instability. Since the advent of MRI, the lesions in both the spinal cord and the ligamentous spinal structures have been readily documented. Nearly all of the lesions have been limited to a single region of the spinal column and usually occur in the upper thoracic and cervical spine. Lower thoracic lesions, when they do occur, are typically in older children.

Two recent case reports have brought attention to the fact that bifocal lesions can occur. One occurred in a 3-year-old boy, who was an unrestrained back-seat passenger involved in a motor vehicle accident and sustained a bifocal lesion at the lower cervical spine and the thoracolumbar junction. Another was in a 2-year-old boy who was knocked down by a car and sustained a bifocal lesion at both the C2 and T2 levels.

Another case report has described a lower thoracic lesion in a younger child. A 3-year-old girl, who was an unrestrained back-seat passenger seated on her mother's lap, was involved in a head-on motor vehicle accident and sustained a lower thoracic SCIWORA. This was believed to be a traction injury, because the mother's hands acted as a lap-belt restraint. The recommended acute treatment for SCIWORA is the administration of steroids and spinal immobilization.

Injury Mechanisms

Vertebral fractures in the immature spine have been studied in porcine and human cadaver spines. The cartilage end plate is the weakest point to pure compression in both adolescent porcine and human specimens. Fractures rarely are seen on plain radiographs; when they are seen on radiographs, they appear as a typical lumbar apophyseal fracture-separation in adolescents. These "injuries" usually are seen on MRI and always are documented histologically, with a failure at the end plate-bone junction.

Child Abuse

Child abuse is an unfortunate etiology of spine fractures in the younger child, with several recent reports continuing to remind physicians of this mechanism. Most of the recent reports have focused on the cervical spine. Because the history of trauma usually is not given, the physician is misled and pursues other diagnoses, such as infection/inflammatory processes or neoplasia (either primary or metastatic), in the differential diagnosis of the infant or toddler with a sudden recent onset of quadriplegia.

These spinal cord injuries result from severe hyperflexion caused by violent shaking. It is an atypical form of the shaken baby syndrome, in that retinal and cerebral hemorrhages are absent. Any young child with a recent and/or sudden onset of spinal cord dysfunction should be considered a possible victim of child abuse. The child at high risk is one with an implausible history, especially if the child has other inadequately explained injuries of various ages.

The child often is brought in as a floppy infant without external signs of injury, with or without respiratory failure. Retinal hemorrhages are infrequent, leading the physician away from considering shaking in the differential diagnosis. Bone scans are very useful to assess for other osseous injuries. Radiographs of the spine may be normal with only MRI demonstrating the neural injury—a SCIWORA picture. The etiology becomes apparent only after both MRI (which determines the neural injury) and the bone scan (which often reveals other skeletal injuries from the violent shaking) are obtained.

The thoracolumbar spine may also be involved in child abuse. Again, there is a rapid-onset paraplegia that often mimics sepsis or other inflammatory/neoplastic processes. CT studies of these children have demonstrated circumferential growth-plate fracture patterns. A separation of the vertebral centrum from the neurocentral synchondrosis occurs in a Salter I fashion. It is a bilateral separation, allowing the freed centrum to rotate and subluxate posteriorly, resulting in cord compression. The mechanism is most likely a combination of axial loading, flexion, and rotation. CT scans with three-dimensional reconstructions delineate the bony anatomy, and MRI scans delineate the neural injury and cord impingement. This fracture pattern usually needs an anterior open reduction/decompression and external immobilization.

Diving Injuries

Diving injuries are a significant cause of spinal cord injuries in older children and adolescents. Recreational diving accounts for 70% of all acute sports-related spinal cord injuries. Most diving injuries are the result of direct head impact on the pool bottom. In spite of these alarming statistics, most children receive little or no instruction in proper diving techniques.

Safe water diving depths recommended by the YMCA for dives off the deck are 2.74 m when learning and 1.5 m after having learned how to dive. The American Red Cross recommends the same depths for deck dives and also recommends a depth of 1.52 m for block dives. The National Collegiate Athletic Association prefers a depth of 2.13 m and certainly no less than 1.22 m for dives off starting blocks at the collegiate level. However, translation of those depths into velocities of the diver in the water were not known for children. This information is crucial because the momentum of head impact at a velocity of 0.6 m/s is enough to dislocate the adult cervical spine, and the momentum of head impact at a velocity of 1.2 m/s is enough to crush the adult cervical spine. These threshold velocities are likely less in children because of the increased spinal laxity in children.

Australian investigators studied 26 children aged 6 to 8 years and looked at body velocities as a function of water depth and dive type. They found that for children performing a standing deck dive, 23% reached a velocity of 0.6 m/s, 11% reached a velocity of 1.2 m/s, and 3.5% reached a velocity of 2.4 m/s at a water depth of 1 m. These numbers were increased for dives off of blocks, with 31% reaching 0.6 m/s, 20% reaching 1.2 m/s, and 12% having reached 1.8 m/s. They concluded that a water depth of at least 2 m should be required for all diving instruction, because some of the children traveled through a depth of 1.5 m at potentially dangerous velocities (> 0.6 m/s).

This same group also studied first-year college students to obtain normative diving data in the age range most likely to sustain a spinal cord injury while diving. The students were unaware that the dive was the focal point of the study. The three most important factors in determining dive depths were: (1) distance from the starting point at maximum depth, (2) flight distance, and

(3) angle of entry into the water. It is therefore recommended that diving instructors at the high school and college levels reinforce so-called "steering-up" techniques, which are used to surface in as short a distance as possible. The diver should also strive to surface as soon as possible by maximizing flight distance and aiming for a low entry angle.

Car Restraint Systems

There is no doubt that the use of lap belts has significantly decreased deaths of both adults and children from motor vehicle crashes. However, it is also well known that lap belts can produce specific injury patterns. The pediatric lap-belt complex consists of both intra-abdominal and lumbar spine injuries. The spine injury is typically a Chance variant: a flexion-distraction injury resulting in either ligamentous or bony disruption of the posterior column with or without anterior compression.

In one report of 28 children with lap-belt lumbar spine injuries, seven children were noted to have anterior compression without posterior disruption. Although the compression ranged from 14% to 40%, the average was 20% and there were no acute kyphotic deformities. All seven children were neurologically intact and all were treated nonsurgically. A brace or body jacket was recommended if the anterior compression was 33% or more. It was postulated that the increased elasticity of the pediatric spine resulted in this new variant of lap-belt injury. The ligamentous elasticity in children allowed for the lap-belt forces to be dissipated in the posterior elements without disruption, with the anterior bony column then failing in flexion.

Abdominal injuries still remain a significant problem in the pediatric lap-belt complex. In the above study, four of the seven children sustained intra-abdominal injuries, with two requiring laparotomy. Another report described three children, all wearing lap belts, in the rear seat of a four-wheel-drive vehicle. All three sustained abdominal injuries and Chance fractures. Each spinal injury was a different pattern. These data substantiate the need for shoulder harnesses to prevent these injuries. Also, the lap belt should always fit over the proximal thighs and not the abdomen to reduce this type of injury.

Air bags are a significant mechanism of injury to children occupying the front seats of cars equipped with them. The trauma inflicted to infants and small children during deployment of the air bag can be lethal, often from craniocervical trauma. Two case reports of small children with fatal spinal injuries from air-bag deployment warrant discussion.

The children were ages 2 and 5 years and both were front seat passengers restrained by lap/shoulder belts. One car was rear-ended at a speed of 30 mph and the other hit a parking barrier at 5 to 10 mph. The air bags deployed in both instances, resulting in death of the two children. The 5-year-old boy, who was riding in the car that hit the parking barrier, sustained a complete C2-3 dislocation and severe skull injury. The 2-year-old girl sustained a transection of the spinal cord at the junction of the medulla oblongata and spinal cord when the car in which she was riding was rear-ended. The mechanism of injury was considered to be a violent hyperextension of the neck (similar to that for judicial hanging). These injuries are not prevented by the shoulder/lap belt but rather arise by direct impact of the rapidly expanding air bag on the child's head with resultant extreme hyperextension of the cervical spine. Thus, no child should be in a seat in which an air bag is present.

Cervical Spine Injuries

General teaching has been that pediatric cervical spine injuries usually involve the upper cervical spine (above C4) in children younger than age 8 years and the lower cervical spine (below C4) in children 8 years of age or older. The report of a recent series of 34 children between 16 months and 16 years of age with cervical spine injuries has questioned this concept. No difference was noted in injury level by age; 50% of those children younger than 8 years of age had injuries below C4. This study also confirmed the high association of head injuries with cervical spine injuries and subsequent mortality due to the head injury; 14 of the 34 children died.

It was postulated that these lower cervical spine injuries are occurring in children between ages 5 and 9 years as a result of inadequate car restraint systems. In these younger children, the shoulder belt impinges on the neck during accelerated hyperflexion, resulting in lower cervical spine injury. This injury could be prevented only by raising the child such that the shoulder belt actually traverses the shoulder and not the neck, which would require a booster seat type of system.

Odontoid fractures in children have also been studied. The report of a recent series covered 15 children, all younger than 6 years of age (average age, 2 years 6 months). Eight fractures were the result of a motor vehicle crash while the child was in a forward-facing car seat, emphasizing the need for all children to be maintained in rear-facing seating systems as long as possible. Eight of the children sustained an associated spinal cord injury, which is a much higher prevalence than in previous series. All but one of the spinal cord injuries were at neurologic levels lower than C2, with MRI scans showing the injury at the cervicothoracic junction. Thus, any pediatric spinal cord injury at the cervicothoracic junction suggests the possibility of a C2 fracture and appropriate evaluation should be performed. Nonsurgical therapy was recommended for these odontoid fractures.

In two other series from Europe, the authors studied four children, ages 18 months to 2 years, with odontoid fractures. In three of these four children, surgical treatment was selected because of major instability or associated head injury. Anterior screw fixation was used in some of the children; a cannulated scaphoid screw system with different thread pitch on opposite screw ends was used. This system has not been given appropriate approval by the United States Food and Drug Administration, however.

The biomechanics of odontoid fractures in children has been studied in a 3-year-old child dummy model restrained by a 4-point system while facing forward. A simple shearing force of 600 N at the moment of maximum anterior flexion of the head is enough to cause a fracture through the synchondrosis of the odontoid. This bending force causes dislocation of the odontoid during accelerated flexion of the cervical spine. This accelerated flexion is not possible if the child is facing backward in a seating system. Backward facing car seats are thus recommended as long as possible during infancy and toddlerhood.

Pediatric Sacral Fractures

Three cases of traumatic sacral fractures in adolescents have been described recently. All occurred at the S1-S2 level. All were due to violent trauma, with a forward force on the sacrum while the rest of the pelvis was fixed. The fractures are a shear fracture, Denis type III, Salter type IV, resulting in a traumatic spondylolisthesis of S1 and S2 at the level of the neural foramen. The inferior sacrum becomes more vertical with an S1-S2 junctional kyphosis. This fracture pattern is a result of the unique development of the sacrum. The sacrum develops from five independent vertebrae that do not completely fuse until age 25 to 30 years. It begins to fuse at S4-S5 and progresses proximally; thus the S1-S2 cartilage junction in adolescents is susceptible to the development of a physeal fracture under the appropriate conditions.

Stress fractures of the sacrum may also occur in older children or adolescents who are athletic. The typical complaints are buttock and low back pain. Other differential diagnoses are spondylolysis/listhesis, inflammatory or infectious disorders, or neoplasia. Plain radiographs are typically negative. A bone scan will demonstrate increased uptake. If a stress fracture is in the differential diagnosis after obtaining the bone scan, then a CT scan is recommended. The CT scan will demonstrate linear band-like high attenuation areas

parallel to the sacroiliac joint with band-like radiolucent regions and cortical buckling. In this instance, MRI is confusing and does not reliably differentiate a stress fracture from neoplasia.

Atlantoaxial Rotatory Subluxation/Fixation

Atlantoaxial rotatory subluxation (AARS) is seen as torticollis in the child. Common etiologies of childhood AARS are postinfectious (for example, the common upper respiratory infection), postoperative (for example, after tonsillectomy), ligamentous laxity (for example, Marfan syndrome), and trauma. In children, the ligaments and joint capsules of the C1-2 facets are sufficiently elastic to allow a subluxation without disruption of the joints. Also, the C1-2 facet joints are more horizontally oriented in children than in adults, allowing for easier subluxation. After the subluxation, a persistent muscle spasm (such as seen after a clavicle fracture) or synovitis of the C1-2 joints (such as seen after an upper respiratory infection) will prevent reduction; then the AARS becomes fixed with the development of atlantoaxial rotatory fixation (AARF).

Recently it has been described that AARS can be masked after a clavicle fracture. Two children with clavicle fractures developed AARS; the torticollis remained after union of the clavicle fracture, with development of AARF. Both children had sustained falls onto their neck and complained of prolonged torticollis and neck pain. Thus an association should always be considered in children who have a clavicular fracture and an acute torticollis. This consideration is important because the early treatment of AARS often will prevent the development of AARF. The initial early treatment of AARS is immobilization and/or traction and is likely to be curative if undertaken early. In a series of 15 children with AARS who had traction or immobilization as the inital therapy, nine were cured and six developed a recurrence. The average duration of the AARS was much less in those children in whom there was no recurrence (14 versus 70 days). If there is a recurrence or nonsurgical therapy fails, then a C1-2 fusion is needed after halo-traction to achieve straightforward alignment of the head and neck.

Management of Traumatic Injuries in the Pediatric Spine

Halo Use

Halo use for the managment of traumatic injuries in the pediatric cervical spine allows for more rigid immobilization than a Minerva cast and allows for mobilization of the child, which is so important in the presence of polytrauma or paralysis so that respiratory complications are minimized. The pediatric skull is thinner than the adult skull and can be quite variable, especially before the age of 6 years. There is, however, a trend toward thicker skulls after 10 years of age. In children younger than 10 years of age a preapplication CT scan has been recommended to accurately assess skull thickness. Because of this skull thinness, more than four pins are recommended when placing a pediatric halo in order to allow for the application of less torque per pin to achieve fixation. The pins should be placed anterolaterally and posterolaterally where the skull is the thickest, using the CT scan as a guide. Complications related to a halo vest are more common in children than in adults. The most common complication is pin site infection. If a pin complication occurs, having multiple pins allows for simple removal of a pin without having to reinsert another pin because the other pins will likely be adequate.

Immobilization During Transport

Because of the large head size of infants and young children, the standard adult backboard, when used for children, places the cervical spine in kyphosis. To avoid this problem, the torso must be raised or the head lowered such that the external auditory meatus is in line with the shoulder.

Difficulties in obtaining neutral cervical spine positions have been further documented recently. A group of 118 children with an average age of 7.9 years who sustained potential cervical injuries was studied. All had been transported on standard adult boards using three different types of immobilization: cervical collar, backboard, and towels; cervical collar, backboard, and blocks; and cervical collar, backboard, with other devices. All were blunt trauma victims and all received lateral radiographs of the cervical spine upon arrival in the emergency department before removal from the board. The cervical Cobb angles ranged from 27° kyphosis to 27° lordosis; only 11% were in the neutral position and 61% had more than 5° of flexion or extension. None of the three different types of immobilization was superior in consistently protecting the cervical spine from angulation.

Annotated Bibliography

Blanksby BA, Wearne FK, Elliott BC: Safe depths for teaching children to dive. *Aust J Sci Med Sport* 1996;28:79-85.

Blitvich JD, McElroy GK, Blanksby BA, Douglas GA: Characteristics of "low risk" and "high risk" dives by young adults: Risk reduction in spinal cord injury. *Spinal Cord* 1999;37:553-559.
These two articles discuss safe diving depths and velocities for both children and young adults. It is recommended that a water depth of 2 m or more be required for all diving instruction. Divers also should be taught to maximize flight distance, minimize entry angle, and use steering swimming techniques to minimize dive depth.

Carrion WV, Dormans JP, Drummond DS, Christofersen MR: Circumferential growth plate fracture of the thoracolumbar spine from child abuse. *J Pediatr Orthop* 1996;16:210-214.
Children who are victims of child abuse were found to have a newly described fracture pattern: a separation of the vertebral centrum from the polar growth centers above and below, analogous to a Salter I fracture. The posterior elements were also separated by a fracture through the neurocentral synchondrosis, allowing the centrum to rotate into the neural canal as a free fragment.

Cooper JT, Balding LE, Jordan FB: Airbag mediated death of a two-year-old child wearing a shoulder/lap belt. *J Forensic Sci* 1998;43:1077-1081.

Willis BK, Smith JL, Falkner LD, Vernon DD, Walker ML: Fatal air bag mediated craniocervical trauma in a child. *Pediatr Neurosurg* 1996;24:323-327.
These two articles discuss the pathology and pathomechanics of recent pediatric deaths caused by deployment of airbags.

Curran C, Dietrich AM, Bowman MJ, Ginn-Pease ME, King DR, Kosnik E: Pediatric cervical-spine immobilization: Achieving neutral position? *J Trauma* 1995;39:729-732.
A review of 118 patients with an average age of 7.9 years who required spinal immobilization demonstrated that only 12 were in a neutral position on lateral cervical spine radiographs. Greater than 5° of kyphosis and lordosis was observed in 60%. No single device provided superior protection from angulation of the cervical spine.

de Vries E, Robben SG, van den Anker JN: Radiologic imaging of severe cervical spinal cord birth trauma. *Eur J Pediatr* 1995;154:230-232.

These authors describe the usefulness of ultrasound to evaluate and diagnose spinal cord lesions in the neonate. It should be considered as the initial imaging technique.

Dormans J, Criscitiello AA, Drummond DS, Davidson RS: Complications in children managed with immobilization in a halo vest. *J Bone Joint Surg Am* 1995;77: 1370-1373.

In 37 children ages 3 to 16 years who were managed in a halo vest, the complication rate was 68%; pin-site infections were the most common complication (occurring in 22 of 25 children). Those children with more than four pins had a similar rate of complications as those managed with a standard four-pin construct. In spite of the high complication rate, all children were able to wear the halo until successful fracture union or arthrodesis had occurred.

Duprez T, De Merlier Y, Clapuyt P, Clement de Cléty S, Cosnard G, Gadisseux JF: Early cord degeneration in bifocal SCIWORA: A case report. *Pediatr Radiol* 1998; 28:186-188.

This article discusses a 2-year-old boy with flaccid high-level paraplegia after being knocked down by a car. There were two focal lesions within the spinal cord (C7 and T2). These two locations likely represent the sites of impact of the posterior arches on the spinal cord.

Givens TG, Polley KA, Smith GF, Hardin WD Jr: Pediatric cervical spine injury: A three-year experience. *J Trauma* 1996;41:310-314.

A review of 34 children from 16 months to 16 years of age with cervical spine injuries demonstrated that 50% of the children younger than 8 years of age had injuries below the C4 level. Overall mortality was 41%, and 12 of the 15 vehicle occupants were unrestrained or improperly restrained.

Herzka A, Sponseller PD, Pyeritz RE: Alantoaxial rotatory subluxation in patients with Marfan syndrome: A report of three cases. *Spine* 2000;25:524-526.

Two patients with Marfan syndrome developed AARS after surgery, and one after minor trauma. The cervical and bony ligamentous abnormalities seen in Marfan syndrome may increase their risk for AARS. Special attention during surgery should be given to this patient population.

Karlsson L, Lundin O, Ekström L, Hansson T, Swärd L: Injuries in adolescent spine exposed to compressive loads: An experimental cadaveric study. *J Spinal Disord* 1998;11:501-507.

Lundin O, Ekström L, Hellström M, Holm S, Swärd L: Injuries in the adolescent porcine spine exposed to mechanical compression. *Spine* 1998;23:2574-2579.

These two articles demonstrated that in both the juvenile pig and human adolescents cartilaginous end plate failure was the most likely point of failure to compressive loads.

Keiper MD, Zimmerman RA, Bilaniuk LT: MRI in the assessment of the supportive soft tissues of the cervical spine in acute trauma in children. *Neuroradiology* 1998; 40:359-363.

The authors reviewed 52 children with cervical spinal trauma. MRI was positive in 16 of the 52; posterior soft-tissue or ligamentous injury was the most common finding in the 10 patients with mild trauma. MRI clearly identified the spinal cord injuries and transcanalicular hemorrhage in the six children with more severe trauma. No child with a normal MRI or any of the 10 with radiographically stable MRI scans positive for soft-tissue injury developed delayed clinical or radiographic instability.

Odent T, Langlais J, Glorion C, Kassis B, Bataille J, Pouliquen J-C: Fractures of the odontoid process: A report of 15 cases in children younger than 6 years. *J Pediatr Orthop* 1999;19:51-54.

This retrospective review of 15 children younger than 6 years of age demonstrated a high level of neurologic injury (8, or 53%). The level of neurologic injury was at the cervicothoracic junction rather than at the fracture.

Pollina J, Li V: Tandem spinal cord injuries without radiographic abnormalities in a young child. *Pediatr Neurosurg* 1999;30:263-266.

This article describes the case of a 3-year-old boy who was an unrestrained back seat passenger involved in a motor vehicle crash. A SCIWORA at both the lower cervical and thoracolumbar spinal cord occurred.

Sturm PF, Glass RB, Sivit CJ, Eichelberger MR: Lumbar compression fractures secondary to lap-belt use in children. *J Pediatr Orthop* 1995;15:521-523.

Seven children with seat belt injuries seen over a 10-year period sustained an anterior compression fracture alone, rather than the expected flexion-distraction injury. Nonsurgical care was recommended; four of the seven children suffered associated abdominal injuries.

Trumble J, Myslinski J: Lower thoracic SCIWORA in a 3-year-old child: Case report. *Pediatr Emerg Care* 2000; 16:91-93.

The case of a 34-month-old girl who sustained a SCIWORA after a motor vehicle crash is described. The neurologic level was T12-L1, which was different from the more common cervical level in young children.

Classic Bibliography

AL-Etani H, D'Astous J, Letts M, Hahn M, Yeadon A: Masked rotatory subluxation of the atlas associated with fracture of the clavicle: A clinical and biomechanical analysis. *Am J Orthop* 1998;27:375-380.

Blauth M, Schmidt U, Otte D, Krettek C: Fractures of the odontoid process in small children: Biomechanical analysis and report of three cases. *Eur Spine J* 1996;5:63-70.

Felsberg GJ, Tien RD, Osumi AK, Cardenas CA: Utility of MR imaging in pediatric spinal cord injury. *Pediatr Radiol* 1995;25:131-135.

Godard J, Hadji M, Raul JS: Odontoid fractures in the child with neurological injury: Direct anterior osteosynthesis with a cortico-spongious screw and literature review. *Childs Nerv Syst* 1997;13:105-107.

Letts M, Kaylor D, Gouw G:A biomechanical analysis of halo fixation in children. *J Bone Joint Surg Br* 1988; 70:277-279.

Martin J, Brandser EA, Shin MJ, Buckwalter JA: Fatigue fracture of the sacrum in a child. *Can Assoc Radiol J* 1995;46:468-470.

Novkov HV, Tanchev PJ, Gyorev IS: Severe fracture-dislocation of SI in a 12-year-old boy: A case report. *Spine* 1996;21:2500-2503.

Piatt JH Jr, Steinberg M: Isolated spinal cord injury as a presentation of child abuse. *Pediatrics* 1995;96:780-782.

Rooks VJ, Sisler C, Burton B: Cervical spine injury in child abuse: Report of two cases. *Pediatr Radiol* 1998; 28:193-195.

Sapkas G, Makris A, Korres D, Kyratzoulis J, Meleteas E, Antoniadis A: Anteriorly displaced transverse fractures of the sacrum in adolescents: Report of two cases. *Eur Spine J* 1997;6:342-346.

Subach BR, McLaughlin MR, Albright AL, Pollack IF: Current management of pediatric atlantoaxial rotatory subluxation. *Spine* 1998;23:2174-2179.

Thomas NH, Robinson L, Evans A, Bullock P: The floppy infant: A new manifestation of nonaccidental injury. *Pediatr Neurosurg* 1995;23:188-191.

Voss L, Cole PA, D'Amato C: Pediatric Chance fractures from lapbelts: Unique case report of three in one accident. *J Orthop Trauma* 1996;10:421-428.

Chapter 32

Surgical Treatment of Degenerative Cervical Disc Disease

John G. Heller, MD

Introduction

Degenerative cervical disc disease comprises a spectrum of disorders ranging from internal disc disruption to focal soft-disc herniations to spondylosis with its osteophyte formation. The process may be isolated to a single level in the cervical spine or involve multiple levels, most commonly in the subaxial cervical spine. This process, frequently referred to as spondylosis, is a by-product of normal age-related changes. Asymptomatic individuals older than 60 years of age have a high prevalence of radiographic evidence of disc degeneration. By age 70 years, 70% of women and 95% of men can be anticipated to have such radiographic changes, most of which are asymptomatic. The process is most prevalent at the C5-6 level, followed by C6-7 and C4-5. As the aging process proceeds, a person's physiologic lordosis diminishes, as does the active range of motion. In 10-year follow-up studies of those asymptomatic patients in whom degenerative changes existed there was a fourfold greater likelihood of progression than in those with normal initial films. Also, 15% of the originally asymptomatic study population required surgical intervention during the 10-year follow-up interval. Degenerative spondylolistheses were much more likely to occur in patients older than age 70 years, almost exclusively at C3-4 or C 4-5 (Fig. 1).

If spondylosis is a manifestation of aging, clinically significant cervical disc degeneration must be defined as those symptoms and signs arising as a manifestation of either spondylosis or other disc pathology. Exactly what symptoms and signs are evident will depend on which neurologic structures are being compressed, such as the spinal cord, nerve root(s), or sinuvertebral nerve. Moreover, there are mesodermal structures in the cervical spine that are innervated with afferent nociceptive fibers. These structures include the anulus, the posterior longitudinal ligament, the facet capsule, and possibly the ventral aspect of the dura. Each of these structures may give rise to pain, and the clinical presentation of a patient will depend on which structures are compro-

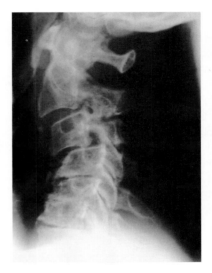

Figure 1 Lateral cervical radiograph of a 63-year-old man who recently developed myelopathy. He had minor neck pain complaints and reduced motion for years before the onset of neurologic signs and symptoms, which were ultimately caused by the degenerative spondylolisthesis at C3-4. Note the typical changes of advanced spondylosis in the subaxial region: Decreased disc height, sclerosis, osteophyte formation, and kyphosis.

mised. Because of variability in afferent circuits and multiple cross-connection variations, protean symptom patterns are the rule, not the exception.

Patterns of pain may be appendicular from a compromised root or in the distribution of the spinal cord. Among the appendicular patterns, orthopaedists must look beyond the standard familiar dermatomal charts to myotomal and sclerotomal patterns that are quite common. Awareness of these other embryologic patterns helps explain why such a small percentage of patients with single root pathology conform to the dermatome maps committed to memory by medical students. The clinician must also be aware of variations in the formation of the brachial plexus. Because of a pre- or post-fixed plexus pattern, the patient's clinical symptoms may actually be caused by an anatomic lesion that is one level above or below the anticipated level. When the imaging studies reveal a lesion that is not specific or exactly consistent with what would be expected on the basis of the history and physical examination, selective nerve root blocks may be helpful in confirming the source of the pain and a brachial plexus anomaly.

Surgery is indicated in the treatment of degenerative cervical disc disease when the patient has failed medical management. It is conceptually appealing to separately consider those patients who have disorders of nerve root function (radiculopathy), those with spinal cord lesions (myelopathy), and those with primarily axial pain. The natural history of an acute radiculopathy is favorable. Most patients will improve with time as the acute inflammatory cycle initiated by the compressive lesion resolves. It also is reasonably likely that most of the objective signs will improve with time. Surgery for radiculopathy is reserved for those patients who have sufficient and intractable pain or functional neurologic deficits that interfere with their professional or personal function. Some judgment must be used in this situation because people have varying tolerance for pain, and the impact of a given neurologic deficit will have different implications for different individuals. The symptoms and signs must be viewed within the context of the patient's functional needs.

The natural history of myelopathy is generally unfavorable with a tendency toward stepwise worsening over time. However, with a particular episode of symptoms and signs, a patient should be advised that a rule of thirds applies. One third of patients will improve, another third will remain unchanged, and the final third will continue to deteriorate. Predicting what will happen to a given patient is the challenge. At the time of evaluation, it is reasonable to recommend surgical care if signs of myelopathy exist and there has been a history of clinical progression over the preceding weeks or months. Also, if the degree of spinal cord dysfunction, such as an unsteady gait, hand dysfunction, or neurogenic bowel/bladder disturbance impairs daily activities, then surgical treatment is appropriate. Patients with lesser degrees of dysfunction and those with minor clinical signs may be treated medically and observed over time. They should be advised of the symptoms, which signal progression of spinal cord dysfunction, because the symptoms can be subtle and readily confused with signs of aging by the patient and family.

The surgeon should exercise considerable restraint in recommending surgical care for axial pain. The outcomes of surgery for this indication have been unpredictable and limited successes. The surgery is more likely to be successful in the event that a discrete lesion exists, especially if it can be established as the probable source of the pain. For example, a good outcome could reasonably be assured for an isolated disc herniation in an otherwise normal neck or for focal facet arthropathy that was confirmed by a fluoroscopically guided facet block. Due restraint is appropriate when multiple levels are abnormal, as is often the case in spondylosis or following acceleration injuries (whiplash) when the precise source(s) of the pain is not clear, especially when

mitigating psychosocial influences may be at work. If a course of surgical treatment is chosen by mutual agreement between patient and surgeon, the patient must clearly be aware that the degree of relief can be unpredictable, and that a major practical risk of the procedure could be failure to relieve the original complaint.

If the surgeon is called on to design an operation to relieve the patient's complaints and/or neurologic deficit, familiarity with the pathologic processes and their influence on the local structures guides a rational choice among the available surgical alternatives. The surgeon must address a number of questions. (1) Which neurologic structure is compromised (spinal cord, nerve root[s], or both)? (2) Is the source of the compression a soft-disc herniation, an osteophyte, ossification of the posterior longitudinal ligament (OPLL), ossification of the ligamentum flavum, or a facet ganglion cyst? (3) From what direction is the structure being compromised: anterior, posterior, or both? (4) How many levels are involved in the pathologic process? (5) What is the patient's cervical alignment? (6) Are there coexistent patterns of segmental instability? (7) Has the patient had any prior cervical spine or head/neck operations or radiation therapy? (8) What relevant medical comorbidities exist that might influence the choice of treatment?

Armed with the answers to these questions, the surgeon can select operations performed from an anterior approach, posterior approach, or a combination thereof. The first objective is to decompress the compromised neural elements. While performing the decompression, tissue (bone, disc, ligament, and so forth) may be excised to such a degree that segmental stability is lost. In such cases, the question of reconstruction or fusion needs to be addressed and the need for internal and/or external fixation must be determined.

Soft-Disc Herniation

Anterior Cervical Discectomy and Fusion

Disc herniations in the cervical spine may occur into the central part of the spine canal, out through the neuroforamen, or anywhere in between (Fig. 2). The location of the herniated fragment itself will determine whether the spinal cord, nerve root, or both are compromised. Accordingly, the patient's symptoms and signs should reflect which of these structures are involved. Currently, anterior cervical discectomy and fusion is the most prevalent operation used for treatment of cervical disc herniation. Anterior cervical discectomy alone was popular for a brief period but fell into disfavor because of persistent postoperative axial pain and the tendency for the disc space to settle into kyphosis.

The anterior surgical approach to the cervical spine

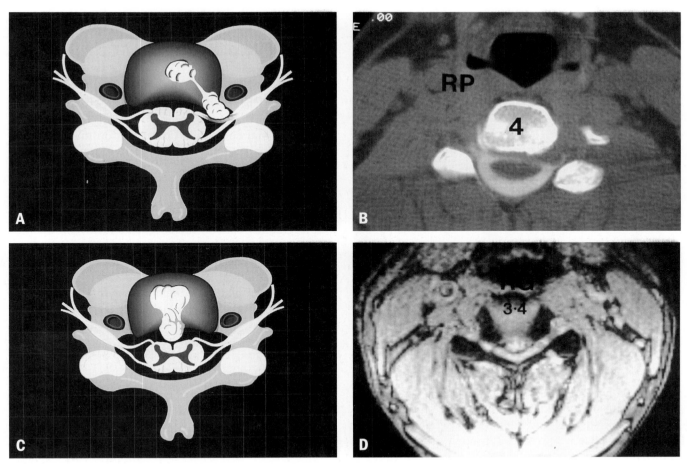

Figure 2 An axial schematic representation of a right posterolateral 'soft' disc herniation **(A)** with a corresponding CT/myelogram image **(B)** from a patient with a left C4-5 disc herniation causing a C5 radiculopathy. This pathology could be effectively treated with either an anterior cervical discectomy and fusion or a posterior keyhole laminoforaminotomy. In contrast, **C** and **D** illustrate a central cervical disc herniation with severe cord compression and advanced myelopathy that should be treated with an anterior excision to avoid manipulation of the spinal cord. Indirect decompression via a laminoplasty might also be considered. Attempts to remove the disc fragment via a posterior exposure would risk further spinal cord injury.

has been well described and is not within the scope of this chapter. However, some comments are in order regarding speech and swallowing disturbance after such exposures due to the risk of injury to the recurrent laryngeal nerve. Often a right-handed surgeon will favor the convenience of an approach through the right-hand side, whereas a left-handed surgeon will select the converse. It was believed that the likelihood of recurrent laryngeal injury was considerably less when approaching from the left-hand side. However, recent investigations have led surgeons to question whether clinically apparent nerve injuries are any more likely on either side. New data suggest that the injury may often be endolaryngeal and that an endotracheal tube may play a role in the pathogenesis. The role of the superior laryngeal nerve in postoperative dysphagia and speech abnormalities has received increasing attention. Therefore, note should be taken of the possibility of prior nerve injury before planning revision anterior cervical

surgery. Preoperative consultation may be appropriate to assess vocal cord function before committing to the side of approach.

An anterior exposure readily affords complete evacuation of the nuclear material and cartilaginous end plate. Defects in the posterior anulus and posterior longitudinal ligament (PLL) must be carefully sought and any sequestered fragments retrieved. If the amount of disc material removed at the time of surgery does not correspond with the size and location of the fragments on the preoperative imaging studies, the surgeon should incise or remove the PLL and possibly a few millimeters of the posterior vertebral margins to ensure that the epidural space has been adequately decompressed (Fig. 3).

Following a discectomy, an anterior interbody fusion must be achieved. A high-speed burr is typically used to remove the superficial portion of the vertebral end plates, thus rendering two parallel graft recipient surfaces. In

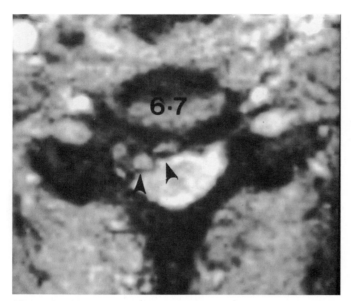

Figure 3 This axial MRI demonstrates multiple herniated disc fragments in the epidural space. The operating surgeon must be satisfied that all clinically relevant sources of neural compression have been removed. Correlation of the preoperative imaging and the intraoperative findings is essential. Removal of the PLL and additional bone can help ensure an adequate decompression in such circumstances.

selecting between the use of autologous iliac crest graft and allograft, the surgeon should recognize the trade-off that exists for surgeon and patient alike. Patient and surgeon convenience is maximized through the use of allograft. Time in surgery is reduced and the potential complications associated with the bone graft donor site are avoided. However, this enhanced convenience comes at the expense of a reduction in the probability of graft healing and the speed with which such a graft heals. The choice can be made all the more complicated by other variables, such as the presence or absence of tobacco product use, the use of adjunctive internal fixation, and the selected means of postoperative immobilization. There is a lack of reliable data in this important debate because of the absence of controlled and independent comparisons of different grafting techniques. Thus, surgeons must make judgments based on limited information, their training and experience, and patient preference.

The use of anterior cervical plates is still in question. Legitimate differences of opinion exist on whether or not internal fixation is appropriate for a single-level anterior cervical discectomy and fusion. As the procedure is performed at greater numbers of levels, more compelling data exist in favor of rigid internal fixation because of the increasing likelihood of bone graft nonunion.

For a single-level anterior cervical discectomy and fusion, satisfactory results should be obtained in approximately 90% to 95% of patients. Nonunion rates will range from 2% to 10% depending on the authority quoted, the host, and probably, the method of implant preparation and graft selected.

Laminoforaminotomy

If a soft-disc herniation occurs in a relatively lateral position, one that compromises the nerve root rather than the spinal cord, then consideration may be given to a posterior keyhole laminoforaminotomy (Fig. 2, *A* and *B*). This procedure is being reevaluated by surgeons as newer retractor systems and less morbid muscle-splitting approaches evolve. The ability to adequately observe the nerve root and safely remove the herniated disc fragments rests on the surgeon's facility in managing the epidural venous plexus surrounding the nerve root. Elevating the head above the thorax (in sitting or reverse Trendelenburg position) reduces epidural venous pressure and bleeding, but engenders some risk of an intraoperative air embolus. With appropriate anesthesia monitoring techniques, this method can be quite safe and a viable alternative to an anterior cervical discectomy. At least 50% and preferably as much as 75% of the facet joint surfaces should be preserved to maintain segmental stability.

Stenosis Secondary to Osteophyte Formation

If a patient's symptoms are caused by spinal canal or neuroforaminal compromise from osteophytes, the technical aspects of the treatment may change. Most often, such osteophytes arise from the margins of the vertebral body along the floor of the spinal canal, especially at the posterolateral corner of the uncovertebral joint (Fig. 4, *A* and *B*). As with all osteophytes, they occur at the point of attachment of a ligament (the anulus) to bone (the vertebral body). Occasionally foraminal stenosis will be caused by facet arthropathy compromising the foramen from behind. Sometimes both processes occur in combination with anterior osteophytes, resulting in a pincer effect (Fig. 4, *C*). If the neural compromise is anterior, adequate decompression of the spinal cord and/or nerve roots can be achieved through anterior decompression.

Anterior Surgery

An anterior decompression for narrowing caused by osteophytes begins with a discectomy as described previously. In this situation the disc is usually quite degenerated. Disc height is usually lost as the patient's spondylosis progresses. After removing the degenerative nuclear material and what remains of the cartilaginous end plates, it is often useful to further distract the

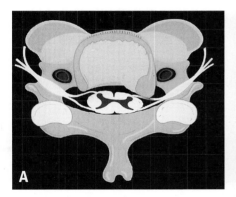 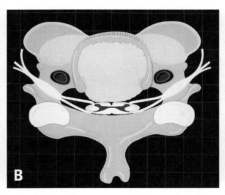 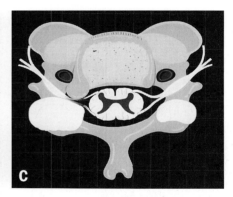

Figure 4 Axial schematics of the spectrum of potential compression due to osteophyte formation with spondylosis. Most often the clinically relevant problem is due to anterior compromise of the nerve root from osteophytes growing from the margins of the uncovertebral joints **(A)**. Less commonly central stenosis and myelopathy will be caused by osteophytes spanning the floor of the spinal canal, especially when underlying congenital stenosis is present **(B)**. The combination of facet arthropathy and uncovertebral osteophytes may exert a pincer effect on a given root **(C)**.

disc space by gently prying it open with a small periosteal elevator. Distraction can be maintained by any one of a number of available instrument systems. Any soft material that has protruded posterior to the vertebral margins can then be evacuated and the PLL seen.

The osteophytes themselves are removed by first removing the portion of the vertebral body from which they arise. A high-speed burr with a carbide cutting tip or a coarse diamond tip can be used to remove the necessary number of millimeters of the upper and lower vertebrae, proceeding in a ventral to dorsal direction. Once the necessary amount of vertebral bone has been removed, the osteophytes may be either peeled off the PLL, or further polished away with the burr. Some surgeons prefer to change to a lower friction diamond burr for the latter portion of the excision. Occasionally, the spondylosis process gives rise to excessive thickening of the PLL. In such patients, it may be wise to remove the PLL across the floor of the spinal canal to ensure full decompression. Supplemental decompression of the neuroforamen may be achieved with the use of 1- and 2-mm punches or fine angled curettes.

Fusion follows the decompression. The same arguments discussed previously exist with regard to selection of graft, trauma, and so forth. The graft is usually 2 to 6 mm taller than a single level interbody graft as a result of the resection of bone that is required.

In the event that multiple levels of spinal cord compression are caused by cervical spondylosis, the surgeon will be faced with the choice of performing a series of adjacent interbody decompressions or corpectomies. If interbody decompressions are performed, multiple interbody grafts will be required to reconstruct the segments. Statistically, the likelihood of one or more graft surfaces failing to heal is greater in the multiple interbody graft approach. Whether this is a by-product of

the number of graft-host interfaces, differential biomechanics, or some other as yet unknown influence is unclear. Many authors favor performing corpectomies to ensure complete decompression of the spinal canal over the involved segments. Reconstruction then requires a bone graft strut spanning the interval. The use of a carefully fitted allograft strut, supplemented by local cancellous autograft saved from the corpectomy(s) (Fig. 5) currently offers the best of both worlds. The freeze-dried allograft provides the necessary vertical support for the spinal column, while the local bone graft from the corpectomy offers the osteoinductive properties necessary to accelerate healing.

Instrumentation of single or multilevel corpectomies is under discussion. Anterior cervical plates once were believed to be a substantial step forward in the management of multilevel corpectomies. However, growing clinical and biomechanical evidence suggests that a rigid plate spanning from the vertebra above to the vertebra below a strut graft actually may negatively influence graft healing. Such static or constrained plates may inhibit the degree of settling and axial loading appropriate to the healing process (Fig. 6). In an attempt to improve on this situation, buttress plates have been used, principally at the caudal end of the strut graft where displacement is most likely (Fig. 7). Also, devices have been designed to allow for a degree of settling to avoid stress shielding.

As the end plates are removed in preparation for insertion of a strut graft, the surgeon must attempt to preserve a cortical lip of bone at the dorsal aspect of the upper and lower vertebral bodies. This lip acts as a check to posterior displacement of the strut graft. As the recipient surfaces are prepared, the surgeon should seek to fashion them parallel to one another, typically by removing more of the posterior aspect of the caudal vertebral body because of the physiologic lordosis of

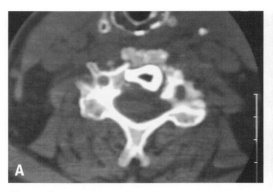
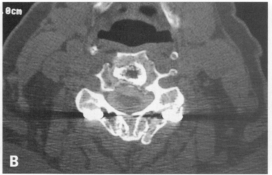
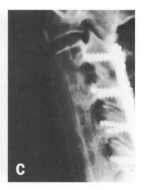

Figure 5 A postoperative axial CT image demonstrating how local cancellous autograft bone and a fibular allograft appear shortly after surgery **(A)**. A postoperative axial CT made 4 years later **(B)** demonstrates the remodeling of the autograft, as well as the effects of vascularization and creeping substitution within the allograft. The remodeling of the cancellous allograft is usually more rapidly identifiable on the postoperative plain radiographs **(C)** than clear evidence of healing of the allograft strut.

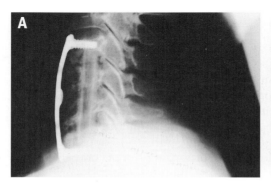
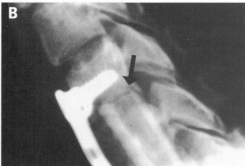

Figure 6 Lateral postoperative radiograph of a two-level corpectomy reconstructed with allograft fibular strut and local cancellous autograft with a rigidly constrained spanning anterior plate **(A)**. Careful inspection of the flexion-extension films demonstrated a nonunion (arrow), which was then managed with a posterior fusion **(B)**.

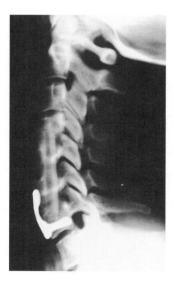

Figure 7 An illustrative radiograph of a patient whose reconstruction used an inferior buttress or kick plate. Such plates are placed at the caudal end of the fusion, which is the most likely place for graft displacement.

the cervical spine. Failure to align the host surfaces may predispose the graft to dislodging anteriorly, especially with longer decompressions.

OPLL was initially described in Japan because its population has a uniquely high prevalence of the disorder. With greater awareness of the condition and its imaging characteristics, OPLL is more frequently being diagnosed in the North American population. Aware-

ness of the differences between OPLL and normal cervical osteophytes is important. The source of compression in OPLL generally extends beyond the margins of the vertebra, behind the posterior wall of the vertebral body. Therefore, when anterior decompression is selected, subtotal or complete corpectomies are required. Corpectomy for OPLL is a reasonable choice when one to three motion segments are involved. The relative morbidity statistics favor a posterior surgical approach as the number of levels of compression increases. In patients with OPLL that is particularly long-standing, with severe spinal cord compromise, it is not unusual for the dura mater to be eroded or replaced by the bone-forming process. In this situation, the absence of dura often will make an anterior decompression more difficult. This problem is managed by placing an appropriate patch graft behind the bone graft as it is inserted. A lumbar cisternal drain is then required to divert the cerebrospinal fluid for a period of 3 to 5 days postoperatively. The patient's head is kept in an elevated position in the interim to minimize intrathecal pressure near the cervical spine.

Posterior Surgery

Posterior decompression for cervical spondylosis is indicated with increasing numbers of levels of compression.

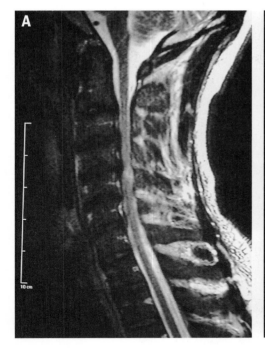

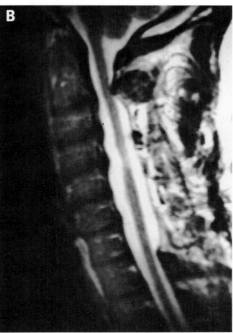

Figure 8 Pre- **(A)** and postoperative **(B)** sagittal MRIs of a patient with cervical spondylotic myelopathy who underwent a C3-7 laminoplasty. Note the generous expansion of the subarachnoid space and posterior shift of the spinal cord.

Posterior operations also require, for the most part, a nonkyphotic cervical alignment. Indirect decompression of the cord can be achieved by a laminectomy or laminoplasty in the presence of cervical lordosis (Fig. 8). The relative effectiveness (clinical and neurologic outcomes) of laminoplasty versus corpectomy for a multilevel cervical myelopathy is equivalent for the two approaches. The total number of complications associated with either strategy favor a laminoplasty. Similarly, other investigators compared laminectomy, laminoplasty, and multilevel anterior cervical discectomy and fusion for cervical spondylosis. Outcomes for their patients were equivalent for the anterior interbody fusion group and laminoplasty. However, the number of complications was greater among the anterior surgery group, principally in the form of nonunions.

Posterior decompression of the cervical spine consists principally of either a laminoplasty or a laminectomy with plating and fusion. Each surgical approach has proponents. Laminoplasty, though held to be technically difficult by some, has the advantage of providing adequate decompression of the spinal cord while simultaneously preserving bone surface for attachment of erector spinae and maintaining at least 50% of the preoperative range of motion. Others note that the laminectomy is much easier to perform than a laminoplasty, and that plating and fusion add little time or risk to the operation. However, lateral mass plating is not free of complications, nor is it technically simple. In addition, autogenous cancellous iliac crest autograft should be used for the fusion. This bone grafting is not

needed for laminoplasty. Finally, the laminectomy, plating, and fusion obliges the surgeon to surrender motion over the operated segments, which has the theoretical disadvantage of accelerating the rate of adjacent segment degeneration.

When performing a laminoplasty, it is important to place the location of the hinges at the junction of the lamina and the medial third of the lateral mass. The hinge should be created so that it is slightly stiff, rather than a loose hinge consisting only of the medial portion of the ligamentum flavum. The hinge portion is created after the division of the laminae on the open side or in the midline. Careful and gradual thinning of the bone will create a hinge that plastically deforms as if creating a greenstick effect. Whether the surgeon selects an open door or French door approach, the laminoplasty can be held open by a variety of techniques. The simplest is suturing the laminar roof to the paraspinal muscles. The surgeon also may suture the laminae to small suture anchors placed in the lateral masses ipsilateral to the hinges. Other techniques involve the use of short bone grafts or spacers to prop open the door (Fig. 9). Miniature plates and screws may be used to achieve the same effect.

After surgery, a patient who has had laminoplasty may be allowed active range of motion as comfort permits, and early neck and shoulder muscle rehabilitation is encouraged to minimize residual neck pain. Complaints of axial pain proportional to activity can be anticipated in approximately 25% of patients undergoing laminoplasty. The degree of impairment is generally

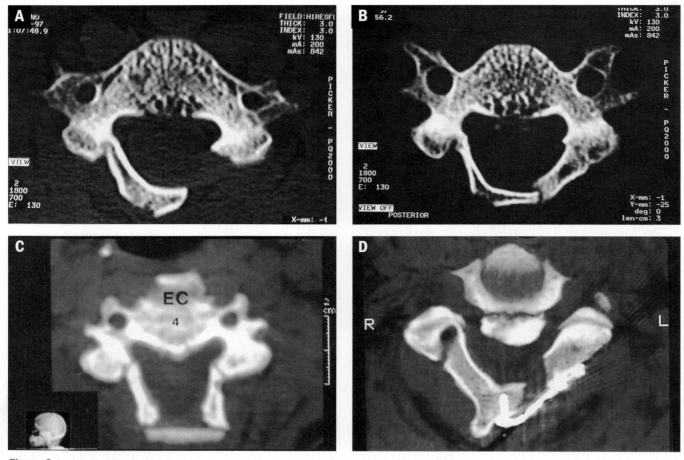

Figure 9 Postoperative CT scans that illustrate various methods of maintaining the hinge position after a laminoplasty: suturing the laminae to the paraspinal muscles **(A)**, propping the 'door' open with a spinous process bone graft **(B)**, holding a French door open with a split spinous process graft after a T-saw laminoplasty **(C)**, and using a miniplate and screws to prop open the door **(D)**.

mild. Activity-related interscapular pain may also be noted among patients undergoing multilevel anterior cervical fusions.

Patients undergoing laminectomy, plating, and fusion require immobilization until their arthrodesis has healed. At that point active rehabilitation of the neck and shoulder muscles can proceed. The likelihood of a successful fusion is improved by the use of autogenous iliac crest bone graft placed ventral to the lateral mass plates and within the decorticated facet joints.

Combined Anterior and Posterior Procedures

In unusual circumstances, the surgeon may decide that the patient's needs will best be served with a combination of anterior and posterior surgery. Typically, such circumstances arise when the surgeon judges that the primary surgical goals, such as decompression and/or correction of kyphosis, will be achieved most effectively by a multilevel anterior operation. The patient's healing potential, bone integrity, or behavioral issues may lead

the surgeon to judge that a supplemental posterior fusion would greatly enhance the overall likelihood of a successful recovery. In these circumstances, the surgeon accepts the trade-off of the increased time in surgery, blood loss, and risks of intraoperative morbidity, for the higher likelihood of graft union during a single convalescence (Fig. 10). Circumstances in which a surgeon might consider this option include patients with advanced osteopenia (three or move level corpectomies and slow fusion), impaired healing potential (patients with rheumatoid arthritis, renal failure, organ transplant), excessive use of tobacco or nicotine products, or anticipated inability to comply with postoperative restrictions (eg, psychopathology, movement disorders). In circumstances that are particularly unusual (eg, athetoid cerebral palsy and behavioral disorders associated with compromised cognition), the surgeon might feel obliged to immobilize the patient's cervical spine with a halo-vest in addition to the combined anterior and posterior surgeries.

Complications

To be forewarned is to be forearmed. Knowledge of what pitfalls are inherent to a given procedure is essential to minimize adverse occurrences and to recognize and effectively manage them should they occur. Successful treatment must begin with an accurate diagnosis. The diligent spinal surgeon must carefully assess the patient's history and physical examination in light of the entire differential diagnosis that applies. Common traps to avoid include mistakenly diagnosing a cervical disorder in the face of carpal tunnel syndrome or other peripheral entrapment neuropathies, thoracic outlet syndrome, primary shoulder pathology, acute brachial neuritis, or degenerative disorders of the central nervous system.

Persistence of neurologic symptoms and signs may be the result of irreparable damage sustained prior to surgery, inadequate decompression, or wrong-level surgery. The latter can be avoided with intraoperative radiographic confirmation of the surgical level. In patients with high riding shoulders, morbid obesity, or anomalous anatomy, the surgeon should extend the exposure so that a marking needle can be placed at an identifiable level, then carefully count and mark the levels from the known reference. Remember to account for any Klippel-Feil lesions, especially at C2-3. When faced with persisting symptoms, do not hesitate to image the patient's cervical spine perioperatively to ensure a technically adequate procedure. A myelographic CT scan with 1.0- to 3.0-mm slice thicknesses is likely to yield the most accurate information postoperatively, because it is less susceptible to metallic artifact and will yield more precise information about the neuroforamen.

Neurologic deficits may be acquired during or shortly after surgery. Careful attention to detail will minimize direct intraoperative trauma. Indirect removal of spinal cord compression, as with partial or complete corpectomies, will reduce any manipulation of the cord. Introducing an instrument between a compromised cord or root and the source of compression risks further harm. The surgeon must consider the possibility of graft or implant malposition or displacement. Plain radiographs yield reasonable information about anterior graft position, but they cannot provide reliable three-dimensional information about screw position, posterior bone grafts, or displaced hinges after a laminoplasty. Therefore, the surgeon should proceed with a thin-section myelographic CT with sagittal and coronal reformations. In the best of circumstances, some acquired deficits are simply a matter of misfortune. This appears to be the case with motor root lesions, which occur most often following laminoplasties but may also occur after anterior decompressions. In the case of severe spinal cord

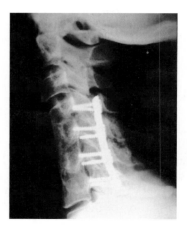

Figure 10 Lateral postoperative radiograph of a patient following a combined multilevel anterior and posterior decompression and reconstruction. Though quite effective, such extensive procedures are warranted in a limited set of circumstances.

compression, some patients can develop progressive paralysis perioperatively, presumably as a result of local inflammatory and/or microvascular changes precipitated by the decompression of a chronically deformed and atrophic spinal cord.

Nonunions of fusions will occur in the best of circumstances. The likelihood increases with increasing numbers of levels fused, the use of allograft bone, tobacco product and/or nicotine use, and primary or drug-induced metabolic bone disease. The key to treating the problem is diagnosis, which rests upon a willingness to consider the possibility. Most often the patient will describe a 6-week to 6-month interval of clear improvement followed by progressive recurrence of axial pain, with or without neurologic symptoms. Careful interpretation of postoperative images, especially lateral flexion-extension films and reformatted CT scans, will establish the diagnosis. The presence of internal fixation devices tends to mask subtle amounts of segmental motion. A supplemental fusion procedure is required, which may be either anterior or posterior, depending on the presence or absence of neurologic compression, reactive sclerosis around the failed graft, and surgeon preference.

Certain problems unique to cervical spine surgery may be associated with anesthesia and airway management. The anesthesiologists should be apprised of spinal cord compromise so that due caution may be exercised during intubation. If the surgeon requires exposure above C4, or if the patient is obese, a nasotracheal intubation will permit full dental occlusion, keeping the mandible from inhibiting the line of sight. Also, postoperative airway management must be discussed. The possibility of acute postoperative airway compromise tends to increase with the extent of dissection and duration of anesthesia. Supplemental intravenous steroids are favored by some to reduce edema. The surgeon should consider maintaining the patient on a ventilator with the head and trunk elevated overnight, with extubation to proceed after confirmation of a patent airway. Acute airway compromise can also occur due to a hematoma. In this instance re-intubation is very difficult. Immediate release of the sutures and digital evacuation of the hematoma will decompress the airway. Once the airway is secured, the wound can be explored in the operating room to identify and control any appreciable sources of hemorrhage.

Speech or swallowing disturbance may complicate anterior cervical surgery. As mentioned previously, it appears that the side of surgical exposure may not be the whole story regarding vocal cord dysfunction. If the endotracheal tube itself is a cause of an endolaryngeal injury, then deflation and re-inflation of the balloon cuff after positioning of self-retaining retractors may reduce the incidence. Patients should be advised that they will experience throat pain and difficulty swallowing for a period after surgery. For patients whose symptoms persist or pose a risk of aspiration, consultation with a knowledgeable speech therapist or otolaryngologist is in order.

Summary

Some syndromes of degenerative cervical disc disease may be successfully treated through surgical intervention, provided that the procedure is tailored to the unique circumstances of the patient's pathoanatomy and overall clinical presentation. Options include anterior and posterior procedures, some of which oblige a fusion. It is incumbent on the spinal surgeon to be familiar with the spectrum of options and their known indications and limitations. Finally, because data are lacking with regard to important areas of uncertainty, the responsible surgeon must continue to apprise himself or herself of the evolving state of knowledge with regard to the tactical details of these cervical spine operations.

Annotated Bibliography

An HS, Vaccaro A, Cotler JM, Lin S: Spinal disorders at the cervicothoracic junction. *Spine* 1994;19:2557-2564.

The authors provide a helpful description of the surgical anatomy and reconstructive challenges posed by the cervicothoracic junction.

Apfelbaum RI, Kriskovich MD, Haller JR: On the incidence, cause, and prevention of recurrent laryngeal nerve palsies during anterior cervical spine surgery. *Spine* 2000;25:2906-2912.

This is a thought-provoking look at an alternative explanation for some of the vocal cord dysfunction seen after anterior cervical surgery. There may be more than one mechanism at work in this complication.

Curylo LJ, Mason HC, Bohlman HH, Yoo JU: Tortuous course of the vertebral artery and anterior cervical decompression: A cadaveric and clinical case study. *Spine* 2000;25:2860-2864.

This extensive analysis of cervical skeletons describes the types and frequency of variations in the size and course of the vertebral arteries. This is essential information for those undertaking anterior cervical procedures.

DiAngelo DJ, Foley KT, Vossel KA, Rampersaud YR, Jansen TH: Anterior cervical plating reverses load transfer through multilevel strut-grafts. *Spine* 2000;25:783-795.

This is one of a pair of articles from the authors' laboratory that provide understanding of the influence of anterior plates on the loads applied to strut grafts.

Do Koh Y, Lim TH, Won You J, Eck J, An HS: A biomechanical comparison of modern anterior and posterior plate fixation of the cervical spine. *Spine* 2001;26:15-21.

This is a useful comparison of contemporary cervical internal fixation options. Keep in mind the scope of the procedure required to implement and/or combine these methods versus their relative clinical success rates.

Emery SE, Bohlman HH, Bolesta MJ, Jones PK: Anterior cervical decompression and arthrodesis for the treatment of cervical spondylotic myelopathy: Two to seventeen-year follow-up. *J Bone Joint Surg Am* 1998;80:941-951.

The authors provide useful perspective on the success rates of anterior decompression and fusion with respect to clinical outcome, union rates, and reoperation rates over time.

Emery SE, Bolesta MJ, Banks MA, Jones PK: Robinson anterior cervical fusion: Comparison of the standard and modified techniques. *Spine* 1994;19:660-663.

The clinical and radiographic results of anterior fusion are compared for two different methods of end-plate preparation.

George B, Gauthier N, Lot G: Multisegmental cervical spondylotic myelopathy and radiculopathy treated by multilevel oblique corpectomies without fusion. *Neurosurgery* 1999;44:81-90.

This is a thought-provoking report of a large group of patients treated with anterior corpectomies that do not require subsequent fusion. This technically demanding technique originally was performed in the 1960s.

Hilibrand AS, Yoo JU, Carlson GD, Bohlman HH: The success of anterior cervical arthrodesis adjacent to a previous fusion. *Spine* 1997;22:1574-1579.

As anterior fusions have become a standard of care, patients and surgeons are increasingly likely to experience the need for revision procedures at adjacent levels. Thus it is wise to learn about the potentials issues to be managed and the likely success rates.

Isomi T, Panjabi MM, Wang JL, Vaccaro AR, Garfin SR, Patel T: Stabilizing potential of anterior cervical plates in multilevel corpectomies. *Spine* 1999;24:2219-2223.

Panjabi MM, Isomi T, Wang JL: Loosening at the screw-vertebra junction in multilevel anterior cervical plate constructs. *Spine* 1999;24:2383-2388.

Wang JL, Panjabi MM, Isomi T: The role of bone graft force in stabilizing the multilevel anterior cervical spine plate system. *Spine* 2000;25:1649-1654.

This trio of publications from the authors' laboratory compare the biomechanics of single-level versus three-level corpectomies with an emphasis on the effects of fatigue testing and the dramatic differences that may be observed in comparison to static tests. Their observations have important clinical implication.

Riew KD, Sethi NS, Devney J, Goette K, Choi K: Complications of buttress plate stabilization of cervical corpectomy. *Spine* 1999;24:2404-2410.

In reporting their experience with this method of instrumentation after multilevel anterior corpectomies, the authors describe a unique but noteworthy complication. Additional reports of series with this technique, which avoids the stress-shielding of anterior locking plates, are needed before its role will be adequately understood.

Saunders RL, Pikus HJ, Ball P: Four-level cervical corpectomy. *Spine* 1998;23:2455-2461.

This is a clinical report of the successes and failures of extensive anterior decompressions and fusion spanning five motion segments.

Schultz KD Jr, McLaughlin MR, Haid RW Jr, Comey CH, Rodts GE Jr, Alexander J: Single-stage anterior-posterior decompression and stabilization for complex cervical spine disorders. *J Neurosurg* 2000;93(suppl 2):214-221.

The frustrations with anterior multilevel grafts have led some authors to favor combined anterior and posterior procedures. The reader should keep an open mind as to whether the risks and costs of greater amounts of surgery outweigh those of potential graft dislodgement or nonunion repair.

Vaccaro AR, Falatyn SP, Scuderi GJ, et al: Early failure of long segment anterior cervical plate fixation. *J Spinal Disord* 1998;11:410-415.

The authors report the clinical failures that may occur following anterior locking plate instrumentation for multilevel strut grafts, with emphasis on the likelihood of failure in relation to the number of motion segments being fused.

Vanichkachorn JS, Vaccaro AR, Silveri CP, Albert TJ: Anterior junctional plate in the cervical spine. *Spine* 1998;23:2462-2467.

The authors report combined anterior and posterior procedures for multilevel fusions, yet still experience graft complications.

Zdeblick TA, Hughes SS, Riew KD, Bohlman HH: Failed anterior cervical discectomy and arthrodesis: Analysis and treatment of thirty-five patients. *J Bone Joint Surg Am* 1997;79:523-532.

The authors provide some perspective on the options for and the results following treatment of symptomatic anterior cervical nonunions.

Classic Bibliography

Anderson PA, Budorick TE, Easton KB, Henley MB, Salciccioli GG: Failure of halo vest to prevent in vivo motion in patients with injured cervical spines. *Spine* 1991;16(suppl 10):S501-S505.

DePalma AF, Rothman RH, Lewinnek GE, Canale ST: Anterior interbody fusion for severe cervical disc degeneration. *Surg Gynecol Obstet* 1972;134:755-758.

Farey ID, McAfee PC, Davis RF, Long DM: Pseudarthrosis of the cervical spine after anterior arthrodesis: Treatment by posterior nerve-root decompression, stabilization, and arthrodesis. *J Bone Joint Surg Am* 1990;72:1171-1177.

Fernyhough JC, White JI, LaRocca H: Fusion rates in multilevel cervical spondylosis comparing allograft fibula with autograft fibula in 126 patients. *Spine* 1991;16(suppl 10):S561-S564.

Riley LH Jr, Robinson RA, Johnson KA, Walker AE: The results of anterior interbody fusion of the cervical spine: A review of ninety-three consecutive cases. *J Neurosurg* 1969;30:127-133.

Robinson RA, Walker AE, Ferlic DC, Wiecking DK: The results of anterior interbody fusion of the cervical spine. *J Bone Joint Surg Am* 1962;44:1569-1587.

White AA III, Southwick WO, Deponte RJ, Gainor JW, Hardy R: Relief of pain by anterior cervical-spine fusion for spondylosis: A report of sixty-five patients. *J Bone Joint Surg Am* 1973;55:525-534.

Yonenobu K, Hosono N, Iwasaki M, Asano M, Ono K: Laminoplasty versus subtotal corpectomy: A comparative study of results in multisegmental cervical spondylotic myelopathy. *Spine* 1992;17:1281-1284.

Zdeblick TA, Ducker TB: The use of freeze-dried allograft bone for anterior cervical fusions. *Spine* 1991;16:726-729.

Chapter 33

Thoracic Discopathy and Stenosis

Srdjan Mirkovic, MD

Thoracic disc herniations (TDHs) and clinically significant stenosis due to spondylosis, ossification of the yellow ligament (OYL), and/or ossification of the posterior longitudinal ligament (OPLL) are relatively unusual diagnoses among patients seeking care from spine-care specialists. Although clinical manifestations are uncommon and often unrecognized, the existence of such pathology has been observed much more commonly since the advent of MRI and other advanced imaging techniques. Clinical characteristics of patients with these disorders are varied, so the spine-care specialist must remain highly suspicious to properly identify patients who are suffering effects from these lesions and must be very cautious to avoid overtreatment of patients whose thoracic spine pathology is not the cause of their symptoms.

If there is no neurologic involvement, nonsurgical care is wisest. Surgical intervention is indicated in the presence of neurologic compromise and/or intractable radicular pain. The surgical approach is determined by the nature, location, and level of the pathology and the surgeon's experience.

Thoracic Disc Herniation

History

The first TDH causing a spinal cord injury was reported in 1838. A central T12-L1 disc herniation caused by lifting and leading to paraplegia and subsequent death was described early in the 20th century. The first surgery for a thoracic disc herniation appears to have been performed in 1922; two more surgical cases were reported about 10 years later.

Incidence

Because of difficulties in the clinical diagnosis and flux in the limitations of imaging studies the true incidence of TDH is unknown. Wide discrepancies in the incidence of clinically significant TDH from that observed by advanced imaging studies demand careful definition of

the population when evaluating incidence. Autopsy studies as well as CT myelography indicate an 11% incidence of asymptomatic TDHs. Incidental TDHs were found in 14.5% of 48 patients suspected of having neoplasms of the thoracic spine or spinal cord. Only one person per million per year has objective neurologic findings secondary to TDH. Thoracic discectomies for clinically significant TDH account for 0.2% to 2% of all discectomies.

Classification

TDHs can be classified according to level and location (central, centrolateral, lateral, or intradural), which is helpful in determining surgical approach. Patients with central herniations may have symptoms of myelopathy, whereas lateral protrusions commonly elicit radicular symptoms. Intradural herniations are rare. Seventy percent of all TDHs are either central or centrolateral. The most commonly involved level is T11-12, at which 26% of herniations occur; 75% of herniations occur between T8 and T12. The increased incidence at the thoracolumbar junction may be attributed to increased motion leading to early disc degeneration. Soft and hard disc herniations associated with degenerative changes of the spine should be differentiated, because this difference influences the surgical approach.

Etiology

The true incidence of trauma as a precipitating event in the etiology of TDH is controversial. A 50% incidence of traumatically induced TDH has been reported. Torsional or twisting movements or heavy lifting have been described as precipitating events; falls rarely are implicated. Scheuermann's disease with myelopathy due to thoracic disc calcification can occur in younger patients. In older patients, degenerative processes may be major predisposing factors in the development of TDH, and manifestations of spondylosis, such as discussed later, may increase vulnerability to symptoms from superimposed disc herniation.

In contrast to cervical and lumbar disc herniations, a significant percentage of TDHs undergo calcification, a helpful radiographic feature. The smaller cross-sectional area of the thoracic spine and close proximity of the spinal cord to the posterior margin of the vertebral bodies can lead to progressive spinal cord compression associated with TDH.

Anatomy

The thoracic spinal cord has unique characteristics that must be considered during surgical manipulation. The etiology of clinical signs and symptoms produced by TDH may be vascular and/or mechanical. The variable blood supply between T4 and T9 (watershed zone) is vulnerable because of limited intramedullary and radicular circulations. Ventral lesions, such as disc herniations, produce a ventral compressive force that is greatest at the impact point. These ventral forces dissipate with distance posteriorly and are minimal on the dorsal surface of the spinal cord. Axial tension forces are also created by the ventral compressive force resulting from the disc herniation. Unlike the compressive forces, the axial tension forces are greatest on the dorsal surface of the spinal cord. Axial pain is most likely due to direct neural compression as well as traction on nerve fibers in the posterior longitudinal ligament and anulus fibrosus.

Radicular pain may result from either traction or direct compression of the thoracic nerve roots. Pain may also be a consequence of direct compression of the cord parenchyma and/or interference with the blood supply or venous drainage from the cord.

Laminectomy can alleviate posterior compression forces created by the lamina and ligamentum flavum. Laminectomy, however, does not address the compression indentation forces generated by the anterior impact of a TDH. In addition, dentate ligaments may resist posterior spinal cord displacement, thereby causing persistent traction on the neural elements. Poor results associated with laminectomy are due, in part, to the spinal manipulation required to address the ventral TDH mass.

Clinical Presentation

Thoracic discopathy is difficult to diagnose because of extreme variations in clinical presentation. Eighty percent of patients are in their fourth to sixth decades, with 33% presenting in their fifties. There is a 1.5 to 1 ratio of men to women. Pain, the most frequent initial symptom (Table 1), may be constant, intermittent, dull, sharp, or shooting. Depending on the disc location, pain distribution may be axial, unilateral, or bilateral. Patients also

TABLE 1 | Initial Symptoms of Thoracic Disc Herniations

Initial Symptoms	Occurrence (%)
Pain	57
Sensory	24
Motor	17
Bladder	2

(Reproduced with permission from Arce CA, Dohrmann GJ: Herniated thoracic disks. Neurol Clin 1985;3:383-392.)

may complain of unilateral lower limb pain, which can mimic that of lumbar disc herniation. Circumferential radiating pain around the chest wall is described commonly. Symptoms may be aggravated with coughing, sneezing, or increased activity and are improved by rest.

Atypical radiating pains occur also. Groin and testicular pain caused by a T11 disc herniation may simulate degenerative hip and renal disease. Patients with midthoracic disc herniations may have chest and abdominal pain. Neck pain, upper extremity pain, and Horner's syndrome secondary to a T1 or T2 disc herniation can be attributed mistakenly to degenerative cervical disease. Sensory changes, especially numbness, are the second most common initial symptoms. Paresthesias and dysesthesias also have been reported. In the absence of pain, these symptoms may be the only clues to the diagnosis of TDH. Motor weakness and bladder dysfunction are less frequent.

At the time of presentation (Table 2), 30% of patients with symptomatic TDH may have bladder dysfunction, whereas 18% describe both bowel and bladder disturbances. Motor and sensory involvement occurs in 60% of symptomatic patients.

Given the nonspecific and varied symptoms, delayed diagnosis and misdiagnosis are common. A history of symptoms for many years is not unusual. Other neurologic disorders should also be considered in the differential diagnosis.

Physical Examination

Early in the course of TDH, physical examination elicits few findings. Decreased dermatomal light touch or pinprick sensations may be present. Spinal cord compression secondary to TDH may produce typical upper motor neuron signs: weakness, spasticity, hyperflexion, positive Babinski's sign, gait disturbances, and a decreased sensory reaction to pinprick or light touch testing. An incomplete spinal cord syndrome, such as

	Occurrence	
	Arce & Dohrman	Stillerman & Weiss
Symptoms	**(%)**	**(n = 51) (%)**
Motor and sensory	61	
Motor only	6	
Sensory only	15	39
Weakness		59
Bladder/sphincter	30	
Bowel and bladder		18
Radicular pain only	9	16

TABLE 2 | Symptoms When Patients Present to a Physician

(Reproduced by permission from Garfin SR, Vaccaro AR (eds): Orthopaedic Knowledge Update: Spine. Rosemont, IL, American Academy of Orthopaedic Surgeons, 1997, pp 87-96.)

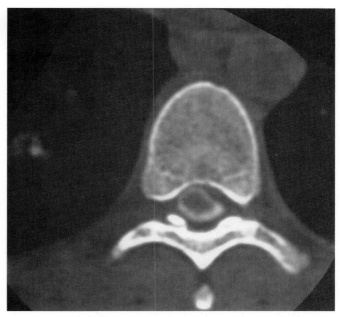

Figure 1 CT myelogram. Soft T8-9 thoracic disc herniation. *(Reproduced with permission from Garfin SR, Vaccaro AR (eds): Orthopaedic Knowledge Update: Spine. Rosemont, IL, American Academy of Orthopaedic Surgeons, 1997, pp 87-96.)*

Brown-Séquard syndrome, may result from a large centrolateral herniation.

Imaging Studies

Osteophyte formation, disc space narrowing, and, occasionally, kyphosis may be seen on radiographs of patients with TDH. The specificity of these findings, however, is low. Disc calcification is seen in 4% to 6% of patients without TDH and in 70% of patients with herniations. The sensitivity of thoracic myelography, although better than plain radiography, is less than 70%.

CT myelography has the advantage of demonstrating accurately encroachment on the spinal cord and presence of lateral herniations (Fig. 1). Disc calcifications also are seen more clearly on CT (Fig. 2). The main disadvantages of CT myelography are that it requires axial cuts at multiple levels and that it is invasive. The sensitivity and specificity of CT myelography are better than that of either technique alone and presently are equal to that of MRI. Myelographic observation of the herniated disc can be particularly beneficial in determining the correct surgical level intraoperatively. The correct level can be determined radiographically during surgery either by counting vertebrae from the fifth lumbar vertebra superiorly on lateral radiographs or by counting ribs from the most inferior rib superiorly on the AP radiograph. The intraoperative radiograph, thus, can be compared to the myelographic AP and lateral films, allowing accurate determination of the level of the TDH.

MRI is the study of choice for screening for suspected

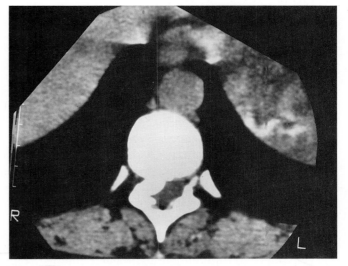

Figure 2 CT scan of lateral calcified thoracic disc herniation. *(Reproduced with permission from Garfin SR, Vaccaro AR (eds): Orthopaedic Knowledge Update: Spine. Rosemont, IL, American Academy of Orthopaedic Surgeons, 1997, pp 87-96.)*

TDH, because it provides sagittal and axial images with excellent anatomic definition (Fig. 3). Imaging studies must be interpreted with awareness of the high prevalence of asymptomatic MRI-documented thoracic spine disease. Sagittal thoracic MRI scans provide visualization of disc degeneration in ways unsurpassed by other conventional techniques. The sensitivity of MRI has

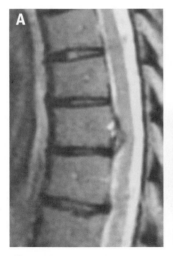

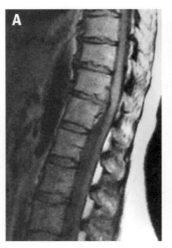

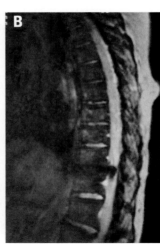

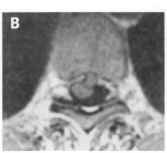

Figure 3 A, Sagittal MRI scan of a T8-9 thoracic disc herniation. **B,** Axial MRI scan of a T9-10 centrolateral thoracic disk herniation. *(Reproduced with permission from Garfin SR, Vaccaro AR (eds):* Orthopaedic Knowledge Update: Spine. *Rosemont, IL, American Academy of Orthopaedic Surgeons, 1997, pp 87-96.)*

Figure 4 A, T1-weighted sagittal MRI scan of isointense T11-12 thoracic disc herniation. **B,** T2-weighted sagittal MRI scan of a T10-11 thoracic disc herniation. *(Reproduced with permission from Garfin SR, Vaccaro AR (eds):* Orthopaedic Knowledge Update: Spine. *Rosemont, IL, American Academy of Orthopaedic Surgeons, 1997, pp 87-96.)*

increased the diagnosis of clinically important TDH and allowed follow-up of smaller lesions. The key features of TDH on sagittal T1-weighted images are extension of disc material beyond the posterior margin of the adjacent vertebral bodies and indentation of the spinal cord.

Herniated disc material is isointense, or slightly hypointense, relative to adjacent disc levels on T1-weighted images (Fig. 4, *A*) and hypointense on T2-weighted images. Sagittal or axial T2-weighted images produce a myelogram effect in which the cerebrospinal fluid is brighter than the spinal cord and, therefore, provides better contrast between the spinal cord and low intensity disc or osteophytes (Fig. 4, *B*). Calcified disc herniations are hypointense on both T1- and T2-weighted sequences. Disc degeneration is observed best on T2-weighted or gradient echo sequences. MRI has the advantages of detecting multiple herniations without the need for multilevel axial imaging and of providing the ability to differentiate neurogenic tumors from disc herniations. MRI may differentiate symptomatic disc herniations based on disc matrix composition. Imaging quality can be compromised by motion artifact, volume averaging, pulsatile cerebrospinal fluid motion, and scoliosis. Conventional myelography with postmyelographic CT scanning may still be helpful in patients with lateral foraminal TDH.

Thoracic discography has been shown to reveal details of pathology of the interior of the disc, disruptions of the outer anulus, and atypical protrusions, including intravertebral herniations (Schmorl's nodes). Evaluating the pain provoked by injection may help distinguish asymptomatic from symptomatic pathology. Clinical usefulness of thoracic discography is limited because it is technically a very demanding, invasive test, and will often reveal morphologically abnormal and sensitive discs that are not the cause of the patient's complaints.

Differential Diagnosis

Given the wide variety of presenting complaints, both spinal and nonspinal origins must be considered. Other neurologic disorders, such as amyotrophic lateral sclerosis, multiple sclerosis, transverse myelitis, spinal cord tumors, and arteriovenous malformations, can present initial symptoms similar to those of TDH, as may compression of neural structures from ligament ossification and spondylosis as discussed below. Cervical disease may refer symptoms to the thorax. Nonspinal disorders with referred symptoms that may mimic those of TDH include cholecystitis, aneurysms, retroperitoneal neoplasm or inflammatory disease, and other intra-abdominal and intrathoracic disorders (Table 3).

Natural History

Although, characteristically, symptoms may progress from pain to sensory disturbances, to weakness and further neurologic compromise, the natural history is variable. Thoracic pain associated with acute traumatic disc herniations in younger patients may precede progressive myelopathy. In the middle-aged population with degenerative disc herniations, the onset of symptoms secondary to spinal cord compression tends to be more gradual.

In the absence of myelopathy, nonsurgical treatment and activity modifications may be warranted. Approxi-

TABLE 3 | Differential Diagnosis of Thoracic Pain

Musculoskeletal
- Infectious
- Neoplastic
- Degenerative
  - Spondylosis
  - Spinal stenosis
  - Degenerative disc disease
  - Facet syndrome
  - Costochondritis
- Metabolic
  - Osteoporosis
  - Osteomalacia
- Traumatic
- Inflammatory
  - Ankylosing spondylitis
- Deformity
  - Scoliosis
  - Kyphosis
- Muscular
  - Strain
  - Fibromyalgia
  - Polymyalgia rheumatica

Neurogenic
- Thoracic disc herniation
- Neoplasms
  - Extradural
  - Intradural
  - Extramedullary
  - Intramedullary
- Arteriovenous malformation
- Inflammatory
  - Herpes zoster
- Postthoracotomy syndrome
- Intercostal neuralgia

Referred pain
- Intrathoracic
  - Cardiovascular
  - Pulmonary
  - Mediastinal
- Intra-abdominal
  - Gastrointestinal
  - Hepatobiliary
- Retroperitoneal
  - Renal
  - Tumor
  - Aneurysm

Sociopsychogenic

(Reproduced with permission from Garfin SR, Vaccaro AR (eds): Orthopaedic Knowledge Update: Spine. Rosemont, IL, American Academy of Orthopaedic Surgeons, 1997, pp 87-96.)

TABLE 4 | Surgical Approaches for Varying Pathologies

Levels	Disc Herniation	Approaches
Soft Discs		
T1 to T4	Central, centrolateral	Transsternal
	Central, centrolateral	Medial clavisectomy
	Centrolateral, lateral	Costotransversectomy
T4 to T12	Central, centrolateral, lateral	Transthoracic
	Central, centrolateral, lateral	Thoracoscopy
	Centrolateral, lateral	Lateral
	Central, centrolateral, lateral	Costotransversectomy
	Lateral	Transpedicular
Calcified Discs		
T1 to T4	Central, centrolateral	Transsternal
	Central, centrolateral	Medial clavisectomy
	Lateral	Costotransversectomy
T4 to T12	Central, centrolateral, lateral	Transthoracic
	Lateral	Lateral
	Lateral, centrolateral	Costotransversectomy

(Reproduced with permission from Garfin SR, Vaccaro AR (eds): Orthopaedic Knowledge Update: Spine. Rosemont, IL, American Academy of Orthopaedic Surgeons, 1997, pp 87-96.)

mately 80% of patients in the nonsurgical group return to their previous activity level. Patients with unrelenting pain and lower extremity complaints are more likely to elect surgery. With bilateral onset of symptoms, progression tends to be more rapid than when the onset is unilateral. The natural history of asymptomatic TDHs is to remain asymptomatic, although they may change in size and also may disappear spontaneously.

Nonsurgical Treatment

Nonsurgical treatment should be considered for patients without long-tract signs or major neurologic deficits. A short trial of bed rest with gradual mobilization and limitation of activities involving axial loading and repetitive flexion, extension, or twisting can be beneficial. Bracing with a thoracolumbar orthosis may be effective. Pain can be managed symptomatically with nonsteroidal anti-inflammatories, acetaminophen, and/or judicious use of narcotics. Physical therapy should involve postural training, extension strengthening, back school, and cardiovascular conditioning.

Surgical Treatment

Surgical intervention is indicated for patients who have myelopathy or who have unrelenting pain and failed a course of nonsurgical treatment.

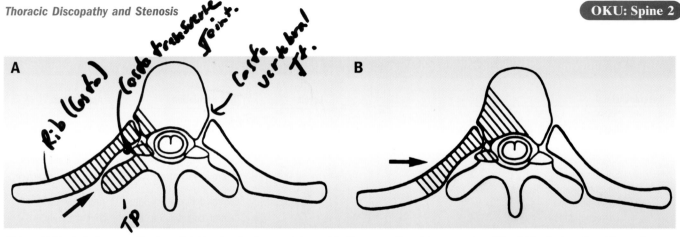

Figure 5 Extent of a bony resection (cross-hatch) and angle of approach (*arrows*) to disc space with costotransversectomy **(A)** and lateral extracavitary **(B)** procedures. *(Reproduced with permission from Cybulski G: Thoracic disc herniation: Surgical technique.* Contemp Neurosurg *1992;14:1-6.)*

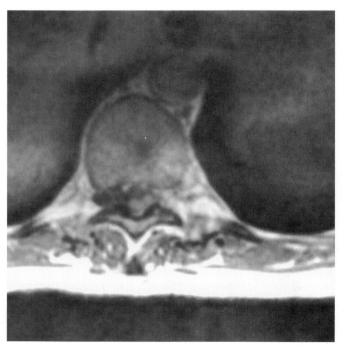

Figure 6 Axial MRI scan of a foraminal T7-8 thoracic disc herniation. *(Reproduced with permission from Garfin SR, Vaccaro AR (eds):* Orthopaedic Knowledge Update: Spine. *Rosemont, IL, American Academy of Orthopaedic Surgeons, 1997, pp 87-96.)*

Decision-making regarding the most appropriate surgical approach should be based on the level of herniation, its location relative to the spinal cord, disc consistency, and the surgeon's experience with the approach (Table 4). The patient's age and medical condition must be considered. Surgical approaches may be either anterior or posterior, as described later.

The correct surgical level commonly is determined by identifying the rib leading to the corresponding level of pathology. Anatomically, the ribs attach to the transverse process and the superior aspect of the same numbered vertebra at the level of the pedicle. The T9-10 disc, for example, can be identified intraoperatively by

AP radiographic determination of the T10 rib costovertebral attachment, located at the superior aspect of the T10 vertebra, delineating the inferior border of the T9-10 disc.

The correct surgical level can also be identified by counting vertebrae from either L5-S1 or T12 proximally on the lateral intraoperative radiograph. The presence of transitional lumbar vertebrae must be ascertained on the AP radiographs and due caution must be taken during counting. Alternatively, the surgical level in high TDHs can be determined on an intraoperative swimmer's view by identifying C1-2 and counting down.

Lateral (Extracavitary) Approach

The lateral (extracavitary) approach (Fig. 5) can be applied to any level of the thoracic spine and is well suited for centrolateral and lateral soft disc (Fig. 6) and lateral calcified disc herniations. The exposure is entirely extrapleural, facilitating thoracolumbar junction exposure without the need to take down the diaphragm. If the pleura is violated, closure should be attempted; otherwise, a chest tube is placed. The procedure requires removal of portions of the rib, costotransverse joint, facet, and pedicle. Additional rib resection allows wider access lateral to the spinal cord, permitting enhanced observation of the nerve root, spinal cord, and disc space without retraction of the cord. This provides additional safety during the decompression. The intercostal nerves generally are not sacrificed. Segmental vessels are dissected off the vertebral bodies and ligated. Multiple levels are exposed easily, as is the thoracolumbar junction. The approach allows anterolateral arthrodesis with rib or strut graft.

The main drawbacks are the paraspinal muscle disruption and the removal of a significant amount of bone, increasing blood loss and time of surgery. Repair of ventral dural tears can be difficult through this approach. Sacrifice of multiple segmental nerves may lead to significant chest wall numbness, which can be particularly bothersome to women.

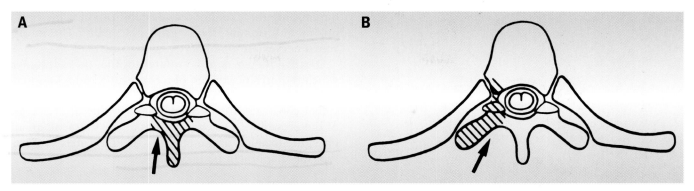

Figure 7 Extent of a bony resection (cross-hatch) and angle of approach (*arrows*) to disc space with laminectomy **(A)** and facetectomy/pediculectomy **(B)** procedures. *(Reproduced with permission from Cybulski G: Thoracic disc herniation: Surgical technique.* Contemp Neurosurg *1992;14:1-6.)*

Costotransversectomy

Costotransversectomy (Fig. 5, *A*) is a posterolateral-extrapleural approach that allows posterior access to a central, centrolateral, or lateral TDH (Fig. 6). The patient is placed prone, and a laterally convex curved paramedian incision is made with its apex about 2 cm from the midline. The posterior medial portion of the rib articulating with the transverse process and the superior aspect of the vertebral body just inferior to the disc herniation is resected. The pleura is mobilized and reflected anterolaterally. The paraspinal muscles either are retracted medially or split transversely. The transverse process and pedicle below the herniated disc are excised and the disc entered laterally. The posterosuperior and posteroinferior vertebral bodies bordering the disc are removed, creating a cavity into which herniated fragments can be pushed ventrally.

Costotransversectomy has the disadvantage of requiring some disruption of the paraspinal muscles as well as more extensive resection of bone. However, it facilitates observation of centrolateral and lateral disc herniations without the need to enter the pulmonary cavity. It may be used for central disc herniations in patients for whom a thoracotomy is contraindicated. It should not be used for large calcified central discs, when large osteophytes are present, or in the presence of transdural herniations. In these conditions, particularly when myelopathy is present, it is the procedure most commonly associated with failure due to incomplete resection.

Transpedicular Approach

For the transpedicular approach, a midline incision is made with the patient prone (Fig. 7). The facet joint and at least the medial portion of the pedicle on the side of the lesion and caudal to the disc are removed. The desired portion of the pedicle is excised flush with the vertebral body. Soft disc material can be removed with curettes. Hard discs are removed by creating a trough with a high-speed burr and delivering the hard disc into

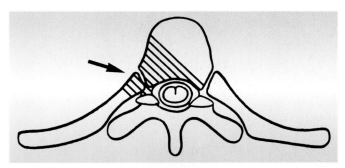

Figure 8 Extent of a bony resection (cross-hatch) and angle of approach (*arrows*) to disc space with transthoracic approach. *(Reproduced with permission from Cybulski G: Thoracic disc herniation: Surgical technique.* Contemp Neurosurg *1992;14:1-6.)*

the trough, thereby minimizing trauma to the neural elements.

The advantage of the transpedicular approach is that it involves a less extensive disc dissection, with potentially decreased bleeding and surgery time, thereby reducing complications. The main disadvantage is the limited view, which renders management of central and centrolateral fragments, as well as osteophytes and calcified discs, difficult and hazardous. Access to dural fistulae and intradural pathology is limited. Furthermore, segmental stability may be compromised following facet, pedicle, and disc removal. This approach is indicated for soft lateral disc herniation in a medically compromised individual. Complications may arise secondary to the limited exposure.

Transthoracic Approach

The transthoracic-transpleural approach (Fig. 8) is the most versatile, allowing excellent central and centrolateral exposure from T4 to the thoracolumbar junction (Fig. 9). Double lumen intubation should be performed. The approach is from the left side for the mid and lower thoracic spine, thereby avoiding manipulation of the inferior vena cava and the liver. A right-sided approach

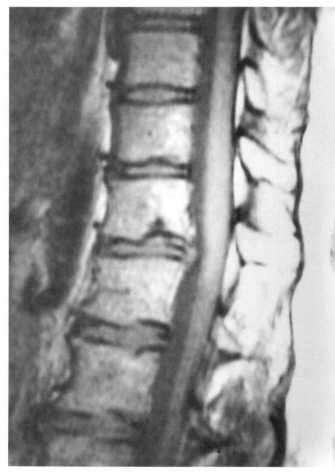

Figure 9 Sagittal MRI scan of a soft thoracic disc herniation. *(Reproduced with permission from Garfin SR, Vaccaro AR (eds): Orthopaedic Knowledge Update: Spine. Rosemont, IL, American Academy of Orthopaedic Surgeons, 1997, pp 87-96.)*

in the upper thoracic spine is preferred in order to avoid the heart and carotid and subclavian vessels. The rib to be resected should be articulating with a vertebral body just caudal to the level of the disc herniation. Following thoracotomy and mobilization of the parietal pleura, the segmental vessels may be ligated if necessary. The base of the rib is excised and the segmental nerves identified. The inferior pedicle is either partially or completely removed and the disc space incised. A partial discectomy is performed. A burr can than be used to create a trough by resecting the posterior portion of each vertebral body. Remaining disc material is then pulled into the trough. Depending on the extent of bone removal, a rib graft fusion may be performed.

Advantages include excellent exposure, anteriorly and anterolaterally, which permits safe decompression and dural manipulation. This approach is preferred for calcified large central discs in the presence of osteophytes or transdural TDH as well as TDH located behind the vertebral body. It entails limited bone removal, thereby diminishing the likelihood of destabilization while optimizing anterior interbody graft placement. The intercostal nerves are minimally traumatized.

Disadvantages mainly relate to the thoracotomy, which requires placement of a chest tube and additional risk of pulmonary complications. The thecal sac and spinal cord are directly in the field in the latter stages of the procedure. Disc herniations at the thoracolumbar level, the location of the majority of TDHs, may require that the diaphragm be taken down.

Laminectomy

Retraction of the thoracic spinal cord through a conventional laminectomy (Fig. 7) is limited by the tethering effect of the intact intradural ligaments and the fragility of the spinal cord. Consequently, exposure is often inadequate, compromising anterolateral access for removing disc material. Poor results for treatment of TDH by laminectomy occur in more than 50% of patients and include a high rate of paraplegia. For most patients, this approach should not be used.

Transsternal/Medial Clavisectomy

Either the transsternal or the medial clavisectomy (Table 4) approach allows access to the upper thoracic spine (T2-T4), which is often difficult to expose using other approaches. Posterolateral costotransversectomy and lateral extracavitary approaches are difficult because of limitations imposed by the scapula. A direct anterior approach should be considered and is indicated in the presence of central and centrolateral disc herniations. Either a transsternal splitting approach or a medial clavisectomy approach extending distally from a cervical Smith-Robinson approach, with the sternum left intact, can be used. Dissection is carried out in the plane between the left common carotid artery and the esophagus, trachea, thyroid, and innominate artery.

Thoracoscopy

Thoracoscopic discectomy is an evolving technique. Advantages include decreased postthoracotomy complications and hospitalization, diminished surgical trauma, less pain, and decreased cost.

The surgical technique is similar to the previously described transthoracic approach. Accurate cannula placement is paramount in optimizing visualization, and the assistance of a thoracic surgeon experienced in thoracoscopy may be useful. In one report of 29 patients with a 1-year follow-up, 75.8% were satisfied, 3.4% unsatisfied, and 20.1% unchanged. Independent postoperative MRI demonstrated adequate resection. The surgical and postoperative complication rate was 13.8%.

A period of practice in a laboratory setting allows familiarization with thoracoscopic orientation and the long instruments required for the procedure. Thoracoscopy may be better suited for far lateral (Fig. 10, *A*) soft disc herniations (Fig. 10, *B*), although treatment of recurrent central calcified disc herniations also has been successful.

Thoracic Spondylopathy and Stenosis

Thoracic stenosis has been defined as narrowing of the AP diameter of the adult thoracic canal to less than 10 mm. The differential diagnosis of the etiology of thoracic stenosis includes causes ensuing from forms of primary spondylopathy, which will be discussed here, and secondary stenosis related to underlying diseases, such as achondroplasia, acromegaly, ankylosing spondylitis, Paget's disease, osteofluorosis, Scheuermann's disease, and vitamin D-refractory rickets, or as complications of trauma, infection, or tumor. Thoracic stenosis only becomes clinically significant if the encroachment on the space available to the spinal cord is sufficient to cause myelopathy.

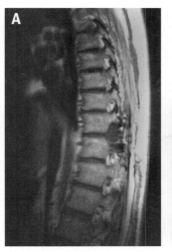
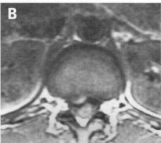

Figure 10 A, Sagittal MRI scan of a far lateral thoracic disc herniation. **B,** Axial MRI scan of a soft thoracic disc herniation. *(Reproduced with permission from Garfin SR, Vaccaro AR (eds):* Orthopaedic Knowledge Update: Spine. *Rosemont, IL, American Academy of Orthopaedic Surgeons, 1997, pp 87-96.)*

Spondylosis

Hypertrophic spondylosis, common to neural compression syndromes of the cervical and lumbar spines, is an uncommon cause of thoracic stenosis of sufficient severity to require surgical care, perhaps because of the limited excursion and coronal orientation of the facet joints and the stability imposed by the rib cage. When clinically significant thoracic stenosis does result from spondylosis, the changes usually have been superimposed on a congenitally small canal in a patient who is likely to have cervical and lumbar stenosis as well. Spondylotic thoracic stenosis is most likely to occur in the lower thoracic spine where the facet joints have a configuration more like that of the lumbar spine. Particularly florid forms of hypertrophic disease, such as diffuse idiopathic skeletal hyperostosis (DISH or Forestier's disease) may place patients at greater risk. However, the hypertrophic changes in that disease are greatest anterior to the vertebrae and are not likely to cause stenosis unless associated with ossification of ligaments within the canal. Synovial cysts arising from spondylotic facet joints can be the cause of myelopathy. Surgical decompression for stenosis secondary to facet arthropathy can be done through a conventional laminectomy, medial facetectomy, and foraminotomy if the imaging studies confirm that the neural compression is purely posterolateral so that retraction of the cord is not necessary.

Ossification of the Posterior Longitudinal Ligament

More than 80% of OPLL occurs in the cervical spine, with the other 20% evenly divided between the thoracic and lumbar spine. The etiology involves a polygenetic autosomal dominant inheritance, with the disorder much more common among Asians, although it has been reported with increasing frequency in North Americans of non-Asian descent. Unlike ordinary spondylosis, mature lamellar bone is juxtaposed with hypertrophic fibers of the posterior longitudinal ligament (PLL), resulting in diffuse boney enlargement of the PLL, which leads to compression of the cord from ventral compromise of the spinal canal. Surgical treatment usually requires anterior or anterior and posterior combined approaches.

Ossification of the Yellow Ligament

Ossification of the ligamentum flavum, or OYL, occurs with about equal frequency in the cervical, dorsal, and lumbar spine. Involvement of the dorsal spine is usually near the thoracolumbar junction, but may occur in the upper thoracic spine as well. The disorder may be associated with metabolic diseases such as diabetes, hemochromatosis, Paget's disease, X-linked hypophosphatemia, and pyrophosphate crystal disease. It may occur along with spondylosis, DISH, and or OPLL. Usually ossification occurs at the laminar attachments of the ligamentum flavum and does not include interlaminar fusion. Evaluation by MRI gives the best view of neural compression, but CT may be more sensitive to the borders of the ossified tissues. Surgical treatment, if the compression is due entirely to posterior disease, can be accomplished through laminectomy and medial facetectomy. In advanced cases, the ossified ligamentum flavum may not be separable from the underlying dura, requiring the surgeon to be prepared to deal with dural defects or fistulae.

Annotated Bibliography

Dickman CA, Rosenthal D, Regan JJ: Reoperation for herniated thoracic discs. *J Neurosurg* 1999;91(suppl 2): 157-162.

The authors reviewed 15 revision TDHs. The posterolateral approach was most commonly associated with failure to excise the disc fragment. In addition, calcified broad-based large and centrally located fragments as well as transdural thoracic discs were more likely to be incompletely resected.

Epstein NE: Ossification of the yellow ligament and spondylosis and/or ossification of the posterior longitudinal ligament of the thoracic and lumbar spine. *J Spinal Disorder* 1999;12:250-256.

Twenty-six patients with lumbar and thoracic stenosis from OYL, OPLL, spondylosis, or combined etiologies were reviewed. Four of the patients had thoracic stenosis, all in the lower thoracic spine; one from OPLL and spondylosis, one from OYL, and two from OPLL, OYL, and spondylosis combined. OPLL/spondylosis patients required anterior/posterior surgical approaches whereas those with OYL alone were approached posteriorly.

Korovessis PG, Stamatakis MV, Baikousis A, Vasiliou D: Transthoracic disc excision with interbody fusion: 12 patients with symptomatic disc herniation followed for 2 to 8 years. *Acta Orthop Scand* Suppl 1997;275:12-16.

A 4-year follow-up of 12 patients who underwent a transthoracic discectomy and fusion is presented. The outcome was excellent to good in 10, fair in 1, and unchanged in 1. Seven patients with incomplete neurologic change recovered at least one grade. There were no approach-related complications.

Kruse JJ, Awasthi D, Harris M, Waguespack A: Ossification of the ligamentum flavum as a cause of myelopathy in North America: report of three cases. *J Spinal Disord* 2000;13:22-25.

The authors' three cases of myelopathy from OYL include one cervical, one upper thoracic, and one lower thoracic.

Lehman RM, Grunweg B, Hall T: Anterior approach to the cervicothoracic junction: An anatomic dissection. *J Spinal Disord* 1997;10:33-39.

Color photographs and excellent anatomic drawings detail the anatomy of the anterior exposure of C4 though T4, along with discussion of the surgical exposure of this region.

Levi N, Gjerris F, Dons K: Thoracic disc herniation: Unilateral transpedicular approach in 35 consecutive patients. *J Neurosurg Sci* 1999;43:37-43.

Of the patients, 74% had a good to fair result. Twenty-three patients presented with myelopathy; in eight the outcome was unchanged.

Regan JJ, Ben-Yishay A, Mack MJ: Video-assisted thoracoscopic excision of herniated thoracic disc: Description of technique and preliminary experience in the first 29 cases. *J Spinal Disord* 1998;11:183-191.

Herniations ranged from T5-6 to T12-L1. Postoperative MRI was obtained in all 29 patients. Twenty-two patients were satisfied, one was not satisfied, and six were unchanged. The complication rate was 13.8%. Follow-up at 1 year showed high patient satisfaction.

Sar C, Hamzaoglu A, Talu U, Domanic U: An anterior approach to the cervicothoracic junction of the spine (modified osteotomy of manubrium sterni and clavicle). *J Spinal Disord* 1999;12:102-106.

Resection of the manubrium sterni and medial clavicle for exposure of the upper thoracic spine and cervicothoracic junction is described and illustrated by a case in which C6 through T2 vertebral bodies were resected and grafted for treatment of tuberculous abscess.

Stillerman CB, Chen TC, Couldwell WT, Zhang W, Weiss MH: Experience in the surgical management of 82 symptomatic HTDs and review of the literature. *J Neurosurg* 1998;88:623-633.

An excellent comprehensive review of the subject, including surgical options and indications is presented.

Stoodley MA, Jones NR, Scott G: Cervical and thoracic juxtafacet cysts causing neurologic defects. *Spine* 2000; 25:970-973.

The authors review 8 cases of juxtafacet spinal cysts, one of which was in the thoracic spine and caused myelopathy. They cite four previously reported cases of cysts arising from the facet joints of the thoracic spine.

van Oostenbrugge RJ, Herpers MJ, de Kruijk JR: Spinal cord compression caused by unusual location and extension of ossified ligamenta flava in a Caucasian male: A case report and literature review. *Spine* 1999;24:486-488.

The authors present and discuss a case of thoracic myelopathy from OYL of the upper thoracic spine.

Wood KB, Blair JM, Aepple DM, et al: The natural history of asymptomatic thoracic disc herniations. *Spine* 1997;22:525-529.

In this study the authors indicated asymptomatic TDHs may exist in a state of flux exhibiting little change while remaining asymptomatic. Small herniations remain unchanged or increased in size while large herniations often decrease in size.

Wood KB, Garvey TA, Gundry C, et al: Magnetic resonance imaging of the thoracic spine: Evaluation of asymptomatic individuals. *J Bone Joint Surg Am* 1995; 77:1631-1638.

Wood KB, Schellhas KP, Garvey TA, Aeppli D: Thoracic discography in healthy individuals: A controlled prospective study of magnetic resonance imaging and discography in asymptomatic and symptomatic individuals. *Spine* 1999;24:1548-1555.

The authors performed four level discography on the thoracic spines of 10 healthy volunteers and 10 nonlitigious thoracic pain patients. Injection of discs at sites of Schmorl's nodes caused intense pain even among the asymptomatic subjects. Discography revealed pathologic changes in thoracic discs that were not seen by MRI.

Classic Bibliography

Arce CA, Dohrmann GJ: Herniated thoracic disks. *Neurol Clin* 1985;3:383-392.

Awwad EE, Martin DS, Smith KR Jr, et al: Asymptomatic versus symptomatic herniated thoracic discs: Their frequency and characteristics as detected by computed tomography after myelography. *Neurosurgery* 1991;28: 180-186.

Bohlmann HH, Zdeblick TA: Anterior excision of herniated thoracic discs. *J Bone Joint Surg Am* 1988;70: 1038-1047.

Brown CW, Deffer PA Jr, Akmakjian J, et al: The natural history of thoracic disc herniation. *Spine* 1992;17 (suppl 6):S97-S102.

Currier BL, Eismont FJ, Green BA: Transthoracic disc excision and fusion for herniated thoracic disks. *Spine* 1994;19:323-328.

el-Kalliny M, Tew JM Jr, van Loveren H, et al: Surgical approaches to thoracic disc herniations. *Acta Neurochir* 1991;111:22-32.

Epstein NE, Schwall G: Thoracic spinal stenosis: Diagnostic and treatment challenges. *J Spinal Disord* 1994;7: 259-269.

Hulme A: The surgical approach to thoracic intervertebral disc protrusions. *J Neurol Neurosurg Psychiatry* 1960;23:133-137.

Kurz LT, Pursel SE, Herkowitz HN: Modified anterior approach to the cervicothoracic junction. *Spine* 1991; 16(suppl 10):S542-S547.

Lesoin F, Rousseaux M, Qautricque A, et al: Thoracic disc herniations: Evolution in the approach and indications. *Acta Neurochir* 1986;80:30-34.

Love JG, Schorn VG: Thoracic-disk protrusions. *JAMA* 1965;191:627-631.

Maiman DJ, Larson SJ, Luck E, et al: Lateral extracavitary approach to the spine for thoracic disc herniation: Report of 23 cases. *Neurosurgery* 1984;14:178-182.

Okada K, Oka S, Tohge K, Ono K, Yonenobu K, Hosoya T: Thoracic myelopathy caused by ossification of the ligamentum flavum: Clinicopathologic study and surgical treatment. *Spine* 1991;16:280-287.

Patterson RH Jr, Arbit E: A surgical approach through the pedicle to protruded thoracic discs. *J Neurosurg* 1978;48:768-772.

Perot PL Jr, Munro DD: Transthoracic removal of midline thoracic disc protrusions causing spinal cord compression. *J Neurosurg* 1969;31:452-458.

Rosenthal D, Rosenthal R, de Simone A: Removal of a protruded thoracic disk using microsurgical endoscopy: A new technique. *Spine* 1994;19:1087-1091.

Simpson JM, Silveri CP, Simeone FA, et al: Thoracic disk herniation: Re-evaluation of the posterior approach using a modified costotransversectomy. *Spine* 1993;18: 1872-1877.

Singounas EG, Kypriades EM, Kellerman AJ, et al: Thoracic disc herniation: Analysis of 14 cases and review of the literature. *Acta Neurochir* 1992;116:49-52.

Stillerman CB, Weiss MH: Management of thoracic disc disease. *Clin Neurosurg* 1992;38:325-352.

Williams MP, Cherryman GR, Husband JE: Significance of thoracic disc herniation demonstrated by MR imaging. *J Comput Assist Tomogr* 1989;13:211-214.

Chapter 34

Lumbar Disc Herniation

Michael G. Johnson, MD, FRCSC

Thomas J. Errico, MD

Epidemiology

Low back pain with or without leg pain has plagued humans for centuries. Approximately 60% to 80% of Americans suffer attacks of low back pain at some time in their lives; however the incidence of sciatica is much less frequent. A symptomatic lumbar disc herniation (LDH) occurs during the lifetime of approximately 2% of the general population. Factors associated with a greater risk of low back disorders and LDH include: male gender, age between 30 and 50 years, jobs requiring heavy lifting, lifting in a twisted or asymmetric posture, stressful occupations, lower income, cigarette smoking, and exposure to prolonged vibrations in the range of 4 to 5 Hz.

The lifetime prevalence of lumbar disc surgery in the United States is approximately 1% to 3%. Significant regional surgical variations exist despite small differences in the incidence and point prevalence of sciatica and low back pain. When the prevalence of sciatica and persistent radiculopathies are considered, surgical treatment should be considered for fewer than 0.5% of the population.

LDH is an important aspect of health care because of the prevalence of symptoms of sciatica and low back pain in the general population, a natural history of resolution of symptoms in most patients, and the dramatic resolution of symptoms that often follows surgical disc excision.

Natural History

A discussion of the natural history of LDH must consider the variable situations in which the disc can herniate. The type of herniation (contained, extruded or sequestered), the canal location (central, posterolateral, foraminal, extraforaminal), the spinal level (high versus low), the inflammatory potential of the herniated material, and coexisting anatomic considerations (stenosis, spondylolisthesis, degenerative scoliosis) can influence the symptoms, signs, and natural history.

Weber's 1983 article is often quoted as a natural history study of LDH. This work describes the first randomized trial comparing surgery to nonsurgical therapy. Two hundred eighty patients with myelographically documented LDHs received 14 days of in-hospital management. After this time the patients who either improved or neurologically deteriorated were excluded, and the rest were randomized to surgical and nonsurgical groups. In the nonsurgical group, 25% were cured and 36% showed satisfactory improvement. Approximately 60% of the patients who underwent surgery may thus have been submitted to an unnecessary procedure. A period of 3 months was sufficient to decide against surgery in four fifths of the nonsurgically treated group who had good and fair results. If all patients were to wait 3 months for a surgical procedure, 40% would spend this time in a painful condition with potential psychosocial consequences. Within the first year after disc excision, surgery was more efficient treatment than nonsurgical therapy. The advantage of surgery faded with time, so that after 4 years there was no difference between the two groups. A 3-month period of observation before performing surgery had no effect on the outcome. Weber concluded that in the absence of cauda equina syndrome or progressive neurologic deficit, the physician can allow some time to pass because the symptoms may resolve spontaneously. After 12 months from the onset of leg symptoms the quality of the surgical result deteriorates.

Important concerns have been raised in regard to Weber's article. Although there had been a long period of follow-up (10 years) and a very low dropout rate, problems include a 25% crossover of the nonsurgically treated group, unclear definition of nonsurgical therapy, inadequate sample size, and an insensitive, author administered, outcome measure.

Pathophysiology

The intervertebral disc is composed of the central nucleus pulposus and the outer anulus fibrosus. The central portion of the disc is avascular, depending on diffusion for nutrition. No healing potential exists.

It is generally believed but not proven that intradiscal fragmentation precedes and is the driving force behind annular rupture. Necropsy studies indicate that structural deterioration begins in the intervertebral disc in early adult life with dehydration, intradiscal fissuring, and fragmentation, which is followed by annular disruption progressing outward from the inner annular layers. The end result is a complete annular tear and, sometimes, herniation of disc material.

During this process, the patient may experience a variety of symptoms. Because the interior of the intervertebral disc is sparsely innervated the process of intradiscal fissure and fragmentation is virtually asymptomatic. When the outer anulus (the innervated portion of the disc) becomes involved, backache frequently becomes a component of the problem. With herniation the pressure that was on the anulus is transferred to the nerve root. In most people this will produce the characteristic radicular pain symptom that defines sciatica. If the anulus finally ruptures completely and the intradiscal fragment completely extrudes into the spinal canal, the back pain and stiffness commonly are relieved, but the sciatica may intensify. However, the entire process of fragmentation, fissure, and herniation can proceed with no back pain or sciatica.

The interaction of mechanical and inflammatory components yielding signs and symptoms of radiculopathy is a generally accepted model for understanding LDH, but the contributions of each are not well understood. In some patients, especially those with excruciating sciatica, there may be a component of local nerve root ischemia.

An extruded lumbar intervertebral disc has inflammatory potential. The specific role of cytokines in symptom generation is a field of evolving study. Local control of inflammation by administration of epidural steroids around the nerve root and dura has resulted in varied success. Some authors report reductions in prescribed analgesic drug consumption and improvements in overall health perception, whereas others have reported increased incidence of epidural abscesses. Further study has the potential to result in clinically relevant treatment options.

Classification and Terminology

LDH classification is based on the relationship of the herniated material to the posterior anulus fibrosus and posterior longitudinal ligament (PLL), the continuity of the herniated material with the remainder of the disc, and the level of the herniation.

All types of disc herniations must be differentiated from a disc bulge, a diffuse symmetrical outpouching of the anulus fibrosus caused by early disc degeneration and collapse, which rarely causes symptoms unless associated with spinal stenosis. A true disc herniation is either a "protrusion," with the base wider than any diameter of the material displaced beyond the disc space, or an "extrusion," in which the displaced portion has a greater diameter than its connection with the parent disc at its base. If an extrusion has lost all connection with the parent disc, it may be characterized as a "sequestration." An extruded disc, whether sequestrated or not, that has been displaced above or below the edges of the disc space is "migrated." Disc herniations can further be characterized by whether they are "contained" or "uncontained," depending on whether the displaced portion is completely enveloped by intact outer anulus or a combination of anulus and PLL, sometimes called "capsule." Disc material contained beneath the PLL is sometimes referred to as "subligamentous," whereas that contained only by peridural membrane can be called "submembranous."

LDHs also are described by their relationship along the circumference of the anulus fibrosus. Herniations along the posterior anulus can be central (midline), posterolateral (most common, along the weaker lateral expansion of the PLL), foraminal (lateral), or extraforaminal (far lateral).

A typical herniation compresses along the lateral border (the shoulder) of the nerve root. Posterolateral herniations will affect the root at the level below the herniation (L5 root with L4-5 LDH). Foraminal and extraforaminal herniations may affect the exiting nerve root at the level of the herniation (the L4 root with L4-5 LDH). An uncontained disc herniation may extend into the axilla of the nerve root residing between the nerve root and the dural sac (an axillary herniation).

High LDHs (L1-2, L2-3) are differentiated from low (L3-4, L4-5, L5-S1) LDHs. The two most common levels of disc herniation are L4-5 and L5-S1. Together these two levels make up 90% of symptomatic disc herniations. The L3-4 level is the next most common. Rare intradural herniations occur predominantly in the higher lumbar levels and account for an extremely small number of the total LDHs.

Clinical Presentations

Sciatica is a sharp pain starting at the hip or proximal portion of the thigh and ultimately progressing distally in a dermatomal pattern. Before the onset of sciatica, a long history of intermittent attacks of low back pain is common. The onset of pain may be sudden and related to a specific innocuous movement that involves bending, twisting, or in some cases a cough or a sneeze.

Radicular pain must be differentiated from referred pain. When mesodermal structures are subjected to abnormal stimuli a deep, dull, aching discomfort is noted that may be referred to the areas of the lumbosacral joint, sacroiliac joint, buttocks, or legs. The pattern of referral is to the area of the sclerotome, which has the same embryonic origin as the mesodermal tissues stimulated. Radicular pain has a dermatomal distribution and usually radiates below the knee.

The sciatica of LDH often is aggravated by sitting and relieved by lying down or by standing. Data regarding intradiscal pressures have demonstrated that pressure varies with position. The L3-4 disc pressure in unsupported upright sitting position is 43% greater than in upright standing. This may help explain the preference for the standing position over the sitting position in some patients.

An understanding of the wide range of presenting symptoms is crucial. Most do not fit the classic presentation of the young patient with an acute onset of unilateral leg symptoms in a dermatomal distribution after a Valsalva maneuver. Very large disc herniations can occupy significant portions of the spinal canal, creating a localized stenotic region that results in symptoms more consistent with stenosis than with true sciatica. In other patients, an LDH can distend the outer, innervated annular structures and cause a significant amount of back pain as well as leg pain. Patients rarely have back pain alone. This pain often is seen with central herniations. The patient may never go on to develop frank sciatica, and few of these patients go on to become surgical candidates. Sciatic pain can occur without any low back pain. In all of these clinical presentations, sciatica due to LDH is suggested because symptoms are accentuated by a Valsalva maneuver.

LDH can present as changes in symptoms in a patient with previous symptoms of lumbar spinal stenosis. Acute radicular symptoms will be superimposed on a chronic history of vague leg pain, dysesthesias, and paresthesias that often are not in a single pure dermatomal pattern and are brought on by activity or spinal postures (extension) that mechanically compromise the size of the spinal canal and neural foramina.

Occasionally the patient may have large midline herniations that compress several or all nerve roots of the cauda equina. Cauda equina syndrome is an uncommon presentation of an LDH but must be recognized because the consequences of delayed recognition and treatment can be disastrous. The incidence is approximately 1% to 2.4% of symptomatic LDHs with no sex differences. It is more likely that a higher lumbar or

intradural herniation will cause cauda equina syndrome. The syndrome is clinically defined by bowel and bladder difficulties, saddle anesthesia, and lower extremity sensory and motor deficits. Difficulty with urination, including frequency or overflow incontinence is common. In males there may be a history of impotence. Compression of the centrally placed sacral fibers to the lower abdominal viscera produce symptoms of perianal numbness, dysesthesias, and loss of the anal reflex or diminished rectal tone. The diagnosis can be difficult if the condition is incomplete or is evolving slowly. The syndrome is considered a reason for prompt surgical intervention because spontaneous recovery has not been reported. Intervention recently has been reported as having the most favorable outcome if done less than 48 hours from onset of symptoms.

Differential Diagnosis

An organized differential diagnosis of sciatica should entertain pathology originating from the spinal cord (myelogenic) and the root as it exits the lateral recess and foramen as well as distally at the plexus level and beyond. Intraspinal pathology, such as lateral recess stenosis, epidural hemorrhage and abscesses, tumors, and facet ganglia, and extraspinal pathology, such as intrapelvic tumors, and local compression of the sciatic nerve in the buttocks, must be considered.

Clinical Examination

The standing patient who declines to sit, with loss of normal lumbar lordosis and paravertebral muscle spasm, suggests a disc herniation. A list (sciatic scoliosis) can suggest the position of the herniated fragment. With an axillary herniation or central herniation the patient will list toward the side of the herniation, and with a posterolateral herniation the patient will list away from the side of the herniation in an effort to decompress the root. Spine range of motion usually is limited, and the patient will describe positions of foreword flexion reproducing the leg pain. Gait is antalagic (painful leg held flexed), and if there is L5 nerve root weakness (gluteus medius) a Trendelenburg gait may be present.

Waddell's signs of nonorganic pathology should be sought. These include tenderness to light touch or in a nonanatomic distribution, low back pain reported with pressure on the patient's head while standing, loss of a positive physical finding by distracting the patient, disturbances of sensation in a nonanatomic distribution, and overreaction. Motor points represent the neuromuscular junction of the involved muscle groups. Patients with signs and symptoms of a radiculopathy have tender motor points in the myotome corresponding to the segmental level of the nerve root involved. In the absence of radicular signs, back pain patients with tender motor points remain disabled nearly three times as long as those patients without tenderness. If a radiculopathy is present with the back pain, the disability is nearly four times as long.

The neurologic examination should include motor and sensory testing as well as reflexes (Table 1). During a straight leg raise maneuver, the L5 and S1 nerve roots either move or passively deform approximately 2 to 6 mm at the level of the foramina. Maximal tension is realized in the sciatic nerve at 35° to 70° of elevation from the supine position. Because deformation in the sciatic nerve after 70° occurs distal to the neural foramina, any radicular symptoms elicited at this elevation should not be attributed to a herniated lumbar disc. The straight leg raise (SLR) test is of most value in lesions of the L5 and S1 roots. A positive SLR test is seen in nearly all patients younger than 30 years old with a symptomatic disc herniation. The absence of a positive SLR in a patient younger than 30 years old makes a disc herniation unlikely. In older patients, the SLR test may be negative in the presence of a symptomatic low lumbar disc herniation.

Classically, the test is performed with the patient supine, one of the examiner's hands on the ilium to stabilize the pelvis, and the other hand on the patient's heel. With the patient's knee straight the leg is slowly elevated, and the patient is asked if this maneuver reproduces leg pain. Only when leg pain or radicular symptoms are produced can the test be considered positive. The test also can be performed with the patient in

different positions. The tripod or flip test is performed with the patient sitting, the hip flexed, and the knee slowly extended. A positive test results in the patient sitting backward, extending the hips, and supporting himself or herself with arms in an effort to relieve tension on the root. The advantage of this test is that the experienced patient may anticipate a supine SLR, and the results may be influenced.

Other variations of the SLR have been described. The knee and hip can be flexed to 90° and the knee can gradually be extended. Both this test and the straight SLR have been attributed to Lasègue. Another variation has the foot dorsiflexed after the knee is extended. The Bowstring sign is another manifestation of tension on the nerve root. The test is performed with the regular SLR, eliciting leg symptoms. At this point, the knee is flexed and symptoms are usually reduced. Finger pressure is then applied in the popliteal space. Reestablishment of the radicular symptoms is considered a positive sign. The contralateral SLR or crossed SLR test is performed in the same manner as the SLR except that the opposite leg is raised. A positive test is indicated by sciatica induced in the contralateral leg. The accuracy of the SLR may be limited by its low specificity, whereas the crossed SLR is more specific of a disc herniation (especially an axillary LDH).

When the roots of the femoral nerve are involved (L2, L3, and L4), the appropriate tension test is the reverse SLR. This usually is performed with the patient in the prone position or laterally with the unaffected hip down with hip extension and knee flexion. As with the SLR, there is a contralateral femoral traction sign. In these cases the pain reproduction is usually in the anterior or lateral aspect of the groin, thigh, knee, or leg.

TABLE 1 | Neurologic Examination Testing of L4, L5, and S1 Nerve Roots

Nerve Root	Motor	Sensory	Reflex
L4	Hip adductors	Posterolateral thigh	Patellar tendon
	Quadriceps	Anterior knee	Tibialis anterior
		Medial leg	
L5	Extensor hallucis longus	Anterolateral leg	Tibialis posterior
	Gluteus medius	Dorsum of the foot	
	Extensor digitorium longus and brevis	Great toe	
S1	Peroneus longus and brevis	Lateral malleolus	Tendocalcaneus
	Gastrocnemius-soleus complex	Lateral foot	
	Gluteus maximus	Web of fourth and fifth toe	

(Adapted with permission from Canale ST (ed): Campbell's Operative Orthopaedics, ed 9. St Louis, MO, Mosby-Year Book, 1998, vol 3, p 3052.)

Imaging

Because of favorable natural history, tests are not mandatory during the first 6 to 8 weeks. Plain radiographs are not helpful for the diagnosis of LDH but are indicated in patients with greater than 6 weeks of low back pain and in patients with a clinical history of significant trauma, constitutional symptoms, or previous cancers. CT scanning is the least expensive and is the best at imaging the osseous elements but is insensitive to lesions of the conus medullaris. MRI provides the best imaging of the disc spaces and neural elements and can image the entire neural canal to the conus. The lateral sagittal MRI cuts can be used to evaluate the neural foramen. Intrathecal contrast (myelography) provides superior detail compared to CT scans, and is indicated if MRI is not available or for patients in whom MRI is contraindicated (due to cardiac pacemakers or brain aneurysm clips).

Accurate interpretation of the imaging is critical because the single best predictor of patient outcome following lumbar discectomy is the size of the protrusion itself. Patients with large protrusions causing nerve compression have a significantly better surgical outcome than do those with less impressive surgical findings. Correlation of imaging findings and clinical examination increases the chance of finding a disc herniation at the time of surgery, decreasing negative surgical explorations.

Correlation of imaging and clinical findings is crucial given the overall incidence of disc abnormalities found in asymptomatic subjects (37%). The ability to predict accurately the presence of a disc herniation is 55% when diagnosis is based on the presence of an objective neurologic finding alone. Accuracy increases to 66% when the clinical finding is an abnormal SLR test. When neurologic abnormality is combined with positive SLR test, the ability to accurately predict the presence of a disc herniation increases to 86%. Finally, when both a positive neurologic finding and a positive SLR are combined with a positive diagnostic image at the level consistent with the observed clinical findings, the chance of finding a disc herniation at surgery is 95%.

Serial CT and MRI scans document overall decreases in the size of the herniated disc material over time, presumably due to dehydration of the disc fragments or vascular inflammatory response. Large extrusions and those that migrate demonstrate the most resorption. The mechanism of resorption is unknown. Once the fragments have been deposited in the vascular environment of the epidural canal, cellular mechanisms may effect resorption. Chemokines have been isolated from macrophages that have infiltrated nuclear herniations. Macrophages may initiate the resorptive process by cytokine expression.

Neurophysiologic Testing

Neurophysiologic testing is not necessary to confirm the presence of radiculopathy and as such is not part of the standard work-up. It is not specific enough to determine the exact spinal root level because multisegmental and/or anomalous innervation patterns often are present. Electrophysiologic testing does not directly evaluate the neurologic mechanism associated with pain generation. It can determine the chronicity and severity of spinal nerve root lesions and differentiate the nervous system level of involvement (ie, cord, root, peripheral nerve, and muscle). Neurophysiologic testing is appropriate when the clinical situation is not clear, or if it is necessary to differentiate a disc herniation from other neurologic disorders such as neuropathy or peripheral nerve entrapment.

Treatment

Nonsurgical Treatment

In most patients a nonsurgical approach is used initially. Weber's findings shape much of the reasoning for nonsurgical management. Although he suggested delaying surgery for 3 months, other authors have lowered this, stating that surgery is not necessary for 6 to 12 weeks.

In the acute setting, an initial period of 2 to 3 days of bed rest may be appropriate. Longer periods of bed rest are detrimental to overall recovery. Useful medications include aspirin and nonsteroidal anti-inflammatory medications. An initial course of oral steroids can be effective in improving the symptoms and signs. Narcotic medication can be used judiciously for short periods of time if the pain is severe. Short-term use of muscle relaxants to control back spasm is appropriate but long-term use of muscle relaxants for primarily radicular complaints is not. Antidepressant medications and antiepileptic drugs have a role in the nonsurgical care of both acute and chronic radicular pain. The long-time use of long acting narcotic medications in acute and chronic disc herniation is a controversial topic, and their exact role remains to be elucidated.

After an initial period of rest, progressive return of daily activities is recommended. A formal program of physical activity may be useful, but a simple set of home exercises and aerobic fitness training is often adequate. Epidural steroid injections may be helpful in improving symptoms although the effects may be temporary. Rat and rabbit animal models have shown varying results, and randomized controlled trials and meta-analysis of epidural steroid use in relief of lumbar radicular symptoms have demonstrated short-term improvements in leg pain and sensory deficit and but no longer-term effects.

Assessing the efficacy of other modalities presents

difficulties because many published studies group different types of patients together. Traction has not been associated with regression of LDH. Some authors report short-term pain relief when traction is applied to patients with sciatica of unclear etiology. Manipulation has been found to be useful in patients with acute low back pain within the first 4 weeks. No data support the use of manipulation in treatment of radiculopathy and LDH. No randomized controlled trials have assessed the efficacy of formal physical therapy. The available data suggest that dynamic, high intensity exercises that build muscle strength and endurance improve the health status of the patient with a lumbar spine disorder. Passive care with bed rest leads to physical deconditioning, loss of motivation, and negative calcium balance. The best predictors of good outcome in nonsurgically treated patients are symptoms less than 6 months in duration, no involvement in litigation, and younger age.

Surgical Treatment

Open discectomy is the standard surgical intervention in patients with LDH whose conservative treatment has failed. Despite over 60 years of experience, the indications for surgery and the expected success rates still are reported variably. Patient selection and surgical procedures also continue to evolve. Surgical excision of the displaced disc tissue removes both the source of pressure and the initiator of the inflammatory response.

Operating before 4 to 6 weeks have passed is too soon, except in the scenario of major muscle weakness, loss of bowel or bladder function, and, in rare instances, of excruciating pain uncontrollable with conservative treatment. Some patients with nerve root symptoms lasting more than 6 months develop chronic nerve pain that is not totally relieved by disc excision. A window of opportunity thus exists. Optimal surgical results can be expected if the period of present attack of sciatica is less than 6 months compared with symptoms of 6 to 12 months or longer than 12 months.

Technique refinements have resulted in numerous variations by which open discectomy may be performed. Current practice includes a small incision, muscle and bone dissection limited to the minimum needed for exposure, and resection of displaced and loose disc material. Adjuncts to the procedure assist in limiting trauma to uninvolved tissue while achieving the goals of decompression with the avoidance of iatrogenic instability. These include a headlamp for high intensity lighting. Vision is enhanced with either loupes (glasses with magnification) or a microscope. The role of the microscope is controversial. Retrospective comparisons of the two methods have shown shorter inpatient stays, less time off work, and better results with microscope

use. Other authors have reported no differences between discectomy with and without the microscope in terms of perioperative bleeding, complications, inpatient stay, time off work, and subjective end result either short term or at 1 year. The incidence of recurrent disc herniation with either technique has been reported to be similar. Overall, the two methods have remarkably similar outcomes. With improved techniques resulting in decreased morbidity, lumbar discectomy has been addressed as a potential outpatient procedure with 88% excellent and good results.

Current rehabilitation protocols after open discectomy vary from several weeks to months of restricted activities. Traditional recommendations regarding return to work are return to light work after 4 weeks, moderate work after 8 weeks, and heavy work after 3 months. The necessity for these restrictions has recently come into question. Lifting the postoperative activity restrictions and promotion of early return to work after discectomy has been reported to allow for shortened sick leave without increasing complications.

Positive prognostic factors of good outcome in lumbar disc surgery have been found to include: no work-related injury, absence of back pain, pain extending to the foot, leg pain with SLR testing, absence of back pain on SLR testing, and size of the disc herniation. Psychosocial factors play a role with social support from the spouse being an independent predictor of pain relief 2 years after surgery. Return to work may be less influenced by clinical findings or MRI-identified morphologic abnormalities and more by psychological factors (depression) and psychological aspects of work (occupational mental stress). Patients who have more than 6 months sick leave before surgery are also less likely to have a good outcome.

Overall, little consensus exists in the literature regarding outcomes of LDH surgery. Whereas retrospective studies show success rates as high as 98%, prospective studies have results in the 73% to 77% range. Conflicting evidence exists as to whether the outcome in appropriately selected patients is maintained at long-term follow-up. Studies have found no differences between surgical and control groups at 10 years. Overall patient responses do tend to show high satisfaction with the outcome of surgery and disability scores at 10-year follow-up are low.

Special Cases

Outcome results in age extremes have been reported. Elderly patients, in both the short and long term, experienced results not significantly different from those of younger groups. Lumbar discectomy in children is reported to have an 80% reoperation rate at 10 years and a 74% reoperation rate at 20 years. Long-term follow-up of children younger than 15 years of age indicated that 40% were totally asymptomatic and 60% had recurring symptoms. Despite these findings, overall long-term outcome in children was subjectively reported as good to moderate in 90%. The amount of disc material to be removed in children is an unresolved issue. Removal of a minimum to maintain the intervertebral disc functions is currently recommended. Leaving the inner anulus intact in the growing child may be important because proteoglycan synthesis is the most active in the anulus of the growing child and leaving the anulus intact may give rise to regeneration of the intervertebral disc material.

The amount of disc to be removed is also an issue in the elite athlete with the trend toward removing the least possible amount of disc. Overall success rates of one-level procedures have been reported at 90% of athletes returning to competition at a highly competitive level, but the results from two-level disease were less favorable.

Multiple studies support suboptimal socioeconomic outcomes for spinal surgery for degenerative conditions in a workers' compensation venue. The literature demonstrates poor outcomes for surgery in workers' compensation patients, with 26% to 43% returning to work. Study groups of patients on workers' compensation consistently show worse outcomes, with less work retention and higher reoperation rates. Legal involvement is associated with poorer outcomes.

Upper lumbar herniations (L1-2, L2-3, L3-4) deserve special mention because the preoperative signs and symptoms have been reported to be highly variable, potentially leading to confusion regarding the level of herniation. Radiographic studies have a high false-negative rate, especially at the higher L2-3 level. The relative medial position of the facet and the pars interarticularis make their violation with even a carefully performed hemilaminotomy more probable. For this reason some authors suggest a bilateral laminotomy for unilateral compression as a safeguard against pars interruption or excessive facet disruption.

Far lateral disc herniations (herniation into or beyond the foramen) occur in 8% to 10% of patients. The nerve root at the same level as the herniation is compressed. Before improved imaging techniques, failure to recognize its presence was responsible for persistent sciatica after surgery. CT and MRI now allow successful identification of the location of the pathology. Varying surgical approaches have been used with the goal being adequate decompression while causing the least amount of muscle and soft-tissue damage and preservation of as much facet joint as possible. Complete removal of a facet joint unilaterally to gain access to a far lateral disc

herniation should be avoided. A better solution is the muscle splitting approach. Proper understanding of the anatomy underneath the intertransverse membrane is critical to the identification of the underlying spinal nerve and ganglion and safe performance of these procedures. In certain instances the disc herniation may occupy a position both intracanal and lateral, and thus an approach from inside and outside the spinal canal may be necessary.

Complications

Failure of disc herniation surgery, known as the failed open discectomy syndrome, is defined by the new onset of leg pain or an increase in low back pain after discectomy. Persisting back pain is sometimes wrongfully looked on as a failure of disc excision surgery. New or increased low back pain does not always constitute an outcome failure because disc excision is intended for relief of sciatic pain rather than back pain.

This syndrome can be classified into two groups: immediate failure and delayed failure. Causes of immediate failure include insufficient neural decompression, surgery at the wrong level, and traumatization of the nerve root. Missed diagnoses are sources of immediate failure: lateral spinal stenosis, 58.5%; recurrent or persistent herniation, 14%; adhesive arachnoiditis, 11%; central canal stenosis, 10.5%; and epidural fibrosis, 7%. Causes of delayed failure include recurrent disc herniation, epidural fibrosis, arachnoiditis, and iatrogenic spinal instability. Infection can play a role either early or late.

The most frequent cause of a poor result is erroneous or incomplete diagnosis. Technical errors, such as removing the wrong disc or failing to remove the offending fragment, explain a small percentage of failures. Worsening of low back pain or onset of low back pain where only leg pain had existed can result from surgery for disc removal. Facet fractures have been investigated as a cause of persisting or recurrent pain. Removal of an entire lamina or of more than 25% of the lamina just above the facet may contribute to this problem.

Recurrent herniations of the same disc may occur because all common techniques leave substantial quantities of disc. There is no consensus of how much disc material the surgeon should remove. Overall recurrence rates of 5% to 8% are quoted with standard discectomy methods.

After excluding infection, stenosis, instability, and arachnoiditis it is important to distinguish between patients with recurrent herniated disc fragments and those with epidural fibrosis because the management of each differs. CT and MRI enhanced with intravenous contrast have accuracy of 75% and as much as 100%, respectively.

Biologic control of inflammation in an effort to decrease the postlaminectomy membrane and decrease postoperative pain has generated considerable interest. The laminectomy membrane is a layer of perineural fibrous tissue. CT and MRI have been used to determine the prevalence of epidural fibrosis in both symptomatic and asymptomatic patients after discectomy, as well as to develop a grading system to quantify the amount of epidural fibrosis. Although many authors have failed to demonstrate a causal relationship between the amount and appearance of epidural fibrosis and patient symptoms, MRI has recently been used to correlate recurrent radicular pain during the first 6 months after surgery and the amount of lumbar peridural fibrosis. Patients having an extensive scar were 3.2 times more likely to experience recurrent radicular pain than those with less extensive peridural scarring. Numerous systemic and local methods currently are used to control the inflammatory response around the nerve root. No single agent has been accepted as a reliable, safe, effective method of eliminating peridural scarring and adhesions.

Current Recommendations

Patients with a definite diagnosis of ruptured lumbar intervertebral disc and sciatic or other radicular pain with neurologic signs and symptoms should be observed carefully and treated by nonsurgical means for 4 to 8 weeks unless there is progressive loss of motor, bladder, or bowel function or if there is excruciating pain that cannot be relieved by nonsurgical treatment. Those who have not improved sufficiently and are not experiencing continued improvement may then be offered treatment by surgical excision of the disc. Such patients should be advised that this is elective surgery, and that delay for longer than 6 months in the face of persistent and severe symptoms may compromise the best ultimate result.

Annotated Bibliography

Ahn UM, Ahn NU, Buchowski JM, Garrett ES, Sieber AN, Kostuik JP: Cauda equina syndrome secondary to lumbar disc herniation: A meta-analysis of surgical outcomes. *Spine* 2000;25:1515-1522.

Preoperative chronic back pain was associated with poorer outcomes in urinary and rectal function, and preoperative rectal dysfunction was associated with worsened outcome in urinary continence. Increasing age was associated with poorer postoperative sexual function. There was no significant improvement in surgical outcome in patients treated within 24 hours from the onset of cauda equina syndrome compared with patients treated within 24 to 48 hours. Significant differences were found in resolution of sensory and motor deficits as well as urinary and rectal function in patients treated within 48 hours compared with those treated more than 48 hours after onset of symptoms.

Albert TJ, Balderston RA, Heller JG, et al: Upper lumbar disc herniations. *J Spinal Disord* 1993;6:351-359.

Preoperative signs and symptoms were highly variable. Sensory, motor, and reflex testing was variable and potentially misleading in suggesting a level of herniation. A high false-negative rate was found for all radiographic studies when considered individually, especially at the higher L2-3 level. Intraoperative radiographs were used with increasing frequency as the level of herniation rose. Six surgical complications (4.3%) were identified, all of which were treated and were resolving at the time of discharge. Follow-up (average, 2.2 years) in 87% of patients by chart review showed no reoperations or late complications.

BenDebba M, Augustus van Alphen H, Long DM: Association between peridural scar and activity-related pain after lumbar discectomy. *Neurol Res* 1999;21(suppl 1):S37-S42.

Activity-related pain 6 months after first surgery for LDH, and the extent of lumbar epidural fibrosis present at the surgical site were assessed by MRI. A significant association between extensive epidural scar and activity-related pain was demonstrated.

Bessette L, Liang MH, Lew RA, Weinstein JN: Classics in spine: Surgery literature revisited. *Spine* 1996;21: 259-263.

This is a review of the criteria for evaluating the quality of clinical trials.

Errico TJ, Dryer JW: Failed disc surgery syndrome, in Kostuik JP (ed): *Failed Spinal Surgery: Spine. State of the Art Reviews 1997*. Philadelphia, PA, Hanley & Belfus, 1997.

This review of the diagnosis and therapeutic options in the patient with failed disc surgery provides an organizational approach to understanding, diagnosing, and managing a difficult patient population.

Kjellby-Wendt G, Styf J: Early active training after lumbar discectomy: A prospective, randomized, and controlled study. *Spine* 1998;23:2345-2351.

Six and 12 weeks after surgery, patients with dominating residual leg pain had significantly less intense pain in the early active training group than those in the control group. Twelve weeks after surgery, range of motion of the lumbar spine was significantly more increased in the early active training group. One year after surgery, there was no significant difference between the groups regarding the duration of sick leave, results in a positive SLR, or pain intensity. Twenty-two patients (88%) in the early active training group and 16 in the control group (67%) were satisfied with the treatment outcome 2 years after surgery.

Klekamp J, McCarty E, Spengler DM: Results of elective lumbar discectomy for patients involved in the workers' compensation system. *J Spinal Disord* 1998;11:277-282.

Outcomes of a control group of patients not involved with compensation or litigation were compared to outcomes from three groups of workers' compensation claimants, those involved in active litigation without compensation, those involved in both compensation and litigation, and those pursuing workers' compensation without litigation. Of the control group, 81% reported good results compared with 29% of patients actively involved in litigation or compensation. Legal involvement was associated with poorer outcome in compensation patients.

Malter AD, Larson EB, Urban N, Deyo RA: Cost-effectiveness of lumbar discectomy for the treatment of herniated intervertebral disc. *Spine* 1996;21:1048-1055.

In a cost-effectiveness analysis of lumbar discectomy based on existing efficacy data and newly gathered cost data, surgery increased average quality-adjusted life expectancy by 0.43 years during the decade following treatment. Reimbursements for surgical patients were $12,550 more than for medical patients. Discectomy's favorable cost effectiveness results from its substantial effect on quality of life and moderate costs.

Maroon JC, Abla A, Bost J: Association between peridural scar and persistent low back pain after lumbar discectomy. *Neurol Res* 1999;21(suppl 1):S43-S46.

Patients with extensive scar reported continuing and debilitating low-back pain more frequently than those with no or minimal scar. Those patients treated with ADCON-L at surgery had significantly less scar than did control patients and had less low back pain than did control patients.

O'Hara LJ, Marshall RW: Far lateral lumbar disc herniation: The key to the intertransverse approach. *J Bone Joint Surg Br* 1997;79:943-947.

The muscle splitting intertransverse approach is described.

Padua R, Padua S, Romanini E, Padua L, de Santis E: Ten-to 15-year outcome of surgery for lumbar disc herniation: Radiographic instability and clinical findings. *Eur Spine J* 1999;8:70-74.

One hundred fifty patients were evaluated by subjective analyses (Roland questionnaire), 68 patients (56.6%) by objective examinations, and 50 patients (41.6%) by radiographic studies to establish the presence of vertebral instability. Radiographic studies showed vertebral instability in 30 patients, but only nine were symptomatic. Recurrences were not observed, and only a few patients suffered from leg pain. The standard procedure for LDH showed good results at 10- and 15-year follow-up.

Papagelopoulos PJ, Shaughnessy WJ, Ebersold MJ, Bianco AJ Jr, Quast LM: Long-term outcome of lumbar discectomy in children and adolescents sixteen years of age or younger. *J Bone Joint Surg Am* 1998;80:689-698.

In this retrospective review of 72 consecutive patients 16 years of age or younger, who had a lumbar discectomy, 20 patients (28%) had one reoperation or more. Fifty-two patients (72%) did not need a reoperation, 92% either had no pain or had occasional pain related to strenuous activity, and 51 patients (98%) could participate in daily activities with no or mild limitations. Survivorship analysis showed that the overall probability that a patient would not need a reoperation was 80% at 10 years and 74% at 20 years. Age, gender, or an arthrodesis performed at the time of the initial surgery were not risk factors for a reoperation.

Postacchini F: Management of herniation of the lumbar disc. *J Bone Joint Surg Br* 1999;81:567-576.

This is a general review with a complete bibliography.

Ross JS, Robertson JT, Frederickson RC, et al: Association between peridural scar and recurrent radicular pain after lumbar discectomy: magnetic resonance evaluation: ADCON-L European Study Group. *Neurosurgery* 1996;38:855-861.

Correlation between recurrent radicular pain during the first 6 months after first surgery for herniated lumbar intervertebral disc and the amount of lumbar peridural fibrosis as defined by MRI was established. Patients having extensive peridural scar were 3.2 times more likely to experience recurrent radicular pain than those patients with less extensive peridural scarring.

Schade V, Semmer N, Main CJ, Hora J, Boos N: The impact of clinical, morphological, psychosocial and work-related factors on the outcome of lumbar discectomy. *Pain* 1999;80:239-249.

Return to work 2 years after surgery was best predicted by depression and occupational mental stress. MRI-identified extent of herniation and depression were significant predictors of a good surgical outcome after lumbar discectomy. Morphologic alterations proved to be significant predictors of postoperative pain relief and improvement of disability in daily activities. Return to work was not influenced by any clinical findings or MRI-identified morphologic alterations.

Silvers HR, Lewis PJ, Asch HL, Clabeaux D: Lumbar microdiscectomy in the elderly patient. *Br J Neurosurg* 1997;11:16-24.

This is a retrospective analysis of 60 patients who had undergone surgical lumbar discectomy at an age of 60 years or older. In the short term, overall pain relief was highly successful and not significantly different in either the elderly (94%) or control group (98%). Long-term follow-up yielded successful outcomes.

Wang JC, Shapiro MS, Hatch JD, Knight J, Dorey FJ, Delamarter RB: The outcome of lumbar discectomy in elite athletes *Spine* 1999;24:570-573.

All 14 patients had improvement of pain with elimination of the radicular component, took less medication than before surgery, and returned to recreational sports. Nine patients returned to varsity sports and five prematurely retired from competitive sports because of continued symptoms. SF-36 scores for bodily pain, physical role, and social and mental health roles were significantly lower in those athletes who retired.

Watts RW, Silagy CA: A meta-analysis on the efficacy of epidural corticosteroids in the treatment of sciatica. *Anaesth Intensive Care* 1995;23:564-569.

Eleven suitable trials involving a total of 907 patients were identified. The use of epidural (caudal or lumbar) steroid in the short term (up to 60 days) increased the chances of pain relief (> 75% improvement) when compared with placebo.

Classic Bibliography

Caspar W: A new surgical procedure for lumbar disc herniation causing less tissue damage through a microsurgical approach. *Adv Neurosurg* 1977;4:74-77.

Lasègue C: Considerations sur la sciatique. *Arch Gen Med* 1864;2:558.

Mixter WJ, Barr JS: Rupture of the intervertebral disc with involvement of the spinal canal. *N Engl J Med* 1934;211:210-215.

Nachemson A: The load on lumbar discs in different positions of the body. *Clin Orthop* 1966;45:107-122.

Weber H: Lumbar disc herniation: A controlled, prospective study with ten years of observation. *Spine* 1983;8:131-140.

Chapter 35

Lumbar Discogenic Pain and Instability

Casey K. Lee, MD

Kenneth J. Kopacz, MD

Lumbar Discogenic Pain

Disorders of the intervertebral disc that may be a source of low back pain include herniation, disruption, resorption, degeneration, instability, and spinal stenosis. Disc herniation and spinal stenosis have been extensively studied and there is a consensus on basic approaches for diagnosis and treatment. However, diagnosis and treatment of disc disruption, disc resorption, and symptomatic degenerative disc disease have been controversial. The main focus of this chapter will be on chronic low back pain (CLBP) caused by internal derangement of the disc (IDD) and on certain aspects of discogenic instability.

The number of fusions of the lumbosacral spine performed in the United States has been steadily increasing during the past 2 decades, and more than 50% of those fusion procedures were for symptomatic degenerative disc disease. Despite the rising popularity of the diagnosis of discogenic pain, diagnosis and treatment have remained controversial because of the lack of consensus on reliable diagnostic methods, lack of knowledge of the natural course of IDD, and insufficient proof of the clinical efficacy of spinal fusion based on randomized controlled clinical studies.

Discogenic Pain

IDD is defined as one or more pathologic conditions within the disc that cause low back pain with no or minimal deformation of the anatomic contour of the disc. Such pathologic conditions include structural disruption of the disc and/or biochemical inflammatory changes (discitis). The possibility that pathologic conditions within the disc were a possible source of low back pain has been overlooked because the disc was believed to have no nociceptive capability and no innervation. More recently, many independent investigators have reported that the outer layers of the anulus and the end plates have innervation from the sinuvertebral nerves and sympathetic nerves, and that various biochemical by-products of injured or degenerated discs or alterations of stress patterns within the disc caused by injury or degeneration may be nociceptive stimuli. Recent reports of immunochemical studies on the possible nociceptive mechanisms within the disc further support the concept of discogenic pain.

With the advancement of basic scientific knowledge, it gradually has been accepted that certain pathologic conditions within the disc may cause low back pain (discogenic pain). However, there are no reliable diagnostic methods that differentiate IDD from an asymptomatic degenerated disc, and no consensus has been reached on indications for and efficacy of spinal fusion for IDD when compared with nonsurgical treatment or to the natural course of disease.

Prevalence and Natural History of IDD

Approximately 10% of patients with acute low back pain become chronic pain sufferers, with either frequent intermittent recurrence or persistent pain. In a recent clinical study approximately 40% of patients with CLBP were found to have IDD. The diagnosis of IDD was confirmed by physical examination, MRI, and discography. Although the pain of most patients with CLBP caused by IDD improves either after nonsurgical treatments or without treatment, a small but significant number of patients have continued disabling pain or worsening symptoms. In recently published studies, only 40% to 60% of patients diagnosed with IDD using physical evaluation and discography had some improvement in pain symptoms with nonsurgical treatments during a 2- to 5-year follow-up period. The remaining 40% to 60% of patients were found to have the same or worse pain, with continued disability.

One or more of the authors or the departments with which they are affiliated have received something of value from a commercial or other party related directly or indirectly to the subject of this chapter.

Diagnosis

Diagnosis of IDD is difficult, and there is no consensus on specific diagnostic criteria. No single finding on clinical examination or imaging studies is diagnostic of IDD. No reliable data are available for sensitivity, specificity, or predictive value of clinical or imaging findings. Diagnosis of IDD is made by correlating clinical information, MRI, and discography and by exclusion of other known pathologic conditions causing CLBP. What follows are some helpful points and possible pitfalls.

Clinical Information

The typical symptom is CLBP in young patients (20 to 50 years old), which either recurs frequently or is persistent. In about 65% of patients it is associated with leg pain to the knee (referred type of sclerotomal distribution). The most common aggravating factor is sitting, and pain often is relieved in the lateral recumbent position. However, no symptom by itself is specific for this diagnosis. Patients have no motor or reflex abnormalities. Some have sensory changes, usually in a nondermatomal distribution. Straight leg raising does not reproduce radicular pain but it often aggravates back pain. All have localized tenderness at the lower back. Pain almost always is reproduced at 20° to 30° of flexion when a standing patient rises from a fully flexed position.

Radiologic Findings

Routine radiographic examination often is negative, without indicating the presence of disc space narrowing, osteophyte formation, or gross instability.

Magnetic Resonance Imaging

There is a decreased or absent T2-weighted signal from the disc that is indistinguishable from that of an asymptomatic degenerated disc (Fig. 1). In addition, a high-intensity zone, defined as an increased signal intensity, is seen within the posterior anulus on T2-weighted images. The presence of a high-intensity zone at the posterior anulus in combination with decreased or absent T2 signal was reported to have a high sensitivity for IDD; however, in other studies, the predictive value was not high enough to consider it as a reliable diagnostic finding. A disc with diffuse disc bulge like a flat tire ("flat tire syndrome" described in the instability section below) or a disc with rotational deformity should be considered under the diagnosis of discogenic instability. These have different clinical presentations and take different clinical courses.

Discography

Discography (Figs. 2 and 3) provides useful information from pain response, patterns of annular disruption, and volume-pressure response during injection of contrast

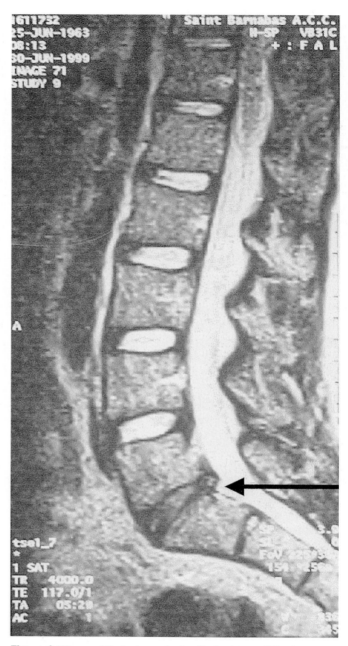

Figure 1 MRI scan of the lumbosacral spine showing decreased T2-weighted signal intensity of the L5-S1 disc. The arrow indicates a small high intensity signal at the posterior area of the disc (high intensity zone).

material. A positive discographic examination consists of a disc with concordant pain reproduction during discography and with an abnormal radiograph demonstrating annular disruption. The value of discography has been and remains controversial. Measurement of quality and quantity of the pain response has been a problem. Between no or little pain response and concordant severe pain response during discography, there is a wide grey zone in which interpretation of patient

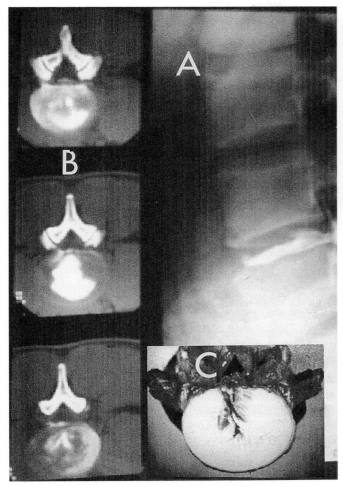

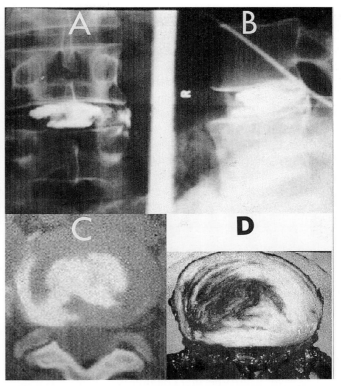

Figure 3 A and **B,** Discograms of AP and lateral views of the lumbosacral spine of a patient with CLBP shows abnormal contrast migration posteriorly and laterally. **C,** Postdiscogram CT scan shows radial and circumferential tear of the anulus. **D,** A similar radial and circumferential tear of the anulus on a specimen obtained from another source.

Figure 2 A, Discogram of a lateral view of the lumbosacral spine of a patient with CLBP shows a radial fissure of the posterior anulus. The patient had a positive concordant pain response during discography. **B,** Postdiscography CT scan shows the posterior midline annular fissure and minimum disc degeneration. **C,** A similar radial tear of the anulus is shown on a specimen obtained from another source, not the patient.

responses is very difficult. Interpretation of pain response in this grey area is further complicated by other factors, such as degree of sedation during the study, the patient's psychological status, and the physician's skill level. Some believe the physician who is most familiar with the patient's history and physical findings should perform discography with preferably no or very little intravenous sedation; others believe an independent person should perform the procedure and assess the pain response.

There are two major concerns in diagnosis of IDD: underdiagnosis and overdiagnosis.

Many physicians are unaware of the nocioceptive capability of the pathologic conditions within the disc and many believe that all patients with IDD get better through the natural course of the disease or with non-surgical treatments. A small percentage, but a significant number of patients with IDD (about 30% to 40%) do not respond satisfactorily to nonsurgical treatments and have continued disabling pain. These patients frequently are denied surgical treatment by this group of practitioners.

Because there is no specific diagnostic clinical or imaging finding for IDD, some physicians make the diagnosis of IDD and perform spinal fusion far too frequently. Not all patients who have low back pain with dark disc on MRI have IDD. Over 30% of normal asymptomatic subjects younger than 40 years old are known to have an abnormal MRI of the lumbosacral spine.

No single clinical finding is reliable for making the diagnosis of IDD. The diagnosis should be made by correlating those clinical findings listed above to MRI and discography and by ruling out other known pathologic conditions.

Treatments

Nonsurgical Treatments
The basic principles of nonsurgical treatments for IDD are activity modification, nonsteroidal anti-inflammatory

medications, epidural steroid injections for the acute stage, and therapeutic exercise. Therapeutic exercises should be directed toward lumbar extension exercises, lumbar stabilization exercises, and isometric and aerobic general conditioning exercises. Lumbar flexion activities such as sit-ups and lumbar torsional exercise often aggravate symptoms. Because the natural history of this condition over a long term has not been well studied, nonsurgical treatments must be actively continued for a minimum of 4 to 6 months or longer. This time frame is not necessarily continuous physical therapy but is active therapy, which includes many treatment options. Maximal compliance and effort to recover through use of nonsurgical methods is a reasonable prerequisite before consideration of surgery.

Surgical Treatments
The results of surgical treatment of IDD depend largely on indication (Table 1), selection of patients, and methods of surgical treatment. Disc excision and other disc decompressive surgeries such as chemonucleolysis, laser disc excision, or percutaneous disc excision usually fail to relieve symptoms for this condition. Symptoms often become worse after disc decompression procedures. Intradiscal electrothermal coagulation (IDET) is a new technique specifically developed for the treatment of this condition. IDET is a minimally invasive procedure in which a percutaneously introduced catheter is used

---

TABLE 1 | Indications for surgical treatment of IDD

Diagnosis of IDD should be made by careful correlation of clinical findings with MRI and discography. Major concerns and pitfalls for diagnosis of IDD are described in the text.

Patients should have continuous, active nonsurgical treatments for a minimum of 6 months or longer. Those who have had very frequently recurring and disabling low back pain more than 2 years or who have persistent severe disabling pain may be considered for surgical treatment after 4 months of active nonsurgical treatments.

Positive MRI findings of disc degeneration with localized tenderness on examination.

Positive discography with annular disruption and positive concordant pain provocation at 1 or at most 2 levels. The positive level should correlate with MRI findings.

No other pathologic findings such as disc herniation, diffuse disc bulge, instability, or spinal stenosis.

Absence of major influence of psychobehavioral factors and symptom magnification.

---

to produce controlled coagulation of the disc collagen in the injured anulus. A preliminary report of a multicenter study indicates successful pain relief in approximately 70% of patients over a 1.5-year follow-up. Any attempts to evaluate its efficacy are premature. Lumbar interbody spinal fusion is the choice of treatment for those patients with IDD who have met the criteria listed in Table 1.

Spinal Fusion Techniques

Lumbar Interbody Fusion Versus Posterolateral Fusion
Many spinal fusion techniques have been used to treat chronic disabling discogenic low back pain. These include posterior fusion, bilateral intertransverse process fusion (lateral fusion), anterior or posterior lumbar interbody fusion, or combined anterior and posterior (circumferential) fusion. Pedicle screw fixation or interbody cage fixation may be used in combination with these fusion techniques. It is impossible from published data to compare these techniques and to draw a conclusion as to which provides better results because there is a wide range of differences in study groups, surgical techniques, and methods of evaluation. However, recent reports indicate that some patients with IDD have persistent low back pain after solid posterolateral fusion. Furthermore, it has been observed that this pain has been relieved by lumbar interbody fusion. It is apparent that lumbar interbody fusion for IDD, either by anterior or posterior technique, provides a better success rate than does posterolateral fusion.

Biomechanical studies on posterolateral lumbosacral spinal fusion showed that reduced but measurable motion was retained across the disc within the segments fused posteriorly. It has been postulated that this retained motion across the disc may be a source of persistent pain. Possible reasons for the advantages of lumbar interbody fusion over posterolateral fusion are: (1) interbody fusion effectively removes nucleus pulposus and the inner anulus, which may be sources of pain (biochemical pain stimulator); (2) interbody fusion with adequate bone graft or bone graft substitutes restores disc height and relieves abnormal stresses within the anulus; and (3) solid interbody fusion completely eliminates motion across the disc.

Anterior lumbar interbody fusion (ALIF) has the advantages of easier exposure and a easier learning curve compared with posterior lumbar interbody fusion (PLIF). ALIF has disadvantages of possible major vessel injury and retrograde ejaculation/impotence. PLIF is difficult to perform and requires manipulation of the nerve roots. A successful fusion rate is highly dependent on the level of surgical skill and experience.

Basic Principles of Lumbar Interbody Fusion

The most important factors for interbody fusion are adequate preparation of the bone graft bed of the host bone (vertebral end plates) and adequate quality and amount of bone graft. The vertebral end plate is very thin and does not contribute significantly to the compressive strength of the vertebral body under axial compressive load (less than 10%). Decortication of the vertebral end plate, therefore, does not significantly increase the chance of migration of the graft into the vertebral body, which is called subsidence. The two most important factors for subsidence are the contact surface area between bone graft and host bone and bone density. The contact surface area must be greater than 6.0 cm^2 for a normal adult lumbar spine (L4-5) with normal bone density to withstand the normal physiologic load without subsidence. The bone graft placed within the disc space for interbody fusion must be strong enough to withstand the physiologic load, or the graft may fracture. Two tricortical iliac crest bone grafts from a person with normal bone density will have sufficient strength to withstand the normal postoperative loading condition (approximately 2 to 2.5 kN) and, if they have 2.5 cm depth, will provide approximately 6.25 cm^2 contact surface area (the average width of two bone grafts is 2.5 cm). Less contact surface area or less bone results in graft failure and/or subsidence. In these situations, supplemental rigid internal fixation is an important addition to help obtain successful fusion. A supplemental rigid internal fixation system is not always necessary at the time of interbody fusion for IDD if the surgeon adheres to the above basic principles (Fig. 4). The use of interbody metallic devices, ie, cages, has gained widespread acceptance. However, as with any fusion method, the basic principles of interbody fusion must be followed. The surgeon must adhere to the basic biologic principles of surface contact area and adequate amounts of bone graft material to achieve fusion.

One common mistake in performing PLIF is to perform total facetectomies for adequate exposure. This iatrogenically created spinal instability requires the use of rigid internal fixation.

The minimum amount of surgery to achieve the maximum results should be the goal for surgical treatments to minimize intraoperative and postoperative morbidity and to maximize cost effectiveness. Training and the level of the surgeon's skill are the most important factors to achieve this goal. An interbody fusion construct (ALIF or PLIF) with adequate bone graft and contact surface is sufficiently stable for obtaining satisfactory fusion without supplemental internal fixation or postoperative rigid external immobilization.

The reported results of interbody lumbar spinal fusion for IDD are satisfactory, ranging between 75% and 90%

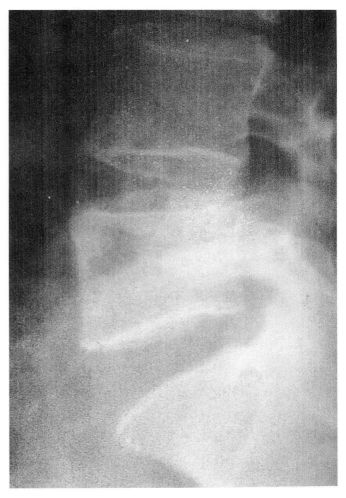

Figure 4 A lateral radiogram of the lumbosacral spine of a patient who was treated with PLIF L4-5 for IDD. No rigid internal fixation or postoperative external support was used. Solid fusion with maintenance of disc height and alignment was obtained with complete pain relief and return to work.

successful pain relief and return to work. The important factors for successful results are proper indication, patient selection, and surgical techniques. The results of interbody spinal fusion for those who have chronic disabling pain beyond 6 months despite active nonsurgical treatments appear to be better for pain relief and return to work than those of nonsurgical treatments or reliance on the natural history of IDD. However, better understanding of the natural history of IDD and randomized controlled studies are needed to evaluate the efficacy of spinal fusion for IDD.

Discogenic Spinal Instability

Spinal instability is a controversial subject because it is difficult to assess clinically. The American Academy of Orthopaedic Surgeons defines clinical spinal stability as "the ability of the spine under physiologic loads to limit patterns of displacement so as not to damage or irritate the spinal cord or nerve root and in addition to prevent incapacitating deformity or pain due to structural changes." This is a very precise definition that is easy to identify when the spine has gross abnormal motion or deformity with symptoms. Many conditions, such as fractures, fracture-dislocations, anterior column infections, neoplasm, spondylolytic spondylolisthesis, and idiopathic scoliosis, may cause gross spinal instability. Degenerative spinal instabilities are another condition caused by progressive disc degeneration that often is more difficult to diagnose. This section will focus on spinal instability caused by a discogenic etiology.

History

Earlier investigators observed gross abnormal translation of a lumbar vertebra in the sagittal plane associated with severe disc degeneration and called it degenerative spondylolisthesis or pseudospondylolisthesis—a new concept for discogenic lumbar instability. Clinical relevance, pathomechanics, and treatments of degenerative spondylolisthesis have been studied extensively, and there is a general consensus for the diagnosis and course of treatments. Discogenic segmental instability, however, has been a most confusing and poorly understood concept.

Macnab in 1971 described traction osteophytes that arise from the vertebral body as osteophytes that are horizontally situated from the vertebral body and originate approximately 2 mm from the anterior end plate of the vertebra. The osteophyte arises at the site of attachment of the outermost annular fibers. Macnab used the term segmental instability to describe the abnormal biomechanics and anatomic changes at the level of the spinal segment. Later reports have shown the traction osteophyte to be an inconsistent finding.

The later work of Kirkaldy-Willis classified the degenerative process into three distinct phases: dysfunction, instability, and stabilization. The degenerative cascade defined an unstable phase characterized by loss of disc height with facet and ligament laxity, creating instability in the motion segment.

Since these early reports, two concepts of instability have evolved. In the first, instability is defined by measurable abnormal patterns of motion seen on routine radiographs. These patterns include degenerative spondylolisthesis defined as greater than 3 mm of anterior displacement of the superior vertebral body in relation to the inferior vertebral body, retrolisthesis, and rotational instability such as degenerative scoliosis.

In the second concept, segmental instability, which was alluded to by Macnab and Kirkaldy-Willis, is defined as abnormal biomechanics of the spinal segment secondary to injury or degeneration of the disc. No measurable changes are seen on routine radiographs.

Many attempts have been made to identify segmental instability in early degenerative disc disease. These include use of centrode patterns or digitized radiographs, and biplanar radiography and biplanar cinefluorography to quantify an unstable segment. None of these techniques has been useful in the clinical setting. Also, a significant rate of late-stage degenerative instability may be seen in an asymptomatic population, adding further to the diagnostic difficulties. The concept of segmental instability evolved before a recent development in IDD in which abnormal biomechanics exist but cannot be measured on routine radiographs. It is probable that many cases considered segmental instability in the past were those of IDD or of the late stage of IDD evolving into gross instability.

Classification

Degenerative instability may be classified depending on the plane of the deformity (Table 2).

Sagittal Plane

In the sagittal plane degenerative spondylolisthesis is the most common discogenic instability (Fig. 5). It occurs when degenerative changes in the facet joints along with laxity in the disc allow anterolisthesis of the superior vertebra on the inferior vertebra. Clinically the patients may complain of CLBP or, in late stages, of symptoms related to spinal stenosis.

Retrolisthesis is posterior displacement of the superior vertebral body. It usually is associated with a

TABLE 2	Classification of Discogenic Lumbar Spinal Instability

Sagittal plane instability

　Degenerative spondylolisthesis

　Degenerative retrolisthesis

　Angular instability

Coronal plane instability

　Rotational instability

　Lateral translational instability (lateral subluxation)

Axial instability

　Circumferential bulge (flat tire syndrome)

　Collapsed disc

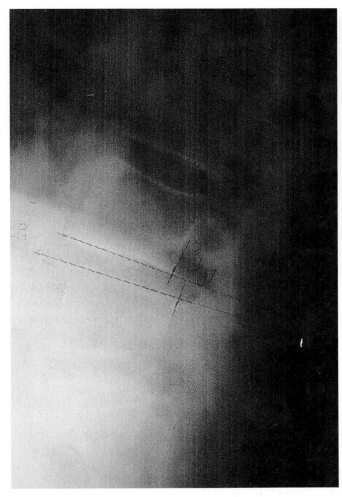

Figure 5 A lateral view of the lumbosacral spine shows anterior translation of L4 on L5 (degenerative spondylolisthesis).

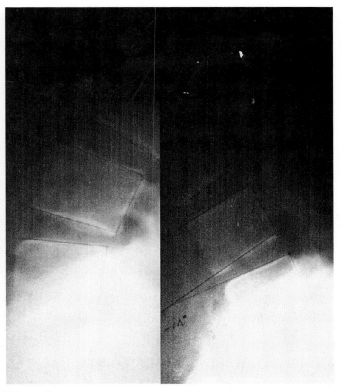

Figure 6 Flexion and extension lateral views of the lumbosacral spine show +13° of a disc-space wedge with opening anteriorly on extension and -14° of a wedge with opening posteriorly on flexion. Slight narrowing of the disc space of L4-5 also is noted.

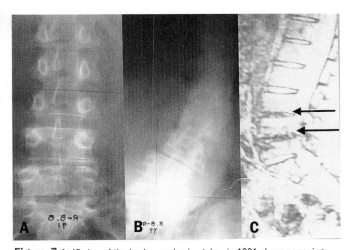

Figure 7 A, AP view of the lumbosacral spine taken in 1991 shows narrowing and slight lateral angulation of the L4-5 disc space and associated minimum rotational deformity of the mid and upper lumbar spine. **B,** Severe degree of disc space wedging, rotation, lateral subluxation of L3-4 and L4-5 with worsened scoliosis are noted 6 years later. **C,** MRI shows severe disc degeneration of L3-4 and L4-5.

severely degenerative disc with disc space collapse and facet degeneration. It may be clinically associated with CLBP and stenosis symptoms.

Angulation deformity in the sagittal plane, which may be seen on flexion-extension radiographs, may occur as a result of postsurgical instability and also of degenerative disc disease (Fig. 6). It is associated with CLBP.

Coronal Plane

The coronal plane deformities include vertebral rotation and translation. Clinically these patients develop degenerative scoliosis, which is the de novo appearance of scoliosis in adulthood (Fig. 7). This condition has become more recognized and prevalent as the population ages.

Axial Plane

In the axial plane, the disc may become unstable, manifesting clinically as the flat tire syndrome (Fig 8). As the annular disruption becomes severe, the anulus bulges

over the vertebral end plates circumferentially. This condition is analogous to a tire bulging over the rim when it loses its air pressure. Some cases of internal disc dis-

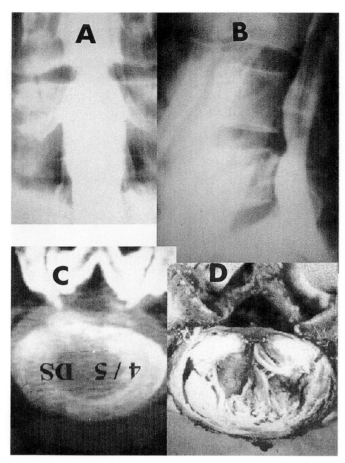

Figure 8 A and **B,** AP and lateral views of lumbosacral myelogram shows bulging disc of L4-5. Slight loss of disc height is also noted. **C,** CT scan of the L4-5 disc shows circumferential bulge of the disc like a flat tire (flat tire syndrome). **D,** A specimen from another source shows severe annular disruption involving the entire disc including periphery that causes circumferential bulge under physiologic axial compressive load.

the disc is severely degenerated it may be difficult to evaluate the pain response because large volumes of fluid are necessary to pressurize the disc.

Treatment

Many patients with instability may be symptomatic or asymptomatic and diagnosed incidentally on radiographs. Patients should be treated only if they become symptomatic. Patients with documented adult scoliosis and rotational deformity should be followed periodically with radiographs. Acute change in the curvature with increased rotation, disc space wedging, and lateral translation may require surgical intervention to prevent further deterioration.

Patients with symptomatic degenerative instabilities initially should be treated with a comprehensive nonsurgical approach. This treatment should include activity modification to avoid rotational loading and reduce the spinal load. Lumbar stabilization exercises and muscle strengthening should be instituted. A trial of nonsteroidal anti-inflammatory medications may also be beneficial.

Surgical Treatments

Any patient who has been fully compliant with and failed nonsurgical treatment and continues to have severe symptoms should be considered for spinal fusion. There are multiple surgical techniques, including posterolateral fusion, PLIF, and ALIF, all of which may be done with or without spinal instrumentation. There is very little information indicating that one technique is superior to another. However, there is information showing that the addition of pedicle screws does increase fusion rates in some series. If there is significant listhesis, disc collapse, loss of lordosis, or rotational deformity, interbody fusion with pedicle screw fixation is preferred because it better corrects and maintains anatomic alignment (disc space height and angle, vertebral translation and rotation, and lumbar lordosis).

Annotated Bibliography

Discogenic Pain Natural History

Lanes TC, Gauron EF, Spratt KF, Wernimont TJ, Found EM, Weinstein JN: Long-term follow-up of patients with chronic back pain treated in a multidisciplinary rehabilitation program. *Spine* 1995;20:801-806.

Of 129 patients with CLBP who completed a multidisciplinary rehabilitation program, 51% had fair or poor job outcome and 47% had the same or worse general well being during a minimum 18-month follow-up period.

ruption evolve into axial instability as the anulus becomes more disrupted, involving a large area of the periphery of the anulus. A symptomatic patient may suffer from chronic discogenic low back pain with morning stiffness and increasing pain at the end of the day. The symptoms are relieved by rest. The disc height decrease may be minimal in early stages, but as the disc collapses further spinal stenosis may develop.

Diagnosis

Patients with discogenic degenerative symptoms should be evaluated with flexion-extension radiographs to rule out measurable instability. MRI is also used to evaluate the discs for any T2 signal changes. Discograms are another diagnostic tool used to evaluate the disc's internal architecture as well as the patient's pain response. If

McCoy CE, Selby D, Henderson R, Handal J, Peloza J, Wolf C: Patients avoiding surgery: Pathology and one-year life status follow-up. *Spine* 1991;16(suppl 6):S198-S200.

Sixty-six patients who had confirmed diagnosis of IDD and indications for spinal fusion because of persistent CLBP after nonsurgical treatments did not have the operation because it was denied by third parties. These patients were followed for 1.5 and 2 years with the following results: 18% returned to work; 20% had increased activity level; 18% retired; and the remainder had the same or worse symptoms.

Smith SE, Darden BV, Rhyne AL, Wood KE: Outcome of unoperated discogram-positive low back pain. *Spine* 1995;20:1997-2001.

Twenty-five patients with CLBP, discogram positive, were followed for a minimum of 3 years. Thirty-two percent had the same or worse symptoms, and 68% had some improvement of pain symptoms. No one became pain free and no one became free of disability at final follow-up evaluation.

Discogenic Pain Mechanisms

Coppes MH, Marani E, Thomeer RT, Groen GJ: Innervation of "painful" lumbar discs. *Spine* 1997;22:2342-2350.

In this investigation of innervation of discographically confirmed degenerated and painful human intervertebral discs, nerve fibers were found in the outer region of 10 discs, and in the inner parts of 8 of 10 discs.

Olmarker K, Blomquist J, Stromberg J, Nannmark U, Thomsen P, Rydevik B: Inflammatogenic properties of nucleus pulposus. *Spine* 1995;20:665-669.

Laboratory tests demonstrated that nucleus pulposus has inflammatogenic properties.

Saal JS: The role of inflammation in lumbar pain. *Spine* 1995;20:1821-1827.

The author identified a high level of an inflammatory enzyme phospholipase A_2 in degenerated discs. This is a probable indication of inflammatogenic capability of the lumbar disc.

Diagnosis

Guyer RD, Ohnmeiss DD: Lumbar discography: Position statement from the North American Spine Society Diagnostic and Therapeutic Committee. *Spine* 1995;20:2048-2059.

Discography is a valuable diagnostic procedure when patients with persistent pain have no confirmative diagnostic imaging studies or when the images need to be correlated with clinical symptoms.

Aprill C, Bogduk N: High intensity zone: A diagnostic sign of painful lumbar disc on magnetic resonance imaging. *Br J Radiol* 1992;65:361-369.

There was an 86% incidence of concordantly painful discography in lumbar disc exhibiting a posterior high intensity zone on T2-weighted MRI of back pain sufferers.

Lumbar Interbody Fusion Biomechanics

Brantigan JW, Cunningham BW, Warden K, McAfee PC, Steffee AD: Compression strength of donor bone for posterior lumbar interbody fusion. *Spine* 1993;18:1213-1221.

Average compressive strength of two tricortical iliac crest bone grafts (2 blocks of $12 \times 1.2 \times 2.5$ cm) was about 2.3 kN.

Closkey RF, Parsons JR, Lee CK, Blacksin MF, Zimmerman MC: Mechanics of interbody spinal fusion: Analysis of critical bone graft area. *Spine* 1993;18:1011-1015.

Bone graft subsidence in lumbar interbody fusion was primarily determined by bone density of the host bone and contact surface area of the bone graft and host bone. The minimum bone graft contact surface area for L4-5 interbody fusion in an adult with normal bone density is about 6.0 cm^2.

Surgical Treatment

Barrick WT, Schofferman JA, Reynolds JB, et al: Anterior lumbar fusion improves discogenic pain at levels of prior posterolateral fusion. *Spine* 2000;25:853-857.

Twenty patients who had solid posterolateral fusion for CLBP and have persistent pain postoperatively, had significant pain relief after anterior interbody fusion at the same level(s) during a 58-month mean follow-up period.

Lee CK, Vessa P, Lee JK: Chronic disabling low back pain syndrome caused by internal disc derangements: The results of disc excision and posterior lumbar interbody fusion. *Spine* 1995;20:356-361.

Sixty-two patients with CLBP caused by IDD were treated with PLIF. Successful pain relief and return to work were obtained in 89% during a 7-year period (minimum, 18-month follow-up).

Discogenic Instability

Bridwell KH, Sedgewick TA, O'Brien MF, Lenke LG, Baldus C: The role of fusion and instrumentation in the treatment of degenerative spondylolisthesis with spinal stenosis. *J Spinal Disord* 1993;6:461-472.

This prospective, randomized study evaluated the role of fusion and spinal fixation in treating degenerative lumbar spondylolisthesis. There was less progression and better fusion rates when using pedicle screw fixation. Furthermore, patient satisfaction was higher if the listhesis did not progress.

Herkowitz HN, Sidhu KS: Lumbar spine fusion in the treatment of degenerative conditions: Current indications and recommendations. *J Am Acad Orthop Surg* 1995;3:123-135.

This article gives an overview of the treatment options in many degenerative lumbar conditions. It describes the diagnosis, indications, and results for many procedures. The authors also review the various techniques of fusion.

Classic Bibliography

Blumenthal SL, Baker J, Dossett A, Selby DK: The role of anterior lumbar fusion for internal disc disruption. *Spine* 1988;13:566-569.

Crock HV: A reappraisal of intervertebral disc lesions. *Med J Aust* 1970;1:983-989.

Farfan HF, Cossette JW, Robertson GH, Wells RV, Kraus H: The effects of torsion on the lumbar intervertebral joints: The role of torsion in the production of disc degeneration. *J Bone Joint Surg Am* 1970;52:468-497.

Kirkaldy-Willis WH, Farfan HF: Instability of the lumbar spine. *Clin Orthop* 1982;165:110-123.

Kirkaldy-Willis WH, Wedge JH, Yong-Hing K, Reilly J: Pathology and pathogenesis of lumbar spondylosis and stenosis. *Spine* 1978;3:319-328.

Lee CK, Langrana NA: Lumbosacral spinal fusion: A biomechanical study. *Spine* 1984;9:574-581.

Macnab I: The traction spur: An indicator of segmental instability. *J Bone Joint Surg Am* 1971;53:663-670.

Posner I, White AA III, Edwards WT, Hayes WC: A biomechanical analysis of the clinical stability of the lumbar and lumbosacral spine. *Spine* 1982;7:374-389.

Rolander SD: Motion of the spine with special reference to the stabilizing effect of posterior fusion: An experimental study on autopsy specimens. *Acta Orthop Scand* 1966;(suppl 90):1-144.

Weinstein J, Claverie W, Gibson S: The pain of discography. *Spine* 1988;13:1344-1348.

Yoshizawa H, O'Brien JP, Smith WT, Trumper M: The neuropathology of intervertebral discs removed for low-back pain. *J Pathol* 1980;132:95-104.

Chapter 36

Surgical Management of Lumbar Spinal Stenosis and Degenerative Spondylolisthesis

Gordon R. Bell, MD

Introduction

The natural history of spinal stenosis and degenerative spondylolisthesis is unclear because there is a lack of longitudinal prospective studies documenting the course of untreated patients. Review of the existing literature suggests that symptoms progress in approximately 20% of patients with spinal stenosis who receive no treatment. However, because most studies are neither randomized nor prospective, it is difficult to arrive at conclusions regarding the natural history of the disease and to compare various treatment options. In one study of the natural course of lumbar spinal stenosis only 15% of patients were improved according to a visual analog scale, 15% were worse, and approximately 70% were unchanged at 4-year follow-up. On clinical examination, 41% of patients were improved, 18% were worse, and 41% were unchanged. The authors concluded that severe progression was unlikely.

Little also is known of the natural history or optimal treatment of degenerative spondylolisthesis. In a recently published meta-analysis of the literature from 1970 to 1993, only 3 of 152 studies adequately addressed the natural history of degenerative spondylolisthesis. Overall, 32% of the patients in these three studies achieved satisfactory results without treatment. In a study of 40 patients who received no treatment for at least 5 years, progressive slip was noted in 12 patients (30%), although no correlation was noted between slip progression and deterioration of symptoms. Clinical deterioration over the course of the study occurred in only four patients (10%), all of whom showed no slip progression over the 4 years. None of the 12 patients who had slip progression deteriorated clinically.

In summary, the natural history of spinal stenosis, with or without associated degenerative spondylolisthesis, is generally favorable, with clinical deterioration in only approximately 10% to 20% of patients with either condition. Clinical improvement seems to occur in approximately one third to one half of patients with either of these two conditions.

Lumbar Spinal Stenosis

Spinal stenosis creates a clinical syndrome characterized by back, buttocks, or leg pain with characteristic provocative and palliative features. The relationship between sciatica and neural compression within the spinal canal was first described in 1900. Subsequent descriptions included etiologies from both congenital narrowing and acquired narrowing by hypertrophied ligamentum flavum or degenerative bony compression. The clinical features of spinal stenosis and its relationship to congenital narrowing, were described in detail by the Dutch surgeon Verbiest who also used myelography to demonstrate mechanical compression of neural structures. Kirkaldy-Willis further defined the pathoanatomy of spinal stenosis and helped to correlate pathologic changes with symptoms.

Surgical Treatment

Surgery for lumbar spinal stenosis may be divided into decompressive procedures without and with concomitant fusion. Surgical decompression may vary from limited procedures, such as single-level unilateral laminotomy for focal neural compression, to global procedures, such as multilevel bilateral laminectomy with bilateral facetectomies and foraminotomies. Fusion procedures include anterior lumbar interbody fusion (ALIF), posterior lumbar interbody fusion (PLIF), posterior fusion, posterolateral (also known as intertransverse or bilateral lateral) fusion, and combinations of these procedures. Indirect neural decompression may occur following ALIF or PLIF if disc space distraction occurs, thereby enlarging the central and foraminal canal. Fusion may be either noninstrumented or instrumented using either nonsegmental or segmental (pedicle screw) spinal instrumentation.

Suitability of the patient for extensive surgical procedures must be assured by having the patient adequately screened by a medical specialist. This screening is particularly important for elderly patients with multiple comorbidities. For extensive surgical procedures the patient usually will donate two or three units of autologous blood before surgery.

The choice of anesthesia depends on the magnitude of the surgery and other medical factors. For routine decompression, spinal anesthesia minimizes both postoperative pulmonary problems such as atelectasis and intraoperative positioning problems that can occur while the patient is asleep. Other intraoperative precautions include the use of prophylactic antibiotics, antiembolic pneumatic compression stockings to reduce the risk of deep venous thrombosis, and intraoperative cell salvage to minimize the need for homologous blood transfusion.

For posterior spinal procedures, it is important to position the patient with the abdomen hanging freely to reduce intra-abdominal pressure, thereby minimizing bleeding from the surgical field. The kneeling position is preferred for routine procedures, such as laminotomy, laminectomy, or single-level noninstrumented fusion. For more extensive surgical procedures, the use of Gardner-Wells cranial tongs with the Jackson table allows the head to hang freely and eliminates the potential for pressure on the eyes. It is extremely helpful to elevate the head of the table in relation to the feet to minimize the amount of facial edema that can occur from prolonged recumbency.

Adequate illumination and magnification are mandatory to assure safe surgery; these may be obtained by the use of either loupes with a headlight or the operating microscope, which permits excellent visualization by both the operating surgeon and the assistant. In addition, the microscope may be tilted to enable observation of the side contralateral to the laminotomy. The use of the microscope also increases surgeon comfort by allowing the surgeon's head to be maintained in a neutral position, thereby eliminating the need for the prolonged neck flexion.

Laminectomy

The standard surgical procedure for spinal stenosis is decompressive laminectomy. Because spinal stenosis is a global degenerative process, encompassing multiple levels and frequently involving nerve roots bilaterally, multilevel bilateral laminectomy commonly is required. For bilateral laminectomy the lamina and ligamentum flavum are removed on both sides of the stenotic level(s) to the lateral recess. Decompression typically begins at the most distal extent of neural compression and proceeds in a caudal-to-cranial manner. Midline decompression is extended laterally until the lateral edge of the nerve root is seen and is determined to be free of compression. Care is taken to preserve the pars interarticularis to minimize the risk of producing insta-

bility by inadvertent sacrifice of the superior articular facet. The surgeon should check for a concomitant disc herniation that might contribute to neural compression.

It is generally best to avoid discectomy in the presence of laminectomy unless the disc herniation contributes to significant neural compression because subsequent instability is more likely to occur when both anterior and posterior supporting structures are violated surgically. When laminectomy is accompanied by discectomy, performance of an arthrodesis at the time of surgery should be considered. Finally, lateral decompression of the foraminae is performed. Decompression is generally complete when a bent probe can easily be passed out the neural foramen both dorsal and ventral to the nerve root, and the root can gently be retracted approximately 1 cm medially.

The question of whether or not to decompress stenotic levels that do not seem to correlate with the patient's symptoms is unresolved. When in doubt as to the symptomatic level, a diagnostic nerve root block may be performed. The risk of producing symptoms at a decompressed but apparently asymptomatic level or side must be balanced against the risk of the degenerative process progressing and symptoms developing at an asymptomatic stenotic site that was not decompressed. Because degenerative changes tend to progress over time, it is probable that asymptomatic stenotic levels eventually will become symptomatic. Indeed, in several studies inadequate decompression has resulted in long-term deterioration in clinical outcome following initially successful surgery.

Hemilaminectomy

Hemilaminectomy involves unilateral, rather than bilateral, removal of bone and ligamentum flavum. It is appropriate for patients with unilateral symptoms from unilateral stenosis. Because the spinous processes, interspinous ligaments, and supraspinous ligaments are preserved medially, normal stabilizing structures are retained, thereby reducing the risk of postoperative instability. Hemilaminectomy also avoids exposure of and potential injury to the contralateral facet joint. The surgeon must take care to preserve the pars interarticularis laterally to minimize the risk of postoperative instability. A disadvantage of this procedure is the relative difficulty of contralateral decompression and of obtaining enough medial exposure to perform an adequate ipsilateral decompression in patients with foraminal stenosis. The presence of an intact spinous process and interspinous/supraspinous ligament complex make it difficult to angle the rongeur laterally enough to enable the jaw of the rongeur to enter the depths of the neural foramen. Under such circumstances, removal of the midline spinous process and interspinous/supraspinous ligament complex may be necessary to allow the proper angulation of the rongeur to perform the foraminal decompression.

Contralateral nerve roots usually can be decompressed through a unilateral hemilaminectomy approach by tilting the operating table away from the surgeon and by angling the operating microscope. The contralateral neural foramen usually can be seen and decompressed, and the more distal portion can be palpated with a long bent probe. Although it preserves normal, noncompressing midline structures and minimizes scar tissue on the opposite side, this technique is more demanding than bilateral laminectomy because decompression is done through a more limited exposure, and the determination of adequate foraminal patency depends more on feel (palpation) than on direct observation. In addition, there is a greater potential for dural laceration from the rongeur when working through such a small opening. Should such a dural tear occur, its repair usually necessitates complete (bilateral) laminectomy with adequate exposure of the dural tear.

Alternatives to Laminectomy
Although some studies report deterioration of standard bilateral decompressive laminectomy over time, more limited alternatives to laminectomy and hemilaminectomy have been espoused to avoid removal of normal, noncompressing structures and thereby to minimize the risk of postoperative instability. Such procedures include hemilaminotomy and laminoplasty. Hemilaminotomy involves a more limited decompression than hemilaminectomy. Rather than removing the entire hemilamina, it removes only the ligamentum flavum and adjacent portions of two hemilaminae. This procedure is done more commonly in younger patients with unilateral focal neural compression. It also may be considered in older patients with localized stenosis. Resection of the distal half of the superior hemilamina is generally required to see and remove the proximal extent of the ligamentum flavum. Hemilaminotomy, therefore, generally involves removal of the inferior half of the superior hemilamina and the superior portion of the inferior hemilamina, together with the intervening ligamentum flavum.

Lateral decompression may also require partial facetectomy. As in hemilaminectomy, contralateral decompression with preservation of spinous processes and midline supraspinous/interspinous ligaments can be done by tilting the operating table away from the surgeon and by removing the midline and contralateral ligamentum flavum with a 45° ronguer.

Laminoplasty was proposed originally as an alternative to laminectomy for active manual workers. This procedure is similar to cervical laminoplasty and involves hinging open the lamina on one side and inserting the excised spinous processes into the open hinge to keep it patent. In a 3-year follow-up study of 10 patients undergoing this procedure, the Japanese Orthopaedic Association mean evaluation score improved an average of 73%, and the size of the spinal canal increased an average of 119% following surgery.

Results of Surgical Decompression
A recent review of the literature for spinal stenosis surgery failed to identify even a single randomized trial comparing surgery and conservative treatment. Authors of an attempted meta-analysis of the literature on surgical outcomes for spinal stenosis concluded that the poor scientific quality of the literature precluded their conducting the intended meta-analysis. Only 74 of 625 articles (12%) identified as potentially relevant actually met the inclusion criteria adopted for this study. None of these were randomized, only three of the 74 articles were prospectively designed and only seven of the 74 had independent rating of outcome. Even using the ratings of the authors of the articles, the average proportion of good-to excellent outcomes was only 72%. This review found no statistically significant relationship between outcome and patient age, gender, presence of prior back surgery, or number of levels operated upon. In the studies reporting only on patients with degenerative spondylolisthesis, the surgical outcome was better. An interesting finding of this attempted meta-analysis was that there was no statistically significant difference in outcome of decompression with or without concomitant fusion. This finding also has been noted in other literature surveys of outcome following lumbar spinal fusion for a variety of diagnoses; it is particularly significant in light of the reported increased morbidity associated with lumbar fusion.

Laminectomy and Laminotomy
In a 1-year prospective, nonrandomized observational cohort study of patients with spinal stenosis treated surgically or nonsurgically in community-based practices in the state of Maine, 87.6% of 81 patients undergoing surgery underwent laminectomy. At 1 year, 55% of these surgical patients reported definite improvement in their predominant symptom, compared with only 28% of the nonsurgical group (Table 1). After adjusting for covariates, surgery was found to increase the relative odds of definite improvement 2.6-fold, compared with nonsurgical treatment. Criticisms of this study include the 1-year follow-up period, its nonrandom nature, and that it examined only 22% of those eligible to be enrolled. In addition, there was no standardization of the type of conservative care or surgery rendered. Although the results of this study should be interpreted with caution,

TABLE 1	One-year Outcome of Surgical and Nonsurgical Treatment of Spinal Stenosis

Outcome Variable	Surgical (%)	Nonsurgical (%)
Low back pain		
Better	77	42
Same	18	38
Worse	5	20
Leg pain		
Better	79	45
Same	15	43
Worse	6	12
Change in predominant symptoms		
Much Better	55	28
Same	42	57
Worse	3	15
Patient satisfaction		
Very good	69	36
Satisfied	68	32
Would have surgery again	88	
Significant improvement in quality of life	81	49

(Adapted with permission from Atlas S, Deyo R, Keller R, et al: The Maine lumbar spine study, part III: 1-year outcomes of surgical and nonsurgical management of lumbar spinal stenosis. Spine 1996;21:1787-1795.)

TABLE 2	Comparison of Surgical Versus Nonsurgical Treatment of Lumbar Spinal Stenosis

Treatment	Worse (%)	Unchanged (%)	Improved (%)
No surgery	10	58	32
Surgery	25	16	59

(Adapted with permission from Johnsson KE, Uden A, Rosen I: The effect of decompression on the natural course of spinal stenosis: A comparison of surgically treated and untreated patients. Spine 1991;16:615-619.)

for 2.8 to 6.8 years (Table 3). Eleven percent of the patients reported poor outcome at 1 year; this increased to 43% at final follow-up. Six percent of the patients had repeat lumbar surgery within the first year, and 17% had additional surgery by the time of the last follow-up. Risk factors for poor outcome included preoperative comorbidities and limited (single level) decompression. The authors concluded that the long-term outlook for patients undergoing decompressive laminectomy for spinal stenosis is not as good as is commonly believed because of progressive deterioration of results over time. They suggested that more extensive decompression should be considered at the time of initial surgery.

The report of a prospective, consecutive, surgical series of 105 patients undergoing laminectomy for lumbar stenosis noted the deterioration of surgical results over time. Although excellent results were reported by two-thirds of the patients at 2-year follow-up, outcome deteriorated to only 52% excellent results by 5 years. During the 5-year period of study, 16% of patients underwent re-operation for severe back pain or recurrent stenosis. A significant correlation was noted between excellent outcome and preoperative duration

it gives some indication of the scope of treatment and expected short-term outcome for patients receiving treatment for spinal stenosis in a rural population.

A study comparing 44 patients with lumbar spinal stenosis who were treated surgically with 19 untreated patients revealed that 59% of the patients (26) who underwent surgery improved, 16% (7) were unchanged, and 25% (11) deteriorated. Thirty-two percent of the patients (6) who did not undergo surgery improved and 68% (13) had the same or worse claudication symptoms at an average follow-up of 31 months (Table 2). Therefore, the percentage of patients in the surgical group that improved was nearly twice that in the nonsurgical group. However, a greater percentage of the surgical group than of the nonsurgical group (25% versus 10%) was worse at follow-up. This study was neither prospective nor random, and it was not clear whether or not the nonsurgical group was truly untreated or had some form of conservative treatment.

Some have reported that long-term outcome following surgical decompression for spinal stenosis is not as good as is commonly perceived. In a large retrospective study, the results were reported for decompressive laminectomy for spinal stenosis in 88 patients followed

TABLE 3	Long-term Results of Laminectomy for Spinal Stenosis

Results	One Year Follow-up	Final Follow-up
Poor outcome	8 of 74 (11%)	31 of 72 (43%)
Severe pain	5 of 74 (7%)	21 of 70 (30%)
Re-operation	5 of 88 (6%)	15 of 88 (17%)
Limited physical function	6 of 74 (8%)	26 of 74 (35%)
Walk < 15 meters	6 of 74 (8%)	15 of 70 (21%)

(Adapted with permission from Katz JN, Lipson SJ, Larson MG, McInnes JM, Fossel AH, Liang MH: The outcome of decompressive laminectomy for degenerative lumbar stenosis. J Bone Joint Surg Am 1991;73:809-816.)

of symptoms of less than 4 years, no preoperative low back pain, and no significant comorbidities.

Laminectomy and Fusion for Spinal Stenosis

The role of fusion in the treatment of spinal stenosis is somewhat controversial. For stenosis not associated with degenerative spondylolisthesis or other deformity, most studies indicate that simple decompression is the preferred method of surgical treatment. For patients with associated degenerative spondylolisthesis, concomitant fusion generally is recommended. The issue of using supplementary spinal instrumentation is yet unresolved.

In a prospective, randomized study of 45 patients undergoing either decompression alone or decompression with fusion for spinal stenosis without associated instability, there were no significant differences in outcome between fused and unfused groups. Patients were randomized to one of three treatment groups: group I, decompression without arthrodesis; group II, decompression with arthrodesis of the most stenotic segment only; and group III, decompression and arthrodesis of all decompressed segments (Table 4). Overall, 78% of patient-reported and 80% of examiner-rated results were satisfactory. When examined by type of procedure performed, there were no significant differences in pain relief among the three groups. Decompression alone produced satisfactory results in 87% of patients. The authors concluded that surgical decompression changed the natural history of spinal stenosis, resulting in generally favorable outcome and improved quality of life in most patients. They further concluded that arthrodesis was not justified in the absence of radiographically proven segmental instability because there was no statistical difference in outcome among the three treatment groups.

The role of fusion for a variety of spinal disorders was examined in a randomized, prospective study of 124 patients undergoing either instrumented or noninstru-

mented fusion. Two types of spinal instrumentation were used: a rigid system and a semirigid system. The overall fusion rate was 65% for the noninstrumented group, 77% for the semirigid fixation group, and 95% for the rigid fixation group. A trend for better clinical outcome with increasing rigidity of fixation also was observed. Seventy-one percent of the noninstrumented patients, 89% of the semirigid group, and 95% of the rigid group reported excellent or good results. A similar trend for higher fusion rates with more rigid fixation was noted for the smaller subgroup of patients with degenerative spondylolisthesis.

Comorbidity and Surgical Outcome

Sick patients have a higher mortality rate, a higher complication rate, and a lower level of function than do healthy patients. Comorbidity typically increases with age and is associated with poor outcome for many medical and surgical conditions. The relationship between age and outcome following lumbar spinal surgery has been investigated. Rates of hospital morbidity and mortality are greater with increasing age of the patient. Complications are more frequent with advancing patient age, increasing complexity of diagnosis, and greater complexity of surgical treatment. In a study of 18,122 hospitalizations in the state of Washington between 1986 and 1988, the overall mortality rate was 0.07%. Mortality increased with age, reaching 0.6% (ninefold increase) in patients older than 75 years of age. This was also true for complications, with an overall complication rate of 9.1%, which increased to 17.7% in patients 75 years of age or older. Similar findings were reported in an administrative database study of 34,418 patients 65 years of age or older from 1986 Medicare claims files. There was an age-related increase in mortality only for patients older than 80 years of age. There was, however, a significant increase in in-hospital and 1-year cumulative mortality associated with an increasing number of comorbidities.

The predictors of outcome following spinal surgery for spinal stenosis have been studied. Authors of a retrospective review of 88 patients undergoing laminectomy for spinal stenosis concluded that long-term outcome was generally less favorable than had been previously reported (Table 3). By 1 year after surgery, 6% of patients had a second operation, and by the time of the last follow-up 17% had a repeat surgery. Although several predictors of poor outcome were identified, such as increasing length of follow-up, single-level decompression, and increased number of comorbidities, only the latter was significant after adjusting for multiple comparisons. Only 40% of patients with the highest comorbidity score had a good outcome at the time of final follow-up compared with 75% of patients

---

TABLE 4 | Comparison of Treatments for Spinal Stenosis

Evaluator	Group I: Decompression Without Fusion (% Satisfactory)	Group II: Decompression and Limited Fusion* (% Satisfactory)	Group III: Decompression and Fusion† (% Satisfactory)
Patient	13 of 15 (87)	12 of 15 (80)	10 of 15 (67)
Examiner	13 of 15 (87)	12 of 15 (80)	11 of 15 (73)

*Only most stenotic segment decompressed
†All levels decompressed

(Reproduced with permission from Grob D, Humke T, Dvorak J: Degenerative lumbar spinal stenosis: Decompression with and without arthrodesis. J Bone Joint Surg Am 1995;77: 1036-1041.)

who had the lowest comorbidity score. The most common comorbidities were osteoarthritis (32%), cardiac disease (22%), rheumatoid arthritis (10%), and chronic pulmonary disease (7%). Data from this study suggested that the effect of comorbidities was additive because no single comorbidity was significantly associated with worse outcome. In a subsequent study by the same authors, comorbidity was found to be second only to preoperative complaints of predominant low back pain as a determinant of disability in lumbar canal stenosis.

Correlation between comorbidities and other measures of outcome have also been examined. Both cost of lumbar spinal surgery and length of stay following surgery have been found to be greater in patients with increased comorbidities. Patients with three or more comorbidities were found to have a 25% longer stay, 36% greater hospital costs, and a 73% higher rate of discharge to a nursing home than those with no comorbidity.

Preferred Surgical Treatment for Spinal Stenois

Decompression without arthrodesis is the preferrred surgical treatment of spinal stenosis unless instability or other structural abnormalities are present, for example, spondylolisthesis or scoliosis. For one- or two-level stenosis, laminectomy is generally preferred, with care taken to minimize damage to the pars interarticularis and the facet joints. If more than one facet joint is sacrificed at any segmental level, then prophylactic fusion should be strongly considered to minimize the risk of development of subsequent spinal instability. Care is taken to avoid discectomy if at all possible. There is a significant risk of postoperative instability if both the disc and posterior structures are surgically violated.

If more than two levels require decompression, multilevel laminotomies are preferred to laminectomy to minimize the risk of development of postoperative instability that may occur with the latter. The laminotomies may be either unilateral or bilateral, depending on the amount of decompression required and the ease with which the decompression can be done from a unilateral approach. Multilevel laminotomies are most appropriate for typical degenerative spinal stenosis, where the narrowing is maximal at the level of the facet joints and disc, but where the canal is otherwise patent. Laminotomies generally are not appropriate with congenital stenosis, where there is global spinal canal narrowing. Under such circumstances, where multilevel stenosis has a significant congenital component and more than two levels require laminectomy, consideration should be given to performing a concomitant fusion to minimize the risk of subsequent instability.

The patient is encouraged to be out of bed by the day after surgery. Bracing generally is not used. The patient

may be as active as the pain will permit, and sitting is not restricted unless there has been a concomitant discectomy. The patient generally is seen 4 weeks after surgery, at which point the patient's activities may be increased further, and aerobic conditioning may be instituted.

Degenerative Spondylolisthesis

Degenerative spondylolisthesis is the term most commonly used to describe the anterior slippage of one vertebral body on another in the presence of an intact neural arch. It may be a source of low back pain and radicular or referred leg pain, and it may produce symptoms of classic neurogenic claudication.

Surgical Treatment

Decompression Without Fusion

Surgical treatment of spinal stenosis associated with degenerative spondylolisthesis involves either decompression alone or decompression with arthrodesis. Only 11 articles reporting the results of decompression without fusion met the inclusion criteria for a meta-analysis of the literature from 1970 to 1993 (Table 5). Overall, only 69% of the patients were found to have satisfactory results following surgery. Thirty-one percent of the patients in the nine studies in which slip progression was recorded showed an increase in the degree of slip. However, there was generally no correlation between clinical outcome and amount of slip progression, except in one study that showed a positive correlation between the two.

In a surgeon-reported, 10-year retrospective review of 290 patients undergoing limited decompression procedures for spinal stenosis with degenerative spondylolis-

TABLE 5	Results of Decompression Without Fusion for Degenerative Spondylolisthesis: Meta-Analysis of Literature 1970-1993 (11 Articles)

Results	Number
Satisfactory	140 of 216 (69%)*
Unsatisfactory	75 of 216 (31%)*
Progressive slip	67 of 216 (31%)**

*Weighted pooled proportion
**Reported in only 9 of 11 articles
(Reproduced with permission from Mardjetko SM, Connolly PJ, Shott S: Degenerative lumbar spondylolisthesis: A meta-analysis of literature 1970-1993. Spine 1994;19(suppl 20):2256S-2265S.)

TABLE 6	Prospective, Randomized Comparison of Decompression Alone Versus Decompression and Noninstrumented Spinal Fusion for Degenerative Spondylolisthesis	
Result	Arthrodesis (No. = 25)	No Arthrodesis (No. = 25)
Excellent	11 (44%)	2 (8%)
Good	13 (52%)	9 (36%)
Fair	1 (4%)	12 (48%)
Poor	0 (0%)	2 (8%)
Mean increase in slip (preoperative to postoperative)	0.5 mm	2.6 mm (*P* = 0.002)

(Reproduced with permission from Herkowitz HN, Kurz LT: Degenerative lumbar spondylolisthesis with spinal stenosis: A prospective study comparing decompression with decompression and intertransverse process arthrodesis. J Bone Joint Surg Am 1991;73:802-808.)

TABLE 7	Results of Decompression with Noninstrumented Fusion: Meta-analysis of Literature 1970-1993 (6 Articles)
Results	Number (%)
Satisfactory	59 of 75 (79)*[†]
Unsatisfactory	16 of 75 (21)*[†]
Fusion	62 of 84 (86)

*Weighted pooled proportion
[†]Data from 5 of 6 articles reported

(Reproduced with permission from Mardjetko SM, Connolly PJ, Shott S: Degenerative lumbar spondylolisthesis: A meta-analysis of literature 1970-1993. Spine 1994;19(suppl 20):2256S-2265S.)

thesis, outcome was reported as excellent in 69%, good in 13%, fair in 12%, and poor in 6%. Because only 2.7% of patients required secondary fusion, the authors concluded that routine concomitant fusion for spinal stenosis with degenerative spondylolisthesis is not warranted.

In a prospective, randomized study comparing decompression alone with combined decompression and noninstrumented fusion for degenerative spondylolisthesis, only 11 of 25 patients (44%) having decompression without fusion had satisfactory results (Table 6). This group had significantly more postoperative low back pain and leg pain than the fused group and had an average 50% increase in the slip from preoperatively.

Decompression With Noninstrumented Fusion

Only six studies that reported the results of decompression with fusion met the inclusion criteria for a meta-analysis of the literature for degenerative spondylolisthesis (Table 7). In these six studies, 79% of patients reported satisfactory outcome following decompression without arthrodesis. Only three of the studies were prospective and randomized; the most widely quoted compared decompression alone to decompression and noninstrumented spinal fusion in the treatment of L3-4 and L4-5 degenerative spondylolisthesis with spinal stenosis (Table 6). The authors reported superior results when concomitant fusion was performed with the decompression: 44% excellent and 52% good results (96% excellent/good) in the arthrodesis group and only 8% excellent and 36% good (44% excellent/good) in the nonarthrodesis group. There was also a significant progression of the slip in patients not receiving an

arthrodesis compared with those undergoing fusion. Although 36% of those undergoing arthrodesis were noted to have a pseudarthrosis, they all had either an excellent or good result. The authors of this study concluded that the results of surgical decompression with in situ arthrodesis were superior to those of decompression alone in the treatment of spinal stenosis associated with L3-4 or L4-5 degenerative spondylolisthesis. They concluded that the decision for arthrodesis should be based purely on the presence or absence of a preoperative spondylolisthesis rather than on other factors, such as the age or sex of the patient, the disc height, or the amount of bone resected during the decompression.

The relationship between bone regrowth following surgical decompression for spinal stenosis and long-term outcome has also been examined. In general, satisfactory outcome has been found to be inversely proportional to the amount of bone regrowth. Although patients with degenerative spondylolisthesis do show some bone regrowth following surgical decompression and fusion, the degree of regrowth is more severe in patients not undergoing arthrodesis. This is reflected in outcome following surgery; outcome was shown to be significantly better in patients undergoing decompression with spinal fusion. Although this study was retrospective and therefore not randomized, it suggested that arthrodesis stabilizes the spine, resulting in less bone regrowth and superior long-term results.

Decompression With Instrumented Fusion

The long-term clinical outcome of surgical decompression with instrumented spinal fusion for degenerative spondylolisthesis is not completely known. A prospective, randomized study examined 124 patients undergoing either instrumented or noninstrumented fusion for a variety of diagnoses. Two types of spinal instrumentation were used: a rigid system and a semirigid system. For the subgroup of patients with degenerative spondylolisthesis, 65% of the noninstrumented group fused compared with 50% of the semirigid fixation group and 86% of the rigid fixation group. Authors of this study concluded that fusion rate and outcome were better in patients undergoing fusion with more rigid fixation systems.

The historic cohort study of spinal fusion using pedicle screw fixation included a retrospective, multicenter study of 2,684 patients with degenerative spondylolisthesis. Solid radiographic fusion was noted in 89% of patients undergoing pedicle screw fixation compared to 70% of those without instrumentation. Clinical outcome was also better in the group of patients undergoing instrumented fusion.

Authors of a recent randomized, prospective study of posterolateral lumbar fusion, with and without pedicle screw instrumentation, for a variety of conditions concluded that the addition of instrumentation did not produce a significant incremental clinical benefit, although there was a slight, nonsignificant trend towards higher fusion rate in the instrumented fusion group. Of the small subset of 10 patients with degenerative spondylolisthesis, five underwent instrumented fusion and five underwent fusion in situ. Four of the five patients (80%) undergoing instrumented fusion achieved excellent/good outcome compared to two of five (40%) of those without instrumentation. Clinical outcome was also better, although this subgroup was too small to determine statistical significance.

Preferred Surgical Treatment for Spinal Stenois With Degenerative Spondylolisthesis

In general, decompression with fusion is recommended for spinal stenosis associated with degenerative spondylolisthesis. For elderly, low demand patients with multiple comorbidities, however, multilevel laminotomies without fusion are sometimes done. This procedure is particularly likely if there is significant collapse of the disc space that makes progression of the slip less likely.

In the younger, healthy, active patient laminectomy with instrumented fusion using pedicle screw fixation is preferable. Autogenous iliac bone is best for posterolateral bone grafting. Alternatives to iliac bone include using the bone from the laminectomy, possibly mixed with a bone graft extender such as demineralized bone matrix. In an attempt to avoid the morbidity associated with harvesting an iliac bone graft, en bloc excision of the intact lamina may be performed with the aid of a high-speed burr and a 2-mm rongeur. The lamina is then cut into small matchstick strips of bone and is mixed with approximately 20 cc of bone marrow aspirated from the iliac crest. The osteoprogenitor cells derived from the bone marrow are believed to increase the bone-forming potential of the bone graft. A PLIF usu-

ally is not done unless a multilevel fusion to the sacrum is required. For this situation a PLIF generally is done at L5-S1.

In the elderly, low demand, but generally healthy patient a laminectomy or laminotomy with a noninstrumented (in situ) fusion frequently is performed, particularly if there is significant collapse of the disc space. Although a pseudarthrosis often occurs, the stability it affords has been shown to be superior to what occurs with only decompression, and outcome is improved over decompression alone.

Summary

There does not appear to be a clear consensus for the optimal surgical treatment of degenerative spondylolisthesis. Most studies show that clinical outcome is better when decompression is accompanied by fusion. It is less clear, however, whether outcome is better with instrumentation than without it. If there is clear evidence of instability on flexion-extension radiographs, the additional time, expense, and potential morbidity associated with the use of instrumentation seems warranted to provide immediate stability. However, the indication for use of instrumentation in the patient with a collapsed disc space, no motion at the spondylolisthetic level, and therefore no clear evidence of instability, is less clear.

Conclusion

Evaluating the results of a treatment requires knowledge of the natural history of the untreated condition. In the case of spinal stenosis, either with or without degenerative spondylolisthesis, the natural history of the untreated condition is not completely understood because there are few long-term studies. The role of fusion in the treatment of spinal stenosis with or without degenerative spondylolisthesis is poorly characterized because there are few controlled, prospective, randomized studies comparing different treatment options.

The available literature suggests that the natural history of spinal stenosis, either with or without degenerative spondylolisthesis, is characterized by improvement in approximately one third of patients and deterioration in a small minority (approximately 10%). Most patients (approximately 50% to 70%) have a generally static clinical course over time with little, if any, improvement.

There seem to be few data to support the routine use of arthrodesis in the surgical treatment of spinal stenosis that is not associated with degenerative spondylolisthesis. Arthrodesis often is recommended when decompression has been excessive or extensive, either by excessive bone removal or by extensive number of levels decompressed. Unfortunately, prospective randomized studies addressing this issue have not been performed.

There is support for decompression and arthrodesis for spinal stenosis associated with degenerative spondylolisthesis. Most studies indicate that the fusion rate is better in patients undergoing instrumented fusion, although the relationship between outcome and fusion rate is less clear. Finally, the future role for bone graft substitutes is only now being addressed, because virtually all clinical studies to date have used autogenous bone graft for arthrodesis.

Annotated Bibliography

Lumbar Spinal Stenosis

Atlas SJ, Deyo RA, Keller RB, et al: The Maine lumbar spine study: Part III. 1-year outcomes of surgical and nonsurgical management of lumbar spinal stenosis. *Spine* 1996;21:1787-1795.

This is a prospective, cohort study of 148 patients with lumbar spinal stenosis recruited from the practices of orthopaedic surgeons and neurosurgeons from the state of Maine. At the 1-year evaluation, surgically treated patients had better outcome than nonsurgically treated patients (55% versus 28%, respectively). The deficiencies of this study include the short (1-year) follow-up and that nearly 80% of patients eligible for inclusion in the study were not enrolled.

Grob D, Humke T, Dvorak J: Degenerative lumbar spinal stenosis: Decompression with and without arthrodesis. *J Bone Joint Surg Am* 1995;77:1036-1041.

Forty-five patients were prospectively evaluated at an average of 28 months following decompression with and without arthrodesis for lumbar spinal stenosis without instability. There was no significant difference in outcome between patients undergoing decompression alone and decompression with fusion.

Hilibrand AS, Rand N: Degenerative lumbar stenosis: Diagnosis and management. *J Am Acad Orthop Surg* 1999;7:239-249.

This is a review article describing the basic science, clinical presentation, diagnosis, and treatments of degenerative spinal stenosis.

Spivak JM: Degenerative lumbar spinal stenosis. *J Bone Joint Surg Am* 1998;80:1053-1066.

This article reviews the definition and classification of lumbar spinal stenosis and details the current knowledge of its pathoanatomy, clinical features, diagnosis, and treatment.

Degenerative Spondylolisthesis

Epstein NE: Decompression in the surgical management of degenerative spondylolisthesis: Advantages of a conservative approach in 290 patients. *J Spinal Disord* 1998;11:116-123.

The authors reviewed 290 of their patients undergoing limited decompression procedures for spinal stenosis with degenerative spondylolisthesis at an average follow-up of 10 years. Outcome was reported as excellent in 69%, good in 13%, fair in 12%, and poor in 6%. Only 2.7% of patients required secondary fusion. The authors concluded that routine concomitant fusion for spinal stenosis with degenerative spondylolisthesis is unwarranted.

Fischgrund JS, Mackay M, Herkowitz HN, Brower R, Montgomery DM, Kurz LT: Degenerative lumbar spondylolisthesis with spinal stenosis: A prospective, randomized study comparing decompressive laminectomy and arthrodesis with and without spinal instrumentation. *Spine* 1997;22:2807-2812.

This is a prospective, randomized study of 76 patients with symptomatic lumbar spinal stenosis associated with degenerative spondylolisthesis who underwent decompression and either noninstrumented in situ posterolateral fusion or instrumented fusion with segmental fixation. There was no significant difference in clinical outcome between the two groups of patients. The authors concluded that the use of segmental (pedicle) fixation in a single-level decompression and fusion for spinal stenosis with degenerative spondylolisthesis does not lead to better clinical outcome.

France JC, Yaszemski MJ, Lauerman WC, et al: A randomized prospective study of posterolateral lumbar fusion: Outcomes with and without pedicle screw instrumentation. *Spine* 1999;24:553-560.

This is a prospective, randomized study of 71 patients undergoing lumbar fusion for a variety of conditions, which included failed back surgery syndrome, degenerative disc disease/disc herniation, isthmic spondylolisthesis, and degenerative spondylolisthesis. Patients were randomized to fusion with pedicle screw instrumentation or fusion without instrumentation. Overall, there was no statistical difference in patient reported outcome between the two groups. In the 10 patients with degenerative spondylolisthesis, 4 of 5 patients with instrumentation had excellent/good outcome compared to 2 of 5 patients without. The authors concluded that their data did not indicate a benefit in outcome from the use of pedicle screw instrumentation.

Classic Bibliography

Deyo RA, Cherkin DC, Loeser JD, Bigos SJ, Ciol MA: Morbidity and mortality in association with operations on the lumbar spine: The influence of age, diagnosis, and procedure. *J Bone Joint Surg Am* 1992;74:536-543.

Deyo RA, Ciol MA, Cherkin DC, Loeser JD, Bigos SJ: Lumbar spinal fusion: A cohort study of complications, reoperations, and resource use in the Medicare population. *Spine* 1993;18:1463-1470.

Fitzgerald JA, Newman PH: Degenerative spondylolisthesis. *J Bone Joint Surg Br* 1976;58:184-192.

Frymoyer JW: Degenerative spondylolisthesis: Diagnosis and treatment. *J Am Acad Orthop Surg* 1994;2:9-15.

Herkowitz HN, Kurz LT: Degenerative lumbar spondylolisthesis with spinal stenosis: A prospective study comparing decompression with decompression and intertransverse process arthrodesis. *J Bone Joint Surg Am* 1991;73:802-808.

Johnsson KE, Uden A, Rosen I: The effect of decompression on the natural course of spinal stenosis: A comparison of surgically treated and untreated patients. *Spine* 1991;16:615-619.

Katz JN, Lipson SJ, Larson MG, McInnes JM, Fossel AH, Liang MH: The outcome of decompressive laminectomy for degenerative lumbar stenosis. *J Bone Joint Surg Am* 1991;73:809-816.

Kirkaldy-Willis WH, Paine KW, Cauchoix J, McIvor G: Lumbar spinal stenosis. *Clin Orthop* 1974;99:30-50.

Macnab I: Spondylolisthesis with an intact neural arch: The so-called pseudo-spondylolisthesis. *J Bone Joint Surg Br* 1950;32:325-333.

Mardjetko SM, Connolly PJ, Shott S: Degenerative lumbar spondylolisthesis: A meta-analysis of literature, 1970-1993. *Spine* 1994;19(suppl 20):2256S-2265S.

Newman PH, Stone KH: The etiology of spondylolisthesis. *J Bone Joint Surg Br* 1963;45:39-59.

Postacchini F, Cinotti G: Bone regrowth after surgical decompression for lumbar spinal stenosis. *J Bone Joint Surg Br* 1992;74:862-869.

Verbiest H: A radicular syndrome from developmental narrowing of the lumbar vertebral canal. *J Bone Joint Surg Br* 1954;36:230-237.

Yuan HA, Garfin SR, Dickman CA, Mardjetko SM: A historical cohort study of pedicle screw fixation in thoracic, lumbar, and sacral spinal fusions. *Spine* 1994;19(suppl 20):2279S-2296S.

Zdeblick TA: A prospective, randomized study of lumbar fusion: Preliminary results. *Spine* 1993;18:983-991.

Chapter 37

Surgical Management of Isthmic and Dysplastic Spondylolisthesis and Spondylolysis

Patrick J. Connolly, MD

Bruce E. Fredrickson, MD

Spondylolisthesis is the forward displacement of one vertebra anterior to the vertebrae below it. The term spondylolisthesis implies anterior translation; however, posterior translation, termed retrolisthesis, can occur. Lateral translation can also occur, usually combined with rotation. The degree of forward translation can be measured as a percent slip or by the Meyerding classification (grades I through IV). The term spondyloptosis has been reserved for cases in which a vertebra is translated 100% and has been displaced anteriorly to the caudal vertebra. The most common classification of spondylolisthesis is that described by Wiltse and Neuman. Type I is congenital or dysplastic spondylolisthesis. There are three subtypes within this classification, including dysplastic facets with axial orientation, dysplastic facets in a sagittal orientation, and other congenital abnormalities of the articulations. Type II is isthmic or spondylitic spondylolisthesis, in which the slip is secondary to a defect in the pars interarticularis. The three subtypes of isthmic spondylolisthesis include a lytic fatigue fracture, elongated intact pars, and an acute fracture of the pars itself. Type III is degenerative spondylolisthesis secondary to loss of integrity of the disc structure and subsequent laxity of the supporting ligamentous structures of the spinal unit. Type IV, traumatic spondylolisthesis, is secondary to traumatic disruption of the facet complex. It is considered separate from an acute fracture of the pars, which is subclassified under type II. Slipping secondary to type II injury may be acute or, more commonly, chronic over a period of weeks and months. Type V is pathologic spondylolisthesis, secondary to destruction of the integrity of the pars, pedicle, and/or facet. There are two subtypes: the first is caused by generalized disease such as osteoporosis or arthrogryposis; the second is the result of a localized pathologic lesion such as tumor or infection. A sixth type of spondylolisthesis added to the original classification includes postsurgical spondylolisthesis in which the bony and/or ligamentous structures have been iatrogenically removed predispos-

ing the development of spondylolisthesis. This chapter will deal exclusively with the first two types of spondylolisthesis: dysplastic and lytic.

Natural History

Dysplastic Spondylolisthesis

Dysplastic spondylolisthesis develops when the posterior facet complexes either are aligned improperly or do not fully develop, allowing gravity to displace the cranial vertebra anteriorly (Fig. 1). The integrity of the ring of bone forming the central canal is maintained. Significant neurologic signs and symptoms can develop rapidly and frequently are the initial complaint. Typically these patients complain of tight hamstrings and may have true neurologic symptoms and signs, such as paresthesias, weakness, and, in the later stages, typical findings of cauda equina syndrome. These symptoms may be present with a relatively small degree of slip because the ring (usually L5) is closed and the canal is truly constricted. Females have been reported to have a higher occurrence, with a ratio of 2:1. The incidence of dysplastic spondylolisthesis relative to spondylolisthesis as a whole is probably less than 15%.

Isthmic Spondylolisthesis

Isthmic spondylolisthesis implies a defect in the pars interarticularis. Displacement of the vertebra is not associated with displacement of the posterior arch, and hence, neurologic sequelae are less common. The incidence of isthmic spondylolisthesis in the general public has varied, depending on the population studied. In general, it has been reported to be 5% to 7% in the United States with a higher incidence in whites than in blacks and an incidence of up to 50% in the Inuit population. The defect has genetic and environmental causes; over one third of affected family members are reported to have a pars defect. Typically, isthmic spondylolisthesis develops by the age of 5 or 6 years, but in some instances

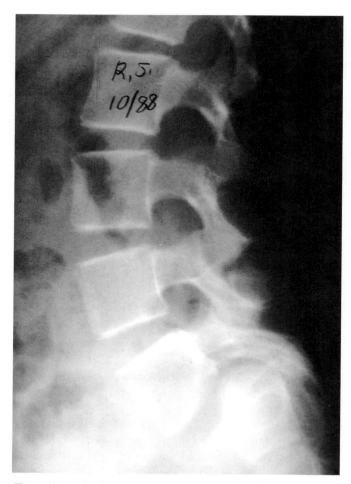

Figure 1 Lateral radiograph of dysplastic spondylolisthesis at L5-S1.

sonnel have not identified spondylolisthesis as a condition that predisposes the individual to greater risk of disability from low back pain than that of the general population.

Radiographic Measurements

The degree of slip of the cranial versus caudal vertebrae can be expressed in two ways. Typically it is expressed as a Meyerding grade I, II, III or IV. The second way is to describe it as a percentage of slip (Figs. 2 and 3).

The lumbar index is a measurement of the trapezoidal shape of the body of L5, represented as the percentage of the posterior height divided by the anterior height (Fig. 4). Although it has been shown that, in individuals with progressive slip, the shape of L5 becomes more trapezoid, this feature has not been predictive of future slips. The slip angle represents the relationship of L5 to the sacrum as measured from a line parallel to the superior surface of L5 and a line perpendicular to the posterior surface of S1 and S2 (Fig. 5). A low angle implies a normal relationship of L5 to the sacrum; whereas a higher angle indicates increasing kyphosis of L5 on S1. Sacral inclination is the degree of verticalization of the sacrum (Fig. 6). Typically in higher-grade slips the sacrum becomes more vertically orientated and L5 assumes a more kyphotic position.

The sagittal pelvic tilt index is a more recent measurement, which evaluates the relationship of the sacrum to L5 and the center of the femoral head (Fig. 7). A normal value is close to 1; decreasing values in a specific individual indicate a change in relationship of the L5 body and sacrum in regards to the femoral head and loss of stability of the lumbosacral junction.

Diagnostic Studies

Serial Radiographs

All radiographs used to measure percent slip and the relationship of L5 to the sacrum should be done in the erect position, if possible, including bending films. A measurement error of up to 10% has been well described and therefore changes of less than 10% should not be considered significant. The frequency of serial radiographs depends on the age of the patient and the presence or absence of symptoms.

Injections can be either diagnostic or therapeutic. Specific to spondylolisthesis, diagnostic blocks include those of the pars interarticularis and selective root blocks usually of L5. Discography is used to determine the location of the pain. Localization of the pain generator through injections can help resolve questions such as whether adjacent degenerative levels are painful.

may not become present until adolescence. Patients rarely have symptoms during development of the defect and its presence usually is identified on radiographs taken for some other cause. A small minority develop progressive spondylolisthesis that rapidly increases from grade I through grade IV and on rare occasions to spondyloptosis.

Symptoms relating to isthmic spondylolisthesis usually consist of low back pain with associated tightness in the hamstrings. Complaints/findings compatible with nerve root irritation, usually the fifth lumbar, may be noted.

Patients with isthmic spondylolisthesis may slowly increase the degree of listhesis over time. Progression of the slip beyond that initially identified is associated with loss of disc height. Some patients have a stable degree of listhesis for many years only to develop further progression during their 30s or 40s. Symptoms may or may not be present during this process. Pregnancy has been associated with progression of the slip.

Large studies of blue-collar workers and military per-

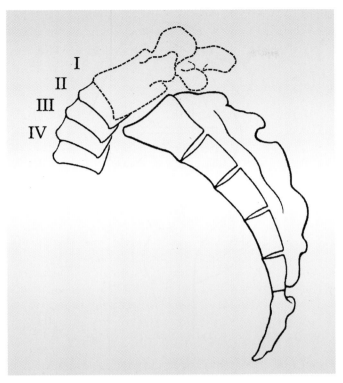

Figure 2 Meyerding grade I, II, III or IV.

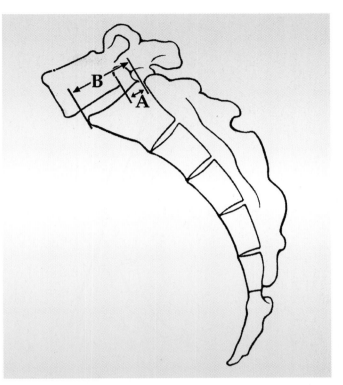

Figure 3 Percentage of slip A/B.

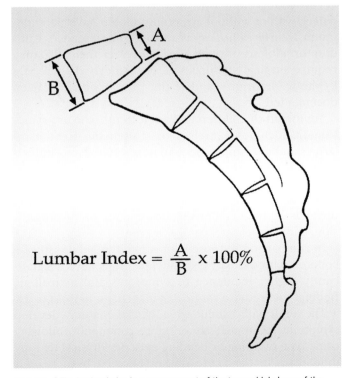

$$\text{Lumbar Index} = \frac{A}{B} \times 100\%$$

Figure 4 The lumbar index is a measurement of the trapezoidal shape of the body of L5; it is represented as the percentage of the posterior height divided by the anterior height.

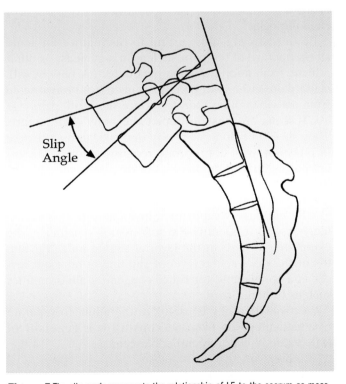

Figure 5 The slip angle represents the relationship of L5 to the sacrum as measured from a line parallel to the superior surface of L5 and a line perpendicular to the posterior surface of S1/2. A low angle implies a normal relationship, an increasing angle indicates a kyphotic deformity.

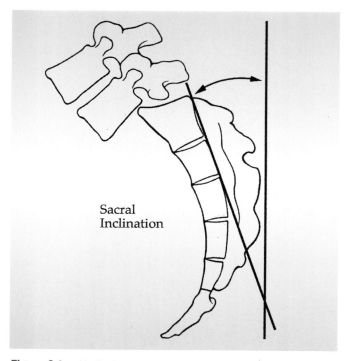

Figure 6 Sacral inclination is the measurement of the degree of verticalization of the sacrum. Typically in higher-grade slips the sacrum becomes more vertically orientated and L5 assumes a more kyphotic position.

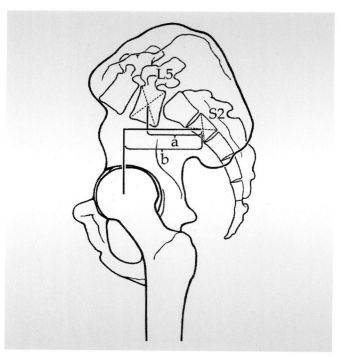

Figure 7 The sagittal pelvic tilt index attempts to evaluate the relationship of the sacrum to L5 and the center of the femoral head. A normal value is close to 1.

Therapeutic blocks can include those of the pars interarticularis, selective nerve root blocks, and epidural or caudal blocks.

Bone scans are most useful to distinguish an acute stress fracture of the pars, such as in a gymnast or other athlete, from a longstanding pars defect. A patient with acute pain and a cold bone scan need not be restricted from activities other than to reduce the acute pain.

CT scans are best to depict the bony architecture. They should be done with very thin cuts across the area in question, with appropriate reconstruction. CT scans are particularly useful in cases of dysplastic spondylolisthesis to define the specific anatomic variance and for surgical planning.

MRI has largely supplanted myelography. It is particularly useful to identify the soft tissues, specifically the exiting nerve roots at the level of slip; to judge the status of the discs at the level of slip and at adjacent levels; and to evaluate for other congenital abnormalities such as tethered cord.

Electromyography is useful, in the adult, to separate true radiculopathy from neuropathy. It is generally of little value in children and adolescents.

Nonsurgical Treatment

Most individuals with isthmic spondylolisthesis are asymptomatic and require no treatment. Activity restrictions are not necessary.

The young child who is discovered to have a pars defect, with or without symptoms, should have, at a minimum, yearly radiographs through adolescence. Children or adolescents with slips of greater than 50% may require surgical stabilization, particularly if there is a kyphotic deformity and if the progression has been documented.

Treatment of children and adolescents who are symptomatic includes exercises to stretch the tight hamstrings and mild analgesics and nonsteroidal anti-inflammatory drugs during acute symptoms. Serial radiographs should be taken more frequently in children having pain. The decision to proceed to surgical stabilization depends on the percent slip, documentation of progression, and the persistence of symptoms.

In comparison to those with isthmic spondylolisthesis, children with dysplastic spondylolisthesis have a significantly higher incidence of symptoms and neurologic findings and require surgical management in most cases.

The adult with isthmic spondylolisthesis may develop symptoms spontaneously or, more commonly, following some type of lifting or bending episode. Physical therapy modalities in the acute phase followed by a regular stretching program and weight control are beneficial. Mild analgesics and nonsteroidal anti-inflammatory drugs during the acute phase can relieve some of the discomfort. Adults generally will have episodic pain that can be controlled with the noninvasive measures. Radicular pain may become a significant factor as the disc degenerates and the neural foramen narrows. Epidural blocks and/or selective nerve root blocks can be both therapeutic and diagnostic. Failure to respond to these measures may be an indication for surgical intervention.

The adult with dysplastic spondylolisthesis may complain only of tight hamstrings and low back pain or may develop symptoms of a full cauda equina syndrome. Those individuals who have true cauda equina syndrome should not be treated conservatively but rather undergo urgent surgical decompression and stabilization.

Factors in Surgical Decision Making

Numerous factors enter into the decision regarding surgical intervention for any spinal disorder. The surgeon must match patient requirements with his or her own skills. The rarity of some severe, problematic spondylolisthesis cases warrants referral to specialty centers.

If the patient's condition warrants surgery, the surgeon must decide whether to perform a neurologic decompression along with a stabilization procedure or stabilization alone. The patient's age, comorbidities, social habits (most important being tobacco use), and chief complaint affect the decision. Adult patients with a history of tobacco use are at a greater risk for pseudoarthrosis and are likely to benefit from supplemental segmental pedicle fixation. Healthy adolescents with grade I slips rarely require pedicle fixation.

In evaluating a patient with radicular pain, the surgeon must sort out whether the nerve simply is being irritated by motion at the pars defect or whether the patient has a significant neurologic deficit that requires decompression. Stabilization alone in the absence of significant neurologic findings is appropriate. The choice of stabilization procedures ranges from a pars interarticularis repair, in situ fusion, reduction fixation with instrumentation, to anterior/posterior reduction fixation.

Plain radiographs along with flexion-extension films and MRI are the imaging studies that aid in selection of the surgical procedure. Additional studies that may be of benefit are pars defect injections, nerve conduction studies, and CT discography.

The slip angle, the specific grade and level of spondylolisthesis, and the health status of the adjacent disc space are all factors in determining the specific surgical procedure. If the slip angle is high, the surgeon may consider performing a reduction with pedicle fixation or elect to extend the fusion cephalad to a more horizontal level.

When the adjacent disc above or below the spondylolisthesis is degenerated it may be associated with the patient's symptoms; the surgeon should consider extending the fusion to include this adjacent level. Although adding an additional level of fusion increases the potential for pseudarthrosis, this action must be weighed against the possibility of a poor result from surgery if the pain generator is not addressed surgically. For the patient with lumbar spondylolisthesis, disabling low back pain, and multilevel disc degeneration, discography along with pars injection can be extremely helpful in formulating a surgical plan that addresses the patient's major pain generator and at the same time limits the number of motion segments that are fused.

Surgical Treatment

Pars interarticularis repair has been discussed in the literature for over 30 years. It is a limited procedure that theoretically does not sacrifice a motion segment. It requires careful patient selection and is limited to patients with a normal disc and a long history of disabling pain from the spondylolysis defect. The surgeon must preoperatively identify the pars interarticularis and rule out the disc as the pain generator. The ideal patient has disabling low back pain exacerbated by lumbar extension, a lumbar disc that looks normal on MRI, and temporary pain relief with pars injection.

Immediate stabilization is necessary for pars interarticularis reconstruction. Although screw fixation across the pars provides immediate stabilization, there has been difficulty with proper placement of this screw. Wire fixation from the transverse process to the spinous process is another method of compression across the pars defect with immediate stabilization. This technique has had excellent results in the hands of a few experienced surgeons; however, others found the technique cumbersome and were concerned about possible nerve root irritation associated with the placement of the wire under the transverse processes. The most recent techniques for pars interarticularis reconstruction involve the use of two pedicle screws and a single rod. The rod is bent into a 'V' shape, placed caudal to the spinous process, and after connection to the pedicle screws, provides compression across the pars defect.

The surgeon initially identifies the pars defect, then clears out the fibrocartilagenous scar, places bone graft in the pars defect, and adds compression/stabilization instrumentation. It is important that the inferior facet above the pars defect (usually L4) be trimmed down to prevent reinjury with hyperextension.

In situ fusion with iliac crest bone graft after decordication of the transverse process is the most commonly performed and described surgical procedure for lumbar spondylolisthesis. In the adolescent patient with a grade 1 or 2 slip it provides a predictably high rate of fusion and pain relief with minimal morbidity. It is also useful in the adult patient who does not use tobacco and has not had extensive surgical decompression or multilevel fusion. Patients with high-grade slips, or those requiring neurologic decompression, have a pseudarthrosis rate as high as 20%. Moreover, patients with a slip angle greater than 50° may have progression of kyphotic deformity after an attempt at posterior fusion.

The roles of reduction fixation techniques have yet to be defined clearly in the literature. The cosmetic result following surgery for high-grade slips is significantly improved with segmental reduction fixation techniques. Unfortunately, the trade-off is a significant increase in neurologic injury associated with the surgical reduction of the lumbar kyphosis. The nerve injury associated with high-grade slip results from stretch of the exiting nerve root from the distraction and posterior translation maneuver associated with a posterior instrumented reduction. A recent trend is toward improvement of the slip angle but incomplete reduction of the high-grade slip, thereby improving the patient's saggital alignment at a reported lower risk of neurologic injury.

The role of anterior column reconstruction in the routine surgical treatment of spondylolisthesis remains controversial. Some surgeons advocate routine restoration of disc height via a posterior lumbar interbody fusion or anterior/posterior fusions. Although this approach does improve the rigidity of the surgically treated motion segment, most literature suggests that this is unnecessary for most low-grade spondylolisthesis.

With the recent introduction of stand alone fusion cages there appears to be a growing interest in treating low-grade slips with an anterior caged fusion device. Although for a number of years, the Asian literature has reported successful treatment of spondylolisthesis with anterior lumbar interbody fusion, the role of fusion cages in treating spondylolisthesis has yet to be fully defined.

Spondyloptosis provides one of the more challenging lumbar reconstructions. The surgeon must decide between fusing the patient in situ or attempting a reduction. The fusion rate for in situ fusion is significantly improved with an anterior and posterior fusion. Because of the nature of the deformity (complete or near complete slip), anterior spinal column fusion is obtained by reaming across the slip (via an anterior or posterior approach) and then placing a fibula graft across the slip into the bodies of L5 and S1 with no attempt to reduce the spondyloptosis. An alternative approach to the surgical treatment of spondyloptosis or severe slips is a two-stage Gaines procedure to surgically reduce the spondyloptosis. The first stage is an anterior resection of the slipped L5 vertebral body along with the adjacent discs. The second stage requires excision of the loose L5 posterior elements, reduction of L4 to the sacrum, and

fusion. This is a difficult procedure that, even in experienced hands, has a high risk for neurologic injury.

Complications

In spondylolisthesis surgery there are four groups of complications. The first, common to any surgical procedure requiring general anesthesia, is related to patient age, nutritional status, duration of anesthesia, and intraoperative blood loss. Pneumonia, urinary tract infection, deep venous thrombosis, pulmonary embolism, and wound infection are examples.

Complications related to the surgical approach include epidural scarring, nerve root injury, dural tear, great vessel injury, bowel injury, and injuries to the ureter, superior hypogastric plexus (causing retrograde ejaculation), and genitofemoral nerve. The third group of complications is related to fusion, specifically pseudarthrosis, graft extrusion or subsidence, accelerated degeneration of adjacent discs, and donor-site morbidity. Finally, reduction/fixation related complications include implant failure, pedicle or vertebral body fracture, and nerve root/cauda equina injury. More difficult cases have a higher percentage of complications with severe slips having up to a 25% rate of neurologic injury.

Postoperative Care

The general trend in postoperative care is toward early mobilization. Except in unusual circumstances of instability, long periods of bed rest are unnecessary and counterproductive. Patients fused without instrumentation are usually braced with a thoracolumbosacral orthosis with a thigh extension. Patients with pedicle fixation do not routinely need prolonged, rigid bracing. A program for ambulating is initiated on discharge from the hospital. Generally speaking, at approximately 12 weeks, a general fitness and back-strengthening program is introduced. The decision to return to work or sports depends on the patient's postoperative course and specific job requirements. In general, the goal is a return to all normal activities between 4 and 6 months after surgery.

Annotated Bibliography

Carragee EJ: Single-level posterolateral arthrodesis, with or without posterior decompression, for the treatment of isthmic spondylolisthesis in adults: A prospective randomized study. *J Bone Joint Surg Am* 1997;79: 1175-1180.

The author reports a prospective randomized study of adults surgically treated for single level isthmic spondylolisthesis. In this study all patients were fused posteriorly. The addition of routine laminectomy to surgical treatment did not improve results.

Deguchi M, Rapoff AJ, Zdeblick TA: Posterolateral fusion for isthmic spondylolisthesis in adults: Analysis of fusion rate and clinical results. *J Spinal Disord* 1998; 11:459-464.

This is a retrospective review of adults treated surgically for isthmic spondylolisthesis. This study demonstrated a strong positive correlation between radiologic fusion and clinical success. In multilevel procedures a higher rate of fusion was obtained with a rigid pedicle screw fixation system.

Esses SI, Natout N, Kip P: Posterior interbody arthrodesis with a fibular strut graft in spondylolisthesis. *J Bone Joint Surg Am* 1995;77:172-176.

This is a retrospective review of adults with severe slip treated surgically with a posterior fibular strut graft. The technique is described, and the authors demonstrated significant clinical improvement in pain.

Fabris DA, Costantini S, Nena U: Surgical treatment of severe L5-S1 spondylolisthesis in children and adolescents: Results of intraoperative reduction, posterior interbody fusion, and segmental pedicle fixation. *Spine* 1996;21:728-733.

This is a retrospective review of teenagers with severe slip treated surgically with a posterior reduction, interbody fusion, and segmental fixation. The results were significant for high fusion rate, no loss of reduction, and minimal complications.

Gillet P, Petit M: Direct repair of spondylolysis without spondylolisthesis, using a rod-screw construct and bone grafting of the pars defect. *Spine* 1999;24:1252-1256.

The authors present their experience with a new pedicle screw-rod technique for pars repair.

Hu SS, Bradford DS, Transfeldt EE, Cohen M: Reduction of high-grade spondylolisthesis using Edwards instrumentation. *Spine* 1996;21:367-371.

This is a retrospective review of patients with severe slip treated surgically with a posterior decompression, reduction, fusion, and segmental fixation. The average follow-up is over 3 years. Overall clinical results are good but a significant complication rate (25%) is reported.

Kim NH, Lee JW: Anterior interbody fusion versus posterolateral fusion with transpedicular fixation for isthmic spondylolisthesis in adults: A comparison of clinical results. *Spine* 1999;24:812-817.

This is a retrospective review of 40 adults who were surgically treated for isthmic spondylolisthesis. Anterior interbody fusion was performed in 20 patients and posterior fusion with transpedicular fixation was performed in 20 patients. There was no statistically significant difference in the results between the two groups.

Muschik M, Zippel H, Perka C: Surgical management of severe spondylolisthesis in children and adolescents: Anterior fusion in situ versus anterior spondylodesis with posterior transpedicular instrumentation and reduction. *Spine* 1997;22:2036-2043.

This is a retrospective review of children and adolescents surgically treated for severe isthmic spondylolisthesis. Two groups were compared: one with anterior fusion alone and one additionally treated with a posterior reduction and transpedicular fixation. The authors demonstrated superior results with the group who underwent the additional posterior procedure.

Ricciardi JE, Pflueger PC, Isaza JE, Whitecloud TS III: Transpedicular fixation for the treatment of isthmic spondylolisthesis in adults. *Spine* 1995;20:1917-1922.

Seventeen consecutive adult patients with symptomatic low-grade isthmic spondylolisthesis underwent the identical surgical procedure consisting of Gill laminectomy, L5 nerve root decompression, Luque pedicle-screw plate instrumentation, and posterolateral arthrodesis at L5-S1 using autogenous iliac crest bone graft. An independent observer reviewed the results. Sixteen had solid fusion using radiographic criteria and had satisfactory clinical results.

Wu SS, Lee CH, Chen PQ: Operative repair of symptomatic spondylolysis following a positive response to diagnostic pars injection. *J Spinal Disord* 1999;12:10-16.

Patients with back pain symptoms and spondylolysis of the lumbar spine were reviewed. Only those whose symptoms failed nonsurgical measures, showing negative bone scan and positive pars injection, were regarded as candidates for surgical management. Patients then received autogenous bone grafting and internal fixation of the pars interarticularis defect. After a follow-up averaging 30.4 months, fusion results were 87%. Clinical results of 85 patients (91.3%) were excellent to good; eight patients were fair; no outcomes were poor.

Classic Bibliography

Boxall D, Bradford DS, Winter RB, Moe JH: Management of severe spondylolisthesis in children and adolescents. *J Bone Joint Surg Am* 1979;61:479-495.

Buck JE: Direct repair of the defect in spondylolisthesis: Preliminary report. *J Bone Joint Surg Br* 1970;52: 432-437.

Burkus JK, Lonstein JE, Winter RB, Denis F: Long-term evaluation of adolescents treated operatively for spondylolisthesis: A comparison of in situ arthrodesis only with in situ arthrodesis and reduction followed by immobilization in a cast. *J Bone Joint Surg Am* 1992;74: 693-704

Fredrickson BE, Baker D, McHolick WJ, Yuan HA, Lubicky JP: The natural history of spondylolysis and spondylolisthesis. *J Bone Joint Surg Am* 1984;66: 699-707.

Lehmer SM, Steffee AD, Gaines RW Jr: Treatment of L5-S1 spondyloptosis by staged L5 resection with reduction and fusion of L4 onto S1 (Gaines procedure). *Spine* 1994;19:1916-1925.

Peek RD, Wiltse LL, Reynolds JB, Thomas JC, Guyer DW, Widell EH: In situ arthrodesis without decompression for grade-III or IV isthmic spondylolisthesis in adults who have severe sciatica. *J Bone Joint Surg Am* 1989;71:62-68.

Chapter 38

Pediatric Spinal Deformity

Peter O. Newton, MD

Dennis R. Wenger, MD

Childhood and Adolescent Scoliosis

Pediatric spinal deformity generally is categorized into frontal plane deformity (scoliosis) and sagittal deformity (kyphosis). However, scoliosis includes both sagittal plane deformity and torsional malalignment. Idiopathic scoliosis is a common and potentially severe musculoskeletal disorder of unknown etiology that, in its milder forms, may produce only trunk shape change, but when severe can be markedly disfiguring and can produce cardiac and pulmonary compromise. The etiology of a scoliotic deformity (idiopathic, congenital, neuromuscular, syndrome-related) largely dictates its natural history, including the risk for and rate of curve progression and the effects the curve will have on cardiopulmonary function, mobility, and appearance.

Etiology

Although the etiology of scoliosis remains unknown, there has been substantial research on areas ranging from genetic factors to disorders of bone, muscles, and disc; growth abnormalities; and central nervous system causes.

Genetic Factors

Several studies have demonstrated an increased incidence of scoliosis in the family members of affected individuals, which suggests a polygenic inheritance pattern. Examination of scoliosis in birth twins has led to further confirmation of genetic etiologic factors. However, the genes and gene products responsible for its development remain unknown.

Tissue Deficiencies

Competing theories propose that the primary pathology of scoliosis is centered in each of the structural tissues of the spine (bone, muscle, ligament/disc). There are known conditions in which each of these tissues is pathologic and associated with scoliosis. For example, fibrous-dysplasia (bone collagen abnormality) resulting in dys-plastic, misshaped vertebrae, muscle disorders such as Duchenne muscular dystrophy leading to a collapsing scoliosis, and soft-tissue-collagen disorders such as Marfan syndrome, each have clear associations with the development of scoliosis.

In Marfan syndrome there is a defective gene coding for fibrillin, which is found in many soft tissues including ligament, cartilage, and periosteum. The fibrillin abnormality found in Marfan syndrome is associated with scoliosis in 55% to 63% of patients. Although fibrillin has been ruled out as a cause, similar subtle deficiencies in any of the tissues of the spine could result in scoliosis.

Vertebral Growth Abnormality Theories

It has been postulated that the etiology of scoliosis relates to the development of relative thoracic lordosis. The belief is that anterior spinal growth outpaces posterior growth, producing hypokyphosis with subsequent buckling of the vertebral column leading to the rotational deformity of scoliosis; however, the cause for this theorized "mismatch" of anterior and posterior spinal column growth has not been presented and may be secondary rather than primary. Interestingly, it has been documented that thoracic kyphosis tends to decrease in normal children during the normal adolescent growth spurt. Thus, irregularities in the changing sagittal shape of the spine during the rapid period of adolescent growth may be important in the development of scoliosis.

Central Nervous System Theories

Disorders of the brain, spinal cord, and muscles may result in scoliosis; the role of the central nervous system in idiopathic scoliosis has been studied in detail. Greater

One or more of the authors or the departments with which they are affiliated have received something of value from a commercial or other party related directly or indirectly to the subject of this chapter.

asymmetry of the cerebral cortices in patients with scoliosis has been noted. Abnormalities in equilibrium and vestibular function also have been noted in patients with scoliosis; however, it is difficult to know if these findings are primary or secondary. Syringomyelia is associated with an increased incidence of scoliosis, possibly caused by direct pressure on the sensory or motor tracts of the spinal cord. Alternatively, there may be no relation to the dilation of the central canal; instead, brain stem irritation from an associated Chiari malformation or enlargement of the fourth ventricle of the brain may be the cause.

Recently, based on research of pinealectomy in chickens, which results in a high incidence of severe scoliosis, it has been postulated that melatonin and the pineal gland may be related to scoliosis. In these studies, presumably melatonin deficiency led to scoliosis in the chicken. Subsequent studies of human melatonin levels have been conflicting and inconclusive. Lower than normal melatonin concentration has been found in the serum of patients with progressive scoliosis compared to those with stable curves. In contrast, other investigators found no difference in urine melatonin levels between patients with scoliosis and normal control subjects. Another study revealed no difference in serum melatonin levels of patients with scoliosis. Thus, confirmation is lacking that melatonin deficiency in humans is associated with scoliosis.

In summary, the etiology of scoliosis remains puzzling. From a biomechanical standpoint, the vertebral column is a naturally unstable construct, made of multiple mobile segments. There are likely several causes of idiopathic scoliosis, and active research continues in an attempt to find a unifying theory as to its cause.

Classification

By etiology, scoliosis may be broadly classified as idiopathic (or idiopathic-like), congenital, neuromuscular, and syndrome-related. It is important to consider a patient with scoliosis as a patient with a sign (scoliosis) rather than a diagnosis. Most scoliosis (approximately 80%) is idiopathic; however, the remaining instances are associated with a wide variety of disorders in which scoliosis is often the presenting complaint.

Congenital scoliosis and kyphosis may lead to progressive spine deformity. Neuromuscular disorders of either neuropathic or myopathic etiology make up a large proportion of the nonidiopathic causes of scoliosis in childhood. Intra- or extraspinal tumors or abnormalities must also be considered as causes of scoliosis. An awareness of each potentially associated condition helps when analyzing the various proposed etiologic factors, and, more importantly, the diagnosis of idiopathic scoliosis requires the exclusion of these conditions.

Clinical Features

History

History-taking should include questions about family history of scoliosis, recent growth, the physical changes of puberty (onset of menses), and complaints of pain. Despite the common belief that mild idiopathic scoliosis is not painful, a recent study suggests that adolescents with mild curves often report discomfort of a mild fatigue variety. One study found back pain in 23% of 2,442 patients with idiopathic scoliosis. Only 9% of those with pain were subsequently found to have an underlying pathologic condition to explain it (eg, diagnoses such as spondylolysis/spondylolisthesis, Scheuermann's kyphosis, syringomyelia, herniated disc, tethered cord, and intraspinal tumor).

A child or adolescent who has severe back pain and is subsequently found to have scoliosis requires a very careful history, physical examination, and radiographic study (a bone scan and MRI study may be required) because an underlying etiologic cause is more likely. However, the clinician must distinguish between severe pain (requiring further workup) and mild fatigue pain.

Age at onset, rate of curve progression, and the presence of neurologic symptoms and signs are the most useful findings in identifying nonidiopathic scoliosis. In patients younger than 10 years with a neurologic cause, actual neurologic findings on physical examination are often absent, and the spinal curvature itself must be considered the initial sign of a neural axis abnormality. The most common intraspinal abnormality found in this age group is syringomyelia (dilation of the central spinal canal) with an associated Chiari malformation (brain stem below the level of the foramen magnum).

Rapid development of a severe curve suggests nonidiopathic scoliosis. Neurologic symptoms such as weakness, sensory changes, and balance/gait disturbance suggest intraspinal pathology (eg, syringomyelia, tethered cord, tumor) as the cause of spinal curvature.

Physical Examination

Physical examination of a patient with scoliosis includes evaluation of trunk shape, trunk balance, the neurologic system, limb length, skin markings, associated skeletal abnormalities, and Tanner stage of pubertal development. An inability to bend directly forward at the waist or decreased range of forward/side bending may be caused by pain, lumbar muscle spasm, and/or hamstring tightness, any of which should suggest underlying pathology. These findings plus abnormalities in straight leg raise testing suggest irritation of the lumbar roots caused by spondylolysis, disc herniation, infection, neoplasm, or other causes.

The neurologic examination should evaluate balance, motor strength in the major muscle groups of all four extremities, and sensation. Reflex testing includes upper and lower extremity deep tendon reflexes and abdominal reflexes, which are obtained by lightly stroking the abdominal wall with a blunt instrument (eg, key, end of reflex hammer) adjacent to the umbilicus with the patient supine and relaxed. The expected brisk and symmetrical unilateral contraction of the abdominal musculature pulling the umbilicus toward the side being stroked indicates normalcy. When persistently abnormal (reflex absent on one side and present on the other), intraspinal disorders, particularly syringomyelia, should be considered and an MRI study ordered.

Radiographic Assessment

The ideal screening radiograph for scoliosis is an upright (standing) posteroanterior (PA) projection of the entire spine exposed on a single cassette. When surgical treatment is being considered, lateral bend radiographs to assess curve flexibility as well as a standing lateral view are required. Controversy remains regarding the best method for obtaining bending films. Supine AP views (patient maximally bent to the right and left) are standard at many institutions, whereas others believe that a standing bend film is a better indicator, particularly in the lumbar spine. Lateral bending over a bolster provides somewhat greater correction and has been proposed as a more accurate predictor of the correction obtained with the more powerful modern surgical instrumentation methods. In curves greater than 60° to 70°, longitudinal traction films may also be helpful in evaluating curve flexibility.

Curve measurement by the Cobb method quantifies the curve. Skeletal maturity should be assessed radiographically (Risser sign) to estimate remaining spinal growth. The status of the triradiate cartilage of the acetabulum also provides a landmark for assessing growth potential. The triradiate growth cartilage usually closes before the iliac apophysis appears (Risser 0) at about the time of maximal spinal growth.

Specialized Imaging Studies

MRI study of the spine is indicated for all patients with infantile and juvenile idiopathic scoliosis, as well as those with congenital bony anomalies if surgical correction is planned. Left thoracic curves and scoliosis in boys have been shown to have increased associations with spinal-cord anomalies and may be indications for MRI study. Indications for routine MRI study in patients with typical idiopathic scoliosis, who have a normal clinical neurologic examination, before corrective surgery, remain unclear. Patients with an abnormality in the neurologic examination or with cutaneous findings suggesting dysraphism or neurofibromatosis should have an MRI study of the spine and/or brain.

Patients with substantial back pain with no obvious cause may require a bone scan to evaluate for possible tumor, infection, or spondylolysis. The bone scan is an excellent test for the patient with painful scoliosis; it allows the physician to screen for conditions ranging from osteoid osteoma to hydronephrosis. A single proton emission CT type bone scan is very useful in identifying spondylolysis and its varying presentations (unilateral, bilateral, cold scan, hot scan, etc). If an area of increased activity is noted on the bone scan, additional imaging (either MRI or CT) may be required. CT studies can be performed with increasing sophistication and provide the best method for imaging the bony anatomy in complex deformities and congenital anomalies. Standard two-dimensional (2-D) transverse images are less helpful in scoliosis than are coronal, sagittal, and three-dimensional (3-D) reformatted images. Additional multiplanar (curved along the deformity) reformatted coronal and sagittal images are particularly helpful in imaging the scoliotic spine when congenital anomalies are suspected (Fig. 1).

Idiopathic Scoliosis

Prevalence and Natural History

The prevalence of idiopathic scoliosis (with a curve of greater than 10°) in a childhood and adolescent population has been reported to be from 0.5 to 3 per 100. The reported prevalence of larger curves (greater than 30°) ranges from 1.5 to 3 per 1,000.

Although, classically, idiopathic scoliosis has been divided into three groups according to the age of onset (infantile, juvenile, adolescent), there is a movement in Britain to simplify this to early onset scoliosis (before age 10 years) and late onset scoliosis (typical adolescent scoliosis). The belief is that only early onset scoliosis has the potential for evolution to severe thoracic deformity with cardiac and pulmonary compromise. This simpler classification has not been fully evaluated, thus the traditional three-age-group division remains the standard in North America.

Adolescent Idiopathic Scoliosis

In adolescent idiopathic scoliosis, the child theoretically develops a curve after the age of 10 years, associated with the rapid growth of adolescence. Roughly 2% of adolescents have a scoliosis of 10° or more, but only 5% of these children have progression of the curve to greater than 30°. The ratio of boys to girls is equal for minor curves but is dominated by girls as the curve magnitude increases, reaching 1:8 for those requiring treatment.

Risk factors for scoliosis progression include gender, remaining skeletal growth, curve location, and curve magnitude. Growth remaining is approximated using

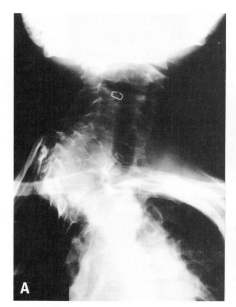 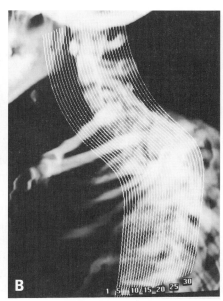 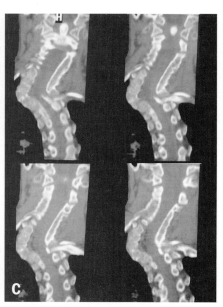

Figure 1 A, AP radiograph of a patient with complex congenital scoliosis. **B,** The lateral scout film for the CT scan using curved 2-D reformatted reconstructions in the sagittal plane. The plane of the coronal images follows the curvilinear path seen in this lateral scout film. **C,** The curved 2-D reformatted images demonstrate the marked angular deformity at the cervicothoracic junction with bar formation from C3 to C7 on the left side.

chronologic age, bone age, menarche (with the onset of menses generally following the most rapid stage of skeletal growth by approximately 12 months), and Risser sign. Closure of the triradiate cartilage of the acetabulum closely approximates the time of peak growth velocity.

Curve pattern is an important variable for predicting the probability of progression. Curves with an apex above T12 are more likely to progress than isolated lumbar curves. Curve magnitude at initial diagnosis appears to predict progression.

Natural History in Adulthood

Not all curves stabilize after growth stops. In long-term studies performed at the University of Iowa, more than two thirds of patients experienced curve progression following skeletal maturity. Curves of less than 30° tended not to progress, and the most marked progression occurred in curves that were between 50° and 75° at the completion of growth (continuing at a rate of nearly 1°/yr). In long-term follow-up studies of untreated patients with adolescent idiopathic scoliosis, the increased mortality rate reported previously has not been confirmed. Estimates regarding the frequency of back pain and associated disability in adults with scoliosis vary, but most studies have demonstrated slightly higher rates of back pain compared with control groups. Disability rates have been higher in some series and similar in others.

Treatment

Nonsurgical Treatment

Because most patients with idiopathic scoliosis have curves of less than 20° and only a few progress to require treatment, most patients simply are monitored. Idiopathic curves of less than 25° should be monitored every 4 to 12 months (depending on the age and growth rate of the patient) with clinical and radiographic examination. Those in the rapid phases of growth are seen at more frequent intervals (every 4 to 6 months).

Indications for Orthotic (Brace) Treatment

In growing children, a spinal orthosis (brace) generally is indicated when a curve progresses to 25° to 30°. Scoliosis braces of many different styles and corrective mechanical principles have been developed, with each having the goal of modifying spinal growth by applying an external force. Because brace treatment depends on spinal growth modulation, treatment is prescribed only for patients with substantial spinal growth remaining (Risser 2 to 3 or less). The upper limit of curve magnitude amenable to brace treatment is approximately 45°. Most studies have confirmed that, even in the most cooperative patients, the final result of brace treatment is maintenance of the curve at the degree of severity present at the onset of bracing. Most surgeons insist that curve progression of more than 5° be documented before bracing curves of less than 30°.

Under-arm braces, (eg, Boston and Wilmington) have replaced the Milwaukee brace in most centers because of increased acceptance by the patients. Despite improvements in brace appearance (brace worn under clothes, no visible neckpiece) many teenagers will not cooperate with brace wear. The Charleston nighttime bending brace, an alternative that attempts to create a more complete correction of the curve, requires a trunk bend so severe that it precludes walking. This brace, therefore, is prescribed only for nighttime wear and is best suited for single curves that are more distal (thoracolumbar and lumbar curves). An elastic strap brace developed in Montreal is currently under investigation as a device without a rigid design that may produce correction.

The effectiveness of bracing for idiopathic scoliosis has been presumed for many years, yet controlled treatment trials with and without bracing had not been completed until recently. Earlier studies reporting high success rates for brace treatment were subsequently noted to have included many patients who were at low risk for progression.

In 1995, the results of a prospective controlled study of bracing were published by the Scoliosis Research Society. The results in 286 patients aged 10 to 15 years with an initial curve of 25° to 35° treated with either observation alone (129 patients), an underarm brace (111 patients), or nighttime electrical stimulation (46 patients) were compared. Curve progression at the end of bracing (skeletal maturity) was limited to less than 5° in 74% of those treated with a brace, compared to 34% of those followed without treatment. The group treated with electrical stimulation had a success rate of only 33%. Although critics cite flaws in this and other studies, most centers have accepted the results and continue to advise brace treatment for progressive curves in skeletally immature adolescents.

Surgical Correction

Introduction and Indications
Goals for surgical treatment of idiopathic scoliosis include improved spinal alignment and balance and prevention of subsequent curve progression. Corrective instrumentation plus arthrodesis (fusion) provides the best method for achieving lasting correction and can be used either anteriorly or posteriorly to restore spinal alignment.

The indications for surgical correction of scoliosis are based on curve magnitude, clinical deformity, risk for progression, skeletal maturity, and curve pattern. In general, thoracic curves of greater than 40° to 50° (Cobb angle) in skeletally immature patients should be corrected surgically, whereas in mature patients (risk of progression decreased), surgical correction is reserved for curves of 50° or more. These Cobb angle ranges are meant as guidelines rather than absolute indications and are based on the natural history of untreated scoliosis in immature and mature patients.

Cotrel-Dubousset and Other Double Rod, Multiple Hook Systems
Nearly 20 years after Harrington's method was introduced, Cotrel and Dubousset introduced a multihook system that allows distraction and compression on the same rod. Sagittal plane contouring of the rods and segmental hook fixation improved curve correction and postoperative stability. Many additional segmental fixation posterior instrumentation systems using similar concepts are now available for surgical correction of scoliosis. Current options for attachment to the posterior spine include hooks (for attachment to the transverse processes, laminae, and pedicles), sublaminar wires (Luque), and pedicle screws.

The introduction of pedicle screw fixation into posterior scoliosis constructs allows greater correction than distal hooks and allows fewer levels to be instrumented caudally. Pedicle screw attachment is highly effective, but the surgeon must have appropriate training and skill to safely improve the stability of corrective scoliosis constructs.

Because with all of these procedures the goal is to obtain fusion, the surgeon must first perform careful subperiosteal exposure of the spine as well as meticulous facet excision. The spine also must be decorticated before adding bone graft. The complexity of modern instrumentation sometimes causes surgeons to pay too little attention to the details required to obtain a successful fusion.

Mechanisms of Correction
Frontal plane realignment of the spine can be accomplished by translating the vertebrae to the concave rod. This translational movement may be performed by connecting the concave rod, precontoured to the desired sagittal profile, to each fixation site along the spine and then rotating the rod into the sagittal plane. This rod rotation maneuver, popularized by Dubousset, remains an effective method for translating the apex of the curve into a more normal position. Another method for translating the apex in space involves locking the concave rod into the position of anticipated correction and then sequentially (with hooks) or incrementally (with sublaminar wires) drawing the spine to the rod. Compression and distraction forces are then added to enhance both frontal and sagittal plane correction.

Anterior Release and Fusion
Indications for a combined anterior and posterior approach in idiopathic scoliosis include patients with large (greater than 75°), rigid (bend correction less than 50°) curves and those at risk for postfusion crankshaft

deformity. Curve flexibility is increased by anterior disc excision, allowing greater correction with posterior instrumentation, and the bone graft used anteriorly leads to a very stable fusion (anterior and posterior).

The crankshaft deformity defines a circumstance in which anterior spinal growth continues despite successful posterior fusion, resulting in worsening rotational deformity. The problem occurs only in skeletally immature patients (Risser 1 or less, triradiate cartilage open). This largely axial rotational deformity is difficult to measure with routine radiography. Recent reports suggest that anterior fusion arrests the anterior growth center and limits the development of this late deformity.

An additional advantage of anterior release and fusion is the increased area for the arthrodesis (vertebral end plates) presumably reducing the risk of pseudarthrosis. The thoracoscopic approach is being developed as a means of doing anterior disc excision and fusion with minimally invasive methods.

Anterior Spinal Instrumentation
At the time of anterior disc excision and fusion, anterior corrective instrumentation with vertebral body screw fixation and a single or double anterolateral rod construct can be considered for some curve patterns.

Rigid solid rod anterior systems have been developed in an attempt to maintain the sagittal alignment, particularly when used for thoracolumbar and lumbar curves. Scoliotic curve patterns that are amenable to corrective anterior instrumentation and fusion generally include those with a single structural deformity (thoracic, thoracolumbar, or lumbar).

Special attention to the sagittal plane is required when anterior compression instrumentation is used distal to the thoracolumbar junction to avoid production of an iatrogenic flat-back deformity (due to loss of desired lordosis). Structural interbody support by use of a structural bone graft or an interbody cage has been advocated as a means of maintaining sagittal alignment (Fig. 2). Double rod, double screw anterior systems have also been introduced as a means of providing additional sagittal plane control. In most cases, anterior instrumentation can achieve similar or greater correction than posterior instrumentation for the same curve, with fewer levels instrumented.

Instrumentation Without Fusion
Instrumentation without fusion, a technique used in young children with curves that progress relentlessly despite aggressive brace treatment includes a subcuta-

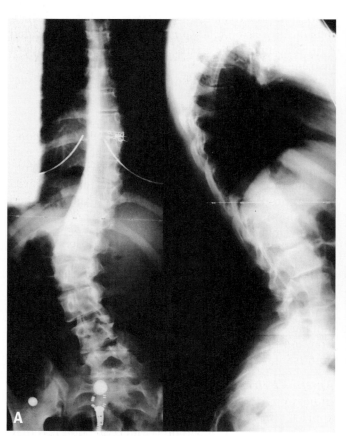
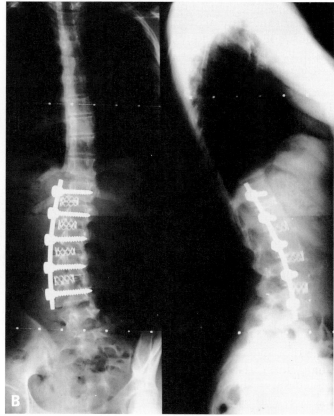

Figure 2 A, Preoperative PA and lateral radiographs of a patient with thoracolumbar scoliosis. **B,** Postoperative radiographs of this patient after undergoing anterior spinal instrumentation and fusion with interbody structural support to maintain lumbar lordosis.

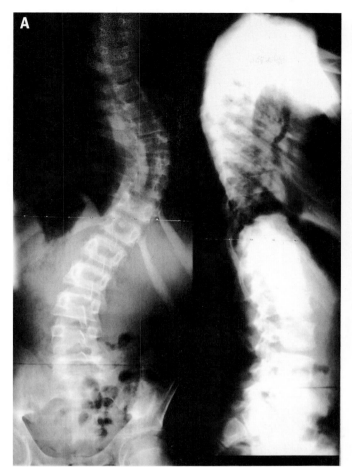

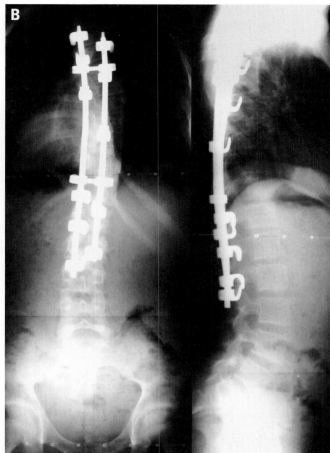

Figure 3 A, Preoperative PA and lateral radiographs of a patient with adolescent idiopathic scoliosis with a right thoracic curve pattern. **B,** Postoperative PA and lateral radiographs of the same patient after posterior spinal instrumentation and fusion.

neously positioned distraction construct that spans the deformity. At the proximal and distal hook sites a limited fusion is performed to decrease the incidence of hook dislodgment. In the intervening segments, the spine is not stripped subperiosteally because exposure alone may lead to spontaneous fusion in a young child (thus the concept of a subcutaneous rod). Sequential distraction is performed every 6 to 12 months during growth until no further correction can be obtained. The height gained with these procedures is usually modest, and complications are common (hook dislodgement, spontaneous fusion, infection); therefore, these systems are presently used in children younger than 5 to 6 years of age in whom there are few other options. The internal splint (spinal rods) requires external protection with a brace throughout the period of sequential rod distraction. Eventually a formal instrumentation and fusion are performed. A short convex hemiepiphysiodesis (anterior and posterior) over the apical levels may also be included in the subcutaneous rod technique.

Surgical Correction According to Curve Pattern: Right Thoracic Curve Pattern

The right thoracic curve pattern most often is corrected with posterior spinal instrumentation and fusion of the thoracic curve. For typical correction, the most distal hook is attached to the vertebra one level proximal to the stable vertebra (vertebra bisected by the central sacral vertical line). Multiple hooks or sublaminar wires on the concave side of the spine are used to draw up the apex of the curve from its lordoscoliotic position into a more normal kyphotic alignment (Fig. 3).

Thoracic curves also can be corrected by anterior instrumentation. Advantages include greater correction, a shorter fusion, and ease of re-creating normal kyphosis in the hypokyphotic thoracic spine. The levels selected for fusion with anterior instrumentation include all vertebrae within the measured Cobb angle. The thoracotomy required for this approach, which results in at least a temporary decrease of pulmonary function, is a disadvantage of the method. Anterior tho-

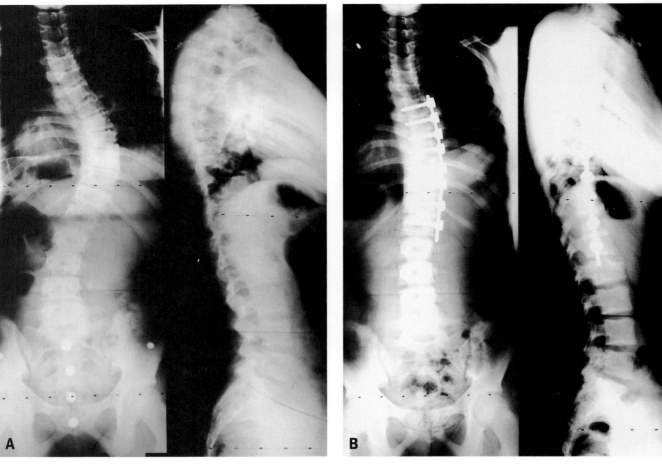

Figure 4 A, A right thoracic curve pattern similar to that seen in Figure 3 *A,* although this patient was corrected with anterior instrumentation. **B,** Postoperative radiographs following anterior spinal instrumentation and fusion over the levels of the measured Cobb angle. This instrumentation was placed using a thoracoscopic approach.

racic corrective instrumentation is being developed for thoracoscopic implantation and in the future may be an option for correction of thoracic scoliosis in some patients (Fig. 4).

Right Thoracic, Left Lumbar Curve Pattern

The lumbar curve (usually convex to the left) that often occurs in association with a right thoracic curve may vary substantially in both magnitude (Cobb angle) and severity of rotation. Either the thoracic or lumbar curve may dominate such a double curve pattern, although the thoracic curve is more often primary. The surgeon must determine which of the curves requires instrumentation and fusion (thoracic, lumbar, or both). When the thoracic curve is larger and/or more rigid than the lumbar curve, selective fusion of the thoracic curve only should be considered. There are situations, however, in which the lumbar curve is large enough to require fusion if a well-balanced spine is to be achieved after correction.

Although universal agreement has not been reached, several authors have provided criteria for selective fusion of the thoracic curve alone. The instrumentation should not end inferiorly just above a junctional kyphosis. If the junction between the thoracic and lumbar curves (approximately T12) is focally kyphotic, the instrumentation should extend distal to the kyphosis. If the lumbar curve is greater than 45° to 50°, vigorous correction of only the thoracic curve with a posterior instrumentation system may result in postoperative truncal decompensation to the left. If selective fusion is elected in these cases, correction of the thoracic curve should be modest to minimize the chance of residual trunk imbalance.

When instrumentation of both the thoracic and lumbar curves is required, the distal extent is usually to the L3 or L4 level. The most predictable spinal balance occurs when the fusion and instrumentation extend distally to the stable vertebra. In patients with limited remaining growth and a left-sided lumbar curve, fusion to L3 may be considered if there is minimal axial rotation of L3 as noted on the bend film to the left and L3 levels above the pelvis with side bending to the right.

Double Thoracic Curve Pattern

The double thoracic curve is indicated by the presence of an elevated left shoulder, whereas an isolated right thoracic curve is typically associated with an elevated right shoulder. If the left shoulder is higher, an upper thoracic curve to the left should be suspected. A left upper thoracic curve that is relatively rigid (reduces to greater than 20° to 25° on bend film) generally requires instrumentation beginning proximally at T1 or T2. If the double pattern is not recognized and the right thoracic curve alone is straightened, the left shoulder elevation is often worse following the surgery.

Left Lumbar or Thoracolumbar Curve Pattern

A primary lumbar or thoracolumbar curve pattern does not have a significant thoracic component and is usually convex to the left with a trunk shift to the left. In these patients, isolated fusion of a lumbar or thoracolumbar curve is appropriate. Correction with posterior hook constructs has not been as successful in achieving derotation of the lumbar curve as has anterior instrumentation. Limited anterior instrumentation of the apical three or four vertebrae or longer anterior constructs, some with the use of bone graft or a structural cage in the disc space, have become popular in the treatment of these curves. Pedicle screw fixation has allowed better control and correction of these curves when posterior instrumentation is used.

Outcomes of Surgical Treatment

The longest follow-up exists for patients treated with Harrington instrumentation and fusion. An average 48% coronal plane improvement of the Cobb angle has been reported. The long-term functional results of long posterior fusions have focused on the prevalence of late onset low-back pain. Conflicting results regarding the prevalence of pain and the correlation of pain with the caudal level of instrumentation have been reported.

The early and midterm (5- to 10-year follow-up) results of Cotrel-Dubousset instrumentation suggest improved coronal and sagittal plane correction when compared with Harrington instrumentation. An average correction of 61% can be expected when considering all curve types. The segmental hook constructs have provided clear improvement in postoperative sagittal alignment, although little improvement in the axial rotation deformity has been seen.

Until recently, anterior correction of scoliosis has been used primarily for the correction of lumbar and thoracolumbar scoliosis. The percentage of frontal plane correction with Dwyer, Zielke, TSRH (Medtronic, Memphis, TN), or Kaneda (Johnson & Johnson, Raynum, MA) instrumentation has been reported between 67% and 98%. Some authors have noticed a loss of sagittal plane lumbar lordosis with anterior compressive systems. Even solid ¼-in rod systems, such as the TSRH system, have not been able to entirely preserve normal lordosis when used without anterior interbody structural support. It has been reported that sagittal alignment in the lumbar spine can be maintained if interbody structural support is added. Two-rod anterior systems are an option that may allow better maintenance of lumbar lordosis, although reported follow-up remains limited.

Anterior instrumentation in the thoracic spine with 3.2- or 4.0-mm threaded rods resulted in coronal plane correction comparable to that achieved with posterior hook systems but was associated with a 31% incidence of rod breakage. The distal level of fusion in the anterior fusion group was, on average, two segments proximal to those in the posterior group. There also appears to be a greater spontaneous improvement of the uninstrumented portion of the lumbar spine when anterior (and shorter) thoracic instrumentation is used (compared with posterior) in treating thoracic curves that had a compensatory lumbar curve pattern. The rate of pseudarthrosis and rod breakage appears to be greatly reduced with the introduction of solid (unthreaded) rods for thoracic curves.

Complications

The complications of scoliosis surgery can be serious, although these procedures have become much safer over the last 20 years as a result of advances in anesthesia, blood loss management, instrumentation systems, and neurologic monitoring.

Continuous electrical spinal cord monitoring has become almost standard in surgical correction of spine deformity. Monitoring of sensory and motor pathways is possible; however, from a technical standpoint, sensory monitoring is simpler and more widely accepted. Somatosensory evoked potentials (SSEPs) are obtained by stimulating distally (legs) and measuring the response proximally (brain). SSEPs have been very reliable in detecting changes in spinal cord function, providing the surgeon relatively rapid feedback as to any effect that deformity correction is having on neurologic function. The lag time between the insult to the spinal cord and the resulting monitoring changes may be 10 to 20 minutes. Factors other than injury to the cord that have been found to affect spinal cord monitoring, resulting in false positive indications of injury, include hypotension, hypothermia, dislodgment of the monitoring leads, and other technical malfunctions in the system. If changes are noted these factors should be evaluated and corrected, and if the monitoring abnormalities persist, a wake-up test should be performed. As soon as a deficit is confirmed, the implants should be loosened to remove any corrective forces or completely removed. Institution of the methylprednisolone steroid spinal cord injury protocol also seems warranted, although the efficacy in this specific group of patients has not been carefully studied.

Congenital Scoliosis

Definition

Congenital scoliosis is the result of abnormally formed vertebral elements, with the altered vertebral shape producing deviations in spinal alignment. These deficiencies occur in the embryonic period of intrauterine development (before 48 days gestation) and are commonly associated with cardiac and urologic abnormalities that develop during the same period. The etiology is unknown in humans; however, in animal studies, congenital scoliosis has been produced by transient exposure to toxic elements during the fetal period.

Classification

Congenital scoliosis classification (based on the developmental anomaly of the spine) includes deficiencies in vertebral formation, segmentation, or a combination of the two (mixed). Failures of formation and segmentation may occur on either the right or left side of the body resulting in pure scoliosis, or in the anterior and posterior elements resulting in pure kyphosis or lordosis, respectively. Combined deficiencies are common, and associated sagittal plane deformity is important to recognize.

Identifying a congenital malformation on the spinal radiographs requires careful assessment of the films. Asymmetry of the size or number of the pedicles may suggest a failure of formation, and an absent rib often is associated with a deficiency of the vertebral elements. An unsegmented bar is suggested when the corresponding ribs and/or pedicles are conjoined. Segmentation defects can also be presumed when the disc space is narrowed. A 3-D CT study often helps to clarify the diagnosis in an older child with a complex deformity.

Natural History

The likelihood of any single patient with congenital scoliosis developing progressive deformity is difficult to state with certainty. There are, however, known anomalies and curve locations that make some generalizations possible. Thoracic curves progress the most, and

curves with multiple hemivertebrae and a convex unilateral bar (failure of segmentation) opposite the hemivertebrae have the poorest prognosis.

Block or wedge vertebrae are associated with a median rate of curve progression of less than 1°/yr and generally do not require treatment. Hemivertebrae, however, increase between 1° and 2.5°/yr and double hemivertebrae increase at roughly twice that rate. Unilateral unsegmented bars progress at rates up to 6° to 9°/yr in the thoracolumbar junction, and the unilateral unsegmented bars with a contralateral hemivertebra are at the greatest risk of progression, at times exceeding 10°/yr.

Careful monitoring of radiographs is required to document and detect progression. The most likely times of increasing deformity match the phases of normally rapid spinal growth (the first 2 to 3 years of life and the adolescent years).

Treatment

Observation

The presence of a congenital spinal anomaly requires close monitoring of spinal growth until maturity. Upright radiographs should be taken. The landmarks used for Cobb angle determination are often difficult to mark and the interobserver error in Cobb angle measurement of congenital scoliosis curves may be as high as 10°.

In general, brace treatment has not been shown to be very effective in managing the primary curve in congenital scoliosis because the curves tend to be short with little flexibility. Certain curves with a long flexible component may be amenable to orthotic management. On occasion, the compensatory curves, which develop above or below a congenital deformity, become problematic, and bracing to aid trunk balance may be helpful.

Surgical Treatment

Surgical management is the standard treatment for progressive congenital scoliosis; however, because of the relative inflexibility of these curves, correction with instrumentation is less feasible than in idiopathic deformities. Surgical treatment options include posterior fusion (in situ or with instrumentation), combined anterior and posterior fusion, convex hemiepiphysiodesis (anterior and/or posterior hemiarthrodesis), and hemivertebra excision.

Preoperative Assessment

The genitourinary system should be screened with an ultrasound examination, looking for a treatable cause of urinary tract outflow obstruction. Before undertaking surgical treatment, an MRI of the entire spinal cord should be considered, especially if distraction instrumentation is planned. Associated intraspinal malformations, such as a diastematomyelia or a tethered cord have been noted in cases of congenital scoliosis.

Goals of Surgery in Congenital Scoliosis

Although the goal for most cases is limiting curve progression, with the use of instrumentation or vertebral excision a surgeon can surgically reduce the degree of deformity in some cases. These procedures carry somewhat greater risk for neurologic injury; the amount of injury varies with the procedure, the curve pattern, flexibility, the location within the spine (cervical, thoracic, and lumbar), and the experience of the surgeon. Thus, many patients with congenital scoliosis are treated with in situ fusion.

Posterior Fusion

The success of posterior in situ arthrodesis in preventing further deformity (increase in the Cobb angle or increase in the rotational deformity) depends on the nature of the malformation and the growth potential of the remaining unfused anterior vertebral bodies. Increased rotational deformity after a posterior spinal fusion (crankshaft phenomenon) was first described in idiopathic scoliosis and also has been documented to occur in skeletally immature patients with congenital scoliosis. The addition of instrumentation to a posterior arthrodesis can be considered in older children. Pediatric-sized instrumentation systems are available for children older than approximately 3 years, which makes limited deformity correction possible in selected cases. Postoperative immobilization may be avoided in juvenile and adolescent patients with secure internal fixation, whereas extended immobilization may be required in the younger group to protect the instrumentation from dislodgment.

Anterior Fusion

Anterior in situ arthrodesis may be required when substantial anterior vertebral growth is expected. Anterior growth potential in congenital deformities appears to depend on the age of the patient (as in idiopathic scoliosis), as well as on the presence and orientation of anterior growth cartilage. The width of the disc space can be used to make inferences regarding growth potential.

Anterior procedures are designed primarily to limit growth of the vertebrae; however, some degree of flexibility may be obtained following discectomies in deformities that do not have a segmentation deficiency. The surgical exposure must allow for complete removal of the disc and end plate growth cartilage of the levels involved. The risk of surgically related paralysis due to vascular insufficiency seems greatest in congenital scoliosis surgery as compared with surgery on other curve types.

Partial Fusion, Growth Modulation, Hemiepiphysiodesis

Convex hemiarthrodesis (hemiepiphysiodesis), a technique that includes performing a fusion only on the convex side of the curve both anteriorly and posteriorly, has led to mixed results. Depending on the growth potential of the concave vertebral elements, the hemiarthrodesis may need to be extended one level above and below the measured curve. This technique has been most useful early in life (before age 5 years). Additionally, it should be used when curves have proven to be progressive yet remain less than 50°. Beyond these levels the results are less predictable. This procedure should not be used if a significant kyphotic component to the deformity exists because the anterior fusion may lead to worsening of the kyphosis.

Hemivertebra Excision

Hemivertebra excision, a procedure that allows for acute deformity correction as well as stabilization with arthrodesis, is associated with greater neurologic risk and is technically much more demanding than the previously discussed options. Resection of a hemivertebra is safest (neurologically) when performed below the tip of the cord (conus) and has the greatest impact on trunk balance when applied to lower lumbar or lumbosacral deformities. Thus, the procedure is most commonly used for lower lumbar hemivertebrae associated with truncal decompensation; although it also has been effectively applied to severe deformities of the thoracic and thoracolumbar spine (Fig. 5). The results of several series suggest that, in experienced hands, excision is a safe and effective approach to the deformity caused by a hemivertebra.

Scheuermann's Disease (Kyphosis)

Scheuermann's disease was initially described as a rigid kyphosis associated with wedged vertebral bodies occurring in late childhood. The condition has been of significant orthopaedic interest since that time, both because the condition is sometimes painful during its relative acute phase and, more importantly, because it causes significant truncal deformity that may be progressive. Subsequently, specific criteria for diagnosis were described in 1964, namely that three adjacent vertebrae must be wedged at least 5° each.

Unlike scoliosis, where any significant lateral deviation in the coronal plane is abnormal, the sagittal alignment of the spine has a normal range of thoracic kyphosis. The Scoliosis Research Society has defined this range as being from 20° to 40° in the growing adolescent. In a study of 316 normal subjects with ages ranging from 2 to 27 years, the upper limit of normal kypho-

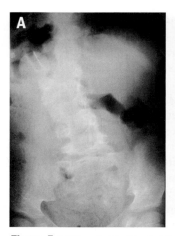 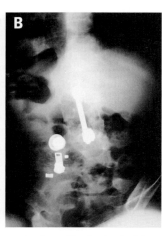

Figure 5 A, This patient had trunk shift secondary to a midlumbar hemivertebra. Given that progression had been documented, the options for treatment included in situ fusion, hemiepiphysiodesis, and hemivertebra excision. **B,** The postoperative radiograph demonstrates alignment after hemivertebra excision by simultaneous anterior and posterior approaches with the deformity corrected with a single posterior compression-rod system supplemented postoperatively by cast immobilization.

sis was noted to be 45°. In addition, it was noted that the average thoracic kyphosis increases with age, from 20° in children, to 25° in adolescents, to 40° in adults.

The subgroup described as lumbar Scheuermann's, type II Scheuermann's, or apprentice kyphosis should also be considered. This condition, most commonly seen in athletically active adolescent boys or those involved in heavy lifting, is characterized by localized back pain and radiographic vertebral changes at the thoracolumbar junction and typically is not associated with increased clinical kyphosis. The Schmorl's nodes and end-plate irregularity may be so severe that lumbar Scheuermann's disease can be confused with infection, tumor, or other conditions. Its etiology is unknown, but strong associations with repetitive activities involving axial loading of the immature spine favor a mechanical cause. Although the radiographic appearance may be similar, lumbar Scheuermann's kyphosis may be a different entity than thoracic Scheuermann's kyphosis.

Etiology of Classic Scheuermann's Disease

The etiology of the rigid roundback seen in type I Scheuermann's disease remains unknown. As a result, it is often categorized using nonspecific and poorly defined terms such as osteochondrosis or epiphysitis. Early theories included osoteonecrosis of the ring apophysis, inhibited enchondral ossification related to intravertebral disc herniations and end-plate perforations, and persistent anterior vascular grooves. Subsequent studies have not verified these theories. Juvenile osteoporosis is also considered as a possible cause of Scheuermann's roundback.

Few studies are available to describe the histologic findings in Scheuermann's disease, and in those that are available the criteria for making the diagnosis are not given. These studies implicate defective cartilage in the vertebral growth plate (end plate), with resultant decreased vertical growth of the anterior vertebral body as a potential cause. Abnormal collagen-proteoglycan ratios have been described in the vertebral body end plate as well. As in all histologic and biochemical analyses of abnormal bone and cartilage, it is not possible to determine if the reported changes are primary or secondary to abnormal loading. An autosomal dominant inheritance pattern with high penetrance and variable expressivity has been described for Scheuermann's disease, suggesting a biologic predisposition in some patients.

Most investigators agree that mechanical factors have a significant role in the pathogenesis of Scheuermann's disease. The reported success of brace treatment lends support to a mechanical etiology. Patients with Scheuermann's disease may have very tight hamstrings, and one biomechanical theory presumes that tight hamstrings prevent anterior pelvic tilt on forward bending, focusing bending stresses on the thoracic spine.

Incidence and Clinical Findings

The incidence of Scheuermann's disease has been estimated at 1% to 8% of the population. The typical occurrence is in the late juvenile age period from 8 to 12 years, with the more severe fixed form commonly appearing between ages 12 and 16 years. Patients with thoracic roundback who have classic type I Scheuermann's disease may have pain in the thoracic spine area, but more frequently come for treatment because of patient and parental concerns related to trunk deformity. In general, boys and girls are involved with equal frequency, although the reported ratios have varied widely.

Natural History

The natural history of Scheuermann's disease remains controversial, with significant pain reported during the teenage years, which later abates. In a long-term follow-up study, pain was noted in the thoracic region in 50% of patients during adolescence, with the number of symptomatic patients decreasing to 25% after skeletal maturity. Later authors offered a contrasting view of the symptoms of untreated Scheuermann's disease, stating that adults with Scheuermann's disease have a higher incidence of disabling back pain than the normal population. Other authors of surgical series have agreed with this, and have described pain unresponsive to nonsurgical treatment as an indication for surgical treatment of Scheuermann's disease.

A recent study was designed to describe the natural

history of Scheuermann's disease. The patients had an average kyphotic deformity of 71°, and the average follow-up was 32 years; an age-matched comparison group was used as control. The authors concluded that patients with Scheuermann's disease may have functional limitations, but these did not result in severe limitations due to pain or cause major interference with their lives.

A subsequent article states that adults with more severe deformities (> 75°) secondary to untreated Scheuermann's disease often have severe thoracic pain secondary to degenerative spondylosis and can be significantly limited by their disease. Thus, the natural history remains controversial.

Deciding on Treatment

The reasons for treatment of Scheuermann's disease can be outlined into five categories: pain, progressive deformity, neurologic compromise, cardiopulmonary compromise, and cosmesis. Neurologic deficits related to Scheuermann's disease have been reported only rarely. These deficits may be related to thoracic disc herniation, epidural cysts, or the hyperkyphosis itself and tend to occur in adult patients.

Deformity is the most common complaint of patients with Scheuermann's disease and is typically the primary reason that younger patients seek medical attention. Unfortunately, the likelihood of progression of a kyphotic curve of any given degree of severity is currently not known. Many girls greatly fear having a dowager's hump by middle age, and boys similarly often are concerned about visual trunk deformity. Unlike scoliosis, for which data are available regarding the risk for curve progression, such studies are not yet available for Scheuermann's disease. Even if the risk of curve progression is not known, some patients may be extremely dissatisfied with their appearance, and the deformity alone may be unacceptable to the patient. Many teenagers and their parents are unwilling to accept permanent fixed roundback deformity, which gives them poor posture and a poor self-image.

Treatment

Initial management of a patient presenting with Scheuermann's disease includes documentation and assessment of the degree of deformity and/or pain, as well as an assessment of the negative impact of the deformity on the patient's life. Physical therapy for postural improvement is often presented, focusing on hamstring and trunk extensor strengthening. There are no conclusive studies documenting improvement in kyphosis with exercises, although one study did note some improvement in patients with moderate degrees of deformity.

Brace Treatment for Kyphosis

The few available studies on efficacy of brace treatment are retrospective, have different inclusion criteria, and do not include control groups. In addition, as previously noted, data are not available to predict which patients are at greatest risk for progression. Despite these shortcomings, bracing is widely regarded as being effective in the treatment of deformity in the skeletally immature patient.

One report on the modified Milwaukee brace for treatment of Scheuermann's disease in 75 patients who had completed treatment documented a 40% decrease in mean thoracic kyphosis and a 35% decrease in mean lumbar lordosis after an average 34 months of brace wear. A later study from the same center, reporting on 120 of 274 patients treated with a Milwaukee brace for Scheuermann's disease, showed a pattern of initial correction of approximately 50% of the kyphosis followed by loss of correction. The average time of brace wear was 14 months full-time and 18 months part-time. At average 5-year follow-up, there was an improvement in the kyphosis of 76 consistent brace wearers, worsening in 24, and no change in 10. Of the 10 patients who were noncompliant with brace wear, two had improvement and eight had worsening of their kyphosis. Other authors have also documented a loss of correction with time out of the brace, decreasing from an initial 21° correction to 6° at final follow-up.

The prerequisites for brace treatment of Scheuermann's disease include a patient with kyphosis of up to 65° and skeletal growth remaining. Curves of greater than 74° have been associated with a higher failure rate; thus, this magnitude of deformity has been declared by some as an indication for surgery.

Complications have not been reported with brace treatment of Scheuermann's disease, although the potential adverse psychological consequences of full-time bracing during adolescence should be considered. Current indications for bracing are evolving, but include patients with kyphosis of greater than 50° and significant pain, cosmetically unacceptable deformity, or documented progression of deformity. A commitment by the patient to wear the brace faithfully for a minimum of 1 year is required. Even with compliant brace wear by the patient, the data available at this point do not allow the prescribing physician to forecast whether brace treatment will result in improvement of deformity, prevention of progression, or failure in any particular patient.

Surgical Treatment

The indications for surgical correction cannot be stated exactly because natural history studies of Scheuermann's disease remain controversial regarding pain, disability, trunk deformity, and self-esteem. Thus, a decision for surgical correction is individual among the surgeon, the patient, and the family. It may depend on the patient's symptoms, self-perception, and sense of self-esteem, as well as the surgeon's training and skill in performing safe, predictable correction. Surgical indications have evolved in the past 2 decades but currently include patients with greater than 75° kyphosis or significant kyphosis (greater than 65°) associated with pain not relieved by nonsurgical treatment. Obviously there is some flexibility in the indications related to the surgeon's and patient's interpretation of natural history data.

The results of surgical treatment of Scheuermann's disease can be considered relative to the two most common indications listed for surgery: relief of pain and correction of deformity. Although pain is listed as the indication for surgery in many studies, results in the published series tend to focus on deformity correction. Relief of back pain related to the deformity after surgery has been reported in all of the patients in many series. Good relief of pain has been reported in 12 of 13 patients treated with combined anterior and posterior fusion. Another report states that 18 of 24 patients treated with staged anterior release and fusion/posterior fusion with L-rod instrumentation had greater than a 75% reduction in pain.

Correction of deformity by posterior spinal fusion alone, using Harrington compression instrumentation, was noted to produce excellent initial correction of deformity, but with loss of correction over time, especially in patients with larger kyphotic curves. Correction of deformity has been reported from a mean kyphotic angle of 72° to 46° at short-term follow-up.

The commonly noted loss of correction after posterior-only surgery has been attributed to the fusion being performed on the tension side of the spine, to inadequate strength and subsequent failure of the implants, to lack of anterior support, and to inadequate initial corrections in severe, rigid deformities. As a result, the surgical approach has been modified to include anterior spinal release and disc excision and fusion in conjunction with instrumented posterior spinal fusion in an effort to improve correction and prevent late deterioration of correction. This approach has been advocated for patients with greater than 75° of deformity, marked wedging of the apical vertebrae, and failure of the kyphosis to correct to less than 50° on a hyperextension lateral radiograph. As surgical techniques and perioperative care have improved, same-day anterior and posterior surgery has become possible and is advocated by some as having less morbidity than staged procedures. Anterior plus posterior surgery has generally resulted in excellent correction of deformity reported in several

published series (mean kyphosis decreasing from 75° to 85° to 40° to 50°).

Complications Associated With Surgical Correction

The complications reported in the literature should be considered carefully. These include death, postoperative neurologic deficit, infection, gastrointestinal obstruction, intraoperative and postoperative hardware failure, pseudarthrosis, prominent hardware, loss of correction, progression of kyphosis, hemothorax, pneumothorax, pulmonary emboli, and persistent back pain.

Which vertebrae to include within the instrumented, corrected segment is important. Despite the early recognition that fusing too short resulted in persistent or recurrent deformity at follow-up, this complication persists in even more recent series. Selection of fusion levels remains a critical part of surgical correction of kyphosis, yet no well-established criteria are available that have been validated with long-term follow-up. It also is not clear whether the failures in series with posterior-only surgery were secondary to the reported deficiencies of this method (fusion on the tension side, lack

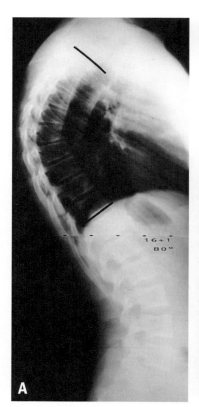
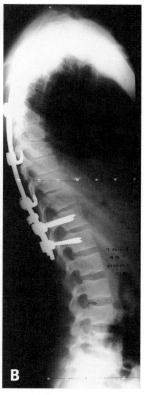

Figure 6 A, This 16-year-old boy had progressive thoracic kyphosis secondary to Scheuermann's disease. **B,** The postoperative lateral radiograph is seen following anterior thorascopic release and fusion followed by posterior spinal instrumentation and fusion. Posterior compression has been the primary mode of correction with pedicle screw instrumentation extending inferiorly into the first lordotic segments in attempts to prevent junctional kyphosis.

of anterior structural support, inadequate initial release) or to improper selection/execution of fusion levels.

The problem of junctional kyphosis at either the proximal or distal end of the fusion mass has received more attention in the recent literature. Some have attributed this complication to Luque methods of spinal fixation, in which disruption of the posterior ligamentous structures for passage of the most cephalad and caudal wires increases the risk of kyphosis; however, the problem was also seen in the earlier Harrington compression constructs. The complication subsequently has been reported with Cotrel-Dubousset instrumentation. The most recent recommendations regarding fusion levels are to include the end vertebra of the kyphosis proximally and to extend the fusion to the first lordotic disc beyond the transitional zone distally. To adequately correct a typical Scheuermann's disease, posterior corrective instrumented fusion from the T3 to the L2 level is necessary. Recommendations also have been made to limit correction to 50% or less of the original deformity in an attempt to prevent later proximal junctional kyphosis. The use of contemporary instrumentation systems has increased the ability to obtain and maintain correction (as compared to the Harrington or Luque systems).

Further developments in surgical techniques and instrumentation include thoracoscopic anterior approaches to decrease the morbidity associated with anterior release and fusion, as well as pedicle screw fixation at the distal aspect of the fusion construct to decrease the incidence of hardware-related complications (Fig. 6). Very long-term studies will be required to analyze the effect of living throughout life with a 65° or 70° kyphosis as compared to having it reduced to 35° with surgical correction, taking into account the potential morbidity of junctional problems between the fused and unfused segments of the spine.

Annotated Bibliography

Idiopathic Scoliosis

Dickson RA, Weinstein SL: Bracing (and screening): Yes or no? *J Bone Joint Surg Br* 1999;81:193-198.

This review article raises issues about nonsurgical scoliosis treatment.

Gupta P, Lenke LG, Bridwell KH: Incidence of neural axis abnormalities in infantile and juvenile patients with spinal deformity: Is a magnetic resonance image screening necessary? *Spine* 1998;23:206-210.

This is a prospective and retrospective review of patients 10 years old or younger with idiopathic scoliosis having MRI scans. Total spine MRIs are recommended for patients with juvenile onset idiopathic scoliosis (greater than 20°) because of the high incidence of neural axis abnormalities.

Lenke LG, Betz RR, Bridwell KH, Harms J, Clements DH, Lowe TG: Spontaneous lumbar curve coronal correction after selective anterior or posterior thoracic fusion in adolescent idiopathic scoliosis. *Spine* 1999;24: 1663-1672.

Spontaneous lumbar curve correction occurs consistently after both selective anterior and posterior thoracic fusion, implying intrinsic ability of the lumbar spine to follow thoracic spine correction. Spontaneous lumbar curve correction was statistically better after anterior thoracic instrumentation and fusion.

Lenke LG, Bridwell KH, Blanke K, Baldus C, Weston J: Radiographic results of arthrodesis with Cotrel-Dubousset instrumentation for the treatment of adolescent idiopathic scoliosis: A five to ten-year follow-up study. *J Bone Joint Surg Am* 1998;80:807-814.

The radiographic results of posterior spinal arthrodesis using Cotrel-Dubousset instrumentation in 76 patients with adolescent idiopathic scoliosis were evaluated. At an average of 6 years (range, 5 to 10 years) postoperatively, the fusion appeared to be solid in all patients.

Nachemson AL, Peterson LE: Effectiveness of treatment with a brace in girls who have adolescent idiopathic scoliosis: A prospective, controlled study based on data from the Brace Study of the Scoliosis Research Society. *J Bone Joint Surg Am* 1995;77:815-822.

In a prospective study, 286 girls with adolescent idiopathic scoliosis, a thoracic/thoracolumbar curve of 25° to 35°, and a mean age of 12.6 years were followed. Brace treatment was successful in 74%; observation only in 34%; and electrical stimulation in 33%.

Noonan KJ, Weinstein SL, Jacobson WC, Dolan LA: Use of the Milwaukee brace for progressive idiopathic scoliosis. *J Bone Joint Surg Am* 1996;78:557-567.

Immature patients with idiopathic scoliosis who were treated with a Milwaukee brace were evaluated. This study raises questions about whether the natural history of progressive idiopathic scoliosis is truly altered by use of the Milwaukee brace.

Sweet FA, Lenke LG, Bridwell KH, Blanke KM: Maintaining lumbar lordosis with anterior single solid-rod instrumentation in thoracolumbar and lumbar adolescent idiopathic scoliosis. *Spine* 1999;24:1655-1662.

Coronal plane correction with preservation of thoracolumbar and lumbar lordosis 2 years after anterior spinal instrumentation was accomplished using a lordotically contoured single solid rod with structural cages in patients with primary thoracolumbar or lumbar adolescent idiopathic scoliosis.

Congenital Scoliosis

McMaster MJ: Congenital scoliosis caused by a unilateral failure of vertebral segmentation with contralateral hemivertebrae. *Spine* 1998;23:998-1005.

Patients with congenital scoliosis caused by unilateral unsegmented bar with contralateral hemivertebrae have the most rapidly progressive type of congenital scoliosis, and require anterior and posterior arthrodesis, preferably in the first year of life.

McMaster MJ, Singh H: Natural history of congenital kyphosis and kyphoscoliosis: A study of one hundred and twelve patients. *J Bone Joint Surg Am* 1999;81: 1367-1383.

Congenital kyphosis and kyphoscoliosis are uncommon deformities with the potential to progress rapidly, resulting in severe deformity and possible neurologic deficits. The natural history is described for these deformities.

Kyphosis

Ponte A, Siccardi GL, Ligure P: Scheuermann's kyphosis: Posterior shortening procedure by segmental closing wedge osteotomies. *J Pediatr Orthop* 1995;15:404.

Forty-six consecutive patients with Scheuermann's disease underwent segmental closing wedge resections. By overcoming selectively unequal resistances, correction can be graduated segment by segment as needed.

Classic Bibliography

Dickson JH, Erwin WD, Rossi D: Harrington instrumentation and arthrodesis for idiopathic scoliosis: A twenty-one-year follow-up. *J Bone Joint Surg Am* 1990; 72:678-683.

Lenke LG, Bridwell KH, Baldus C, Blanke K: Preventing decompensation in King type II curves treated with Cotrel-Dubousset instrumentation: Strict guidelines for selective thoracic fusion. *Spine* 1992;17(suppl 8): 274-281.

Lonstein JE, Carlson JM: The prediction of curve progression in untreated idiopathic scoliosis during growth. *J Bone Joint Surg Am* 1984;66:1061-1071.

Lonstein JE, Winter RB: The Milwaukee brace for the treatment of adolescent idiopathic scoliosis: A review of one thousand and twenty patients. *J Bone Joint Surg Am* 1994;76:1207-1221.

Lowe TG, Kasten MD: An analysis of sagittal curves and balance after Cotrel-Dubousset instrumentation for kyphosis secondary to Scheuermann's disease: A review of 32 patients. *Spine* 1994;19:1680-1685.

McMaster MJ, Ohtsuka K: The natural history of congenital scoliosis: A study of two hundred and fifty-one patients. *J Bone Joint Surg Am* 1982;64:1128-1147.

Mehta MH: The rib vertebral angle in the early diagnosis between resolving and progressive infantile scoliosis. *J Bone Joint Surg Br* 1972;54:230-243.

Murray PM, Weinstein SL, Spratt KF: The natural history and long-term follow-up of Scheuermann kyphosis. *J Bone Joint Surg Am* 1993;75:236-248.

U.S. Preventive Services Task Force: Screening for adolescent idiopathic scoliosis: Review article. *JAMA* 1993; 269:2667-2672.

Weinstein SL: Idiopathic scoliosis: Natural history. *Spine* 1986;11:780-783.

Chapter 39

Adult Scoliosis and Deformity

Oheneba Boachie-Adjei, MD

Munish C. Gupta, MD

Introduction

Deformity of the spine in an adult presents a biomechanical as well as a biologic challenge. In addition to stiffness, an aging spine with a curvature develops degenerative changes of the intervertebral discs and facets, often impinging on neural elements. Decompressing these neural elements removes additional stability and bone surface area for arthrodesis. Determination of the pain generator is also difficult with diffuse degenerative changes in the spine. For example, a patient with a significant lumbar curve who has degenerative changes in the lumbosacral junction presents a diagnostic challenge in determining the pain source and a therapeutic challenge in trying to alleviate the pain with spinal fusion. Arthrodesis, which is unnatural for the spine, is no panacea.

The major categories of adult scoliosis include (1) idiopathic scoliosis without degenerative changes in adults younger than 40 years who have had spinal deformity since adolescence, (2) the patient older than 40 years of age who has adult idiopathic scoliosis with superimposed degenerative changes, and (3) the elderly adult patient who has had no preexisting spinal deformity and has developed de novo scoliosis as a result of degenerative changes of the thoracolumbar spine.

General Surgical Considerations

In general, risk of complications is higher for the adult than for the adolescent patient undergoing surgical treatment for scoliosis. This difference must be taken into consideration in the selection of patients for surgical treatment. The primary goals of surgical treatment for the adult patient with idiopathic scoliosis are to (1) correct and stabilize a progressive spinal deformity, (2) improve or restore coronal and sagittal balance, (3) obtain a solid arthrodesis of the spine, (4) relieve pain, and (5) decompress neural elements associated with spinal stenosis. Factors to be considered in surgical

planning include preoperative comorbidities, patient expectations, and levels to be fused and instrumented based on symptoms and diagnostic imaging. Adults usually do not obtain the same percentage of correction as adolescents, and the goal must be achieving a balanced correction in both sagittal and coronal planes.

The preoperative nutritional status of the older adult patient who may have medical comorbidities should be evaluated and, if needed, preoperative nutritional enhancement should be given. Assessment of nutritional parameters include serum albumin, prealbumin, total lymphocyte count, and transferrin levels. The type of procedure—posterior approach only, anterior approach only, combined anterior and posterior procedures—and whether combined procedures can be performed on the same day under one anesthetic or staged is based on the complexity of the surgery, the surgeon's expertise, and the patient's medical condition. In general, same-day procedures are preferred to staged procedures to reduce complications related to postoperative malnutrition and length of hospital stay.

For patients undergoing staged procedures, studies have shown that there is delay in the normalization of nutritional parameters and that supplementation by total parenteral nutrition will reduce postoperative morbidity associated with infectious complications of the wound, urinary tract, and respiratory systems. Moreover, if same-day surgery is being considered, the surgeon must be prepared to abort the procedure if the patient's hemodynamic status becomes unstable, blood loss exceeds the patient's blood volume, or the operating time is anticipated to go beyond 12 hours.

Adult Idiopathic Scoliosis

Patients with adult idiopathic scoliosis have lived with their deformities for most of their lives. Some have been treated for their deformity, but later developed pain, radiculopathy, neurogenic claudication, or progression of the deformity. Advances in instrumentation, anesthetic techniques, and fusion with graft substitutes, as well as osteoinduction or gene therapy give these patients a better future.

Prevalence and Natural History

The prevalence of scoliosis in patients older than 50 years of age is 6%, including patients with adult idiopathic scoliosis and patients with degenerative or de novo scoliosis. Curves of less than 30° at skeletal maturity tend not to progress; however, curves larger than 50° tend to progress an average of 1° to 2°/yr. For lumbar curves, risk factors such as apical rotation and lateral and rotatory listhesis help in determining prognosis of an individual curve. In double curves, the lumbar components tend to progress more than the thoracic ones. Patients with untreated adult idiopathic scoliosis show no difference in pulmonary function other than age-related changes. Patients with scoliosis tend to have similar incidence of back pain as adults without scoliosis, but those with adult idiopathic scoliosis tend to have more severe pain with more frequent recurrences. Lumbar curves and compensatory lumbosacral curves are associated with more pain.

Clinical Presentation and Evaluation

Pain within the curvature and progression of the deformity are the most common reasons for patients with adult idiopathic scoliosis to seek medical intervention, which they do at an average age of 40 years. Radicular or neurogenic claudication complaints are less common when compared to those of patients with degenerative scoliosis. Compression of the neural elements, if present, usually is found in the concavity of the lumbar curve. Evaluation of these patients requires thorough radiographic and neurologic examination as well as determination of the painful area of the spine with deep palpation.

Radiographic Assessment

Long-cassette, standing radiographs are mandatory for determination of major and compensatory curves. Evaluation of the sagittal as well as the coronal balance should be included. The cervical lordosis and the pelvic alignment or tilt also should be observed to assess contractures around the pelvis. Ideally, the gravity line should pass from C7 through the center of the femoral head. Radiographic assessment should include full standing AP, lateral, and flexibility studies (supine side-bending or traction radiographs). For curves exceeding 60°, traction radiographs have been shown to be more predictive of curve flexibility. In addition, CT scans, MRI scans, or discography can be obtained as indicated

to ascertain the integrity of the distal lumbar discs and facet joints to be included in the fusion. MRI scan is helpful in delineating the internal characteristics of the discs at the lumbosacral junction. The goal should be to preserve as many lumbar segments as possible and avoid fusion to the pelvis whenever possible. Discography may be used to determine where to end the fusion. Mild changes on the MRI scan do not warrant fusion to the pelvis.

Nonsurgical Treatment

Nonsurgical treatment of back pain includes aerobic conditioning, strengthening and stretching, local modalities, and nonsteroidal anti-inflammatory medication. Epidural steroid injections and nerve root blocks can be added to these modalities in patients with associated lumbar radiculopathy or neurogenic claudication. Lumbar corsets for patients with significant lumbar curves or lumbosacral curves may be helpful for pain reduction. Undergoing nonsurgical treatment and improving aerobic conditioning and strength helps patients if they later undergo a surgical procedure.

Surgical Treatment

Successful correction and arthrodesis of patients with adult idiopathic scoliosis has gone through a gradual evolution that started with the Harrington rod and its one-dimensional correction in distraction, which created flattening of the sagittal plane, especially in the lumbar spine, and progressed to multiple-stage anterior and posterior approaches. The sagittal plane has been the definite focus recently, with improvements in segmental instrumentation and interbody strut grafting and use of spacers such as femoral rings or mesh cages. Other areas coming to the forefront of concern because of their intimate relationships to the thoracic and lumbar spine are the cervical spine and the pelvis.

The focus of the correction should be a balanced, stable, and successfully fused spine. Pain alleviation after such an arthrodesis is not complete; the severity of the pain has been shown to be 70% improved but the frequency of pain does not necessarily improve. The patient has to have reasonable expectations of pain relief and deformity correction after these procedures.

Young adults whose lumbar spines have not had the chance to develop moderate to severe degenerative changes can be treated similarly to patients with adolescent idiopathic scoliosis. The major indications for treatment in this population are progression of the curvature to over 50° and pain over the curve that is unresponsive to nonsurgical measures. Patients older than 40 to 50 years, who have had time to develop degenerative changes in the lumbar spine or the compensatory

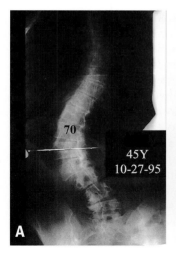
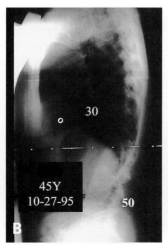
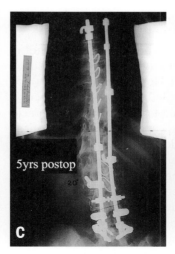
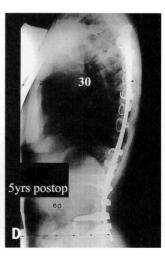

Figure 1 Long cassette, coronal **(A)** and sagittal **(B)** radiographs of a 45-year-old woman with untreated idiopathic lumbar scoliosis with progressive decompensation and back pain. Rotatory subluxations of L2-L3 and L3-L4 with significant osteophyte on the concavity of the fractional curve are noted. Relative sparing of the L5-S1 disc was noted on MRI scan. The radiograph demonstrates sagittal balance; a plumb line from C7 falls through the lumbosacral disc. The patient was treated with same-day, combined anterior-posterior multilevel thoracolumbar discectomies and fusion from T11 to L5 with structural grafts and femoral ring at the L4-L5 level and autogenous morcellized rib graft from T11 to L3. Long cassette, upright, standing coronal **(C)** and sagittal **(D)** radiographs of the patient taken 5 years after surgery. Note the physiologic contour of the rod and the restoration of physiologic sagittal alignment. A plumb line from C7 falls through the lumbosacral disc.

lumbosacral curve, provide a more difficult decision-making process. These patients are more likely to complain of low back pain with referred or radicular pain in the legs. Patients who have pain over the lumbar curvature as well as at the degenerated lumbosacral junction may have coronal or sagittal imbalance and, in addition, may require a fusion to the sacrum with augmentation of the fusion anteriorly.

Selection of Fusion Levels

For the adult younger than 40 years, with thoracic or thoracolumbar deformity without degenerative changes of the lumbar and lumbosacral spine, fusion levels are similar to those for the adolescent patient. The cephalad and caudal levels of the fusion should be stable and neutral. Sagittal profile should be as near normal and physiologic as possible. The young adult with a pristine L5-S1 disc and facet joint can be fused safely to L5. However, the patient must be warned of the potential for progressive degeneration, instability, and pain, requiring extension to the sacrum at a later time (Fig. 1).

In the older adult with extensive degenerative changes, modification of the fusion levels used for the young adult must be considered. Painful joints, translational changes in the lumbar spine, and levels requiring decompression for concomitant spinal stenosis should be included in the fusion.

Current, third-generation spinal instrumentation systems provide a more stable, balanced correction of the spine in the adult patient. Multilevel instrumentation is useful to increase the number of fixation points in order to reduce failures at the bone-metal interface in patients with osteoporosis. Current instrumentation systems that use multiple fixation anchor sites with pedicle screws in the lumbar spine and with hooks offer better curve correction and balance. Maintenance of correction and improvement of compensatory curves below the instrumented levels can also be achieved with distal lumbar pedicle screws. For rigid deformities, sublaminar or sub pars wires may provide better translational corrective maneuvers than do hooks placed at the apices of the deformity.

Specific Surgical Procedures

Posterior spinal fusion with instrumentation is indicated for flexible adult thoracic scoliosis of 60° to 75° and balanced double thoracic and lumbar curves of similar magnitude. The technique usually involves fusion of the thoracic curve to the stable vertebra for single thoracic major curves (King-Moe II or III). The minor compensatory lumbar curves can be left unfused to preserve distal motion segments. However, double major thoracic and lumbar curves may require arthrodesis of both curves through the posterior-only approach.

For thoracic deformities with a rib hump exceeding 3 cm (or 20°), thoracoplasty performed through the same midline posterior incision helps achieve reduction of the prominence and improves the overall cosmetic appearance. It also provides an excellent source of autologous bone graft, which may sometimes obviate the need for iliac graft or be safely combined with allogeneic bone. However, because thoracoplasty may reduce pulmonary function by as much as 23%, persistent 2 years after surgery, it is imperative to consider thoracoplasty procedures only for patients with optimum pulmonary function.

Adults up to age 40 years who have flexible thoracolumbar and lumbar curves up to 60° with mild to moderate thoracic deformity less than 40° that is not painful and not progressive can be treated with anterior spinal fusion with instrumentation to preserve thoracic and distal lumbar motion segments. The surgical approach can be thoracoabdominal, transdiaphragmatic for T10 and above levels, and retropleural, retroperitoneal for lower thoracolumbar and lumbar levels.

Indications for combined anterior and posterior spinal fusion with posterior instrumentation without fusion to the sacrum include (1) rigid thoracic deformities exceeding 75°, (2) decompensated lumbar and thoracolumbar deformity, and (3) a double curve pattern with significant lumbar/thoracolumbar deformity. The lumbar spine usually is approached anteriorly by discectomy and fusion without instrumentation, the thoracic spine usually is corrected to the level that will achieve balance correction of both curves, and both curves are fused and instrumented posteriorly.

Indications to extend the arthrodesis to the sacrum include deformity extending to the L5-S1 level with oblique take-off of the L5 level, stenosis and/or herniated intervertebral disc at L4-5 or L5-S1, presence of spondylolisthesis at the L5-S1 level, or painful lumbosacral facet joints and disc degeneration. Because the pseudarthrosis rate is up to 17.5% in patients with fusion to the sacrum, single posterior approaches are not recommended.

Arthrodesis to the Sacrum

An anterior thoracoabdominal or retroperitoneal procedure with discectomy and fusion of the thoracolumbar spine to the sacrum without instrumentation is performed. Structural grafts with femoral ring allograft, tricortical iliac crest, or metal cages for L4-5 and L5-S1 have been shown to provide anterior column support and to enhance the arthrodesis and spinal stability of long fusions to the sacrum and sacropelvic region. Bicortical sacral screw fixation, Galveston fixation, and intrasacral fixation (Jackson) are used to achieve sacral and/or sacropelvic fixation. Instrumentation across the sacroiliac joint without fusing the joint is not without problems. The Galveston extension or iliac extension sometimes has to be removed because of prominence and pain. Preservation or restoration of lumbar lordosis is critical for sagittal balance for the patient undergoing a long thoracolumbar-sacral fusion.

There is significant blood loss from complex reconstruction of the spine in adult patients. Autologous blood donation helps reduce homologous transfusion and can be combined with intraoperative blood salvaged using the cell saver and hemodilution. Others have advocated preoperative administration of erythropoietin.

Recent advances in anesthetic management and intraoperative blood conservation have also shown the efficacy of antifibrinolytics in the reduction of blood loss during complex adult reconstructive surgery. Agents effective at reducing blood loss have included aprotinin, a polypeptide with serine protease inhibitor activity, and the synthetic lysine analogs, aminocaproic acid and tranexamic acid. In preliminary studies a 30% to 60% reduction has been demonstrated in intraoperative blood loss in patients given these agents one at a time as individual agents.

Because the pseudarthrosis rate is higher in adults than in adolescents, it is imperative that autograft be used, and it may be supplemented with allograft such as femoral head cancellous bone (fresh frozen). For patients undergoing distal lumbar and lumbosacral fusion, structural autografts with femoral ring, iliac crest, or titanium mesh cages have been shown in both biomechanical and clinical studies to provide a more stable construct and reduce the pseudarthrosis rate in the distal motion segments.

Specific Curve Patterns

In adult idiopathic scoliosis, there are thoracic, thoracolumbar, and lumbar curves; double curves in the thoracic and lumbar spine levels; and, finally, curves that require fusion to the sacrum. In progressive thoracic curves, bending radiographs can help delineate the flexibility of the curvature. In general, curves up to 60° or 70° can be approached posteriorly with a single approach (Fig. 2). Segmental instrumentation with multiple hooks or a combination of sublaminar wires and hooks in the thoracic spine and pedicle screws in the lumbar spine have improved the correction of these curves. Anterior thoracic instrumentation with screws and rods also has been shown to be effective in correcting these curves and reducing the number of levels fused. Currently, the posterior approach appears to be more common. The advantages of the posterior approach are that it is more familiar to most spine surgeons and it has been documented by the most long-term follow-up data. Disadvantages of the posterior approach are trauma to the paraspinal muscles and, generally, the need to fuse levels beyond the Cobb measurements. Use of pedicle screws has provided greater correction with the posterior approach and the ability to fuse to levels similar to those fused using the anterior approach.

Curves with flexibility exceeding 35% have been shown to be adequate to obtain final correction exceeding 50% to 60% when treated by posterior segmental instrumentation. The ability to correct significantly the

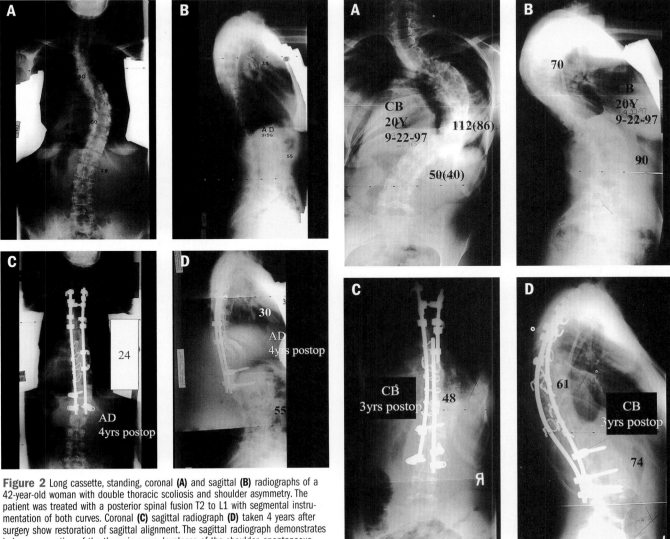

Figure 2 Long cassette, standing, coronal **(A)** and sagittal **(B)** radiographs of a 42-year-old woman with double thoracic scoliosis and shoulder asymmetry. The patient was treated with a posterior spinal fusion T2 to L1 with segmental instrumentation of both curves. Coronal **(C)** sagittal radiograph **(D)** taken 4 years after surgery show restoration of sagittal alignment. The sagittal radiograph demonstrates balance correction of the thoracic curve, levelness of the shoulder, spontaneous improvement of the lumbar curve, and distal lumbar pedicle screws.

Figure 3 A, Long cassette, standing, coronal radiograph of a 20-year-old woman with untreated progressive painful thoracic scoliosis and pulmonary functional capacity (FVC) of 40%. Patient shows a 112° stiff right thoracic scoliosis that bends only to 86°. **B,** Long cassette, sagittal, standing radiograph of the patient with 70° of thoracic kyphosis and 90° of lumbar lordosis. The patient was treated with a same-day, anterior thoracic multilevel discectomy and fusion using the rib as a morcellized graft and internal convex thoracoplasties T6 to T11 and posterior segmental instrumentation, with multiple rods and distal lumbar pedicle screws with thoracic hooks and sublaminar wires for apical translation. Concave rib osteotomies performed at the apical thoracic spine aided correction and alignment. Note the balance correction obtained of the thoracic and lumbar spines with symmetry of the trunk over the level pelvis. Postoperative, long cassette, standing, coronal **(C)** and sagittal **(D)** radiographs taken 3 years after surgery. There is improvement in overall sagittal alignment, thoracic kyphosis, and lumbar lordosis.

thoracic deformity helps with the final correction of the minor compensatory thoracolumbar-lumbar curve. The distal lumbar end-fusion vertebra should be horizontalized as much as possible by use of distal pedicle screws to reduce translational or junctional degeneration, which most commonly occurs if there is significant residual tilt of the lower instrumented vertebrae. Selection of the proper levels for fusion must be made with consideration of the degenerative segments in the distal lumbar spine.

For severe rigid thoracic deformities exceeding 80° to 100° with ankylosis of the concave facets, first-stage anterior discectomy and fusion without instrumentation followed with posterior segmental instrumentation and fusion and convex thoracoplasty with or without concave rib osteotomies, provides best balance correction

of the curve and achieves the highest arthrodesis rate (Fig. 3). The anterior thoracic discectomies can be approached via a traditional thoracotomy incision with removal of a major segment of the rib articulating with the most proximal end-vertebra. Internal thoracoplasties can be performed by this same approach. Convex and concave rib osteotomies can be performed through a second incision in the posterior midline.

Video-Assisted Thoracoscopy

The alternative approach to the open anterior procedure is the use of video-assisted thoracoscopic surgery (VATS) for the anterior thoracic discectomy and fusion. The convexity of the thoracic spine is approached through four to five portals. The portals are usually widely spaced, such that working portals allow an approach to one or two discs. The working portals usually are placed at the anterior axillary line. This procedure requires double-lumen endotracheal intubation and deflation of the ipsilateral lung. The double lumen is continually monitored and tube function checked several times during the surgery. It is imperative that the bronchoscope remain in the operating room for possible intubation and conversion.

With either the open or thoracoscopic approach, segmental vessels can be preserved or can be taken down with coagulation instruments such as the harmonic scalpel. Internal thoracoplasties can be performed using VATS but can make the surgical procedure excessively long, especially if the posterior surgical procedure is to be done under the same anesthetic. Femoral head cancellous allograft has been used as the graft material of choice for VATS so as to be able to complete the two stages. The fusion rate is encouraging in the preliminary reports. Surgical correction is similar to that of open procedures. The traditional convex approach has been used for most thoracoscopic approaches to thoracic scoliosis. The scope camera with a 10-mm diameter, 30° or 0° angle, can provide exposure of the entire thoracic spine distal to the thoracolumbar junction. Long-handled instruments, Cobb elevators, and curettes, used appropriately to remove the intervertebral disc can be carried circumferentially and posterior to the longitudinal ligament. When approaching on the right side care must be taken not to injure the azygos vessel, which can be protected with the fan retractor used to retract the lungs. The end plate can be decorticated with a long-handle burr or osteotomes, and bone graft material from local rib bone or allograft can be used. The conduit for bone graft administration can be a chest tube or a similarly fashioned device to access the spine, thoracic cage, and intervertebral disc spaces (Fig. 4).

Anterior Approach

Adults younger than 40 to 50 years of age with flexible thoracolumbar-lumbar curves up to 60° can be treated with anterior thoracolumbar or lumbar discectomy and fusion with anterior instrumentation. Flexibility studies should demonstrate a flexible lumbosacral fractional curve with horizontalization of the distal-end instrumented vertebra. Criteria used for anterior thoracolumbar-lumbar adolescent deformity can be used with some modification. If the apex falls on the vertebral body, instead of fusion a level above and a level below, an odd number of vertebrae can be fused to include the index curve. If the apex is at the disc, the two levels

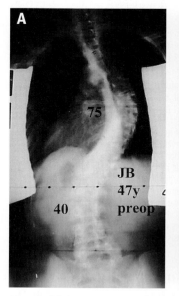 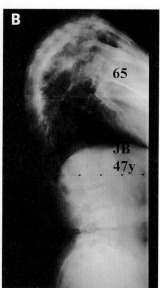 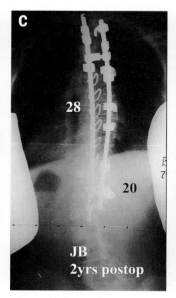 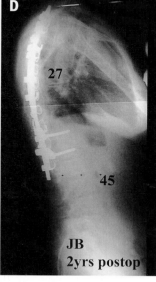

Figure 4 A, Long cassette, standing, coronal radiograph of a 47-year-old woman with progressive painful thoracic kyphoscoliosis and a flexible lumbar compensatory curve. **B,** Long cassette, standing, lateral radiograph of the patient demonstrates thoracic hyperkyphosis. Side bending and hyperextension radiographs demonstrated minimum flexibility of the thoracic curve from 75° to 65°. The patient was treated with a one-stage, anterior, multilevel discectomy and fusion of the thoracic spine from T5 to T12 via VATS, followed under the same anesthetic by posterior segmental instrumentation from T2 to L1. Spontaneous correction of the lumbar curve was obtained. Convex thoracoplasty was performed during the posterior approach, and the ribs were used for bone graft, supplemented with fresh frozen femoral head cancellous allograft. Long cassette, standing, coronal **(C)** and sagittal **(D)** radiographs taken 2 years after the surgery. The sagittal radiograph demonstrates reduction of the thoracic kyphosis to 27° and restoration of sagittal alignment with the plumbline from C7 falling through the lumbosacral disc.

above and two levels below or an even number of segments to encompass the entire index curve can be fused. Patients indicated for thoracolumbar-lumbar fusion should have mild to moderate thoracic curves, which correct to less than 25° on bending radiographs and flexible lumbosacral fractional curves. The compensatory thoracic or lumbosacral curves have been shown to correct roughly 30% to 40%. MRI studies should demonstrate healthy discs at the selected end vertebrae. If there are degenerative changes or translational listhesis at the selected end vertebra, extension to include this level should be considered. It is not advisable to extend the anterior fusion and instrumentation to the fifth lumbar vertebra because of the proximity of the great vessels and the technical difficulty of instrumenting this segment. To avoid the problem of kyphosis, which is common with anterior instrumentation systems such as the Zielke and the Dwyer, rigid rods are preferred for anterior instrumentation. Structural grafts such as femoral ring allograft or titanium mesh cages will aid in preserving the lordotic configuration of the thoracolumbar-lumbar spine and prevent the occurrence of kyphosis within the instrumented segment (Fig. 5).

A preoperative workup for these patients should include bone mineral density (BMD). The presence of severe osteoporosis with BMD more than 2.5 SD below normal would be a contraindication for selective anterior instrumentation. External mobilization for patients undergoing anterior thoracolumbar-lumbar fusion with instrumentation should be based on the integrity of the bony structure and the surgeon's discretion.

Double Curves

Double major thoracic and lumbar curves need to be evaluated for flexibility. For two flexible curves, up to 60° to 70°, a posterior approach that includes both curvatures is adequate. Curves greater than 60° to 70° benefit from release of the larger, stiffer curve. A flexible curve is generally defined as a curve that bends to less than 50% of its original Cobb angle. If there are two large, rigid thoracic and lumbar curves exceeding 70° to 80°, release of both curves and a staged posterior fusion, or release of the lumbar spine for improving the fusion rate and flexibility and concave and convex rib osteotomies in the thoracic spine are alternative approaches to achieve balanced correction (Fig. 6).

Current advances in spinal instrumentation provide modular ways for extending instrumentation into the pelvis and sacrum in multiple ways, improving the ability to place instrumentation in a more user-friendly and timely manner. Multiple rod constructs, segmentally connected to anchors including lumbar pedicle screws, and thoracic hooks with or without sublaminar wires

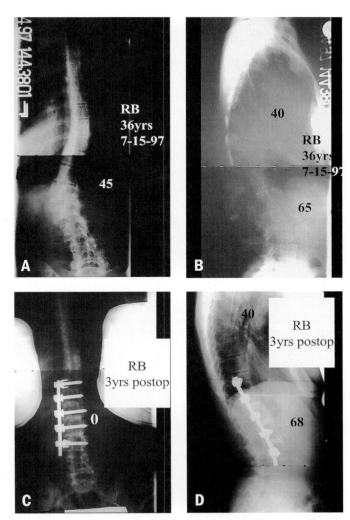

Figure 5 A, Long cassette, standing, coronal radiograph of a 36-year-old woman with progressive lumbar and lumbosacral pain, and failed conservative treatment. **B,** Standing, lateral, radiographs on long cassette film demonstrates normal sagittal alignment with thoracolumbar kyphosis. MRI demonstrates dehydration of the L4-5 and L5-S1 discs with normal hydration of the L3-4 disc. Patient was treated with anterior multilevel discectomies of T11 to L2 and fusion with anterior instrumentation from T11 to L2 with total correction of the primary deformity and horizontalization of the L3 vertebrae. Structural allograft and a femoral ring were used anteriorly with autogenous rib graft. **C,** Long cassette, standing, coronal radiograph taken 3 years after surgery shows total correction of the lumbar primary deformity and horizontal alignment of L3 relative to the pelvis. Complete thigh pain relief with rotational correction was noted clinically. **D,** Long cassette, standing, sagittal radiograph taken 3 years after surgery demonstrates restoration of sagittal alignment and anterior bony incorporation of the lumbar spine from T11 to L3. The plumb line from C7 falls between the lumbosacral disc.

will provide multiplane correction and spinal balance (Fig 7).

Long-cassette radiographs to check intraoperative alignment of the long constructs to the pelvis are essential to avoid unrecognized decompensation. Postoperative immobilization for patients undergoing extensive, long constructs to the sacral pelvic region is individualized, depending on the patient's BMD, integrity of the spinal fixation constructs, and the surgeon's discretion.

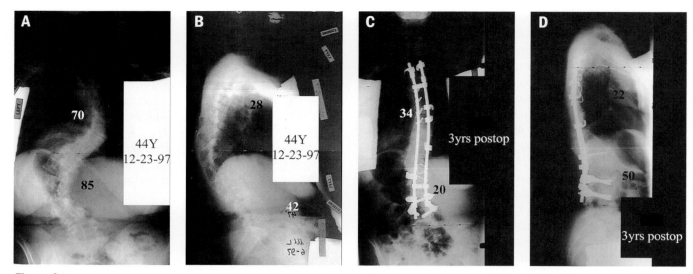

Figure 6 Long cassette, standing, coronal **(A)** and sagittal **(B)** radiographs of a 44-year-old woman with idiopathic scoliosis treated with a brace as a teenager. Patient had progressive lumbar pain, fatigue, and loss of height over the previous 10 years. Double major thoracic and lumbar scoliosis with minimal flexibility was seen on side-bending radiographs. MRI of the lumbar spine demonstrated normal hydration of the L4-5 and L5-S1 discs. The sagittal upright radiograph shows the shortening of the trunk with thoracolumbar kyphosis. The patient was treated using anterior discectomies and fusion performed from T11 to L4 using morcellized rib graft supplemented with femoral head cancellous allograft and posterior segmental instrumentation with dual rods and multiple fixation points. Thoracic hooks and distal lumbar pedicle screws and sublaminar wires for translational correction of the apical thoracic and lumbar deformity were used. Note the improvement in the tilt of L4 relative to the pelvis. Coronal **(C)** and sagittal **(D)** upright standing radiographs taken 3 years after surgery.

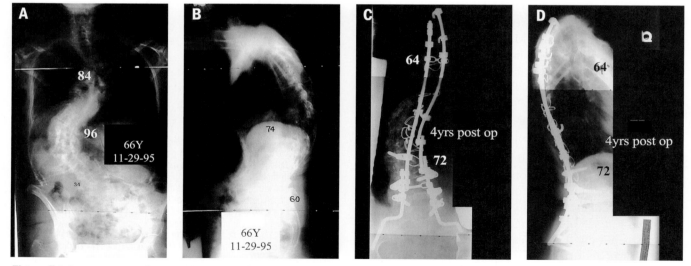

Figure 7 A, Long cassette, standing, coronal radiograph of a 66-year-old woman with untreated idiopathic scoliosis who has developed progressive decompensation, loss of height, and lumbar pain. Shortening of the trunk is noted with the rib cage abutting the iliac crests; the patient has difficulty with eating because of early fullness. **B,** Long cassette, standing, radiograph in the sagittal plane. Note the thoracolumbar kyphosis and shortening of the trunk height. Patient was treated with an anterior multilevel discectomy and fusion via a thoracolumbar approach from T11 to S1, morcellized autograft with a rib and supplemented with femoral head cancellous allograft, and same-day posterior multilevel rod segmental fixation from T2 to the sacropelvis via the use of Galveston rods placed into the ilium. **C,** Long cassette, standing, coronal radiograph taken 4 years after surgery. Note substantial correction of the thoracic and lumbar curves. Balanced correction with plumb line from T1 falling through the middle of the sacrum. **D,** Long cassette, standing, sagittal radiographs showing restoration of sagittal alignment, trunk lengthening, and thoracic and lumbar kyphosis.

Degenerative Scoliosis

Degenerative scoliosis, or de novo scoliosis as it is sometimes called, occurs in a patient who had a straight spine until middle age. When first described, it was thought to occur because of osteoporosis but this theory has not borne out. Degenerative scoliosis results from degeneration of the discs and facet joints and may lead to instability, causing rotation, lateral listhesis, or spondylolisthesis. This problem usually occurs in the mid to low lumbar spine, producing a domino-like effect of rotation and translation into the upper lumbar and sometimes the thoracolumbar spine.

Prevalence and Natural History

Prevalence is reportedly 6%, and the average age of those seeking medical care is in the 60s. The deformity may progress with an average of 3.3° in a year. The full extent of the natural history is not fully delineated. Degenerative scoliosis occurs in male as well as female patients, with a higher percentage of male patients than seen in adult idiopathic scoliosis, which primarily is seen in females. The most common complaint in patients with degenerative scoliosis is related to compression of the neural elements. Neurogenic claudication or radicular symptoms lead these patients to seek medical attention. Back pain may be present but is not the primary symptom. In moderate to severe degenerative scoliosis, decompensation will also be a complaint. A thorough review of systems has to be performed to rule out other conditions that might simulate symptoms of back pain and claudication; for example, smoldering pancreatitis or arterial insufficiency. Assessment of comorbidities such as diabetes, heart disease, or pulmonary disease is essential because they may enter into the treatment decision making.

On physical examination, neurologic deficits may not be present. Coronal and sagittal plane decompensation should be noted. Neurologic examination, including long-tract signs should be checked to ensure cervical myelopathy is not present because of cervical spondylosis, which often is present in patients in this age group.

Diagnostic Evaluation

Full-length radiographs are necessary to evaluate compensatory curves above the usual lumbar curve as well as coronal and sagittal balance. The most common findings are marked facet arthrosis, lateral and rotatory listhesis, and spondylolisthesis. The curve magnitudes are generally smaller than found in adult idiopathic cases. On the lateral radiograph, decrease in disc height at multiple levels, osteophytes at multiple levels, and flattening of the lumbar lordosis are seen. However, the thoracic spine may be spared such changes.

MRI scan provides an excellent screening as well as diagnostic test to assess spinal stenosis, disc degeneration, and marrow abnormalities. Because most of these curves are mild, MRI is frequently adequate. In larger curves, CT myelogram may be necessary to assess the spinal stenosis and bone detail more carefully. Discography has not been found to be as useful in this population because the disc morphologically appears degenerated at multiple levels and does not have a dependable concordant pain response. Bending and supine hyperextension radiographs may be useful in assessing the flexibility of the spine, especially when the surgeon is contemplating a posterior procedure only versus a combined anterior release and posterior fusion and instrumentation.

Nonsurgical Treatment

Treatment with nonsteroidal anti-inflammatory medication, epidural injections, and lumbar corset may help alleviate some of the symptoms. A patient who is not debilitated may benefit from aerobic conditioning exercise in maintaining strength and flexibility of the lower extremities and spine, with an additional long-term benefit of preventing further progression of osteoporosis.

Surgical Treatment

The goals of surgical treatment are decompression of the neural elements and achieving a balanced and stable spine. Decompression alone is indicated in patients who have mild scoliosis with no signs of instability, such as lateral listhesis, rotatory subluxation, or spondylolisthesis. These patients frequently require two-level laminectomy with foraminotomies with careful preservation of the pars interarticularis and facet joints. Patients who have curves greater than 30° and signs of instability require a concomitant posterior spinal fusion and instrumentation.

Most patients who are in good balance can be treated in the above manner. Patients who have sagittal imbalance or, more commonly, are leaning forward imbalanced in the coronal plane, require additional anterior release and fusion. The anterior release improves correction and fusion rates. Anterior procedures extend the ability of the surgeon to create improvement in the lumbar lordosis and obviate extension of the fusion into the thoracic spine.

When long fusions are performed to the sacrum, anterior strut graft at the lumbosacral junction at L4-L5 and L5-S1 levels not only improved the fusion rate but also reduced the biomechanical stress on instrumentation such as the pedicle screws in the sacrum. Distal extension of the instrumentation to the pelvis via Galveston technique, iliac bolts, intrasacral rod placement, or S2 screws also helps reduce the strain on the S1 screws and the rod at the lumbosacral junction. The sacropelvic extension is especially critical in patients with osteoporosis (Fig. 8). Posterior lumbar interbody graft with placement of structural grafts or cages can provide distraction and increase the foraminal height and interpedicular distance at the levels of foraminal stenosis and in the concavity of fractional lumbosacral curves.

Patients who have undergone previous extensive decompression may come to the physician with persistent stenosis and neurogenic claudication because of segmental instability, stenosis, and multiplane deformity. They lack posterior elements and sufficient surface area

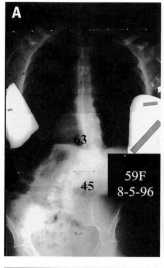

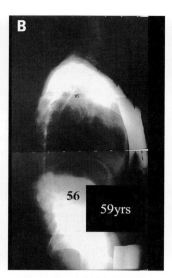

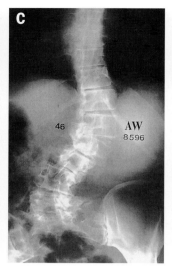

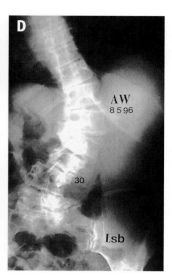

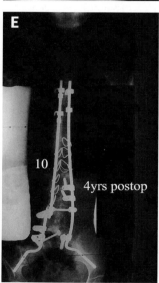

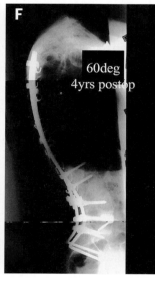

Figure 8 A, Long cassette, standing, coronal radiograph of a 58-year-old woman with painful degenerative lumbar scoliosis and rotatory subluxation of the L2-3 and L3-4 discs. Note the translational decompensation of the trunk relative to the pelvis. **B,** Long cassette, standing, sagittal radiograph shows the loss of lumbar lordosis with thoracolumbar kyphosis and shortening of the trunk. **C,** Supine side-bending radiograph demonstrates moderate flexibility of the lumbar curve. Note the significant rotatory subluxations of L2-3 and L3-4, osteophytes of the facets and intervertebral discs and the concavity of the lumbar and lumbosacral fractional curves. MRI demonstrated significant disc space narrowing and degeneration of the spine. **D,** Left side-bending radiograph shows moderate flexibility of the lumbosacral fractional curve. The subluxations of L2-3 and L3-4 persist on side bending to the left. The patient was treated with a one-stage combined anterior lumbar discectomy and fusion from T11 to the sacrum, and posterior segmental instrumentation and fusion to the sacrum. Femoral ring allografts and AO screw fixation as a graft retainer at L4-5 and L5-S1 and morcellized autologous rib graft were used for the remaining levels. **E,** Long cassette, standing, coronal radiograph taken 4 years after surgery. Note the balance correction and trunk realignment relative to the pelvis with a plumb line from C7 falling to the middle of the lumbosacral spine. **F,** Long cassette, standing, radiograph taken 4 years after surgery demonstrates the sagittal alignment and the significant increase in lumbar lordosis created by lengthening the anterior column with structural grafts and prebending the rod to obtain physiologic sagittal contour.

for fusion and are best treated with a combined anterior and posterior procedure. The morbidity of anterior and posterior surgery in these elderly patients should not be taken lightly. They frequently require Intensive Care Unit care postoperatively, and surgery sometimes has to be staged, especially if there is a long fusion to the pelvis.

Revision and Salvage Deformity Surgery

Revision of previous surgery for spinal deformity provides spine specialists with some of their most complex and challenging cases. Failed spinal deformity surgery can be the result of a pseudarthrosis with failure of instrumentation and progression of deformity, prominence of hardware, degeneration of levels above or below, spinal decompensation, or progressive deformity adjacent to a successful fusion. Each of these scenarios

has its individual challenges. Plain radiographs may not be helpful. CT scan or polytomography can be used to help delineate the fusion mass. CT myelogram or gadolinium-enhanced MRI scan, if titanium has been used for instrumentation, can be used to evaluate the spinal canal. The conditions that need revision and salvage deformity surgery can be divided into three main categories: painful deformity, progressive deformity, and acquired deformity.

Painful Deformity

Painful deformity can be the result of prominent or painful hardware that localizes in one area. A pseudarthrosis can be painful and lead to hardware failure. Oblique radiographs, polytomography, or CT may be helpful in delineating a pseudarthrosis. Finally, the surgeon may have to explore the fusion mass after hardware removal. In general, the periosteum strips easily in the presence of a solid fusion. The pseudarthrosis should be repaired and the spine reinstrumented. Anterior augmentation with bone at the level of the pseudarthrosis should be considered for multilevel pseudarthroses. Degeneration adjacent to the fusion proximally or distally can create pain as well as symptoms of spinal stenosis with hypertrophy of the ligamentum flavum and facet joints. These areas can be evaluated using a CT myelogram or MRI. Decompression and extension of the fusion is all that may be required in such cases. Disc degeneration causing back pain alone without any symptoms of spinal stenosis may be evaluated with MRI or discography and the fusion extended.

Progressive Deformity

Pseudarthrosis may lead to progressive deformity. The deformity, if not acceptable, should be corrected through the area of the pseudarthrosis as an osteotomy site with revision of posterior instrumentation. If the deformity is acceptable, the pseudarthrosis may be repaired, posterior instrumentation revised, and anterior fusion considered for multilevel pseudarthroses.

Junctional kyphosis can occur above and below a previously fused spine, and progressive deformity can result from progression of the unfused compensatory curve. These can be addressed with appropriate extension of the fusion and osteotomies of segments of the previously fused spine to achieve balanced correction (Fig. 9).

Acquired Deformity

The classic example of acquired deformity is a flat back after a successful fusion posteriorly with Harrington rod instrumentation. This condition leads to a crouched position, fatigue in the quadriceps, and degeneration of segments below, with symptoms of spinal stenosis. Flat back can be treated in several ways, including posterior osteotomies, anterior and posterior osteotomies, and pedicle subtraction osteotomy (Fig. 10).

Reconstruction Techniques

Reconstruction techniques are anterior osteotomies and posterior osteotomies, decancellation or pedicle subtraction osteotomies, and vertebral column resection. The most common procedure includes spinal osteotomies. Posterior spinal osteotomies are performed through the area of fusion between the transverse processes. After entering the epidural space with a burr or rongeur, Kerrison rongeurs are used to remove bone from the midline through the intertransverse foramen bilaterally. Posterior osteotomies at multiple levels are excellent ways for achieving correction over a large radius. Anterior osteotomies, if needed, are performed through the area of the ankylosed or fused disc space. The surgeon must identify the foramen and the pedicles before using an osteotome or a high-speed burr to resect down to the posterior cortex. The posterior cortex is removed with Kerrison rongeurs or curettes. Gel

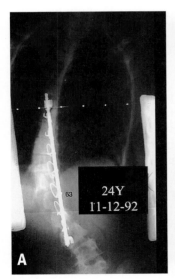
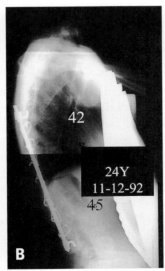
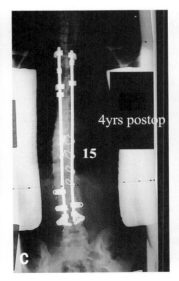
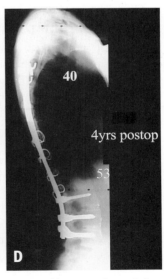

Figure 9 Long cassette standing coronal **(A)** and sagittal **(B)** radiographs of a 24-year-old woman who has undergone previous Harrington rod instrumentation, posterior fusion, and segmental wiring. The patient developed progressive trunk decompensation and low back pain associated with fatigue. Lateral radiograph demonstrated a straightening of the upper lumbar spine and thoracolumbar kyphosis. Note no contouring of the posterior instrumentation. The patient was treated with a same-day combined anterior multilevel discectomy and fusion of the thoracolumbar spine from T11 to L4 followed by posterior fusion mass exploration, removal of the Harrington instrumentation and sublaminar wires, osteotomies at multiple levels of the thoracic and lumbar spine from T11 to L3, and posterior segmental instrumentation from T3 to L4 with restoration of sagittal and coronal plane alignment. **C,** Long cassette, standing, coronal radiograph of the patient taken 4 years after surgery. Note significant improvement of the scoliosis and horizontal alignment of the lower end instrumented L4 vertebra via lumbar pedicle screws. **D,** Long cassette standing lateral radiographs taken 4 years after surgery demonstrates the restoration of sagittal contour and physiologic alignment, with a plumb line from C7 falling through the lumbosacral disc and a solid anterior fusion via use of morcellized autograft with rib and femoral head cancellous allograft.

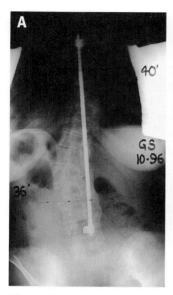
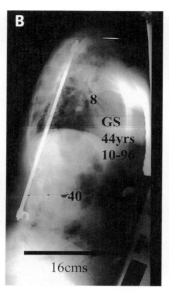
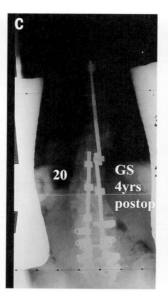
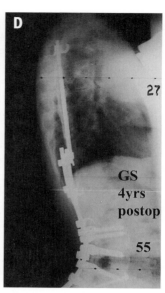

Figure 10 Long cassette, coronal **(A)** and sagittal **(B)** radiographs of a 44-year-old woman who had been treated with posterior spinal fusion from T4 to L4 using Harrington distraction instrumentation. The patient had a progressive painful deformity and loss of lumbar lordosis. Since her surgery, she had been pitching forward with fatigue. Her coronal balance is acceptable. However, the patient is in significant positive balance on the standing sagittal radiographs, with a plumb line from C7 falling 16 cm anterior to the lumbosacral disc. Note straightening of the lumbar spine and lack of contouring of the distraction instrumentation. Patient was treated with same-day anterior multilevel discectomies and fusion from L2 to the sacrum, with femoral ring allografts at L4-5 and L5-S1 with AO screw transfixation as a graft retainer and morcellized local bone and femoral head cancellous allograft for L3-4 and L2-3. The anterior procedure was followed with posterior exploration of the fusion mass, osteotomies at L2-3 and L3-4, and facetectomies at L4-5 and L5-S1, with segmental dual rod instrumentation. The right-sided rod was connected with special connector to the upper half of the Harrington instrumentation, which was imbedded in the fusion mass. Long cassette, standing, coronal **(C)** and sagittal **(D)** radiographs taken 4 years after surgery. The sagittal view shows excellent sagittal alignment, with a plumb line falling from C7 through the lumbosacral disc and restoration of lumbar lordosis.

foam and bone wax can be used to control bleeding. The surgeon may have to go back and forth between multiple osteotomy sites to control bleeding.

Results and Complications

A balanced surgical correction of adult idiopathic scoliosis and deformity with solid arthrodesis will not completely alleviate pain. The severity of pain improves but the frequency does not. The risks of infection, neurologic injury, prominent hardware, fretting and corrosion, and junctional problems such as degeneration and deformity continue to be challenges in this surgery. Improved anesthesia, spinal monitoring, and intensive care medicine advances have markedly improved perioperative care.

The morbidity associated with bone grafting remains a problem. Arthrodesis from autograft is still the gold standard. Allograft supplementation and, in the future, bone graft substitutes such as ceramics or demineralized bone and biologic enhancement with bone morphogenic proteins or growth factors may improve fusion rates, but problems associated with arthrodesis of the spine still will not be eliminated.

The use of segmental instrumentation has decreased the necessity of postoperative casting or bracing. Patients who undergo revision surgery face the risks of

surgery again, but have a better chance of achieving a successful outcome with the revision and salvage techniques complemented by modern segmental instrumentation techniques. Correction of the deformity has positive effects on the self-image, pain, fatigue, and self-confidence of the patient.

Neurologic Complications

In general, neurologic complications in adult scoliosis surgery are uncommon, occurring in less than 1% to 5% of patients. Risks are greater with complex deformity reconstruction that combines anterior and posterior spinal surgery for severe rigid curves and in patients undergoing revision surgery. Direct injury of neural elements can result from instrumentation (hooks, wires, and screws) or from indirect injury caused by ischemic insult or neurapraxia related to distractive forces. The use of the intraoperative wake-up test and intraoperative spinal cord monitoring by somatosensory and motor evoked potentials will help alert the surgeon to the onset of such injuries and limit these complications. For complex procedures such as osteotomies for revision surgery, nerve root or dura entrapment may result if the edges of the osteotomy and the foramina are not carefully undercut to allow adequate space for the neural elements after correction of the deformity.

Pseudarthrosis

Failed fusion is the most common complication related directly to adult spinal deformity surgery. The pseudarthrosis rates vary between 5% and 28%, with high rates occurring after revision spinal surgery. Factors that increase the pseudarthrosis rate include the use of predominantly allogeneic bone, as opposed to the use of autologous bone graft, and the use of nonsegmented spinal instrumentation in the distraction mode.

Wound Infection

Wound infection following spinal deformity surgery in adults varies from 1% to 8%. Infection after anterior surgery alone is very rare compared to infection after the posterior procedures. The use of preoperative broad-spectrum intravenous antibiotics, meticulous wound handling, and nutritional augmentation for patients undergoing staged procedures decreases infection and wound healing complications.

Spinal Decompensation

Spinal decompensation is most commonly related to improper selection of fusion levels. When installing corrective instrumentation for adult deformity, attention must be paid to achieving balance in both coronal and sagittal planes in a standing position for the ambulatory patient. Progressive decompensation and deformity caudal to an arthrodesis may occur if instrumentation is terminated proximal to a stable vertebra or if there is a significant residual tilt of the lower-end instrumented vertebra. One of the most devastating postsurgical deformities is flat back resulting from distraction in the distal lumbar spine. Commonly overlooked aspects of maintaining lumbar lordosis are proper positioning of the patient and correct bending of the rod for lordosis. Another potential complication is termination of instrumentation at the sagittal apex of a curve, most commonly in the thoracolumbar spine, which can result in progressive junctional kyphosis and iatrogenic sagittal decompensation. Failure to fuse all structural curves in double major curves may also lead to postsurgical decompensation. Overcorrection during selective thoracic fusion, especially with rotational maneuvers may also result in progressive coronal plane imbalance. Attempts should be made to correct the thoracic deformity to within the correctability of the lumbar spine to maintain balance.

Posterior Element Failure at the Bone-Metal Interface

Osteoporosis may compromise the stability of instrumentation applied posteriorly, which may lead to fracture of the lamina or transverse process during corrective maneuvers. Evaluation of bone mineral density helps in the choice of implant and fixation points and the amount of corrective force that should be applied to achieve desired balance correction. To reduce the occurrence of bone-metal interface failure, a large number of fixation points may be required. For rigid deformities in the presence of osteopenia, anterior discectomies and fusions combined with posterior arthrodesis and instrumentation will be needed to provide a more supple correctable deformity, reducing the amount of corrective force that needs to be applied at each fixation point. In the osteopenic thoracic spine, the lamina rather than the transverse process or spinous process is the fixation point of choice for hook claw constructs. Pedicle screws at the caudal end of an instrumentation provide for a stronger foundation for long constructs. For fixation to the sacrum, the addition of an intrailiac (Galveston) or intrasacral (Jackson) fixation will help enhance the distal foundation and stability and reduce the risk of sacral screw failure, and anterior structural grafts will increase the longevity and stability of the construct.

Summary and Conclusion

The clinical presentation and surgical indications for adult idiopathic scoliosis with or without superimposed degenerative changes, adult de novo degenerative scoliosis, and postsurgical deformity are generally distinct from those of adolescent scoliosis patients. Most patients complain of pain, progressive deformity, or symptoms of neurogenic claudication related to spinal stenosis. Clinical assessment is more complex and should include CT myelography, MRI scan, discography, bone scan, and bone density assessment. Recovery from surgery for the adult patient usually takes longer, often requiring up to 1 or 2 years for full recovery.

Most adults with flexible thoracic and thoracolumbar balance deformities fare well with posterior spinal reconstruction alone. Selective anterior thoracolumbar and lumbar fusion and instrumentation will also provide balance correction for most adults with moderate curves of the thoracolumbar spine with flexible thoracic curves and lumbosacral fractional curves. Adults with decompensated thoracolumbar-lumbar rigid deformities and large rigid thoracic curves benefit from combined anterior discectomy and fusion and posterior segmental instrumentation. Arthrodesis to the sacrum should be used sparingly and only in adults with significant degenerative changes at the lumbosacral junction with oblique take-off of L5 or complex translational deformities that include the lumbosacral region. Patients who require fusion to the sacrum have the most complications related to nonunion and balance problems.

Outcome instruments for adult scoliosis surgery are still in the process of development. Preliminary outcome studies have shown improved quality of life for most appropriately selected adult patients. A study using the SF-36 for adult patients with spinal deformity showed significant improvement in self-reported health assessment and function and that the beneficial results did not appear to deteriorate with age or in those with more caudal end vertebral levels of fusion. Studies combining disease-specific outcome analysis and generic health surveys to evaluate the end results would be useful for future evaluation of the adult patient considering spinal reconstructive surgery for deformity. Currently under investigation are North American Spine Society and Scoliosis Research Society outcome instruments.

Annotated Bibliography

Adult Idiopathic Scoliosis

Albert TJ, Purtill J, Mesa J, McIntosh T, Balderston RA: Health outcome assessment before and after adult deformity surgery: A prospective study. *Spine* 1995;20: 2002-2005.

This prospective study using SF-36 showed that spinal deformity surgery statistically improved physical function, social function, bodily pain, and perceived health change, with an average follow-up of 22.5 months.

Bradford DS, Tay BK, Hu SS: Adult scoliosis: Surgical indications, operative management, complications, and outcomes. *Spine* 1999;24:2617-2629.

This review article discusses the current treatment methodologies and controversies in the treatment of adult idiopathic scoliosis.

Dick J, Boachie-Adjei O, Wilson M: One-stage versus two-stage anterior and posterior spinal reconstruction in adults: Comparison of outcomes including nutritional status, complication rates, hospital costs and other factors. *Spine* 1992;17(suppl 8):S310-S316.

A prospective review of 24 adults treated with either one- or two-stage combined anterior and posterior surgery showed a high prevalence of postoperative malnutrition in the staged patients, who also had a higher postoperative morbidity, longer hospital stay, and higher hospital costs.

Haher TR, Merola A, Zipnick RI, Gorup J, Mannor D, Orchowski J: Meta-analysis of surgical outcome in adolescent idiopathic scoliosis: A 35-year English literature review of 11,000 patients. *Spine* 1995;20:1575-1584.

The meta-analysis showed that there was a significant correlation between the amount of correction and percentage of patient satisfaction.

Horton WC, Holt RT, Muldowny DS: Controversy: Fusion of L5-S1 in adult scoliosis. *Spine* 1996;21:2520-2522.

A discussion of this controversial topic is presented.

Kostuik JP, Musha Y: Extension to the sacrum of previous adolescent scoliosis fusions in adult life. *Clin Orthop* 1999;364:53-60.

Experience with a large number of patients and an evolution of the techniques are shared.

Lenke LG, Bridwell KH, Blanke K, Baldus C: Analysis of pulmonary function and chest cage dimension changes after thoracoplasty in idiopathic scoliosis. *Spine* 1995;20:1343-1350.

After thoracoplasty, the adult patients showed a decline of 27% in pulmonary function with a residual 23% decrease left at 2-year follow-up.

Weinstein SL: Natural history. *Spine* 1999;24:2592-2600.

This review article discusses the various aspects of natural history for idiopathic scoliosis including curve progression, back pain, pulmonary function, mortality, psychological effects, and pregnancy.

Degenerative Scoliosis

Grubb SA, Lipscomb HJ, Suh PB: Results of surgical treatment of painful adult scoliosis. *Spine* 1994;19:1619-1627.

Seventy percent pain relief after surgery was found in patients with degenerative scoliosis.

Zurbriggen C, Markwalder TM, Wyss S: Long-term results in patients treated with posterior instrumentation and fusion for degenerative scoliosis of the lumbar spine. *Acta Neurochir (Wien)* 1999;141:21-26.

The authors report a homogeneously investigated and surgically treated series of 40 patients with degenerative scoliosis of the lumbar spine. The results suggest that maintenance or correction of lumbar lordosis is more important than the conversion of the scoliotic deformity, which is probably treated sufficiently by partial correction and stabilization.

Revision and Salvage Deformity Surgery

Bradford DS, Tribus CB: Vertebral column resection for the treatment of rigid coronal decompensation. *Spine* 1997;22:1590-1599.

Twenty four patients with fixed coronal imbalance underwent vertebral column resection safely, with 82% improvement in coronal balance and 52% improvement in scoliosis.

Hu SS, Fontaine F, Kelly B, Bradford DS: Nutritional depletion in staged spinal reconstructive surgery: The effect of total parenteral nutrition. *Spine* 1998;23:1401-1405.

Total parenteral nutrition was found to lessen the decrease in albumin and prealbumin in patients requiring staged reconstructive surgery. Patients with nutritional depletion were found to have more perioperative infectious complications.

Rawlins B, Boachie-Adjei O: Revision adult spinal deformity surgery. *Semin Spine Surg* 1997;169-180.

This is a comprehensive review of the major causes of failed adult spinal deformity surgery, patients' clinical appearance, and salvage and reconstruction methods.

Complications

Bridwell KH, Lenke LG, Baldus C, Blanke K: Major intraoperative neurologic deficits in pediatric and adult spinal deformity patients: Incidence and etiology at one institution. *Spine* 1998;23:324-331.

In four patients who suffered major neurologic deficits at one institution, anterior and posterior surgery as well as hyperkyphosis were identified as risk factors for neurologic deficits during spinal deformity surgery.

Myers MA, Hamilton SR, Bogosian AJ, Smith C, Wagner TA: Visual loss as a complication of spine surgery: A review of 37 cases. *Spine* 1997;22:1325-1329.

Twenty-seven cases from a survey of Scoliosis Research Society members and 10 cases from the literature were reviewed in an attempt to determine the etiology or risk factors of this complication. The etiology is still not known.

Classic Bibliography

Byrd JA III, Scoles PV, Winter RB, Bradford DS, Lonstein JE, Moe JH: Adult idiopathic scoliosis treated by anterior and posterior spinal fusion. *J Bone Joint Surg Am* 1987;69:843-850.

Marchesi DG, Aebi M: Pedicle fixation devices in the treatment of adult lumbar scoliosis. *Spine* 1992;17(suppl 8):S304-S309.

Perennou D, Marcelli C, Herisson C, Simon L: Adult lumbar scoliosis: Epidemiologic aspects in a low back pain population. *Spine* 1994;19:123-128.

Simmons ED Jr, Kowalski JM, Simmons EH: The results of surgical treatment for adult scoliosis. *Spine* 1993;18:718-724.

Simmons ED Jr, Simmons EH: Spinal stenosis with scoliosis. *Spine* 1992;17(suppl 6):S117-S120.

Sponseller PD, Cohen MS, Nachemson AL, Hall JE, Wohl ME: Results of surgical treatment of adults with idiopathic scoliosis. *J Bone Joint Surg Am* 1987;69:667-675.

Swank S, Lonstein JE, Moe JH, Winter RB, Bradford DS: Surgical treatment of adult scoliosis: A review of two hundred and twenty-two cases. *J Bone Joint Surg Am* 1981;63:268-287.

Vanderpool DW, James JI, Wynne-Davies R: Scoliosis in the elderly. *J Bone Joint Surg Am* 1969;51:446-455.

Weinstein SL, Ponseti IV: Curve progression in idiopathic scoliosis. *J Bone Joint Surg Am* 1983;65:447-455.

Chapter 40

Surgical Care of Arthritides of the Spine

Jeffrey S. Fischgrund, MD

Ankylosing Spondylitis

Ankylosing spondylitis is an inflammatory spondyloarthropathy that primarily affects the axial skeleton, beginning with sacroiliitis. The hallmarks of advanced disease are formation of syndesmophytes and eventual ankylosis with kyphosis of the spine. The disease is predominant in men and is characterized by chronic low back pain of insidious onset, usually beginning in early adulthood. Since the initial association of HLA-B27 with ankylosing spondylitis in 1972, there has been continued debate regarding the role of this protein in the initiation of a spondyloarthropathy. Molecular mimicry is the oldest theory, describing an autoimmune response initially mounted against a peptide from an infectious agent, which is directed against HLA-B27 itself. Newer studies have theorized that the presence of HLA-B27 could result in defective immunity against certain microorganisms, possibly by influencing T-cell response. Additionally, genetic influences may interact with HLA-B27 to produce a spectrum of spondyloarthropathies.

Although this disease is characterized by back pain and stiffness, there are numerous significant nonspinal manifestations of ankylosing spondylitis. Patients are frequently afflicted with arthritis of the peripheral joints, and acute anterior uveitis is a common finding. Occasionally, serious systemic diseases occur including renal amyloidosis, cardiac conduction disturbances, and cardiac valve dysfunctions.

The most effective measure of trunk deformity in ankylosing spondylitis is the chin-brow to vertical angle. This angle is formed by a line from the brow to the chin, through the vertical, when the patient stands with the hips and knees fully extended with the neck in its neutral or fixed position. Hip flexion contractures can also result in significant sagittal imbalance and may need to be corrected prior to spinal osteotomy.

A difficult clinical scenario often occurs when a patient with ankylosing spondylitis presents following blunt trauma or involvement in a motor vehicle acci-

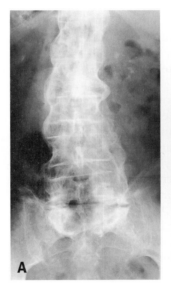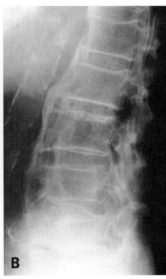

Figure 1 AP **(A)** and lateral **(B)** radiographs of the lumbar spine in a patient with ankylosing spondylitis. This patient presented to the emergency room with increasing back pain following a minor motor vehicle accident. Careful review of the radiographs show a cleft in the fusion mass at L5-S1. A bone scan confirmed increased activity of this level, indicative of a new fracture.

dent. These patients are more prone to spinal injury because of rigidity of the spinal column and osteoporosis. Radiographs are often difficult to interpret because of distortion of the normal anatomy, ossification of the spinal ligaments, and overall kyphotic alignment. Injuries in the lower cervical spine and cervicothoracic region frequently occur, and this is probably the most difficult region to see on plain radiographs. A high index of suspicion must be present, and the entire spine must adequately be seen in any patient who presents with increasing pain or change in their deformity (Fig. 1).

Additional imaging modalities are frequently required following trauma in patients with ankylosing spondylitis. CT scans are not practical when trying to visualize the entire spine, and bone scans are frequently nonspecific, with difficulty differentiating occult fracture from degenerative changes. Recent studies have shown MRI to be a reliable test for detecting occult fractures in patients with ankylosing spondylitis. Although costs and availability remain significant issues, the increased sensitivity of this test greatly improves the clinician's chances of diagnosing an occult fracture. Frequently, a screening MRI involving a single midline sequence using a large field of view can make both the cervical and upper thoracic spine visible in one image, with the lower lumbar spine being imaged in a second film. Diagnostic clues leading toward a diagnosis of occult fracture include intramedullary edema, disc space injury, spinal cord injury, or epidural hematoma. Early diagnosis of occult fracture is important because there is an increased incidence of secondary or late neurologic deficits with missed spinal fractures, compared with those individuals whose fractures were identified on the initial screening.

The management of acute fractures in ankylosing spondylitis follows the same guidelines as the treatment of fractures in patients without ankylosing spondylitis. The fracture should be reduced and realigned to relieve or prevent spinal cord injury, and patient transfers should be minimized because of the risk of further injury. Because of spinal ankylosis, which results in long lever arms, stresses are concentrated at the fracture site and prompt rigid immobilization by either surgical or external means is required. A halo brace can be used for most nondisplaced cervical spine fractures. Patients who present with worsening of their cervical kyphosis may have a gentle awake reduction performed, followed by application of the halo brace. Although correction of a preexisting deformity is possible through a fracture site, extreme caution is mandated during this maneuver because excessive motion at the fracture site could lead to epidural hematoma and resultant neurologic compression. Displaced thoracolumbar injuries frequently require rigid surgical stabilization to prevent further displacement and promote healing.

Surgical Treatment

The surgical treatment of ankylosing spondylitis has shown little change in technique over the past 5 years. The basic technique of cervical osteotomy has changed little since the initial description by Simmons in 1972. Although there have been advances in fixation and monitoring techniques, the basic principles remain relevant.

The predominant indication for an extension osteotomy of the cervical spine is a significant flexion deformity at the cervicothoracic junction that limits the patient's visual field. Significant deformity can also interfere with eating and swallowing because severe flexion can cause a chin-on-chest deformity, thus limiting jaw excursion. Originally, the osteotomy was performed under local anesthesia with the patient in a sitting position. Following a posterior cervical laminectomy, the patient is briefly anesthetized while the spine is fractured anteriorly, followed by rapid return to consciousness. This technique allows for immediate neurologic evaluation as patients can be instructed to move all four limbs. If significant weakness or radicular pain is noted on reawakening, the amount of correction is lessened, thereby relieving neural compression.

Advances in anesthetic and intubation techniques, as well as spinal cord monitoring, have led recent authors to recommend this procedure be performed under a general anesthetic. Somatosensory-evoked potentials, motor-evoked potentials, and spontaneous electromyograms can be used singularly or in combination to monitor the status of the spinal cord and nerve roots during the corrective phase of the procedure. Finally, if doubt remains regarding the neurologic status of the patient because of changes in evoked potentials, a wake-up test can safely be performed.

Most authors of current studies advocate the use of postoperative immobilization, commonly in a halo jacket. The original surgical technique also did not incorporate the use of any cervical instrumentation. Recent advances in spinal instrumentation have been applied to the treatment of patients with ankylosing spondylitis. Options for cervical fixation include rods with Drummond buttons, various types of interspinous process wiring, or more recently, the use of hybrid constructs incorporating screws and/or hooks in the lower cervical and upper thoracic spine (Fig. 2). Caution should be used when placing hooks in the cervical or thoracic spine in the patient with ankylosing spondylitis because the dura is frequently adherent to the undersurface of the lamina.

Although there has been a dramatic increase in the number of spinal implants available over the past 5 years, there have been remarkably few studies describing their use for fixation following cervical osteotomies. The largest single study described 15 patients with ankylosing spondylitis who had severe flexion deformities and underwent extension osteotomies at C7-T1. This report noted a mean correction of 54°, with all patients able to see straight ahead following the surgical procedure. No patients developed quadriparesis immediately following the surgical procedure, although one patient became permanently quadriparetic 1 week after the index procedure. Somatosensory-evoked potentials were used in this study, but this modality failed to detect the occurrence of two cases of C8 radiculopathy following the osteotomy.

Primary thoracic kyphosis can also lead to significant sagittal imbalance. If the thoracic kyphosis is mild or

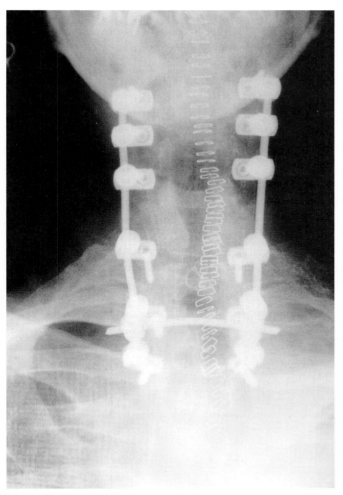

Figure 2 AP postoperative radiograph following cervical osteotomy for ankylosing spondylitis. Lateral mass screws are used in the lower cervical spine, while pedicle screws are used at the cervicothoracic junction. (Courtesy of Alexander Vaccaro, MD, Philadelphia, PA.)

moderate, the overall spinal deformity may be corrected by a compensatory osteotomy in the lumbar spine. In this procedure, the lumbar spine is overcorrected to compensate for the thoracic kyphosis. Correction of the thoracic kyphosis is significantly more dangerous than correction of lumbar kyphosis and, if required, should be performed with multiple osteotomies such that the correction at any one level is minimal.

Osteotomy of the lumbar spine and correction of the kyphotic deformity were first reported in 1945. Multiple techniques of osteotomies have been described, including closing wedge, opening wedge, decancellation procedures, and pedicle subtraction osteotomies. Most authors recommend the osteotomy be performed between the second and fourth lumbar vertebrae.

The largest recent report described 175 patients with a fixed flexion deformity of the lumbar spine resulting from ankylosing spondylitis who underwent surgical

correction. These patients had multiple V-shaped posterior lumbar osteotomies and correction with either a Harrington compression system or a transpedicular segmental fixation system. The authors of this study found that the most common complication occurred when multiple segmental osteotomies were performed, but correction occurred almost exclusively in one segment, resulting in sharply angular lordosis at one level. This complication occurred much more frequently with the Harrington compression system than with transpedicular fixation. The patients who presented in an advanced stage of syndesmophytosis were noted to have a higher incidence of unisegmental correction, with the postoperative paraplegic rate as high as 9%, which reversed after decompression. Multilevel lumbar osteotomies with multisegmental correction of lordosis by transpedicular screw fixation is a safer method of surgery in terms of neurologic and fatal vascular complications. More recent studies have advocated the use of transpedicular closing wedge osteotomy, which avoids the use of sudden forces because it is a closing osteoclasis rather than an opening wedge osteotomy. This eliminates tension forces that are produced anteriorly on the aorta following an opening wedge osteotomy.

Most of the literature concerning the outcomes of lumbar osteotomy in patients who have ankylosing spondylitis focuses on the correction of the deformity and postoperative complication rate. Although it is difficult to measure patient outcome, the Modified Arthritis Impact Measurement Scale measures patient mobility, physical activity, household activity, daily activity, social activity, pain, dexterity, anxiety, and depression. This outcome instrument was used when evaluating 175 patients with ankylosing spondylitis who underwent surgical treatment for fixed flexion deformity of the spine. Postoperatively, 47 of 60 items measured showed significant improvement. Only two of the measured items showed a significant impairment of function. Of all the patients, almost 90% were very satisfied with the outcome of the procedure and more than 60% were able to return to work.

Rheumatoid Arthritis

Rheumatoid arthritis is a chronic, progressive, systemic, inflammatory disease that primarily affects synovial joints throughout the body. The most common sites of involvement are the hands and feet, and the cervical spine is the next most common area of involvement. Resultant instability and pannus formation can lead to spinal cord compromise and neurologic deficits. Involvement in the cervical spine can lead to subaxial subluxation, basilar invagination, or damage to the transverse ligament, alar and apical ligaments, and capsular ligaments of the C1-C2 joints allowing atlantoaxial subluxation (Fig. 3). Basilar invagination is the cranial migration of the odontoid from erosion and bone loss between the occipital condyles and the atlas, as well as erosion between the atlas and axis (Fig. 4). This migration occurs when the cranial tip of the dens is above the transverse diameter of the foramen magnum (McRae's line). Additional radiographic parameters used to define cranial settling include Chamberlain's line, Wackenheim's line, and the Ranawat measurement. Subaxial subluxation occurs from erosion of the facet joints, laxity of interspinous ligaments, and intervertebral disc degeneration. These three radiographic findings can occur as isolated events or in combination, leading to instability and/or neurologic compromise. Neurologic symptoms may be produced by direct compression of bone and soft tissue at the cervical medullary junction, or by ischemia from compression of the vertebral arteries, the anterior spinal arteries, or the small perforating vessels of the brain stem.

The Ranawat classification of neurologic deficit is useful for categorizing patients with rheumatoid myelopathy. Class I defines patients who present with no neurologic deficit. Class II defines patients who have

subjective weakness, dysesthesias, and hyperreflexia on physical examination. Patients who present with objective findings of weakness and long tract signs are classified as class III. Those patients who remain ambulatory are subclassified as IIIa, while those who are no longer ambulatory are classified as IIIb.

To minimize the risk of irreversible paralysis, patients recommended for stabilization of the rheumatoid cervical spine in the presence or absence of neurologic deficit include: (1) patients who have atlantoaxial subluxation with a posterior atlanto-odontoid interval of 14 mm or less; (2) patients who have atlantoaxial subluxation and at least 5 mm of basilar invagination; and (3) patients who have subaxial subluxation and a sagittal diameter of the spinal canal of 14 mm or less.

When myelopathy develops in patients with rheumatoid arthritis caused by cervical spine involvement, the prognosis is often poor. A recent review of continued medical care for this disorder noted that 76% of patients showed deterioration at an average of 6 years of follow-up. Additionally, 100% became bedridden within 3 years of the onset of myelopathy; one third of the patients died suddenly for unknown reasons. Based on this and other studies, patients with rheumatoid

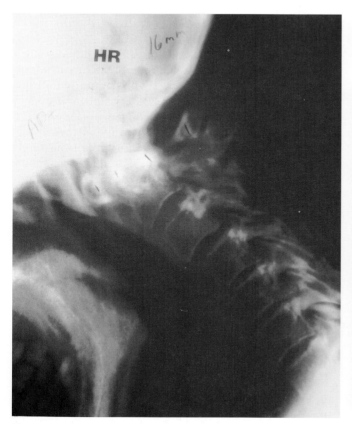

Figure 3 Lateral radiograph demonstrating atlantoaxial instability in a patient with rheumatoid arthritis. Basilar invagination is also present, although it is difficult to visualize on these radiographs.

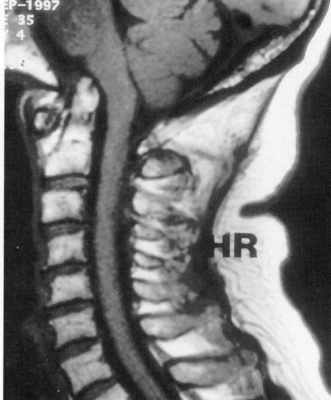

Figure 4 Sagittal MRI study demonstrating basilar invagination in a patient with rheumatoid arthritis.

arthritis and myelopathy should be stabilized surgically as soon as possible to enhance functional recovery. Although patients with myelopathy treated nonsurgically have a poor outcome, surgical procedures have significant complications with a high morbidity and mortality rate in this population.

A recent review of the functional results of the surgical results in patients who were myelopathic and nonambulatory due to rheumatoid arthritis (Ranawat class IIIb) showed an alarmingly high rate of morbidity and mortality. Fifty-five patients underwent either a posterior or a combined transoral and posterior approach for spinal cord decompression and stabilization. The 30-day mortality rate was 13%, rising to 60% by 4 years. Significant neurologic or functional improvement was seen in only 25% of the patients. Earlier treatment with surgery, prior to the permanent loss of function and damage to the neural elements, is important to improve the relatively poor results of this disorder.

Surgical Treatment

As the surgical indications continue to become more defined, surgical options for the patient with cervical spine involvement due to rheumatoid arthritis continue to expand. Over the past 5 years, there have been numerous reports of surgical techniques for occipitocervical fixation. These techniques include various types of smooth or threaded rods secured with sublaminar wires, and more recently, occipitocervical plate and screw fixation.

To obtain immediate fixation and improved fusion rates, various instrumentation options have been explored. The surgeon must remember that patients with severe rheumatoid arthritis frequently have poor bone quality. Fixation techniques that work quite well in the posttraumatic spine may not provide rigid fixation in osteopenic bone. Sublaminar hooks or wires must be used with caution in patients who already have a narrow neural canal. Interspinous wires may not be an option in the patient who also requires a laminectomy. Lateral mass screws may provide poor purchase in weakened bone and although cervical pedicle screws are an option, the procedure is technically challenging with a significant rate of screw misplacement.

Internal fixation at the occipitocervical junction can be achieved by securing a wide diameter, contoured threaded or smooth Steinmann pin, or a contoured rectangular rod. The rod usually is affixed to the occiput with wires placed through drill holes in the skull, while cervical fixation can be obtained with sublaminar wires or cables. Recent long-term follow-up studies have noted successful union rates ranging from 80% to 85%. The advantage of using these pins or rods is that they are readily available and are relatively inexpensive.

However, because they are usually made of stainless steel, they can cause marked metal artifact on MRIs, and subsequent imaging studies of the occipitocervical junction can be difficult. The use of titanium rods can decrease the amount of distortion seen on MRIs, compared to stainless steel pins. However, titanium is more expensive than stainless steel, and care must be taken to avoid a combination of titanium rods with stainless steel wire or cable to avoid the possibility of accelerated corrosion of the hardware. Precise contouring of the rod is a difficult critical component of this procedure. Care should be taken that the final construct lies flush against the occiput and lamina, bilaterally.

The use of sublaminar wires in the cervical spine remains controversial and has the potential for significant neurologic complications. Generally, if the space available for the cord at the C1 arch is decreased, or the patient is known to have a myelopathy, sublaminar wires at C1 should be avoided to reduce the chance of iatrogenic neurologic injury.

Although the placement of contoured rods and sublaminar wires is considered rigid fixation, this does not adequately counteract the forces of cranial settling and compression. Cranial settling can be exaggerated by decompressive procedures, which often are required in this disease process. Additionally, it is impossible to pass sublaminar wires following cervical laminectomy.

Posterior cervical plate fixation, with screw placement in the lateral masses, has the advantage of decreased risk to neural structures because sublaminar cables are not needed with the availability of adequate fixation points, even following laminectomy. Over the past decade, there have been numerous descriptions of custom plates that were designed for occipitocervical fixation. Most of these techniques describe the use of unicortical or bicortical screw fixation to the occiput, with transarticular fixation across the C1-C2 joint and lateral mass screws in the subaxial cervical spine. Significant technical complications have been reported, but they are usually overcome as experience is gained with this challenging technique.

As fixation techniques in the occipitocervical region continue to evolve, the successful fusion rate has been increased, although the nonunion rate remains significant. Traditional methods of fusion involve the use of iliac crest autograft, with morbidities due to graft harvesting ranging as high as 25%. Recently described alternative techniques involve the use of occipital calvarial bone graft. The calvarial graft is membranous, which some authors consider superior to endochondral bone because of its decreased resorption rate. Additionally, the graft can be obtained from the same posterior cervical incision, thus, obviating the need for a second incision, decreasing the incidence of postoperative infection and donor site pain. The largest series to date describing this technique reported a successful fusion rate in 22 of 25 patients, most of whom had rheumatoid arthritis.

Recently, several authors have noted that patients who undergo occipitocervical fusion and instrumentation and develop nonunions seem to do as well as those with successful fusions. This observation led to the publication of a recent report in which 150 patients who underwent posterior occipitocervical stabilization with the use of a contoured metal implant that was affixed by sublaminar wires were examined. One hundred twenty of the patients had internal fixation without bone grafting, while 30 of the patients had the identical internal fixation performed with the use of autogenous bone grafting. After a follow-up of 3 to 11 years, the authors noted there were no differences between the patients managed with a graft and those managed without a graft in respect to survival after the operation, Ranawat class, head or neck pain rating, presence of subaxial abnormalities, radiographic cranial-vertebral motion, or vertical subluxation. The authors believed that much of the clinical improvement was a result of the joint being stabilized rather than an osseous fusion. It was theorized that because patients with rheumatoid arthritis and occipitocervical instability generally do not make the same demands on the skeleton as do active nonrheumatoid age-matched individuals, bone grafting to achieve permanent stability may not be necessary for a satisfactory outcome.

Annotated Bibliography

Apostolides PJ, Dickman CA, Golfinos JG, Papadopoulos SM, Sonntag VK: Threaded Steinmann pin fusion of the craniovertebral junction. *Spine* 1996;21:1630-1637.

Rigid segmental fixation of the craniovertebral junction using a wide diameter, contoured, threaded Steinmann pin with supplemental autograft results in a successful outcome in patients with occipitocervical instability and rheumatoid arthritis.

Casey AT, Crockard HA, Bland JM, Stevens J, Moskovich R, Ransford A: Predictors of outcome in the quadriparetic nonambulatory myelopathic patient with rheumatoid arthritis: A prospective study of 55 surgically treated Ranawat Class IIIb patients. *J Neurosurg* 1996;85:574-581.

Only 25% of patients who were Ranawat class IIIb patients and underwent surgical decompression had a favorable outcome. Preoperative spinal cord area is the major determinant of successful surgical outcome.

Christensson D, Saveland H, Zygmunt S, Jonsson K, Rydholm U: Cervical laminectomy without fusion in patients with rheumatoid arthritis. *J Neurosurg* 1999; 90(suppl 4):186-190.

Laminectomy without simultaneous fusion can be performed in selected patients when rheumatoid changes result in medullary compression in a stable cervical spine.

Finkelstein JA, Chapman JR, Mirza S: Occult vertebral fractures in ankylosing spondylitis. *Spinal Cord* 1999;37: 444-447.

Twenty-one patients with ankylosing spondylitis had an occult fracture that was unrecognized primarily or occurred as a second noncontiguous fracture of the spinal column.

Gran JT, Skomsvoll JF: The outcome of ankylosing spondylitis: A study of 100 patients. *Br J Rheumatol* 1997;36:766-771.

One hundred patients with ankylosing spondylitis were reviewed and functional outcome was noted to correlate with the occurrence of peripheral arthritis and development of a bamboo spine.

Halm H, Metz-Stavenhagen P, Zielke K: Results of surgical correction of kyphotic deformities of the spine in ankylosing spondylitis on the basis of the modified Arthritis Impact Measurement Scales. *Spine* 1995;20: 1612-1619.

The modified Arthritis Impact Measurement Scales noted excellent overall improvement of health status in patients following surgical correction of the kyphotic spine in patients with ankylosing spondylitis.

McMaster MJ: Osteotomy of the cervical spine in ankylosing spondylitis. *J Bone Joint Surg Br* 1997;79:197-203.

A mean correction of 54° was noted in patients who underwent osteotomy of the cervical spine for ankylosing spondylitis, with fixation having been obtained using a Luque rectangle and wiring.

Mori T, Matsunaga S, Sunahara N, Sakou T: 3- to 11-year followup of occipitocervical fusion for rheumatoid arthritis. *Clin Orthop* 1998;351:169-179.

Relief of the neurologic deficit from irreducible atlantoaxial dislocation in rheumatoid arthritis was noted in 25 patients who underwent occipitocervical fusion using a rectangular rod accompanied by a decompressive laminectomy of the atlas.

Moskovich R, Crockard HA, Shott S, Ransford AO: Occipitocervical stabilization for myelopathy in patients with rheumatoid arthritis: Implications of not bone-grafting. *J Bone Joint Surg Am* 2000;82:349-365.

Patients with rheumatoid arthritis who presented with vertical instability and multiple level involvement were treated with posterior occipitocervical stabilization, with the use of contoured occipitocervical loop and sublaminar wire fixation, without bone grafting.

Reveille JD: HLA-B27 and the seronegative spondyloarthropathies. *Am J Med Sci* 1998;316:239-249.

This article presents a review of the current knowledge regarding HLA-B27 and disease, especially in the seronegative spondyloarthropathies.

Robertson SC, Menezes AH: Occipital calvarial bone graft in posterior occipitocervical fusion. *Spine* 1998;23: 249-255.

Split-thickness autologous calvarial bone graft with contoured loop and cable instrumentation was used for a posterior occipitocervical stabilization and fusion in patients with rheumatoid arthritis and occipitocervical instability.

Sunahara N, Matsunaga S, Mori T, Ijiri K, Sakou T: Clinical course of conservatively managed rheumatoid arthritis patients with myelopathy. *Spine* 1997;22:2603-2608.

Surgical treatment was recommended for patients with rheumatoid arthritis and myelopathy, as those treated without surgery had a poor outcome, with deterioration noted in 76% of patients.

Vale FL, Oliver M, Cahill DW: Rigid occipitocervical fusion. *J Neurosurg* 1999;91(suppl 2):144-150.

The technique of rigid occipitocervical fusion using occipitocervical plates and screws in 24 patients with occipitocervical instability was described.

Classic Bibliography

Boden SD, Dodge LD, Bohlman HH, Rechtine GR: Rheumatoid arthritis of the cervical spine: A long-term analysis with predictors of paralysis and recovery. *J Bone Joint Surg Am* 1993;75:1282-1297.

Clark CR, Goetz DD, Menezes AH: Arthrodesis of the cervical spine in rheumatoid arthritis. *J Bone Joint Surg Am* 1989;71:381-392.

Simmons EH: The surgical correction of flexion deformity of the cervical spine in ankylosing spondylitis. *Clin Orthop* 1972;86:132-143.

Chapter 41

Primary Spinal Cord Disorders

Randall W. Porter, MD

Volker K.H. Sonntag, MD

This chapter discusses the two most common primary spinal cord abnormalities and their surgical treatment.

Syringomyelia

In 1824 Olivier d'Angers described a spinal cord cavity in continuity with the fourth ventricle, which he called syringomyelia. In Greek, syringomyelia means tubular cavitation of the spinal cord. Initially, spinal cord lesions were classified into syringomyelia and hydromyelia. Syringomyelia was believed to result from a traumatic cystic dilatation of the spinal cord as a result of central cord hematomyelia, chronic trauma, or both. The defect was believed to be a fluid-filled cavity without an ependymal lining and therefore was termed noncommunicating. The fluid was believed to consist of necrotic breakdown products. A syrinx that forms after trauma is believed to be noncommunicating. Pathologically, a central area of hemorrhagic necrosis and spinal cord infarction start, and eventually a cystic lesion results from liquefaction necrosis. In contrast, hydromyelia has been used to describe a syndrome in which the central canal becomes obstructed by a tumor, inflammation, or mechanical process that causes hydrocephalus of the spinal cord. The distinction, however, has become less important because the latter entity has not been associated uniformly with an ependymal lining. The important distinction is the origin of the cystic dilatation, which has profound implications for treatment. Currently, the term syringomyelia is used for all cysts of the spinal cord, whether lined by ependymal or glial tissue.

Syringes of the spinal cord associated with intramedullary tumors are believed to result from proteinaceous fluid secreted by the tumor, much akin to a cystic tumor of the cerebral hemispheres or cerebellum. The most common tumors associated with cysts are ependymomas and hemangioblastomas. After spinal cord tumors are removed, intra- or extradural scarring can occlude the central canal. Syringobulbia, which is occasionally associated with syringomyelia, describes a cystic dilation in the brain stem.

Pathophysiology

Once a cystic lesion of the spinal cord has been identified, its cause must be determined. For example, 30% to 70% of Chiari type I malformations are frequently associated with syringomyelia and can be acquired or congenital. Chiari type I malformations are characterized by downward displacement of the cerebellar tonsils and medulla into the cervical spine (Fig. 1). Patients who have Chiari type I malformations without syringomyelia have better outcomes than patients with syringomyelia alone. Chiari type II malformations, which are almost always associated with spina bifida, are identified by caudal displacement of the vermis, fourth ventricle, and brain stem into the cervical canal. Even more rare is the descent of the entire cerebellum into the upper cervical canal, which is classified as Chiari type III. The latter, most common in infants, appears to be lethal if left untreated. Many other craniovertebral junction abnormalities, such as tumors (extradural, intradural, intramedullary), Dandy-Walker syndrome, and basilar invagination, also can be associated with syringomyelia.

The features of Chiari malformations that predispose an individual to develop syringomyelia are poorly understood. Chiari proposed embryonic hydrocephalus as the cause, and Gardner favored the hydrodynamic theory in which the central canal becomes distended from a Chiari malformation. In 1972, it was proposed that cerebrospinal fluid (CSF) dissection along the Virchow-Robin spaces resulted from obstruction at the foramen magnum by tonsillar impaction. Recently, Oldfield and associates have theorized that CSF flows through interstitial spaces within the external surface of the spinal cord during systole. They believe that the fluid flows into the central canal because it has nowhere else to go when the fourth ventricle is obstructed. This theory is supported by cine MRI studies. Others claim that inflammatory-induced outlet obstruction causes central cavitation when CSF is produced by the ependymal surface. Finally, traumatic hematomyelia not only causes cystic central canal dilatation but also subarachnoid scarring with cen-

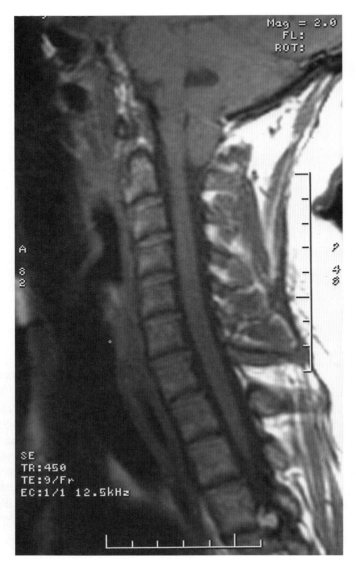

Figure 1 A 34-year-old woman experienced dysesthesia in her left arm and headaches for 3 years. Her symptoms worsened with coughing. MRI of the cervical spine showed herniation of the cerebellar tonsils 2 cm below the foramen magnum. MRI of the brain revealed mild hydrocephalus. She underwent a suboccipital craniectomy, C1 and C2 laminectomies, and lysis of the fourth ventricular adhesions. A fourth ventricular-to-subarachnoid shunt was placed, and a bovine dural patch graft was used for closure. At a 6-month follow-up examination, she was doing well except for nystagmus on leftward gaze and some mild neck discomfort.

tral canal occlusion and propagation of syringomyelia by the same mechanism. This situation can occur years or even decades after seemingly insignificant trauma. Furthermore, tethering can obstruct the flow of CSF around the spinal cord. A similar mechanism may be responsible for the central canal dilatation observed in cervical spondylitic disease.

Pathology

Different pathologic findings have been reported to predispose individuals to develop a syrinx. Any process at the craniovertebral junction that obstructs the flow of CSF may make a patient susceptible. In particular, in type I Chiari malformations, a thickened outer layer of dura (the so-called dural band, which can be three to five times thicker than that of control subjects) can be present. In posttraumatic syringomyelia, the most characteristic initial finding is hemorrhagic infarction followed by the development of a cystic lesion from liquefaction of the spinal cord hematoma. The syrinx is lined by collagen and may be separate from the central canal. Arachnoiditis can contribute to the development of delayed spinal cord ischemia and subarachnoid blockage. The cavity is lined by thick-walled blood vessels and reactive astrocytes or ependyma. The fluid within the syrinx is usually low in protein and clear or xanthochromic. The most common location of a syrinx is the cervical region followed by thoracic and lumbar regions. The surrounding white matter is often compressed. Histologic changes in collagen fibrils include an irregular polarity, hyalinous nodules, fiber splitting, calcification, or ossification.

Natural History

Valsalva-like maneuvers can cause a dissection with a concomitant increase in symptoms and the size of the cavity. Coughing episodes, for example, have been associated with neurologic deterioration. Most patients who are diagnosed with syringomyelia undergo a neuroimaging study prompted by their symptoms. Because it is unusual to discover this disease incidentally, the natural course of an untreated syrinx is poorly defined. All types of syringomyelia, including the so-called posttraumatic types, can progress. Delayed neurologic deterioration is a well-documented clinical presentation. Cystic cavitation associated with spondylitic disease is often stable, but patients must be monitored closely for neurologic deterioration. These patients can remain in the arrested state for quite some time; periodic evaluation with MRI likely will detect an enlarging cavity before serious symptoms can progress.

Clinical Presentation

The classic presentation of a suspended sensory deficit still is observed in various forms. Clinically, syringomyelia can be confused with intramedullary spinal cord tumors, traumatic myelopathy, postirradiation myelopathy, infarction, cervical spondylosis, or cervical necrotizing myelitis. It has been described as a syndrome of segmental sensory dissociation with brachial amyotrophy. Weakness and atrophy of the hands with loss of pain and temperature sensation and sparing of light touch are common. Thoracic kyphoscoliosis is often present. In addition to the syrinx, the presence or absence of hindbrain herniation influences the symptomatology. Most series have not distinguished these two disorders, syringomyelia and hind brain herniation making it difficult to characterize each in isolation.

The condition can manifest from the first year of life until the seventh decade. The most common symptoms are headache, followed by sensory disturbance or numbness. Other relatively common symptoms include neck pain, limb pain, ataxia, spasticity, blurred vision or diplopia, dysphagia, tinnitus, emesis, dysarthria, or oscillopsia. A suboccipital headache, which worsens with straining or a Valsalva maneuver, can exacerbate symptoms in those with an isolated hindbrain herniation. Lower cranial nerve palsies are more likely to be associated with Chiari II malformations or more severe forms of type I. Syringomyelia, with or without hindbrain herniation, can cause spinal pain due to dural stretching from the enlarging intramedullary cyst. Patients with a prior spinal cord injury can develop delayed posttraumatic syringomyelia or may be completely asymptomatic. The time to symptomatic presentation has ranged from 3 to 48 years.

Neuroimaging

MRI, the best modality for radiographic documentation of syringomyelia, reveals such abnormalities at the cranioverterbal junction as Chiari malformations or cranial settling. The extent and degree of the syrinx, along with any associated points of tethering, can be observed. Plain radiography identifies bony findings, including basilar impression or atlantoaxial instability. If MRI is contraindicated, CT-myelography can be performed. Occasionally, the iodinated contrast fills the intramedullary cyst, which may be multiloculated. This feature, which has implications for treatment, may be revealed on MRI, but is not always revealed. A discrete area of focal scarring can point the surgeon to the pathology. Cine MRI synchronized with cardiac systole may also help evaluate CSF flow patterns. Lower velocities of flow, preferential cranial flow of CSF, and shorter periods of caudal CSF flow are all present in those whose CSF flow is obstructed by a tonsillar herniation of more than 5 mm. Syringomyelia associated with pulsatile flow is more likely to respond to surgical decompression.

Intramedullary tumors associated with syringes are seen most readily with contrast-enhanced MRI. Samii and Klekamp reported that 4% of 100 patients with intramedullary tumors had associated syringes. Interestingly, the syrinx is more likely to be found above than below an intramedullary tumor, and the higher the location of the tumor, the more likely it is to be associated with a syrinx. Traumatic syringomyelia usually manifests

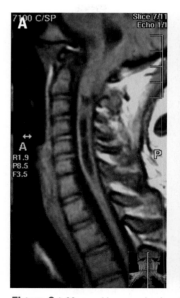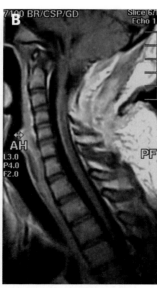

Figure 2 A 28-year-old woman developed a limp in her left leg followed by progressive leg weakness and vertigo. Ultimately, she required a walker and a wheelchair. She also complained of headaches that were exacerbated by turning her head to the left. **(A)** MRI revealed a Chiari malformation down to the vertebral body of C3 and a syrinx with multiple septations from C2-3 to T1. She underwent a suboccipital craniectomy, C1 to C3 laminectomy, duraplasty, syringomyelotomy, and placement of a fourth ventricular-to-subarachnoid shunt. **(B)** MRI 2 months after surgery showed a dramatic decrease in the syrinx and a newly created cisterna magna.

many years after spinal cord injury and may involve 3 to 20 segments. The syringes tend to be paracentral at their rostral end and central at their caudal end.

Treatment

If the cause of syringomyelia is assumed to be obstruction of CSF flow, the goal of surgery should be to restore the flow. If the cause is hindbrain herniation, a posterior fossa decompression is the procedure of choice (Figs. 2 and 3). If the cause is an intramedullary spinal cord tumor, its excision should make the cavity into a pouch and at the same time restore CSF communication with the central canal. In fact, the association of a syrinx with a spinal cord tumor favors its resectability, suggesting that it may be displacing rather than infiltrating tissue. If disorders of the craniovertebral junction such as basilar invagination are causing anterior compression, a transoral odontoidectomy followed by a posterior C1 to C2 fusion or occipital cervical fusion is the preferred treatment. Why a compressive extramedullary or extradural process can cause syringomyelia and its removal resolve the syrinx is poorly understood.

Infants with a severe hindbrain herniation and associated syrinx present difficult challenges. Some surgeons question the long-term efficacy of a posterior fossa decompression while others support it steadfastly. In

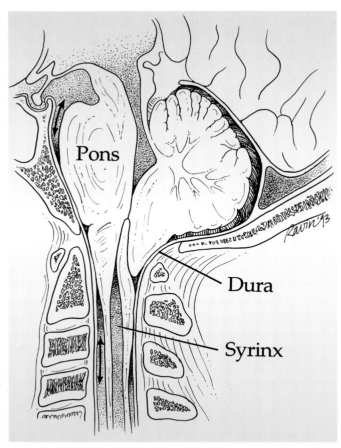

Figure 3 Artist's rendition of a Chiari malformation with an intramedullary syrinx. (*Reproduced with permission from the Barrow Neurological Institute.*)

Syringopleural and syringoperitoneal shunts can be placed with the patient in the lateral decubitus position. Alternatively, the patient can be placed in the prone position for the spinal portion of the procedure. The catheter is then placed in the subcutaneous space in the midaxillary line. In a second stage, the patient is placed supine and the catheter is tunneled to the peritoneum or pleural cavity.

Various shunt catheters have been used. Straight, K-shaped, and T-shaped configurations are the most popular. Regardless of the tube chosen, once it is in the syrinx, it should be sewn to the dura. The peritoneal catheter should have no valve, and it should open at the end.

Complications can include delayed tethering, shunt dislodgement, infection, incomplete drainage of a multi-loculated cyst, or occlusion of the shunt tubing from reactive gliosis. Furthermore, spinal cord injury can result from the myelotomy. Consequently, a shunting procedure should be considered only after suboccipital decompression has failed.

Many techniques of posterior fossa decompression have been described, but the goals of surgery are uniform: to decompress the foramen magnum and to restore CSF flow through the foramen of Magendie. Typically, the suboccipital craniectomy is 2 cm wide by 3 cm high. Recently, however, a suboccipital craniotomy has been performed with a craniectomy of the posterior foramen magnum. At the end of the procedure the remaining bone is replaced in an inverted fashion with the concave side exterior. The dural graft is tacked to the bone to create a new cisterna magna. If the tonsils descend to that level, the posterior arch of C1 and the lamina of C2 and C3 are removed.

The dura is opened in an inverted Y-shaped configuration, with the vertical limb on the paramedian area extending into the cervical region and either limb over the cerebellar hemispheres. The arachnoid is kept intact until hemostasis is achieved to prevent blood from contaminating the subarachnoid space. If the hindbrain herniation is mild, the arachnoid does not have to be opened. If the dura is opened, a patch may or may not be needed. The dura can be tacked back and the arachnoid covered with fibrin glue. A lumbar drain minimizes the chance of CSF leak, but this technique is not recommended if there are intradural membranes such as fourth ventricular outlet obstruction. Alternatively, a dural patch graft can be placed over the opening. A Gore-Tex® (W.L. Gore & Associates, Inc, Flagstaff, AZ) graft may minimize the chance of scarring. However, the suture holes do not seal well and are prone to CSF leakage. No untoward effects have been observed with use of bovine pericardium, and fascia lata is another reasonable alternative.

After excellent hemostasis has been achieved, the

either case, the diversion of CSF in the presence of hydrocephalus is always indicated. In fact, this procedure alone occasionally resolves a Chiari type I malformation and syrinx. If the origin of a syrinx is posttraumatic, the obstruction is relieved by decompression. Detethering and pouch formation continue until the previously scarred cavity communicates with the subarachnoid space.

For years surgeons have shunted the syrinx cavity into the subarachnoid space but the long-term efficacy of this strategy is tenuous. Fluid diversion should not be the primary or only treatment of syringomyelia. Alternative destinations of cyst fluid have been sought. The peritoneum and pleural spaces are the most common sites; relative to the cyst, they create a negative pressure that may be favorable for drainage dynamics.

During the posterior approach to the syrinx, a one- to two-level laminectomy is performed over the most inferior portion of the cyst. The myelotomy can either be midline or in a root entry zone that corresponds to an area of anesthetic. Intraoperative ultrasonography can be invaluable during this portion of the procedure.

arachnoid can be opened and tacked to the dural edges. The tonsils are elevated and the foramen of Magendie is opened. If the foramen is extremely scarred, dissection should be conservative. An overzealous approach to dissection can damage the lower brain stem. Some authors recommend placing a fourth ventricular catheter that drains into the cervical subarachnoid space. To increase the space around the foramen magnum, the tonsils can be coagulated with bipolar coagulation or resected in a subpial fashion. Plugging the obex with muscle has been suggested but is not advocated because it does not address the pathophysiology of the disease and because the brain stem can be injured in the process.

After sewing the patch, fibrin glue or its equivalent should be applied, and a Valsalva maneuver performed to determine if the closure is watertight. The patch must be large and fit loosely enough to allow room for a newly created cisterna magna. If the dura is left open, nausea and vomiting can result from a posterior fossa syndrome.

In the case of posttraumatic or postinflammatory syringomyelia, a laminectomy should be performed over the scarred area and adhesions should be lysed. A dural patch graft usually is placed, but Williams has advocated creating a meningocele without a dural closure and with a watertight fascial closure.

Outcomes

Surgical outcomes have been difficult to interpret. Some authors report the results of both syringomyelia and a Chiari malformation, and some report the results of primary forms of syringomyelia. In general, symptoms improved in two thirds of patients with hindbrain herniation and syringomyelia after decompression of the posterior fossa. Dyste and associates treated 32 patients with foramen magnum decompression, obex plugging, a dural graft, and fourth ventricular drainage: 28 (87.5%) improved, 3 were unchanged, and 1 worsened. Matsumoto and Symon found no difference in the reduction of hydromyelia after decompression of the posterior fossa, but those without a duraplasty had significantly worse outcomes.

Munshi and associates reviewed 11 patients who underwent posterior fossa decompression and C1 laminectomy without a dural opening. Symptoms improved in eight (73%), and seven had hydromyelia. An increase in the volume of the posterior fossa correlated with clinical improvement. Of those who underwent foramen magnum decompression with duraplasty and a C1 laminectomy, 87% experienced clinical improvement. Radiographic follow-up was available in nine patients with hydromyelia; the syrinx decreased in all

and eight improved clinically. Complications included seromas, superficial wound infections, CSF leaks, aseptic meningitis, and occipital nerve pain. Of patients with primary syringomyelia, 50% to 80% improve.

Excellent results have also been reported with the use of subarachnoid shunting. In a series by Hida and associates, 11 of 14 patients with posttraumatic syringomyelia underwent surgical intervention. A syringosubarachnoid shunt was placed in six patients, a syringoperitoneal shunt in four, and a ventriculoperitoneal shunt in one. Only the ventriculoperitoneal shunt and three of the four syringoperitoneal shunts failed. At follow-up, motor function, pain, numbness, and sensory symptoms had improved in all patients.

Intramedullary Spinal Cord Tumors

The first spinal cord tumor was removed in 1887, and the patient's neurologic status improved. The first large series of intradural spinal tumors treated surgically was reported in 1925. Intramedullary spinal cord tumors account for about 20% of all intraspinal neoplasms and are readily treatable. Traditional therapy has consisted of biopsy and radiation. As surgical techniques and instrumentation have improved, however, surgery has become the most effective form of therapy, and long-term survivals and good neurologic outcomes can be expected. Improved neuroimaging techniques have afforded early diagnosis, and the relative ineffectiveness of radiation has led to an increasing and earlier role for surgical resection.

Incidence

Most intramedullary spinal cord tumors are benign glial tumors, about 5% are hemangioblastomas, and less common tumors include lymphomas, intramedullary metastatic tumors, lipomas, and cavernomas. The thoracic spine may be the site most frequently involved, but tumors tend to be distributed evenly throughout the spinal axis. In a series of patients younger than 2 years, about half of glial spinal tumors were astrocytomas, a quarter of which were malignant. Of the remaining half, 27% were gangliogliomas, 12% were ependymomas, 6% were mixed gliomas, and 9% were other types (ganglioneurocytomas, ganglioneurofibromas, and primitive neuroectodermal tumors). In a series of adults, 50% of intramedullary spinal cord tumors were ependymomas and 30% were astrocytomas. Histologically, ependymomas tend to be benign and to grow slowly; most involve the lumbar region (either cauda equina or filum terminale). Myxopapillary tumors are the most common in this location. Spinal cord astrocytomas tend to manifest in patients between 25 and 40 years of age. About 75% are low grade, occur most commonly in cervical and thoracic regions, and are infiltrative along multiple segments. Sensory complaints are the most common initial symptoms; motor deficits can follow. The progression of symptoms tends to be faster with malignant tumors.

MRI of intramedullary tumors may reveal enlargement of the spinal cord, cysts, peritumoral edema, and even intratumoral hemorrhage. Gadolinium-enhanced images of ependymomas typically reveal uniform enhancement compared with variable enhancement with astrocytomas. Plaque from multiple sclerosis should be considered in the differential diagnosis if the lesion does not enhance. Hemangioblastomas are solid and homogenously enhancing, or they are associated with a cyst and a mural nodule. Cavernous malformations show a classic mulberry appearance with variable ages of blood products and a surrounding ring of hemosiderin. In most cases, CSF reveals elevated levels of protein.

Symptoms in patients with intramedullary spinal cord tumors can be insidious, delaying diagnosis. Dysesthesia or radicular pain from compression of a radicular nerve or surrounding structures may be the only symptom. Weakness or loss of coordination, bowel or bladder disturbances, loss of pain and temperature sensation, loss of position sense, or sexual difficulties are some of the problems associated with intramedullary spinal cord tumors. Syringes can be located above or below the tumor. Motor impairment or regression was the most common symptom in 63% of 164 patients younger than 21 years. Pain was present in 46%, gait abnormality in 37%, dysesthesia in 33%, and progressive kyphoscoliosis in 32%. The earliest symptom was usually pain. Dysfunction of the dorsal columns, numbness, and paresthesia are observed in almost all patients. Patients' satisfaction with treatment is greatly improved if they are warned of these anticipated deficits before surgery.

Treatment

Given the infiltrative nature of astrocytomas, their treatment is controversial. Some advocate surgical treatment alone whereas others believe radiation therapy plays a significant role. The treatment of ependymomas is less controversial. Complete surgical resection is the ideal treatment; radiation therapy is reserved for malignant or incompletely resected lesions after several surgical attempts.

In general, surgical resection is the mainstay of therapy for intramedullary tumors. Adjuvant therapy should be used if the histology is malignant or if more than 20% residual is present. The goal of surgery is to preserve neurologic function; however, patients should not necessarily expect restoration to normal neurologic function if preoperative deficits are profound because

the degree of preoperative neurologic deficit is an important predictor of postoperative outcomes.

The patient, under general endotracheal anesthesia, is placed prone in a Mayfield headholder. The head is elevated and the neck is flexed. Antibiotics and steroids are administered preoperatively. Somatosensory-evoked potentials and motor-evoked potentials (MEPs), if available, are monitored. A significant change in MEPs indicates that further manipulation of the spinal cord should be staged. A laminoplasty is performed with the craniotome foot plate one level above and below the level of the tumor. Excellent extradural hemostasis is achieved. The dura is opened in the midline under microscopic observation while the arachnoid is kept intact, if possible, to prevent contamination of the subarachnoid space. The arachnoid can then be opened and tacked to the dural edges with hemoclips.

If the dorsal surface of the spinal cord is thinned or bulges, a myelotomy can be made. If the location of the tumor is not obvious on first inspection, intraoperative ultrasonography can be a useful adjunct. The myelotomy can be made in the posterior median fissure or in the root entry zone. Bipolar coagulation, followed by a No. 11 blade, is used to start the myelotomy on the white, glistening fibrocartilage. The pia should be opened over the entire extent of the tumor. The glial tissue is then spread apart with microdissectors. Prolene (6-0) (Ethicon; Johnson & Johnson, Somerville, NJ) can be used to gently tack the pia laterally.

Hemangioblastomas may be associated with enlarged pial veins and an orange hue. Cavernous malformations may have an exophytic mulberry appearance or may be completely intramedullary. A grayish-fleshy appearance with a clear interface with the yellow myelin is characteristic of ependymomas. Astrocytomas are often discrete in the center, but the margins become less distinct as the interface with the spinal cord is approached.

The ultrasonic aspirator can be used to debulk the center of larger tumors, and the fibrous and vascular attachments can be cauterized and divided sharply. The exceptions, of course, are hemangioblastomas, which should not be debulked internally because of their vascularity. Hemangioblastomas must be dissected circumferentially, devascularized, and removed en bloc. Some authors advocate the use of a laser; others do not believe that a laser is superior to sharp dissection performed under high magnification.

After the tumor is resected, the tumor bed should be inspected for residual tumor and then irrigated. The pial sutures are removed, but the spinal cord should not be sutured together. The dura is closed under the microscope, and fibrin glue or tissue sealant is placed over the suture line. A dural patch can be placed over a spinal cord expanded by an unresectable tumor.

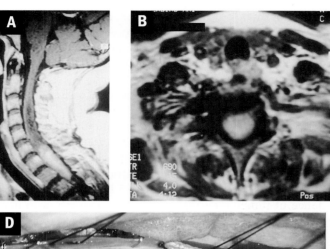

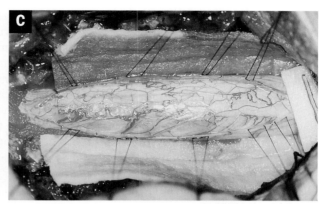

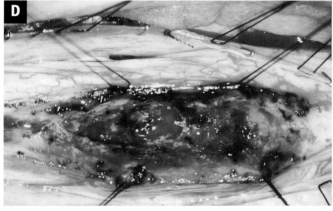

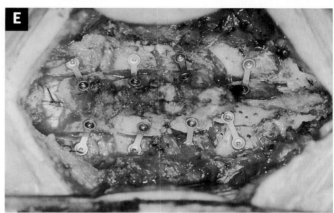

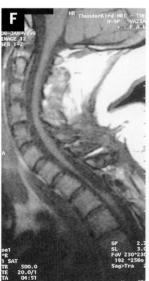

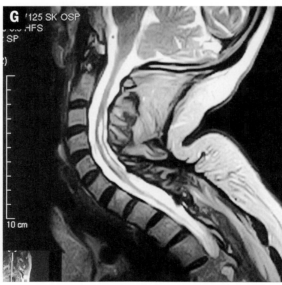

Figure 4 A, Sagittal T1-weighted MRI with contrast showing an intramedullary enhancing lesion with cystic components in a 41-year-old woman with a 12-year history of hand numbness and paresthesia and a 7-year history of urinary difficulty. She had undergone a prior carpal tunnel release on the right. She presented with a hemiparesis, clonus, and decreased sensation in the right upper extremity. **B,** Axial T1-weighted MRI with contrast demonstrates homogenous and enhancing intramedullary tumor. **C,** Intraoperative photograph demonstrates diffuse expansion of the spinal cord and congestion of the pial vessels. Bilaterally, the dura is tacked up with retention sutures. Cotton pledgets are placed on both sides to prevent blood from entering the surgical field. **D,** Resection cavity after the tumor is removed. **E,** Osteoplastic laminoplasty is replaced with miniplates at the end of the procedure. Sagittal **(F)** T1- and **(G)** T2-weighted MRI scans demonstrate complete resection of the tumor. At a 15-month follow-up examination, the patient had decreased sensation on the left side of the body and right-sided weakness. Her strength was 5/5 distally and 4/5 proximally. She complained of an electric feeling in her right hand but was exercising three to four times a week.

The most important factor in obtaining good surgical outcomes is to define and maintain the tumor-spinal cord interface (Fig. 4). The location of a tumor should not influence the extent of resection unless the lesion is in the conus medullaris. In that case, if the cauda equina is extensively involved, only debulking is possible. Ependymomas and hemangioblastomas are considered benign lesions with a clear interface between tumor and spinal cord. Astrocytomas are much less likely to have a clear tumor-spinal cord interface, and their histology is more likely to be variable. Although most astrocytomas are infiltrative, a few astrocytomas seem to have distinct margins. The surgical goal with astrocytomas is therefore less clear; extent of resection has not always correlated with outcome. Intramedullary spinal lipomas are embryologic rests that can enlarge with time. Complete resection is rarely possible or necessary given their benign histology. Conservative debulking is more prudent and usually adequate to control the symptoms long-term. Cavernous malformations are well-circumscribed benign lesions prone to recurrent hemorrhage. Although they usually are associated with a good dissection plane, they often have an associated surrounding hemosiderin ring that should be considered part of the normal myelin. Intraoperative biopsy should be considered because a malignant histology portends a poor prognosis regardless of the extent of resection.

Surgical Outcomes

If good technique and judgment are exercised, the rate of morbidity associated with the surgical treatment of spinal cord tumors should be low. Based on contemporary series, the risk of deteriorating more than one Frankel grade is about 10%. Constantini and associates reviewed their large experience with the surgical resection of intramedullary spinal cord tumors in children and young adults. Gross total resection was achieved in 77% of the patients, and a subtotal resection was achieved in 20%. Three months after surgery, 60% of the patients were the same compared with their preoperative neurologic function, 16% improved, and 24% were worse. Thirteen patients deteriorated more than one grade. Those with minimal or mild preoperative deficits rarely worsened after surgery. Those with subtotal resection had worse outcomes than those with gross total resections. Previous surgery, chemotherapy, and radiation did not influence outcome nor did extent of resection, age, or histologic composition. The need for ventriculoperitoneal shunting was higher in patients with malignant tumors than in those with benign lesions and correlated with a worse prognosis. Histologic grade was the most important determinant of outcome. The 5-year progression-free survival rate was 30% for high-grade tumors and 78% for low-grade tumors. Overall, the 10-year survival rate was about 70%.

The progression-free survival for all tumors was 80%, 71%, and 54% for 3-, 5-, and 10-year intervals, respectively. The most common cause of death was local recurrence or leptomeningeal metastasis. In this same study, the most important factor in survival was tumor pathology. The 5-year survival for low-grade tumors was 88% compared with 18% for high-grade tumors.

Tumors recurred in 35% of the patients, usually at a local site or in the form of leptomeningeal metastasis. The mean time of recurrence was 38 months. With a mean follow-up of about 13 years, more than 60% of the patients had functioned independently. Kyphoscoliosis was present in 71%, 37% required an orthopaedic procedure, 40% had urinary problems, 26% were incontinent, and 61% had dysesthesias.

Epstein and associates treated 25 intramedullary astrocytomas with radical excision: 19 were low-grade and six were malignant. Five patients with malignant tumors died within 2 years and the disease progressed in the sixth. Of the patients with benign tumors, three had gangliogliomas and 16 had astrocytomas. At a mean follow-up of more than 4 years, 15 had no clinical evidence of tumor recurrence. All seven patients who had undergone prior radiation had tumor progression.

Others, however, maintain that conservative surgery followed by radiation has a significant role in the control of astrocytomas. Minehan and associates reported their experience with astrocytomas and radiation in 79 patients who underwent surgery; 54% were classified as having pilocytic astrocytomas, 32% as having diffuse fibrillary astrocytomas, and 14% as having astrocytomas only. The 10-year survival rate was 81% for those with pilocytic astrocytomas and 15% for those with diffuse fibrillary astrocytomas. The extent of resection did not appear to influence survival, but radiation appeared to improve outcomes in the diffuse fibrillary type of astrocytomas.

Conclusion

Multiple surgical procedures are available to treat syringomyelia either directly by shunting or indirectly by establishing normal CSF flow. Despite attempts at nonsurgical treatment, surgery remains the mainstay of therapy of benign intramedullary tumors. Aggressive, early, and complete removal of these tumors offers the best chance of obtaining clinical and radiographic cure. Therefore, discrete residual tumors should probably be removed in an early second-stage operation. Adjuvant therapy should be reserved for patients with significant recurrent tumors or those with a malignant histology.

Annotated Bibliography

Blagodatsky MD, Larionov SN, Alexandrov YA, Velm AI: Surgical treatment: Chiari I malformation with or without syringomyelia. *Acta Neurochir* 1999;141: 963-968.

The authors reviewed 102 patients with or without syringomyelia who underwent Arnold-Chiari suboccipital decompression. Indications and retrospective results are discussed.

Constantini S, Miller DC, Allen JC, Rorke LB, Freed D, Epstein FJ: Radical excision of intramedullary spinal cord tumors: Surgical morbidity and long-term follow-up evaluation in 164 children and young adults. *J Neurosurg* 2000;93:183-193.

This landmark article reviews the results of 164 patients younger than 21 years of age who underwent surgical decompression of intramedullary spinal cord tumors. Only 13 patients deteriorated more than one Frankel grade. The rate of long-term survival depended on the histology of the tumor in the 5-year period. Of patients with a low-grade glioma, 78% had stable disease compared with 30% of those with a high-grade glioma. Patients with less than 80% of the tumor resected fared significantly worse that those with 80% or more resected.

Hida K, Iwasaki Y, Imamura H, Abe H: Posttraumatic syringomyelia: Its characteristic magnetic resonance imaging findings and surgical management. *Neurosurgery* 1994;35:886-891.

The authors reviewed 14 patients with posttraumatic syringomyelia, 11 of whom were symptomatic. The period of spinal cord injury ranged from 3 to 33 years; 11 patients had good outcomes. This small series of patients offers an interesting review of the radiographic features of posttraumatic syringomyelia.

Hida K, Iwasaki Y, Koyanagi I, Sawamura Y, Abe H: Surgical indication and results of foramen magnum decompression versus syringosubarachnoid shunting for syringomyelia associated with Chiari I malformation. *Neurosurgery* 1995;37:673-679.

The authors compared the results of foramen magnum decompression (33 patients) to those of syringosubarachnoid shunting (37 patients). Subarachnoid shunting was used in patients with large syringes. Syrinx size decreased in almost all patients in both groups. Neurologic improvements were observed in 82% of those who underwent decompression and in 97% of those who underwent shunting. Overall the symptoms and radiologic findings improved more quickly in the shunted group.

Jyothirmayi R, Madhavan J, Nair MK, Rajan B: Conservative surgery and radiotherapy in the treatment of spinal cord astrocytoma. *J Neurooncol* 1997;33:205-211.

The authors reviewed their experience with 23 patients. The presence of both malignant and low-grade tumors makes it difficult to draw sweeping conclusions. All patients received radiation (45 Gy in 25 fractions over 5 weeks). Survival rates were 55% at 5 years and 39% at 10 years. The median survival of patients with high-grade tumors was 10 months. The main weakness is that this retrospective review does not necessarily compare two identical groups.

Levi ADO, Sonntag VKH: Management of posttraumatic syringomyelia using an expansile duraplasty: A case report. *Spine* 1998;23:128-132.

The authors reported a patient who developed syringomyelia 34 years after an L2 fracture, the most delayed onset of symptoms from a posttraumatic syrinx reported to date. The patient was managed by lysis of adhesions, fenestration of the cysts, and expansile duraplasty. The patient's symptoms improved, and MRI showed that the size of the syrinx had decreased.

Minehan KJ, Shaw EG, Scheithauer BW, Davis DL, Onofrio BM: Spinal cord astrocytoma: Pathological and treatment considerations. *J Neurosurg* 1995;83:590-595.

The authors reviewed 79 patients who underwent surgery for spinal cord astrocytomas with or without radiation therapy. Of the patients, 54% had pilocytic and 32% had diffuse tumors; 14% could not be classified other than astrocytoma. None had malignant histology. The overall 10-year survival rate was 50%, but was 81% for pilocytic compared with 15% for diffuse astrocytomas. The extent of surgical resection did not significantly affect survival. Postoperative radiotherapy improved survival more for those with a fibrillary astrocytoma than for others.

Munshi I, Frim D, Stine-Reyes R, Weir BKA, Hekmatpanah J, Brown F: Effects of posterior fossa decompression with and without duraplasty on Chiari malformation-associated hydromyelia. *Neurosurgery* 2000;46: 1384-1390.

The authors reviewed 34 patients. Of the 23 patients who had a posterior fossa decompression with duraplasty, 87% improved. Of the 11 who did not have duraplasty, 73% improved, and the size of the syrinx decreased in 50%. Two patients worsened, and one underwent a reoperation for a duraplasty. The authors concluded that duraplasty probably leads to a more reliable reduction in the volume of hydromyelia.

Nakamura N, Iwasaki Y, Hida K, Abe H, Fujioka Y, Nagashima K: Dural band pathology in syringomyelia with Chiari type I malformation. *Neuropathology* 2000; 1:38-43.

The authors undertook a pathologic investigation of patients with Chiari type I malformations and found dural bands and an increase in the number of collagen fibers. These changes were not observed in the four control cases. The authors suggested that the thickening of the dura may be a causative factor in syringomyelia.

Newton HB, Newton CL, Gatens C, Herbert R, Pack R: Spinal cord tumors: Review of etiology, diagnosis, and multidisciplinary approach to treatment. *Cancer Practice* 1995;3:207-218.

The authors comprehensively reviewed intradural, extradural, intramedullary, and extramedullary spinal cord tumors in terms of radiographic evaluation, management, and outcomes.

Oldfield EH, Muraszko K, Shawker TH, et al: Pathophysiology of syringomyelia associated with Chiari I malformation of the cerebellar tonsils: Implications for diagnosis and treatment. *J Neurosurg* 1994;80:3-15.

The authors reported a novel imaging technique known as phase contrast cine-MRI, intraoperative ultrasonography for examining the anatomy, dynamics, and movement of the cerebellar tonsils and of the CSF during respiratory and cardiac cycles. These studies revealed an abrupt downward movement of CSF and syrinx fluid during systole, an upward movement during diastole, but limited movement of CSF across the foramen magnum. During systole ultrasonography revealed downward movement of the tonsils that occurred concomitantly with a sudden constriction of the spinal cord and syrinx. After decompression, syringomyelia resolved within 1 to 6 months of surgery.

Samii M, Klekamp J: Surgical results of 100 intramedullary tumors in relation to accompanying syringomyelia. *Neurosurgery* 1994;35:865-873.

The authors reported their experience with 100 intramedullary tumors in 94 patients. There were associated syringes in 45%. Syrinx was more likely to be found above than below the tumor and was most frequently found with ependymomas or hemangioblastomas. This review of a large surgical series specifically considers syringes and their relation to tumor resectability and outcomes.

Classic Bibliography

Barbaro NM: Surgery for primary spinal syringomyelia, in Batzdorf U (ed): *Syringomyelia: Current Concepts in Diagnosis and Treatment*. Baltimore, MD, Williams & Wilkins, 1991, pp 183-198.

Batzdorf U: Syringomyelia, Chiari malformation, and hydromyelia, in Youmans J (ed): *Youman's Neurological Surgery*, ed 4. Philadelphia, PA, WB Saunders, 1996, pp 1090-1109.

Cohen AR, Wisoff JH, Allen JC, Epstein F: Malignant astrocytomas of the spinal cord. *J Neurosurg* 1989;70: 50-54.

Dyste GN, Menezes AH, VanGilder JC: Symptomatic Chiari malformations: An analysis of presentation, management, and long-term outcome. *J Neurosurg* 1989;71: 159-168.

Enzmann DR: Imaging of syringomyelia, in Batzdorf U (ed): *Syringomyelia: Current Concepts in Diagnosis and Treatment*. Baltimore, MD, Williams & Wilkins, 1991, pp 116-139.

Epstein FJ, Farmer JP, Freed D: Adult intramedullary astrocytomas of the spinal cord. *J Neurosurg* 1992;77: 355-359.

Gardner WJ, Abdullah AF, McCormack LJ: The varying expressions of embryonal atresia of the 4th ventricle in adults: Arnold-Chiari malformation, Dandy-Walker syndrome, "arachnoid" cyst of the cerebellum, and syringomyelia. *J Neurosurg* 1957;14:591-605.

Guidetti B, Mercuri S, Vagnozzi R: Long-term results of the surgical treatment of 129 intramedullary spinal gliomas. *J Neurosurg* 1981;54:323-330.

Matsumoto T, Symon L: Surgical management of syringomyelia: Current results. *Surg Neurol* 1989;32: 258-265.

McCormick PC, Torres R, Post KD, Stein BM: Intramedullary ependymoma of the spinal cord. *J Neurosurg* 1990;72:523-532.

Menezes AH, Smoker WRK, Dyste GN: Syringomyelia, Chiari malformations, and hydromyelia, in Youmans JR (ed): *Neurological Surgery*, ed 3. Philadelphia, PA, WB Saunders, 1990, pp 1421-1459.

Menezes AH: Chiari I malformations and hydromyelia. *Pediatr Neurosurg* 1991;92:146-154.

Milhorat TH, Miller JL, Johnson WD, Aldler DE, Heger IM: Anatomical basis of syringomyelia occurring with hindbrain lesions. *Neurosurgery* 1993;32:748-754.

Rossitch E Jr, Zeidman SM, Burger PC, et al: Clinical and pathological analysis of spinal cord astrocytomas in children. *Neurosurgery* 1990;27:193-196.

Sandler HM, Papadopoulos SM, Thornton AF Jr, Ross DA: Spinal cord astrocytomas: Results of therapy. *Neurosurgery* 1992;30:490-493.

Simeone FA: Spinal cord tumors in adults, in Youmans JR (ed): *Neurological Surgery*, ed 3. Philadelphia, PA, WB Saunders, 1990, pp 3531-3547.

Sonneland PR, Scheithauer BW, Onofrio BM: Myxopapillary ependymoma: A clinicopathologic and immunocytochemical study of 77 cases. *Cancer* 1985; 56:883-893.

Williams B: Surgical treatment of syringobulbia. *Neurosurg Clin N Am* 1993;4:553-571.

Williams B: Syringomyelia. *Neurosurg Clin N Am* 1990; 1:653-685.

Chapter 42

Musculoskeletal and Metastatic Tumors

Albert J. Aboulafia, MD

Alan M. Levine, MD

Introduction

Of all the patients who seek medical attention for symptoms originating in the spine, those with tumors comprise only a small percentage. Delays in diagnosis may occur if the physician is not familiar with typical features that differentiate the manifestations of primary and metastatic tumors from those of more common, nonneoplastic spinal disorders.

Optimal treatment of patients with spinal tumors requires a merging of the knowledge and techniques developed by spine surgeons with principles of oncologic surgery. Orthopaedic oncologists have dealt most commonly with neoplastic conditions in the nonaxial skeleton, while spine surgeons have dealt primarily with nonneoplastic conditions of the spine. Neoplastic conditions of the spine with which spine surgeons deal are usually vertebral metastases or benign bone tumors.

In the past, few treatment strategies were available for patients with primary malignant tumors of the spine. The surgical techniques appropriate for patients with fractures or metastases, aimed at achieving short-term functional results, were often inappropriately applied to patients with primary malignant tumors. Over the past decade, spine surgeons with an understanding of the principles of orthopaedic oncology have developed newer classifications for spinal tumors and introduced treatment modalities based on sound oncologic principles, leading to a better understanding of the goals of surgery for patients with primary bone tumors and a common language for describing surgical margins. Advances in imaging modalities, surgical techniques, and spinal instrumentation, and a better understanding of spinal stability have added to the surgical treatment options for treating patients with either primary or metastatic tumors of the spine.

Incidence

The most common neoplastic conditions affecting the spine are skeletal metastases resulting from carcinomas and lymphoproliferative diseases (myeloma and lymphoma). The skeleton is the third most common site of metastasis from carcinomas (following the lung and liver), and the spine is the most common site of skeletal metastasis. It is estimated that there will be 1.2 million new carcinomas diagnosed in the United States in the year 2000, with greater than 75%, or 800,000, of these in the breast, prostate, or lung. Along with renal and thyroid carcinomas, these account for most metastases to the spine. Gastrointestinal and gynecologic tumors and melanoma less commonly metastasize to the spine. In as many as 10% of patients with bony metastases, the primary site will not be identified before the patient's demise. In women, breast carcinoma is the most frequent primary lesion, and accounts for more than half of all metastatic lesions to the spine; in men, lung and prostate carcinomas are the most common primary lesions.

As many as 90% of patients who die of cancer may have spinal metastases at autopsy. Only half of all patients who die with metastatic carcinoma will have symptoms from a spinal metastasis. The reported incidence of spinal metastasis for any given tumor type varies dramatically depending on whether only symptomatic lesions are reported or the incidence is based on autopsy studies. Fewer than 10% of patients with symptomatic spinal metastases are treated surgically. With recent advances in understanding of the mechanisms of pain production in spinal metastatic disease, spinal instability, and spinal instrumentation, and with longer survival of patients with metastatic disease, the percentage of patients that may benefit from treatment is increasing.

The most common location for skeletal metastases is the thoracolumbar region, which accounts for approximately 70% of all lesions. The lumbar and sacral spine accounts for approximately 20% of spinal metastases, and the cervical spine the remainder. However, recent studies have suggested that the cervical spine may account for up to 20% of spinal metastases. In the cervical spine, spinal cord compression is more common when tumor involvement is in the subaxial area as opposed to the atlantoaxial region where, because of increased space available for the cord, symptoms are usually pain or instability.

It is estimated that there are only 2,000 primary bone sarcomas and 6,000 soft-tissue sarcomas diagnosed annually in the United States, with involvement of the spine accounting for less than 10%. The incidence of benign bone tumors affecting the spine is unknown. Lesions such as hemangiomas and enostoses (bone islands) frequently are asymptomatic and remain undiagnosed until discovered as an incidental finding during an imaging study. The incidence of hemangioma and enostoses of the spine has been estimated as 11% and 14%, respectively, in the general population. Recognizing the ubiquitous nature of these lesions and their benign clinical course is important to avoid costly and unnecessary procedures. Most benign tumors of the spine (ie, osteoid osteoma, osteochondroma, and aneurysmal bone cyst) occur in the second and third decades of life, often causing pain or radicular symptoms. More aggressive tumors, such as giant cell tumors and osteoblastomas, although relatively rare, may be present from the second decade onward, causing pain, occasionally paraparesis, and severe spinal compromise and requiring differentiation from infection and metastatic disease.

Evaluation

History and Physical Examination

For most patients with tumors involving the spine, the history and physical examination will provide clues to the possibility, but the physician must be aware of the common symptoms and findings in patients with spinal tumors. More than 85% of patients with spinal tumors come for treatment with a chief complaint of back pain. Patients may associate the onset of symptoms with a traumatic episode, which may be the case when trauma has caused a fracture in compromised vertebrae. Useful clues that may suggest an underlying neoplasm include slow, gradual onset of pain that has become progressively worse, persistent pain at night, and symptoms unrelated to mechanical stress. Pathologic fracture should be considered when patients complain of acute onset of pain in the absence of a clear history of significant trauma. Patients may develop radicular symptoms as the result of compression of nerve roots either by the tumor or as the result of vertebral fracture. The history of the onset of pain and neural deficit is critical to the prognosis for recovery from spinal cord compression. If the patient has progressed from neurologically intact

(but with pain) to high-grade paraplegia in 24 h or less, the chance of recovery to functional ambulation is much worse than in the patient with gradual onset of weakness over 5 to 7 days before admission. The age of the patient is helpful in delineating the type of tumor, because spinal metastasis and lymphoproliferative disorders are the most common neoplasms affecting the spine in patients older than age 40 years. In patients younger than 18 years of age benign tumors such as hemangioma, Langerhans' cell histiocytosis, osteoid osteoma, osteoblastoma, aneurysmal bone cyst, giant cell tumor, and osteochondroma predominate. The most common primary malignant spine tumors affecting the young are osteosarcoma and Ewing's sarcoma.

When a patient is evaluated for spinal pain, the physician should inquire into any prior history of cancer, no matter how remote. Patients with breast cancer may have a disease-free interval of greater than 10 to 20 years before requesting treatment of a spinal metastasis. Some patients may not recall or think it significant that they had removal of a skin lesion that may have been a melanoma. Patients who have undergone prostate or breast biopsy have the exact pathology documented. Patients should be asked specifically about radiation treatments and/or exposure to carcinogens. The social history should include questions regarding tobacco and alcohol use as well as a sexual history and transfusion history that may predispose a person to the human immunodeficiency virus. The review of systems should include specific questions regarding respiratory, endocrine, genitourinary, and constitutional symptoms of cancer. Women older than age 40 years should be asked about their last breast examination or mammogram. A family history of cancer should be solicited. In elderly adults, the physician must resist the tendency to attribute symptoms such as pain and weakness to degenerative processes.

The most common primary bone tumors affecting the spine in adults, other than multiple myeloma, include chordoma, chondrosarcoma, osteosarcoma, Ewing's sarcoma, and malignant fibrous histiocytoma. In such instances the history usually does not provide clues to suggest a specific primary tumor, and no systemic complaints can be elicited. Although earlier studies suggested that as many as 70% of patients with spinal tumors had evidence of neurologic dysfunction at the time of diagnosis, more recent reports suggest that the incidence of neurologic deficit at the time of request for treatment is now less than 10%.

Patients with spinal tumors are more likely to have a specific site of focal tenderness compared to patients with mechanical or discogenic back pain. Spinal deformity (typically kyphosis) may be seen in patients with pathologic fractures. The entire spine should be pal-

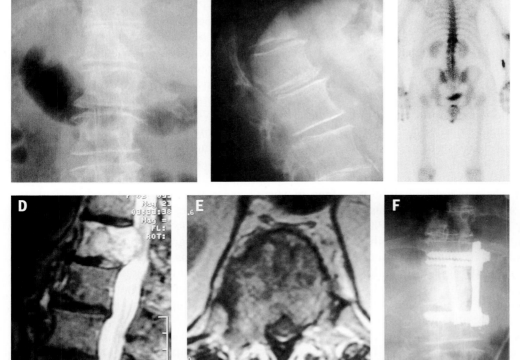

Figure 1 This 82-year-old woman had an invasive ductal carcinoma of the breast 9 years prior to admission without recurrence. She has a 3-month history of back pain and began having numbness, tingling, and weakness in her lower extremities 5 to 6 days before admission. AP **(A)** and lateral **(B)** radiographs did not show significant findings. Bone scan **(C)** demonstrated a lesion at T12. On MRI, the spin echo sagittal image **(D)** showed involvement of the T12 body with a posterior soft-tissue mass compressing the dural sac. The axial T2 images **(E)** showed involvement of the entire vertebral body with compression of the anterior portion of the dural sac. The patient underwent an anterior corpectomy with decompression of the dural sac and stabilization using methylmethacrylate and a plate **(F)**.

pated to identify areas of tenderness or paraspinal masses. Benign spinal tumors in children may appear as painful scoliosis in the thoracic or lumbar spine and painful torticollis in the cervical spine. If a spinal tumor is being considered, a complete physical examination including evaluation of the breasts, thyroid, abdomen, rectum, and prostate should be performed. If the surgeon does not feel confident in his or her skills in evaluating these anatomic sites, appropriate referral should be made. As part of the rectal examination the prostate should be palpated for masses, and a stool guiac performed. More than half of all patients with sacral chordomas have a palpable presacral mass identifiable on rectal examination.

Imaging Studies

Plain radiographs are recommended for any patient with prolonged back pain that fails to improve over a period of 6 weeks. Plain radiographs will identify 80% of benign bone tumors involving the spine as well as a significant proportion of primary or metastatic spinal lesions. If negative, depending on the index of suspicion, further imaging studies may be warranted, especially

for patients with a previous known primary carcinoma. Plain radiographs, even with two orthogonal views, lack sensitivity in identifying lesions without cortical bone changes or fracture. It is estimated that only 40% of patients with metastatic spine disease have changes that can be initially detected using plain radiographs (Fig. 1, *A* and *B*). As much as 50% of trabecular bone loss is necessary before changes can be seen on plain radiographs; therefore, tumors that involve the vertebral marrow, especially the lymphoproliferative disorders, may not be seen on plain radiographs until late in the course of the disease. Primary bone tumors such as chondrosarcoma or osteosarcoma are likely to be associated with a radiodense mass extending beyond the vertebral body.

Metastatic lesions may be osteolytic, osteoblastic, or mixed osteolytic or blastic. Prostate and breast carcinomas often incite a blastic or mixed lytic and blastic response, whereas renal cell carcinoma most often is associated with a lytic lesion. Metastatic lesions usually involve the vertebral body and may be associated with vertebral collapse, simulating an osteoporotic compression fracture. The vertebral body is seven times more likely to be involved than the posterior elements in cases of metastasis. Although metastases usually originate at the base of the pedicle, extension into the body and into the pedicle at the time of diagnosis is not uncommon. Destruction of the pedicle, which is mostly composed of cortical bone, can be seen on an AP view in many cases. In patients with neural deficit, 70% of the lesions are anterior in the body, and 10% are in the posterior elements. Lesions involving the posterior elements, especially in patients younger than age 30 years, are more likely to be benign than malignant.

The plain radiograph can be very helpful in distinguishing conditions such as Paget's disease and infection from tumor. In the case of infection there is often destruction of adjacent vertebral end plates and disc involvement, whereas these usually are preserved in cases of tumor. Plain radiographs may not be helpful in differentiating osteopenic compression from neoplastic compression that can occur in the same patient. Plain radiographs are useful for assessing spinal stability. Although defining spinal stability in metastatic disease has been difficult and not uniformly agreed upon, loss of 50% of vertebral height or increasing angular deformity have been recommended as parameters used to assess spinal stability. Plain radiographs are especially useful in identifying angular, translational, and kyphotic deformity and are, in fact, superior to CT or MRI in assessing these parameters.

Technetium (^{99m}Tc) bone scan is most commonly used as a screening examination for patients with known malignancy. Bone scintigraphy can identify skeletal metastases 2 to 12 months before plain radiographs can detect them (Fig. 1, *C*). Patients diagnosed with either breast, prostate, lung, kidney, or thyroid carcinomas should undergo bone scintigraphy as part of initial staging studies. Technetium bone scan provides a method of evaluating the entire skeleton for areas of increased bone activity. Because most patients with spinal metastasis often have other sites of skeletal involvement at the time of diagnosis, it may be useful in distinguishing a primary bone tumor from a metastatic lesion. Depending on age and history, a solitary bone lesion in the spine may suggest the possibility of a primary bone sarcoma. Additionally, for patients with spinal metastases of unknown origin who need a tissue diagnosis, a safer site for biopsy may be identified if other lesions are identified on bone scan.

Bone scans lack sensitivity and specificity in certain conditions. A scan may fail to identify tumors that lack osteoblastic activity and tumors such as myeloma or aggressive osteolytic metastasis from a renal primary tumor, and it may fail to distinguish neoplastic from nonneoplastic conditions involving the spine. Nonneoplastic conditions that commonly demonstrate increased activity on bone scan include osteoporotic compression fracture, insufficiency fracture of the sacrum, infection, and degenerative arthritis.

To improve specificity, single positron emission computed tomography (SPECT) with high resolution has been used to acquire better localization of bone activity within the vertebral body. Using this technique, the presence or absence of pedicle involvement has been used as a diagnostic criterion to predict vertebral metastasis. The sensitivity and specificity of SPECT in identifying vertebral metastases are 87% and 91%, respectively, compared with 74% and 81% for planar imaging. The positive and negative predictive values of SPECT imaging were 82% and 94%, respectively, compared with 64% and 88% for planar imaging. Although SPECT imaging provides a more detailed view of the area of vertebral involvement compared with planar technetium scans, it has not been shown to be superior to MRI in assessing pedicle involvement.

Positron emission tomography (PET) using 2-deoxy-2[F-18]fluro-D-glucose has the theoretical advantage over other imaging modalities currently in use of being able to assess pulmonary and lymphatic sites for disease as well as osseous sites not identified using conventional bone scintigraphy, CT, or MRI. Previous reports have demonstrated improved accuracy for technetium-labeled phosphonates compared to planar scintigraphy using sodium fluoride F 18. However, with the use of PET scanners in lieu of standard gamma cameras, sodium fluoride F 18 may prove useful in the future. Recently, PET F 18 has been shown to be more sensitive than technetium bone scan in detecting benign and malignant bone lesions. In some tumors such as lung cancer it may provide a single test to detect all sites of metastatic disease. Its biggest current limitation is the inability to discern lesions less than 1 cm in diameter.

CT is superior to MRI for assessing bone detail in patients with benign or malignant tumors. For patients in whom an intralesional procedure is anticipated, the quality and quantity of anticipated remaining bone following surgery can be assessed. Additionally, accurate measurements of the vertebral body and pedicle can be obtained if spinal instrumentation is anticipated. CT is also helpful in evaluating patients with pathologic fractures for canal compromise and osseous impingement on the spinal cord. MRI is superior to CT for identifying spinal lesions, especially those with just marrow replacement as well as documenting neural compression; however, there is a small subset of patients who are unable to obtain an MRI scan in whom CT or CT myelography is indicated.

MRI is useful both for screening of patients with known primary tumors and spine pain and for critically evaluating a lesion seen on plain radiographs or bone scan. MRI is also useful for evaluating soft-tissue masses adjacent to the spine, as well as marrow characteristics at the site of the lesion and along the entire spine (Fig. 1, *D* and *E*). With sagittal images the entire spine can be assessed for potential sites of disease. If noncontiguous sites of spinal involvement are identified, the diagnosis of metastatic tumor is almost certain. Conversely, if only a single spinal lesion is identified, additional studies in search of a primary lesion should begin. If subsequent studies fail to identify a primary carcinoma, the lesion should be considered primary until proven otherwise. MRI of the entire spine is indicated in assessing spinal cord compression. Studies have demonstrated that 10% of patients with spinal cord compression will have multiple levels of compression, and a much higher number will have additional areas of vertebral involvement without compression. In most patients (73%), more than one region of the spine (cervical, thoracic, or lumbosacral) is involved.

Of particularly important clinical significance is the use of MRI to distinguish osteoporotic compression fractures and pathologic compression fractures. Although several recent studies have been published attempting to differentiate the two entities, there is not a set of parameters that can be relied on to distinguish one from the other. Even in osteoporotic fractures the normal marrow signal is dramatically altered, and thus the ability to discriminate on the basis of MRI is not absolute. Pathologic fractures often exhibit low signal intensity on T1-weighted images and high signal intensity on T2-weighted images. Benign or osteoporotic vertebral fractures demonstrate normal marrow signals on both T1- and T2-weighted images. Metastatic lesions may easily be confused with healing fractures based on signal intensity (Fig. 2). In these patients, it is important to study the pattern of marrow signal. Pathologic lesions often involve the pedicle and posterior elements and exhibit diffuse marrow infiltration. The addition of gadolinium can delineate spinal cord compression and distinguish extradural, intradural or extramedullary, and intramedullary tumors. Extradural metastatic tumors are the most common. Most intradural lesions are nerve sheath tumors. In the lumbar spine, the most common intramedullary lesion is the ependymoma.

In using MRI to differentiate tumor versus infection, it is useful to remember that vertebral osteomyelitis is located adjacent to the end plates and often involves the intervertebral disc space. Infection produces decreased signal intensity in both the bone and disc on T1-weighted images and increased signal intensity on T2-weighted images. Diffusion-weighted MRI of bone marrow helps differentiate benign from pathologic vertebral compression fractures. Whereas most benign vertebral compression fractures are hypo- or isointense to adjacent vertebral bodies, most pathologic fractures are hyperintense. Benign vertebral fractures have negative bone marrow contrast ratios with diffusion-weighted imaging, whereas pathologic fractures have positive values. This difference is not elicited with T1-weighted spin echo and STIR imaging.

CT with intrathecal contrast (CT-myelography) is a useful alternative when MRI is unavailable or cannot be tolerated. Cerebrospinal fluid for analysis may be obtained during the dural puncture. CT is especially useful for determining the bony characteristics of the lesion and the amount of bony destruction. The amount of bony destruction is a critical factor in deciding to treat a lesion surgically or nonsurgically, and CT is superior to MRI for this evaluation. CT-guided needle biopsies of soft tissue associated with spinal lesions has proven to be a safe and useful modality, and the use of transpedicular biopsies allows sampling of the vertebral body.

Angiography may be used as a diagnostic tool in identifying the vascular supply of a tumor or the regional neural elements. It also can be used for preoperative embolization of very vascular metastatic tumors, such as thyroid or renal carcinomas, as well as prior to resection of some primary tumors. With cervical tumors that involve the vertebral artery, a trial occlusion of the vertebral artery may be done with a balloon, with the patient awake to assess its effect before occluding the artery with coils.

Tumor Staging

The Enneking surgical staging system for benign and malignant primary bone tumors has been used for more than 20 years. Malignant tumors are staged according to histologic grade, intra- or extracompartmental location of the tumor, and the presence or absence of metastases. Benign tumors are staged using an Arabic numeric system (1-3). The stage of the tumor describes the biologic characteristics of the tumor. Stage 1 tumors remain stable or heal spontaneously. They remain confined to bone and are therefore intracompartmental. Stage 2 lesions are characterized by progressive growth that is limited by natural barriers and are characterized radiographically as being contained within bone. Stage 3 tumors are biologically aggressive tumors that destroy natural barriers as they grow; they are characterized radiographically by cortical destruction and extraosseous extension of tumor into surrounding soft tissue.

Malignant tumors are designated with roman numerals, again into three stages. Each stage is further subdivided into A and B, designating whether the tumor is intracompartmental (A) or extracompartmental (B). Stage I tumors are low grade, whereas stage II tumors are high grade. Stage III tumors are any grade tumor with regional or distant metastases.

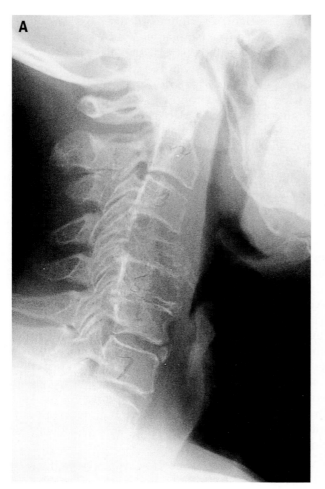

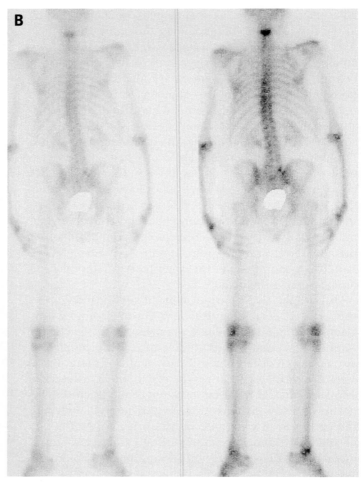

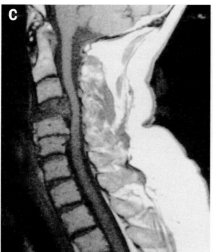

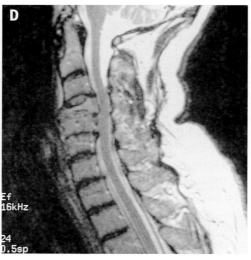

Figure 2 This 76-year-old man had prostate cancer 9 years prior to admission with a recurrence in the bed of the prostate 6 years prior to admission and had been well subsequently with a stable PSA. He was involved in a motor vehicle accident with the acute onset of neck pain approximately 5 months before admission. The pain slowly improved and then began to get worse again. The lateral radiograph showed compression of C4 **(A)** with relative osteopenia. The bone scan **(B)** showed activity only in C4 compatible with either osteopenic fracture or pathologic fracture. A T1 sagittal MRI scan **(C)** showed hypointense compressed body and the T2 sagittal scan **(D)** showed decrease in height but no soft-tissue mass and slightly hyperintense lesion compared with the surrounding vertebrae. Needle biopsy was definitive for metastatic prostate carcinoma.

The Enneking staging system has proven useful in a variety of ways for staging pelvic and extremity bone and soft-tissue tumors. However, the application of this system to the staging of bone tumors in the spine has not been established. This is, at least in part, due to the unique and complex anatomy of the vertebrae and the spinal cord. According to the Enneking system, malignant bone tumors are classified as stage A or B depending on the presence or absence of soft-tissue extension. In the spine, however, the direction of soft-tissue extension, that is, extraosseous intradural versus extraosseous paraspinal soft tissue, is important for surgical planning and may affect prognosis. In an effort to develop a staging system that takes into account some of the unique considerations related to the anatomy of the spine, Weinstein, Boriani, and Biagini developed the WBB staging system. This system divides the vertebra into 12 sectors in a clock-face arrangement, distinguishing right from left and anterior from posterior. Also, five tissue layers are defined, allowing distinction between extension into the paraspinous region from canal extension. Some recent studies, at least preliminarily, show that this system may be superior in developing treatment algorithms and in assessing outcome in patients with benign and malignant primary bone tumors.

For patients with metastatic carcinomas of the spine, predicted survival is important for selecting appropriate treatment. Tokuhashi and associates outlined a prognostic scoring system (Table 1) to predict length of survival for patients with spinal metastases. The scoring system uses six parameters. Within each category patients receive a score from 0 to 2 with increasing scores for more favorable conditions. Thus, a maximum score of 12 would indicate a patient with a more favorable prognosis. Enkaoua and associates found that patients with a score of seven or less had a median survival of only 5.3 months compared with patients with a score of eight or more who had a median survival of 23.6 months.

Surgical Margins

The terminology used for describing surgical margins for spine tumors has been used loosely, without regard to accepted oncologic terminology. Thus, terms such as resection, excision, radical, vertebrectomy, and spondylectomy have been used without defined reproducible definitions. The need for exacting terminology is paramount for preoperative planning and to assess outcomes. The Musculoskeletal Tumor Society has adopted a system of defining surgical margins. Surgical procedures are defined as intralesional, marginal, wide, or radical.

An intralesional procedure is one in which the plane of dissection is through the tumor. This includes curettage within the tumor as well as the total resection of a tumor by breaking it up into pieces. Piecemeal resections or corpectomies therefore always are classified as intralesional, irrespective of whether or not gross tumor is left behind. Curettage, by definition, is an intralesional procedure. Thus, most procedures done for metastatic disease of the spine are piecemeal corpectomies and are intralesional. This type of tumor removal does not affect the prognosis of the patient with metastatic disease because local recurrence after use of adjuvant radiation treatment and/or chemotherapy is rarely a problem except in selected tumors such as renal cell carcinomas.

A marginal resection is one in which the plane of dissection proceeds through the reactive zone of the tumor. This technique is of use in aggressive nonmalignant lesions and occasionally in metastatic lesions.

A wide margin is one in which the plane of dissection is through normal tissue. In a wide resection, normal tissue surrounds the entire tumor. In this case there must be an intact normal margin at all surfaces, and this may be limited by the presence of the dura. Even when the entire tumor is removed as a single block, it is not considered a wide resection if any margin is contaminated. A radical resection is one in which the entire compartment involved by tumor is removed. This resection generally is not feasible for tumors of the spine. Therefore, an en bloc resection may be marginal or wide depending on the plane of dissection achieved when the tumor was removed. It is understood that for primary high-grade sarcomas local control is optimized when a wide

---

TABLE 1 | Tokuhashi's Evaluation System for Prognosis of Metastatic Spinal Tumors

Symptoms	Score*		
	0	**1**	**2**
General condition performance status	Poor (PS 10% to 40%)	Moderate (50% to 70%)	Good (80% to 100%)
No. of extraspinal skeletal metastases	> 3	1 to 2	0
Metastases to internal organs	Unremovable	Removable	No metastases
Primary site of tumor	Lung, stomach	Kidney, liver, uterus, unknown	Thyroid, prostate, breast, rectum
Number of metastases to spine	> 3	2	1
Spinal cord palsy	Complete	Incomplete	None

*Total Score versus survival period:
  9 to 12 points: >12 months survival;
  0 to 5 points: < 3 months survival
(Reproduced with permission from Tokuhashi Y, Matsuzaki H, Toriyama S, Kawano H, Ohsaka S: Scoring system for the preoperative evaluation of metastatic spine tumor prognosis. Spine 1990;15:1110-1113.)

or radical margin can be obtained. In the spine, there is no procedure that will provide a radical margin and maintain the integrity of the spinal cord as defined by the criteria listed above. However, attempts should be made to achieve a wide margin when possible. As such, a high-grade sarcoma involving the vertebral body without involvement of the pedicles or extraosseous extension can be removed with a wide margin. To achieve a wide margin for a tumor that extends to the dura, the dura needs to be resected in continuity with the tumor. It is important to establish that a complete resection removing the tumor piecemeal does not achieve the same result as an actual wide resection.

Making the Diagnosis

After completing an appropriate history and physical examination and obtaining selected imaging studies a tissue diagnosis may be necessary. Before proceeding to biopsy, the differential diagnosis should be considered based on the results of the clinical, radiographic, and laboratory data.

Patients with metastatic disease are likely to have one of two clinical scenarios. The first involves a patient with a lesion involving the spine, as the first appearance of metastatic disease, without a known primary lesion. In this case the evaluation should include a complete physical examination; CT of the chest, abdomen, and pelvis; a bone scan; and blood work (complete blood count, chemistry panel, serum and urine protein electrophoresis). The primary site of disease will be identified in approximately 80% of patients. In some patients a more accessible site for biopsy, other than the spine, will be identified. If the evaluation does not identify the primary site or a more accessible site for biopsy, a CT-guided biopsy of the spine lesion should be performed to differentiate the metastatic lesion from a primary tumor. In the second scenario the patient has a known history of primary carcinoma, but remotely in the past, and the spine lesion is the first presumed recurrence after a long disease-free interval or the characteristics of the lesion do not match those commonly associated with a metastatic lesion from the original primary. A needle biopsy should be performed.

In the small group of patients with suspected primary tumors of the spine, a CT-guided needle biopsy of the lesion should be done, avoiding an open biopsy. For many primary tumors of the spine, surgery is not the first phase of treatment; for example, osteosarcoma and Ewing's sarcoma are best treated with preoperative chemotherapy. Open biopsy is indicated if adequate tissue cannot be obtained with a needle biopsy. If a patient is taken to the operating room for either a needle biopsy or an open biopsy, frozen section analysis of a portion of the tissue should be performed to ensure adequacy of the biopsy before completion of the procedure.

Although the biopsy may be a technically simple procedure, it requires significant cognitive skills and may be associated with high complication rates. The principles of tumor surgery require that the biopsy be performed in such a way as to minimize local contamination and be placed so that the biopsy tract can be excised with the definitive surgical resection. The surgeons who will perform the definitive resection, in the event the tumor proves to be primary, should be consulted before performing a biopsy. Once the decision to proceed with a biopsy has been made, the team of physicians, including radiologists, pathologists, and surgeons, need to decide on the most appropriate biopsy technique.

The techniques available include fine needle aspiration, percutaneous core needle biopsy, and open biopsy. The most appropriate technique will depend on the location of the tumor, the extent of the tumor, and the suspected diagnosis, as well as the expertise of the surgeon, radiologist, and pathologist. Fine needle aspiration is reserved for situations where only a small sample is required and an experienced pathologist and/or cytologist is available. Fine needle aspiration may be useful in confirming a metastatic site when the primary site is unknown, but definitive diagnosis is difficult and core biopsy or open procedure is more appropriate in that instance. It is generally recommended that, if a lymphoma or sarcoma is suspected, a core needle biopsy or open biopsy should be performed. It is impossible to prove a negative, and in the context of the biopsy, it should be remembered that a negative biopsy (no tumor seen) is not the same as proving that a patient's condition is not secondary to a neoplastic process. If a needle biopsy fails to provide a histologic diagnosis and the clinical suspicion is high that there is an underlying neoplastic process, an open biopsy is indicated.

Benign Primary Tumors

The most common benign primary tumors of the spine are osteoid osteoma, osteoblastoma, osteochondroma, giant cell tumor (GCT), hemangioma, Langerhans' cell histiocytosis (previously referred to as eosinophilic granuloma), aneurysmal bone cysts (ABC), and neurofibroma. Benign, primary tumors are far less common than malignant primaries in the spine. The age of the patient and the location of the tumor are very important prognostic indicators. In patients older than 21 years, most spinal tumors are malignant, whereas most spinal tumors in patients younger than 21 years are benign. Furthermore, tumors involving the posterior elements tend to be benign, whereas those in the anterior elements or body are more likely malignant. Pain is by far the most common symptom that may be associated with radicular symptoms; neurologic deficits are generally less common. There are subsets of benign tumors that either can have a high rate of local recurrence (GCT, ABC, osteoblastoma) or can be extremely locally destructive. Their treatment differs from that of other benign, less aggressive tumors because they may require either marginal resection or use of adjuvants to extend the margin of resection.

Osteochondromas of the spine are treated much as they are in the extremities. They generally arise from the posterior elements and, therefore, neurologic compromise is uncommon. When an osteochondroma extends into the spinal canal or impinges on a nerve root, it may become symptomatic and require treatment. Persistently painful lesions or those that cause neurologic deficit can be excised. The risk of local recurrence depends on the patient's age and whether or not the cartilage cap is completely excised. In adults, the risk of local recurrence is negligible irrespective of the extent of the surgery. In skeletally immature patients the lesion may recur if the cartilage cap is not excised with the entire lesion.

Osteoid osteomas are probably the most common primary benign vertebral tumors. They generally occur in teenagers or young adults and most commonly involve the pedicles, transverse processes, or facets. Painful scoliosis or pain that is worse at night and relieved by anti-inflammatory medications suggests this diagnosis. Symptoms may adequately be controlled in some patients with the use of anti-inflammatory medications. Ultimately, the symptoms will resolve as the lesion spontaneously resolves. For patients who cannot tolerate long-term anti-inflammatory medications, surgical excision is recommended. In patients who develop scoliosis associated with the tumor, the tumor tends to be located at the apex of the concavity of the curve. If the tumor is excised at a young age and within 15 months of onset of symptoms, the scoliosis generally resolves. Surgical goals should include excision of the nidus of the tumor. Intralesional procedures with removal of the entire nidus are associated with excellent relief of symptoms and local control.

Osteoblastomas tend to have many of the same clinical characteristics as osteoid osteoma; however, they are larger (greater than 2 cm), and pain is not relieved as predictably with anti-inflammatory medications. They also often have a larger soft-tissue component and have a higher incidence of neurologic involvement secondary to spinal canal invasion than osteoid osteomas. The spine is the most common site of involvement, accounting for 40% of all cases. Osteoblastomas have a propensity for involvement of the posterior elements of the spine. The treatment of osteoblastomas involving the

spine depends on the stage and location of the tumor. For stage 2 lesions, intralesional procedures may suffice, but, when possible, marginal resection should be performed. For stage 3 lesions marginal resection is more likely to achieve local control than intralesional curettage. Radiation has been used as an adjuvant in recurrent stage 3 lesions.

Hemangiomas of the spine usually first come to attention after they are discovered as an incidental finding. It is important to recognize the condition so as to avoid unnecessary interventions. Autopsy studies indicate that more than 10% of the population have asymptomatic hemangiomas involving the spine. Although the vast majority of lesions remain asymptomatic, they can cause pathologic fractures and cord compression. Radiographically, hemangiomas of the spine appear as parallel, vertically oriented striations without vertebral enlargement. The vertically oriented lines have been referred to as having a corduroy cloth appearance. On CT scan the thickened trabeculae, viewed in cross section, give a polka dot appearance. Hemangiomas may be confused with Paget's disease on plain film, but the vertebral enlargement associated with Paget's disease is not seen in hemangiomas. In most cases patients with hemangiomas require no treatment.

Hemangiomas of the thoracic or lumbar spine may become symptomatic in the third trimester of pregnancy. If neural symptoms or severe pain ensue, embolization may provide symptomatic relief until after the pregnancy is complete. In rare cases of progressive vertebral collapse and/or nerve root or cord compression, surgery may be indicated. Angiography and preoperative embolization are recommended prior to curettage.

ABCs can occur anywhere in the spine but are most commonly found in the thoracolumbar region and in the posterior elements. Multiple levels of adjacent vertebral involvement are common. Affected patients are rarely younger than 5 years of age but 85% are younger than 20 years. Radiographically, ABCs produce cortical expansion with osteolysis. Within the central lytic area septations may give a soap bubble appearance. MRI may reveal fluid/fluid levels within the lesion. Cortical destruction with soft-tissue tumor extension is not uncommon. Treatment may include curettage, wide local excision (if possible), embolization, and radiation. Embolization may lead to resolution of the cyst. In cases where the cyst does not resolve, embolization at least reduces intraoperative blood loss associated with curettage. Recurrence rates of up to 25% have been reported.

GCTs typically are seen in patients during the third or fourth decade of life. Any level or column of the spine can be affected, especially the sacrum. Local control is especially difficult to achieve for large lesions involving the spine that may be associated with a large soft-tissue component (stage 3) (Fig. 3, *A* to *D*). Surgical treatment usually involves extended intralesional curettage or in selected cases a marginal en bloc resection(Fig. 3, *E*). Curettage alone results in a 50% recurrence rate of GCTs, and some form of adjuvant treatment such as liquid nitrogen, phenol, or methylmethacrylate is necessary for improved control. Radiation has been used as an adjuvant for patients

with tumors that cannot be resected. Before deeming a tumor unresectable a surgeon experienced in the treatment of spinal tumors should be consulted. Local recurrences are especially difficult to treat and, despite the tumor being benign, local progression of tumor may result in the patient's demise.

Langerhans' cell histiocytosis (previously eosinophilic granuloma) is seen in the first and second decades of life. It usually is located in the vertebral body and is

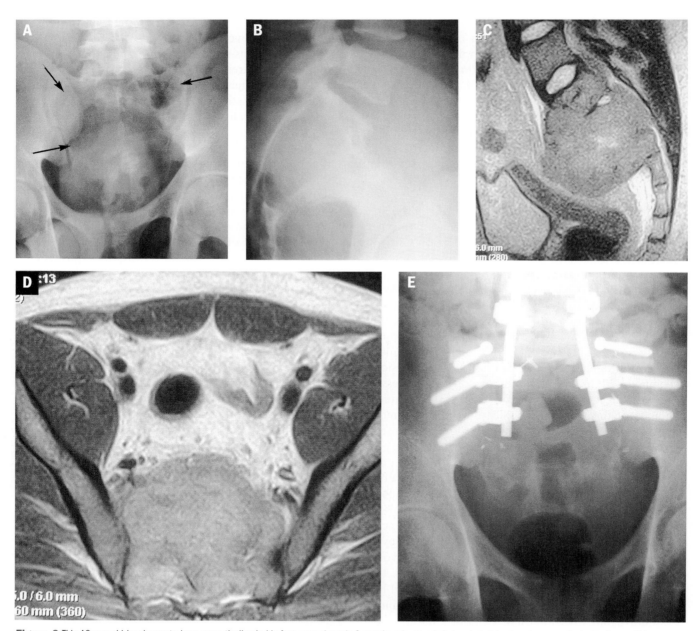

Figure 3 This 18-year-old boy began to have some tingling in his foot approximately 6 months prior to admission, but did not seek any medical attention until he was involved in a motor vehicle accident and had back pain with increased weakness in his foot. The AP radiograph **(A)** of his pelvis shows an expansile lesion of the sacrum (*arrows*). The lateral radiograph of the sacrum **(B)** also shows an expansile lesion with midsagittal MRI demonstrating an involvement of S1 through S3 **(C)** with a large anterior soft-tissue mass. The axial cuts **(D)** show the extent of the soft-tissue mass and the compromise of the sacral roots. The patient underwent a combined anterior and posterior resection of S1, S2, and S3. Reconstruction **(E)** was done with a humeral strut from one side of the ilium to the other and fusion of the lumbar spine into the ilium bilaterally.

classically discovered as vertebra plana. Observation is the mainstay of therapy because this lesion is generally self-limited. Bracing can be used to prevent kyphosis as the vertebral height reconstitutes. Low-dose radiation, steroid injection, and occasionally curettage are alternate therapies. Langerhans' cell histiocytosis of the spine may represent an isolated lesion or one of multiple lesions comprising a spectrum of disease. Surgical intervention rarely is warranted and biopsy, when indicated, usually can be performed with a needle.

Neurofibromas generally arise from the nerve root or its associated sheath. They tend to exist both intradurally and extradurally. They have a classic dumbbell shape when they extend out through the neuroforamen. Scoliosis is a complication, and these patients must be treated early and aggressively. Malignant degeneration occurs in up to 20% of patients. Symptomatic lesions should be resected, preferably en bloc in noncritical nerve roots. Otherwise, they should be resected with microsurgical techniques.

Primary Sarcomas of Bone

There are three major types of primary sarcomas of bone. These are osteosarcoma, Ewing's sarcoma, and chondrosarcoma. Both osteosarcoma and Ewing's sarcoma are more common in young adults, whereas chondrosarcoma is more commonly seen in the age group from approximately 30 to 70 years. These primary sarcomas of bone can involve any areas of the spine.

Ewing's sarcoma generally is seen in the youngest age group of the three, commonly between the ages of 5 and 20 years. This tumor can be mistaken for infection (Fig. 4) because patients may have a history of local pain, slightly elevated sedimentation rate, and occasionally, fever. In the early stages, a soft-tissue mass may not be evident. Approximately 5% of all Ewing's sarcomas occur in the spine, and it also is common in the pelvis. The radiologic picture for Ewing's sarcoma is a motheaten appearance of the involved vertebra. A major differentiating factor is the preservation of the disc spaces. Most spine infections in children begin in the disc space and involve the end plates and then adjacent vertebrae; with Ewing's sarcoma the end plates are preserved until late in the disease and a soft-tissue mass can often be seen adjacent to the vertebra early in the disease (Fig. 4).

Ewing's sarcoma has a well-defined treatment program that has been shown to be reasonably effective for patients with tumors in the extremities and pelvis.

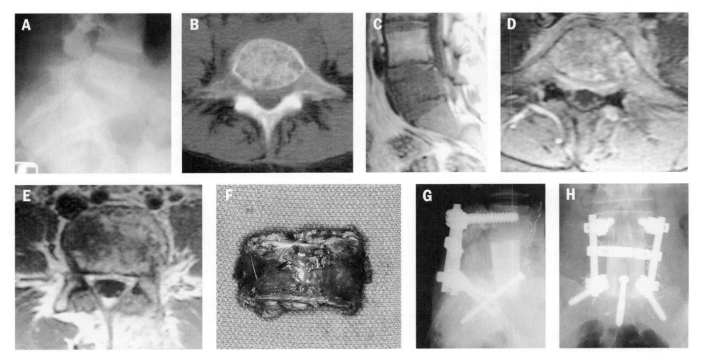

Figure 4 This 16-year-old girl began having severe low back pain with a slight elevation of her white blood cell count and sedimentation rate. The lateral radiograph **(A)** showed some sclerosis of the vertebral body but preservation of the end plates. Initial diagnosis was of osteomyelitis, although no organisms were grown, and she was treated with antibiotics without improvement for approximately 6 weeks. The CT scan axial cuts of L5 **(B)** demonstrate a motheaten appearance with a soft-tissue mass anterior to the body. Sagittal T1 MRI scan **(C)** demonstrated an involvement of the L5 vertebral body with an anterior soft-tissue mass. Axial images with gadolinium enhancement **(D)** accentuated the vertebral body involvement and the paraspinal mass. Percutaneous needle biopsy was nondiagnostic and a transpedicular biopsy was diagnostic of Ewing's sarcoma. She subsequently underwent chemotherapy, and a postchemotherapy gadolinium-enhanced axial MRI scan **(E)** demonstrates complete regression of the tumor mass and loss of enhancement. After completion of the initial four cycles of the chemotherapy the patient underwent an en bloc resection **(F)** with the disc serving as soft-tissue margin superiorly and inferiorly and the periosteum as the margin both anteriorly and posteriorly. Reconstruction **(G and H)** was done after the initial posterior stage with posterior instrumentation and strut grafts from L4 to the sacral ala and anteriorly after removal of the body using a femoral allograft with fixation into the sacrum. Pathology demonstrated essentially complete necrosis of the tumor.

For satisfactory results, it is critical to translate that treatment regimen as closely as possible to tumors of the spine. Use of this multimodality regimen currently yields an average 5-year survival rate of 75%. The treatment regimen includes initial biopsy, generally CT-guided. Usually the soft-tissue component of the tumor rather than the bone can be biopsied (Fig. 4, *B* to *D*). Ewing's sarcoma is most easily defined with biopsy into the adjacent soft-tissue mass. Occasionally a transpedicular biopsy is necessary. The biopsy tract should be placed in line of the subsequent resection. Preoperative chemotherapy is then instituted. Depending on the protocol, several cycles of chemotherapy are administered and the staging studies repeated. Ewing's sarcomas are generally very sensitive to chemotherapy, and the soft-tissue component of the tumor should dramatically decrease in size or resolve completely (Fig. 4, *E*). Pain response is generally immediate within the first cycle, with resolution of pain and stabilization of any compression fractures that have occurred.

In the extremities, chemotherapy can be followed by radiation alone for tumors in nonexpendable bones that have not fractured. A radiation dose of 6,000 cGy is necessary for a cure of Ewing's lesions. For expendable bones, resection of the tumor has been used as a very effective modality, with radiation reserved for only those patients who have a positive margin. In the spine, the use of 6,000 cGy of radiation therapy is not conventionally undertaken. Above 5,000 cGy, the incidence of radiation myelitis is prohibitive. Thus, it was believed that Ewing's sarcoma of the vertebrae was less effectively treated than that in the extremity; however, using the same principles as in the extremity, an en bloc resection of the vertebrae should be undertaken. If the soft-tissue mass has shrunk completely with chemotherapy, the vertebral body can be resected in toto (Fig. 4, *F* to *H*). If the margins are negative, no radiation therapy is indicated. With the use of proton beam radiation, higher doses can be achieved around the spine, and with the use of brachytherapy, effective doses can be used to attempt to sterilize positive margins. Adequate doses of radiation (> 6,000 cGy) can be delivered with close proximity to the spinal cord by either the implantation of iodine I 125 seeds or catheters for brachytherapy. Subsequent to the en bloc resection, the chemotherapy is completed and follow-up is undertaken in a fashion similar to that for extremity sarcomas.

Although osteosarcoma is the second most common osseous malignant tumor, it is extremely infrequent in the spine. Less than 2% of all osteosarcomas occur primarily in the spine. Although most patients with osteosarcoma are seen in either the second or third decade of life there is another peak at approximately the sixth decade of life, which sometimes but not always is

related to the presence of Paget's disease. The treatment of osteosarcoma involving the spine should parallel that seen for osteosarcomas within the extremity. Current treatment with multiagent chemotherapy for two cycles preoperatively followed by resection of the tumor and four cycles postoperatively can give very encouraging results. If the degree of necrosis within the resected tumor specimen demonstrates 90% tumor kill or better, the expected survival of the patient at 5 years is 85%. However, if there is less than 90% tumor kill and the chemotherapy regimen is not changed, the survival rate mirrors the prechemotherapy era of 5-year survival at approximately 25%.

The biopsy tract should be placed in an area that is conducive to resection of the tract with the definitive tumor resection. The work-up should mirror that of extremity osteosarcomas, with CT scan of the chest, bone scan, and accurate delineation of the lesion by MRI and CT scan. High dose chemotherapy should then be initiated using the same multiagent regimen as for extremity osteosarcomas. A satisfactory response to chemotherapy radiographically often is indicated by heavy calcification within the previously seen soft-tissue mass adjacent to the spine or extremity structure.

The principles of resection for osteosarcoma of the extremity are clear and should be adhered to when considering resection of osteosarcomas of the spine. The tumor must be taken out as a single block with a negative margin. Positive margins in osteosarcoma routinely result in recurrence of the tumor. In the spine it is clearly more difficult to obtain a true wide resection. The resection margins should be through the disc, proximal and distal to the lesion and, if the end plates have been destroyed, through the bodies of the uninvolved vertebrae adjacent to the lesion. Anteriorly, the resection should be extraperiosteal and the posterior margin for lesions involving the vertebral body should be the posterior longitudinal ligament. In most sarcomas, the posterior longitudinal ligament is respected by the tumor. For posterior lesions, en bloc resection is somewhat easier because the paraspinous musculature can be used as a margin, with the pedicles resected through their bases and the entire posterior aspect of the spine removed as a single block.

Postoperatively, the same consideration should be used in evaluating the response of the tumor to chemotherapy, with additional cycles of the same chemotherapy if an adequate tumor response is noted in the specimen and with a change in chemotherapy for inadequate responses. The role of radiation therapy is not clearly defined in the treatment of osteosarcoma of the spine. Long-term survival has now been reported for patients with osteosarcoma of the spine.

Chondrosarcoma occurs with a higher relative frequency than the other sarcomas. In comparison to both Ewing's sarcoma and osteosarcoma, chondrosarcomas are neither radiosensitive nor chemosensitive. Therefore the primary modality is surgical treatment. Again, as in extremity chondrosarcoma, the goal is to achieve a wide surgical margin.

Chordomas are malignant tumors that are believed to arise from residual notochordal tissue within the vertebrae. They arise strictly within the axial skeleton, although occasional tumors arise within the sinuses. They most commonly are seen in the fifth to seventh decades of life, although they can occur as early as the second decade. Approximately 60% of all chordomas arise in the sacrum, followed by 25% in the clivus and the remainder (15%) distributed among the cervical, thoracic, and lumbar spine with predominance in the lumbar spine.

Chordomas account for nearly half of all solitary sacral tumors. In the sacrum they tend to be central in location and involve the distal sacrum (S3 and below). Symptoms of sacral chordomas include an insidious onset of pain that may be associated with constipation, coccydynia, hemorrhoids, and, ultimately, changes in bowel and bladder function. More than 50% of sacral chordomas are palpable by rectal examination initially. Radiographically, chordomas are lytic but are very difficult to see in the sacrum. Delays in diagnosis of chordomas and other sacral tumors occur often because the radiographic changes are too subtle and obscured by the overlying bowel gas. The most effective modality for visualizing these tumors is MRI, because they generally have a large soft-tissue mass, effectively delineating the tumor.

Treatment of these tumors is predominantly surgical. Because of the relatively slow growth of the lesions there are no effective chemotherapeutic modalities. The tumors can be metastatic to both bone and lung. Preoperative evaluation should include a CT scan of the chest. Tumors of the sacrum are usually relatively amenable to an en bloc resection. Sacral tumors can be divided into two groups: tumors at S3 and below, which can usually be resected from a posterior-only approach with sparing of continence. If both S2 roots are preserved, continence will be present in most patients. Tumors that extend above S3 generally require a sequenced anterior and posterior resection to control the mass anteriorly prior to removing it posteriorly. With lesions involving S1 and S2, sacral stability is a potential problem. With sacral chordomas survival is generally long, with a mean survival in excess of 7 years in spite of presence of tumor, in contrast to tumors of the mobile spine where survival is much more limited (generally less than 5 years).

Although it has been difficult, removing the entire vertebral segment as a single bloc with negative margins is the goal for treatment of chordomas of the mobile spine. It has been well demonstrated in a recent series from the Rizzoli Institute that attempts at debulking or piecemeal corpectomy, as opposed to removing the entire vertebral body en bloc, routinely result in recurrence of the disease. Proton beam radiation has been shown to be a helpful adjunct in tumors of the clivus and cervical spine. The tumor is generally not sensitive to doses under 6,000 cGy, thus a standard external beam does not achieve high enough doses to stabilize the tumor; however, proton beam radiation allows higher doses in close proximity to the spinal cord without unreasonable risk of radiation myelitis. Thus in patients with positive margins at their initial resection or at the time of recurrence after debulking of recurrent tumor, the use of either brachytherapy or proton beam treatment may be indicated.

Surgical Techniques for Treatment of Primary Tumors of the Spine

Benign Primary Tumors

For most benign primary tumors of the spine, curettage with bone grafting, using either autologous or allograft bone is sufficient. Occasionally, as with stage II osteoblastomas, a corpectomy is indicated using standard piecemeal techniques. Preoperative embolization in highly vascular tumors, such as osteoblastomas, GCTs and ABCs, may diminish the morbidity of the procedure.

Care must be taken when planning surgical procedures in children to prevent secondary deformities after removal of segments that may affect spinal stability. Children who have undergone laminectomies in either the thoracic or the cervical spine may develop secondary kyphotic deformities. The incidence is extremely high in children younger than age 10 years; therefore, concurrent short fusions should be considered to prevent excess kyphosis.

More aggressive benign lesions may require either adjunctive techniques or more extensive resections. GCTs can be approached by an intralesional technique when there is a sufficient remnant of cortical margin; however, curettage and bone grafting alone should result in a 50% recurrence rate as in extremity GCTs. Thus adjuvant techniques, using either phenol, methylmethacrylate, or liquid nitrogen, should help to decrease the recurrence rate. Methylmethacrylate can be used in the anterior portion of the spine for stability as well as an adjunct in prevention of tumor recurrence. When methylmethacrylate is used anteriorly, a posterior fusion over the same levels should be undertaken. The second approach for large, aggressive tumors such as GCTs is a marginal resection, which obviates the need for an adjuvant and is most effective in large tumors with a ballooned cortex and a significant soft-tissue mass, even though the mass is rimmed by a very thin reactive bone margin in the periosteum. Reconstruction, especially in the sacrum, can be challenging (Fig. 3).

Malignant Primary Tumors

Malignant primary tumors of the spine present a much greater challenge to the surgeon. Techniques for resection of the sacrum (initially described by Stener) have been refined over a long period of time. Posterior resection of the distal portion of the sacrum (S3 and below) has the common problem of adequacy of the proximal margin (Fig. 5). Resection of more proximal lesions can be done through a simultaneous anterior and posterior resection, although that often is more morbid than a sequenced anterior and posterior resection. The ante-

rior portion, done first, frees the rectum from the anterior portion of the tumor or resects the rectum and adds colostomy. Control of all the feeding vessels is critical. Initial separation of the anterior portion of the sacroiliac (SI) joints and resection of the L5-S1 discs makes later posterior removal of the tumor feasible. The second stage posterior procedure resects either through the SI joints or just lateral to the SI joints. Prior control of both the nerves and the vessels anteriorly makes the posterior resection a less morbid procedure.

En bloc vertebrectomy, originally reported by Raymond Roy-Camille, differs slightly between the thoracic and the lumbar spine. In either case the vertebral body is resected as an entire piece. A recent modification by Tomita uses a saw to transect the pedicles. En bloc resection in the lumbar spine begins with resection of the posterior elements all the way down to the posterior aspect

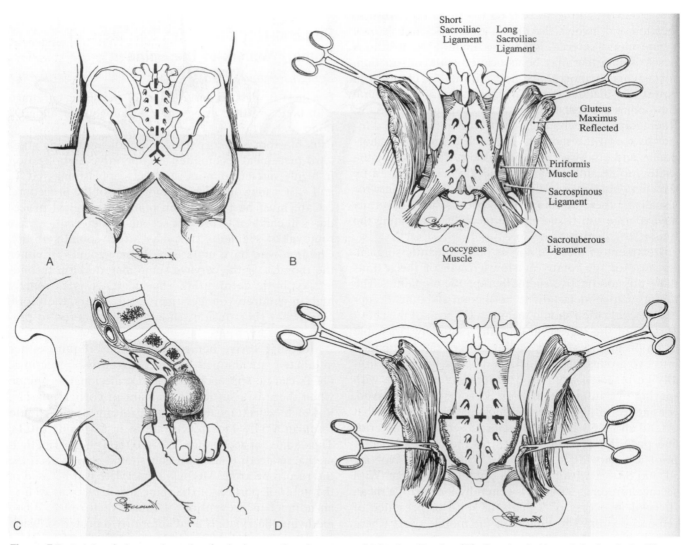

Figure 5 The technique for low sacral resection of a chordoma or other primary tumors distal to the midportion of L3. *(Reproduced with permission from Levine AM, Crandall DG: Treatment of primary malignant tumors of the spince and sacrum, in Bridwell KH (ed): The Textbook of Spinal Surgery, ed 2. New York, NY, Lippincott-Raven, 1997, pp 1983-2006.)*

of the vertebral body, leveling the pedicles flush to the back of the vertebral body (Fig. 4). The transverse processes must be resected and the nerve roots under them freed. If there is tumor within one of the pedicles, the pedicle can be left long and the end of it plugged with methylmethacrylate to keep from spilling tumor or resected just short of the margin of the tumor. As part of the posterior stage, the posterior aspects of the anulus of the discs above and below the vertebrae that are to be resected are transected as widely as possible. If one pedicle is left long, there is an increased chance of damaging or removing the adjacent nerve root, which adds some additional complexity to the resection. If tumor does penetrate into the posterior elements, transecting the pedicles and removing the posterior elements en bloc will leave a contaminated margin. Even with the Tomita technique of transecting the pedicles using a T-saw, if there is tumor back into the pedicle, the margin will be contaminated although the vertebra is taken out in two large pieces. Once all of the resection is done posteriorly, stabilization is inserted, generally at a level above and below the area of resection.

Anteriorly, resection is done in an extraperiosteal fashion because, at all levels, the aorta and vena cava lie directly on the vertebral body and must be immobilized. Therefore, the margin is generally no greater than the periosteum. An intact margin can be maintained even in the face of a small soft-tissue mass. Reconstruction is done with various techniques depending on the level and the need for additional treatment. Methylmethacrylate can be used as an anterior spacer, which in the face of radiation, may be the preferable reconstruction if a posterior fusion is done. For those patients not requiring radiation therapy, use of either a cage or a femoral or humeral allograft is generally effective.

En bloc vertebrectomy has been shown to be effective for the treatment of chordomas as well as other malignant tumors in the lumbar spine. The modification of this technique for the thoracic spine can be done in several different ways, as described by Raymond Roy-Camille; the entire procedure can be done extrapleurally from a posterior approach. The posterior elements are resected, and the costovertebral junctions are either disarticulated or the ribs are resected, leaving the rib head with the specimen. If the segmental vessels and nerve roots are sacrificed on one side, the entire specimen can be removed posteriorly and the reconstruction also done extrapleurally posteriorly. This is possible in tumors that are completely intraosseous, but less preferable in those with a soft-tissue mass where the pleura may be the margin and anterior resection and reconstruction are necessary.

Resection of primary tumors of the cervical spine presents the greatest challenge. Frequently the tumor

involves the vertebral artery on at least one side, and achieving a margin is extremely difficult. Authors of a recent small series have outlined the technique of sacrifice of the vertebral artery to obtain a wider margin in tumors of the cervical spine (Fig. 6). Advanced radiation therapy techniques such as brachytherapy and proton radiation still need further investigation.

Metastatic Disease

The most commonly encountered tumor of the spine is a metastasis. The goals of treatment for metastatic tumor to the spine must be clearly identified. In most tumors, the treatment of the metastatic lesion does not prolong the patient's survival except to prevent quadriplegia and paraplegia, which can markedly diminish a patient's life expectancy. The goals of treatment are to control pain, restore neural functioning, correct instability, and prevent pathologic fracture. The methods by which these goals are accomplished are based on the histology of the tumor, the extent of spine involvement, the presence of other metastatic disease, the sensitivity of the primary tumor to radiation and/or chemotherapy, and the patient's remaining life expectancy.

Patients are found to have spinal metastases in one of three ways: as an incidental finding during routine initial evaluation or in subsequent follow-up evaluations, as a result of a symptomatic back lesion (either at the initial manifestation of an undiagnosed primary or at some interval after diagnosis of the original primary tumor), or after seeking medical evaluation as a result

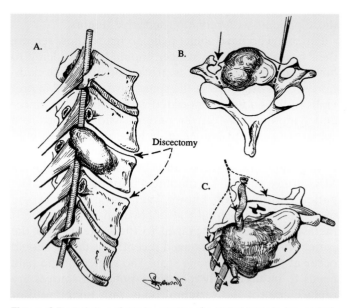

Figure 6 The technique of anterior resection of a cervical tumor having vertebral artery involvement. *(Reproduced with permission from Levine AM, Crandall DG: Treatment of primary malignant tumors of the spince and sacrum, in Bridwell KH (ed): The Textbook of Spinal Surgery, ed 2. New York, NY, Lippincott-Raven, 1997, pp 1983-2006.)*

of neurologic deficit.

The patient with an incidental finding of a metastatic lesion should carefully be examined to make sure there are absolutely no symptoms. It is critical to know the amount of pain medication that the patient is receiving and what the clinical course with relation to the level of pain management has been in recent weeks. There are patients who state that they are pain free but have escalated their reliance on pain medicine. Thus, the patient who clearly is taking no significant narcotic pain medication and is doing well is truly asymptomatic; whereas, the patient taking increasing doses of opiates may be having significant spinal pain masked by the amount of pain medication. If the patient is asymptomatic and the radiographs do not show any findings, the patient simply can be followed without further radiologic evaluation. If obvious destruction of the vertebra is evident on plain radiograph, a CT or MRI scan is indicated to assess the degree of destruction of the vertebral body. Attempts have been made to predict which patient will go on to pathologic fracture based on the degree of destruction (Table 2). More than 50% destruction of the vertebral body on CT in the lumbar spine along with any disruption of the posterior elements generally suggests further collapse of the vertebra. In the thoracic spine, destruction of the costovertebral junction and a significant portion of the vertebral body suggests potential for pathologic fracture. Several point systems and methodologies have been suggested but they are, at best, helpful and not clearly diagnostic (Table 2). If significant new structural compromises occur in the vertebral body, radiation may be a reasonable alternative for those patients with radiation-sensitive tumors.

Patients who have spinal pain, no matter how remote their history of primary cancer, should be considered to have a metastasis until it is proven otherwise. In addition, second primaries in the spine have occurred in previous radiation fields associated with both breast cancer and lymphoma. A cancer patient who has localized spinal pain should immediately have radiographs with no delay for a trial of nonsurgical treatment. If the plain radiographs are negative and the pain is radicular an MRI study should be obtained initially as well. The patient with other known metastatic disease and mechanical pain should also have an MRI study. If metastatic tumor is localized to the vertebra and the patient has not been restaged recently, restaging should occur at least with a bone scan. The source of the pain needs to be accurately identified; potential sources are replacement of the vertebral body with tumor with or without microfracture, root and/or cord compression, or instability because of structural deformation of the vertebral body.

The plan for treatment is then based significantly on

TABLE 2	Risk Factors for Collapse With Metastatic Disease of The Thoracic And Lumbar Spine

Thoracic Spine
Risk factors
    Costovertebral joint destruction
    Percent of body involvement

Criteria for impending collapse
    50% to 60% body involvement alone
    25% to 30% of body with costovertebral involvement

Lumbar Spine
Risk factors
    Pedicle destruction
    Percent of body involvement

Criteria for impending collapse
    35%to40% of body involvement alone
    25% with pedicle and/or posterior element destruction

(Reproduced with permission from Taneichi H, Kaneda K, Takeda N, Abumi K, Satoh S: Risk factors and probability of vertebral body collapse in metastases of the thoracic and lumbar spine. Spine 1997;22:239-245.)

the life expectancy and overall condition of the patient, along with the desires and wishes of both the patient and his or her family, on the sensitivity of the tumor to radiation and chemotherapy, and on the cause of pain. Assuming reasonable longevity, if the source of pain is simply tumor invasion without compression of neural structures and radiation is possible, radiation therapy is generally the first line of treatment. Change in chemotherapeutic regimen or initiation of chemotherapy in tumors such as lymphoma, myeloma, and breast cancer may also be instituted. If neural compression without frank neurologic deficit is the source of pain, radiation is indicated for a radiosensitive tumor; however, in tumors such as renal cell carcinoma the effect of radiation is at best equivocal. The physician must consider the potential for surgery, because if a port being used for radiation is subsequently needed for surgery the potential for secondary wound healing problems is increased especially in the face of steroid use or malnutrition. In such situations, a combined modality may be used first, followed by radiation therapy to minimize subsequent complications. If the pain is from gross instability or from actual fracture of the vertebra, radiation therapy generally will not be effective.

In tumors such as lung carcinoma and renal cell carcinoma the potential for a fracture to heal within the residual life span of the patient is often minimal. Even in tumors such as breast carcinoma only 50% of patients will have pathologic fractures heal within their life expectancies. Myeloproliferative tumors, such as myeloma and lymphoma, are preferentially treated with radiation unless there is gross instability or pain secondary to instability in those with radioinsensitive tumors or without chemotherapy options and a sufficient life expectancy. In that case posterior instrumentation or anterior vertebral body resection and stabilization could be performed based on the nature of the instability.

A new alternative for treatment of patients with a pathologic fracture with minimal deformity is vertebroplasty. This technique is effective for patients with mechanical pain, or intact posterior wall and no dural or root compression. The vertebral body is percutaneously stabilized by a bipedicular injection of methylmethacrylate. Short-term results are encouraging, and complication rates are acceptable. In most cases if tumor needs to be removed, a piecemeal corpectomy or partial removal of a tumor generally achieves the goals of the surgery.

For patients with neurologic deficit, an MRI is used to assess the mechanism for production of the deficit and localize the area of compression to either anterolateral or posterior and to evaluate the entire spine for additional areas of disease. Recent studies have demonstrated that more than 10% of patients with neurologic deficit will have a second area of cord compression. It is catastrophic if a patient undergoes surgery for a lesion in one area and wakes up with additional neurologic deficit because of manipulation of an unstable lesion in another area. Generally, patients with two levels of significant epidural compression have a shorter life expectancy than patients with single-level compression, so treatment alternatives other than surgery may be indicated.

When considering treatment for patients with neurologic deficit, the factors discussed for other metastatic disease to the spine are important. First the patient's general condition and the overall wishes of the patient and the family must be considered. Rating scales, while of limited value, may give some guidance. An extremely critical feature in making a decision on the patient who has neurologic deficit secondary to epidural compression is the histology of the tumor. Patients with myeloma and lymphoma are much more likely to have quick resolution of their neurologic symptoms with the use of radiation therapy; whereas, patients with renal cell carcinoma, prostate carcinoma, and breast and lung carcinoma are less likely to have such rapid resolution. After initial assessment, the patient should be started on dexamethasone. Randomized studies have demonstrated that no additional effects of steroids are achieved with doses in excess of 10 mg administered

intravenously every 6 hours.

The rate of onset of neurologic deficit has a significant effect on prognosis. A recent study looking at the effectiveness of radiation therapy for patients with motor deficits from spinal cord compression demonstrated that approximately 90% of patients with a slow onset of motor deficit (longer than 2 weeks) had improvement of motor function when treated with radiation. In contrast, only 12% of patients who developed a more rapid onset of motor deficit (between 1 and 13 days) had improvement of motor function. Only 6% of patients who developed severe deterioration of motor deficit in less than 48 hours showed any improvement. After radiation, patients with a very slow onset of deficit had a result that was stable over a 3-month period; whereas, 50% of patients with an intermediate rate of onset showed further deterioration within the next 3 months, and 65% who rapidly developed deficit showed further deterioration at 3 months. Interestingly, the median survival for that series was only 4 months.

The controversy between the use of surgical intervention and radiation therapy has been long and persistent. The data overall seem to favor a more rapid and complete response in patients undergoing surgical intervention for one level of isolated neural compression due to metastatic disease.

The other controversy that has been evident in the treatment of metastatic disease is the mode of decompression. For the last 20 years a large number of studies have been published looking at both anterior and posterior decompression. Of patients having neural deficit, 70% have anterior tumor pressing on the dural sac, 20% have predominantly lateral tumor depressing the dural sac, and only 10% have posterior tumor. Generally, the studies have demonstrated that anterior decompression for anterior tumor is superior.

Several recent studies have looked at the quality of the improvement. In one series of 76 patients the postoperative mean survival was 13.1 months and the mean time at home after the spinal surgery was 11.1 months. Of the patients, 93% were able to walk postoperatively and pain relief was noted in 89%, with 67% of the patients achieving moderate or good health as shown by the Karnofsky Index and 80% being satisfied with their surgical intervention. However, postoperative complications occurred in about 20% of the patients, and local tumor recurred in 20% of those in a series looking at all tumor types.

Renal cell carcinoma recurs in approximately 50% of patients at 6 months if no adjuvant modalities to radiation and surgery are used. Intraoperative radiation therapy has been attempted for spinal tumors but the technique needs further verification of its effectiveness. A recent report of 101 patients undergoing surgery, with

80% of them operated on from a posterolateral approach, demonstrated local recurrence of 70% after 1 year; only 22% of patients who were unable to walk before the surgery regained that ability within the first 3 months. Thus, overall, the neurologic recovery rates have not been as high in patients having surgery from a posterior approach as in those having surgery from an anterior approach. Some patients have had only laminectomy while others have had laminectomy and stabilization, neither of which adequately decompresses the patient with anterior tumor. The transpedicular approach to decompression is technically more difficult and does not allow as adequate a decompression as is done from anterior.

Method of Reconstruction of Patients Undergoing Decompression and Stabilization for Metastatic Disease of the Spine

For those patients undergoing anterior decompression in either the cervical or the thoracic spine, methylmethacrylate, autologous bone, and allograft bone have been used for reconstruction. The mean life expectancy of these patients is approximately 14 months, and most of the patients will have received radiation therapy either preoperatively or postoperatively; therefore, the probability of obtaining a solid arthrodesis with bone graft placed anteriorly is not significant. Reconstruction with methylmethacrylate as a spacer anteriorly with the use of other adjunctive stabilization (a rod within the methylmethacrylate or a plate spanning the construct) has been shown to be durable (Fig. 1). The overall consideration for these patients is rapidity of mobilization by means of a construct that will allow them to return to function as rapidly as possible. Postoperative immobilization using a shell or brace should be avoided if possible to maximize remaining quality of life.

The evaluation of patients with autologous graft in place to look for recurrent disease may be more difficult than the evaluation of patients with methylmethacrylate. In the cervical spine of a patient with presumed long life expectancy (breast cancer, thyroid carcinoma), a posterior arthrodesis can be done easily; it adds only a short duration to the surgery and generally will be out of the radiation field. In the thoracic spine and especially in the lumbar spine, when there is both anterior and posterior destruction, an anterior decompression and reconstruction may be augmented by a posterior procedure. If anterior disease alone is evident, anterior reconstruction may be sufficient.

Summary

Tumors of the spine need to be divided into primary benign tumors, primary malignant tumors, and metastatic tumors. Goals of treatment must be clearly delineated and the oncologic principles for effective tumor treatment must be merged with emerging techniques in spinal surgery. It is understood that, in the spine, it may be difficult to obtain a true wide resection. However, negative margins can be obtained, especially in tumors that involve only the posterior elements or only the anterior elements. Obtaining a negative margin is critical to the long-term survival of patients with osteosarcoma, chondrosarcoma, Ewing's sarcoma, and chordoma. Contaminated margins may require adjuvant treatment. Finally, metastatic disease of the spine has a wide spectrum of manifestations. In considering the appropriate treatment not only the manifestation but also the patient's condition, survival, histologic type, response to adjuvant modalities, and reason for symptoms must clearly be delineated. When treating these patients, techniques that require prolonged immobilization should be avoided, with the goal of treatment being rapid mobilization and return to function.

Annotated Bibliography

Boriani S, Weinstein JN, Biagini R: Primary bone tumors of the spine: Terminology and surgical staging. *Spine* 1997;22:1036-1044.

The authors review oncologic staging and terminology and describe surgical procedures for benign and malignant primary bone tumors of the spine. They introduce a tumor classification for the spine, based on the principles of the Enneking system.

Cook AM, Lau TN, Tomlinson MJ, Vaidya M, Wakeley CJ, Goddard P: Magnetic resonance imaging of the whole spine in suspected malignant spinal cord compression: Impact on management. *Clin Oncol (R Coll Radiol)* 1998;1039-1043.

Data from 127 patients with suspected cord compression secondary to tumor who underwent MRI of the whole spine were reviewed. The authors recommend that patients with suspected spinal cord compression resulting from tumor should undergo MRI evaluation of the entire spine.

Katagiri H, Takahashi M, Inagaki J, et al: Clinical results of nonsurgical treatment for spinal metastases. *Int J Radiat Oncol Biol Phys* 1998;42:1127-1132.

The authors of this prospective study evaluated 101 patients with spinal metastasis who were treated with radiation and/or chemotherapy. They found that responsiveness of the primary tumor was a reliable predictor of neurologic outcome.

McPhee IB, Williams RP, Swanson CE: Factors influencing wound healing after surgery for metastatic disease of the spine. *Spine* 1998;23:726-733.

The authors reviewed the records of 53 patients who underwent 75 surgeries for metastatic tumor involving the spine to determine the risk factors associated with wound complications. They found that poor preoperative nutritional status and perioperative administration of corticosteriods were statistically significant factors predisposing patients to wound complications.

Rades D, Blach M, Nerreter V, Bremer M, Karstens JH: Metastatic spinal cord compression: Influence of time between onset of motoric deficits and start of irradiation on therapeutic effect. *Strahlenther Onkol* 1999;175: 378-381.

In a retrospective review of patients with spinal metastasis and motor deficit, the authors found that patients who had a slower onset of neurologic deficit before starting radiation therapy had a better response to therapy and a better functional outcome than patients who developed deficits over a period greater than or equal to 14 days. Patients who developed severe motor deficit within 48 hours before starting radiation fared poorly.

Weill A, Chiras J, Simon JM, Rose M, Sola-Martinez T, Enkaoua E: Spinal metastases: Indications for and results of percutaneous injection of acrylic surgical cement. *Radiology* 1996;199:241-247.

The authors report their experience with 37 patients with metastatic disease involving the spine who underwent 52 percutaneous injections of acrylic cement into a vertebra (vertebroplasy) Complications occurred in five patients and included transient radiculopathy in three due to cement extrusion, and two with transient difficulty swallowing.

Wise JJ, Fischgrund JS, Herkowitz HN, Montgomery D, Kurz LT: Complication, survival rates, and risk factors of surgery for metastatic disease of the spine. *Spine* 1999;24:1943-1951.

Eighty patients who underwent surgery for metastatic disease of the spine were evaluated. The risk of complications was associated with significant neurologic deficits and preoperative radiation.

Classic Bibliography

Abdu WA, Provencher M: Primary bone and metastatic tumors of the cervical spine. *Spine* 1998;23:2767-2777.

Boriani S, Biagini R, De Iure F, et al: En bloc resections of bone tumors of the thoracolumbar spine: A preliminary report on 29 patients. *Spine* 1996;21:1927-1931.

Bushnell DL, Kahn D, Huston B, Bevering CG: Utility of SPECT imaging for determination of vertebral metastases in patients with known primary tumors. *Skeletal Radiol* 1995;24:13-16.

Cotten A, Boutry N, Cortet B, et al: Percutaneous vertebroplasty: State of the art. *Radiographics* 1998;18: 311-323.

Enkaoua EA, Doursounian L, Chatellier G, Mabesoone F, Aimard T, Saillant G: Vertebral metastases: A critical appreciation of the preoperative prognostic tokuhashi score in a series of 71 cases. *Spine* 1997;22:2293-2298.

Galasko CS, Norris HE, Crank S: Spinal instability secondary to metastatic cancer. *J Bone Joint Surg Am* 2000;82:570-594.

Hart RA, Boriani S, Biagini R, Currier B, Weinstein JN: A system for surgical staging and management of spine tumors: A clinical outcome study of giant cell tumors of the spine. *Spine* 1997;22:1773-1783.

Jenis LG, Dunn EJ, An HS: Metastatic disease of the cervical spine: A review. *Clin Orthop* 1999;359:89-103.

Missenard G, Lapresle P, Cote D: Local control after surgical treatment of spinal metastatic disease. *Eur Spine J* 1996;5:45-50.

Roy-Camille R, Bisserie M, Derlon JM: Technique de vertebrectomie totale, in *Troisiemes Journees d'Orthopedie de la Pitie*. Paris, France, Masson, 1983.

Schirrmeister H, Guhlmann A, Elsner K, et al: Sensitivity in detecting osseous lesions depends on anatomic localization: Planar bone scintigraphy versus 18F PET. *J Nucl Med* 1999;40:1623-1629.

Stener B: Complete removal of vertebra for extirpation of tumors: A 20 year experience. *Clin Orthop* 1989;245: 72-82.

Stener B: Resection of the sacrum for tumors. *Chir Organi Mov* 1990;75(suppl 1):108-110.

Stener B, Gunterberg B: High amputation of the sacrum for extirpation of tumors: Principles and technique. *Spine* 1978;3:351-366.

Sundaresan N, Steinberger AA, Moore F, et al: Indications and results of combined anterior-posterior approaches for spine tumor surgery. *J Neurosurg* 1996; 85:438-446.

Tokuhashi Y, Matsuzaki H, Toriyama S, Kawano H, Ohsaka S: Scoring system for the preoperative evaluation of metastatic spine tumor prognosis. *Spine* 1990;15:1110-1113.

Tomita K, Kawahara N, Toribatake Y, Heller JG: Expansive midline T-saw laminoplasty (modified spinous process-splitting) for the management of cervical myelopathy. *Spine* 1998;23:32-37.

York JE, Berk RH, Fuller GN, et al: Chondrosarcoma of the spine: 1954-1997. *J Neurosurg* 1990;90(suppl 1):73-78.

Yuh WT, Quets JP, Lee HJ, et al: Anatomic distribution of metastases in the vertebral body and modes of hematogenous spread. *Spine* 1996;21:2243-2250.

Chapter 43

Infections of the Spine

David Jacofsky, MD

Bradford L. Currier, MD

Since the description of tuberculous spondylitis by Hippocrates circa 400 BC, infections of the spine have remained a formidable challenge to even the most learned of spine specialists. Despite undeniable improvements in diagnostic modalities, antibiotic therapy, and surgical techniques, as well as reduction of surgical morbidity, the spine infection continues to demand great respect from the clinician. Diagnosis and treatment may be elusive as a result of the often insidious onset and frequent paucity of symptoms and of the tendency for these infections to affect the elderly, debilitated, immunosuppressed, or postoperative patient.

Pyogenic Vertebral Osteomyelitis

Pathogenesis

There are as many theories regarding the route of disc space inoculation as there are synonyms for the disease, which also is known as adult discitis, septic discitis, or disc space infection. The traditional belief that Batson's plexus and venous drainage from the pelvis act as conduits for bacterial dissemination has fallen out of favor. The pressures required to cause retrograde flow in these systems are not encountered clinically, and the location of the insult implicates the end-arteriole as the culprit. Most authors now agree that the infection begins at the vertebral end plate. As the cartilaginous end plates of childhood mature, blind loops of vascular anastomoses remain. These low-flow conduits provide an access route for septic emboli and bacterial seeding. Local end plate inflammation and lysosomal activity cause weakening and destruction of the subchondral plate and subsequent disc penetration. The avascular nature of the nucleus pulposus in the adult has been postulated to contribute to the ability of bacteria to flourish in the region of the disc space. Intuitively this seems reasonable because a lack of vascularity should imply a relative lack of immunity. The rich anastomoses of the posterior spinal arteries about the disc likely aid in spread from one level to the next. The disc is rapidly destroyed, leading to reduced disc height. Conceptually, pyogenic vertebral osteomyelitis can be considered to be primarily a lesion of the disc and its osseous margins.

Demographics

Vertebral osteomyelitis comprises about 2% to 5% of all pyogenic osteomyelitis. Risk factors include increased age (likely not an independent risk factor), obesity, smoking, malignancy, irradiation, malnutrition, diabetes, immunodeficiencies, recent infections, trauma, or surgical procedures. The demographics of vertebral osteomyelitis are quite different in many respects than those of pyogenic osteomyelitis of the extremities. For example, the median age of patients with vertebral osteomyelitis is 66 years as compared to 16 years for appendicular osteomyelitis. The ratio of males to females is near 1:1 as compared to 2:1 for the extremities. The number of males with pyogenic vertebral osteomyelitis is markedly higher and the average age is lower in populations in which there are large numbers of intravenous drug abusers (IVDA).

Microbiology

Historically, *Staphylococcus aureus* was considered to be almost an exclusive pathogen in pyogenic vertebral osteomyelitis. Today it remains the most common, accounting for about 30% to 55% of such infections in adults (80% to 90% in the pediatric population). However, the incidence of gram-negative bacteria as the offending flora has increased markedly over the last decade. The source of these pathogens includes the genitourinary tract, the respiratory tract, soft-tissue infection (for example, diabetic foot ulcers), or the normal flora in the immunocompromised host. Some authors investigating pyogenic osteomyelitis in IVDA found the etiologic pathogen to be *Pseudomonas* in up to 65% of affected patients. *Escherichia coli*, *Enterococcus*, *Propi-*

onobacterium acnes, Streptococcus viridans, Streptococcus agalactiae, Staphylococcus epidermidis, Diptheroids, and Proteus have all been identified with this disease.

Clinical Presentation

The clinical presentation of pyogenic vertebral osteomyelitis is highly variable. Extent of symptoms may be related to host factors and immunocompetence, virulence of the offending pathogen, and the duration of the disease process. It is helpful to consider or classify presentation as acute, chronic, or subacute. In almost all series, over half of the patients are diagnosed more than 3 months after onset of symptoms because the patient did not seek earlier medical care or the physician did not arrive at a diagnosis. The advent of MRI and simple laboratory tests in the last decade have helped the physician expedite proper diagnosis.

Most patients will have back (or neck) pain. A high index of suspicion is imperative. The patient's pain usually will be relentless and present at rest. Night pain often is present, and workup initially may be undertaken because of concern regarding possible malignancy. Muscle spasm can be seen, and in the cervical spine it may lead to frank torticollis. Loss of lumbar lordosis, hamstring tightness, and hip flexion should be recognized as possible associated findings.

There is a predilection for the lumbar spine to be the site of disease within the vertebral column. Although the cervical spine is affected less than 10% of the time, about half of the incidence of pyogenic vertebral osteomyelitis in most studies is in the lumbar spine. Extension of the infection into the paravertebral region is seen frequently, but frank abscesses are rare. When present, however, they may track significant distances along tissue planes. In the cervical spine, an abscess may cause airway obstruction or may extend into the mediastinum to cause a life-threatening situation.

In most series neurologic findings occur in 15% to 20% of patients. In Rezai and associates' recent series of 57 consecutive patients with pyogenic vertebral osteomyelitis, 98% of the patients complained of pain, 68% demonstrated motor weakness, 55% demonstrated gait difficulty, 49% had sensory complaints, 46% had fever, and 25% had sphincter disturbance. The percentages of neurologic findings in this group are higher than in other series, most likely because of the referral pattern associated with the authors' neurosurgical practice. Moreover, a high number of IVDA correlates with a higher number of cervical or cephalad lesions, which are themselves risk factors for neurologic compromise. Other risk factors for neurologic compromise at the time of diagnosis include diabetes, rheumatoid arthritis, increased age, and systemic steroid use. The etiology of

neurologic compromise may include direct compression from the disc or osseous structures, from epidural pus or abscess, from instability, from scar tissue, and/or from edema. Local thrombosis caused by inflammation and resulting in phlebitis or arteritis can cause deficit from ischemia. Septic emboli can cause vascular occlusion as well. In addition, direct extension of the infection/inflammation (for example, meningitis) can cause neurologic findings.

The discovery of epidural abscesses, either isolated or as an extension of vertebral osteomyelitis, is increasing, in part because of improved imaging with MRI. Seven percent of spine infections are associated with an epidural abscess. The incidence of epidural abscesses at a given location is roughly proportional to the amount of epidural space (fat and loose areolar tissue) available. Epidural abscesses of the cervical spine are fairly rare (6% to 18% in most series). However, the incidence of cervical epidural abscesses may be markedly higher in the populations of IVDA who use the upper extremity for injection. Epidural abscesses usually are found anteriorly in the cervical spine and posteriorly in the thoracic and lumbar spine. They can communicate with the retropharyngeal space, mediastinum, or the retroperitoneum via the intervertebral foramen. Patients with acute epidural abscesses tend to be the most symptomatic. As in pyogenic vertebral osteomyelitis, the presentation of epidural abscess is highly variable. Although neurologic findings may be present with pyogenic vertebral osteomyelitis alone, clinical signs of myelopathy or radiculopathy should strongly alert the physician to the possibility of abscess formation. Untreated, the disease may progress through five stages of variable duration. Local spine discomfort will precede radiculopathy, weakness, paralysis, and ultimately toxemia and death. Admittedly, the clinical relevance of stages of disease as well as the importance of acute versus chronic infection remains unproven.

Fortunately, subdural abscesses are uncommon. Since described in 1927 by Sittig as spinal subdural empyema, only about 50 cases have been reported in the literature. Wallerian degeneration, which is more common in patients with diabetes and pregnant women, occurs in the presence of liquefaction necrosis and minimal inflammation. The pathogenesis of neurologic injury may be secondary to ischemia or compression. Differentiation of subdural and epidural abscesses may be difficult, but percussion tenderness usually is absent with subdural infection.

Meningitis also may clinically mimic epidural abscess; both can cause nuchal rigidity, meningeal irritation signs, and similar clinical pictures. Toxemia may be more apparent in the patient with true meningitis. Another rare affliction is intramedullary spinal abscess, which

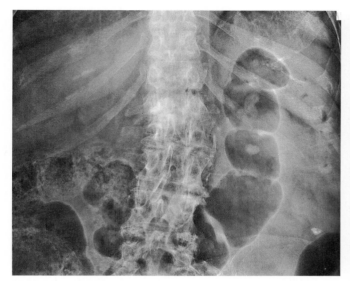

Figure 1 AP radiograph demonstrating destruction of the L1 vertebral body.

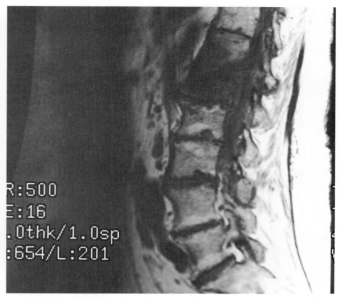

Figure 2 Sagittal MRI T1-sequence. The entire L1 vertebral body shows low signal intensity due to replacement of marrow fat and replacement of marrow elements. The end plates are noted to be indistinct.

unlike epidural abscesses, affects patients who are healthy before onset of symptoms. In one series of 93 patients, only 3% had diabetes and only 2% were IVDA. In this series, the male:female ratio was 3:1.

Diagnostic Evaluation

Definitive diagnosis may be challenging. Obtaining tissue for culture is ideal. The differential diagnosis includes granulomatous infections, metastatic disease, multiple myeloma, degenerative disease, trauma, osteoporotic fracture, destructive spondyloarthropathy, focal Scheuermann's disease, and, rarely, primary neoplasm. Laboratory studies are helpful, yet undeniably nonspecific. The complete blood count shows leukocytosis in 40% to 50% of patients, but may be normal. As in all chronic disease states, the leukocyte count may actually be low if nutritional reserves are depleted.

The erythrocyte sedimentation rate (ESR) is elevated in 90% of patients and, in most series, the mean falls between 50 and 55 mm/h. However, its specificity for infection is poor. The C-reactive protein is slightly more sensitive and specific and may be elevated sooner than the ESR. Both of these markers of inflammation will be elevated after surgical procedures, including such minimally invasive tests as a lumbar puncture. Therefore, a single result often is not helpful; instead, a rising trend (or the absence of improvement) is required to make these tests valuable clinically. Both are of great value in following the course of treatment. A rapid decline in ESR of greater than 50% in the first 4 weeks of treatment is almost always indicative of a successful response to management, although a persistently elevated or even rising ESR does not necessarily portend a bad

result. In one series, 40% of patients without improvement in ESR after 1 month continued on to cure with continuation of their nonsurgical therapy. The C-reactive protein tends to correlate to treatment response in a closer temporal manner than does the ESR; however, because this is a relatively new test, good comparative studies specific to vertebral osteomyelitis are lacking.

Both of these tests must be interpreted in the context of the patient's clinical response to treatment. Blood cultures are helpful if the patient is in the group of 20% to 25% who have positive cultures in the face of active disease. A negative blood culture should lend no support to the presumption of an aseptic state.

Plain radiographs will be negative for at least 2 to 4 weeks after onset of disease. The physician can then first see loss of disc space height and blurring of prevertebral soft-tissue contours followed by osteolysis, reactive bone formation in the subchondral region, and endplate haziness (Figs. 1 and 2). Late in the pathophysiology of the disease, deformity, structural changes, and/or fracture may be seen. Loss of the psoas shadow may indicate retroperitoneal abscess, and retropharyngeal edema or widened mediastinum are obviously worrisome findings.

Radionuclide studies often provide positive findings long before plain radiographs are diagnostic. These studies typically survey the entire skeleton and therefore can detect multifocal involvement, which is present 3% to 5% of the time. Although indium In 111 white blood cell scans are very helpful in the diagnosis of appendicular osteomyelitis and septic arthritis, their usefulness is limited in axial osteomyelitis. Although approaching 100% specificity, the scan's sensitivity for pyogenic vertebral osteomyelitis is only 15% to 20%. Both technetium Tc 99m bone scans and gallium Ga 67 scans have about a 90% sensitivity and an 85% accuracy. The specificity of gallium Ga 67 is 85%, which is slightly superior to the 78% specificity of technetium Tc 99m. Moreover, gallium Ga 67 scans seem to turn positive more quickly than do technetium Tc 99m scans. Gallium Ga 67 scans will return to normal within a few weeks of eradication of infection, and technetium Tc 99m scans will remain positive for months and occasionally longer than 1 year while remodeling of osseous structures ensues. The value and accuracy of both scans increases with the use of single-photon emission CT (SPECT) studies to assist with three-dimensional localization. In one series gallium Ga 67 scans were reported to be abnormal in only 11% of occult vertebral osteomyelitis, whereas in another study of 41 patients gallium Ga 67 scans were reported to be 100% sensitive, specific, and accurate. The authors of the latter report recommended that a positive scan should prompt biopsy, while a negative scan indicated no need for further investigation into the evaluation of infection. All tests must be interpreted in light of the clinical examination.

MRI is the modality of choice for evaluating infections of the spine. Edema will cause an increase in T2-weighted signal intensity in both the disc and the vertebral body. T1-weighted signal will be decreased in the disc and vertebral body due to the replacement of the marrow fat. Indistinct disc margins and loss of the disc's intranuclear cleft will help confirm disc space involvement. Gadolinium can be helpful in differentiating infection from postoperative change. MRI is approximately 95% accurate and allows simultaneous evaluation of soft-tissue involvement. MRI also allows the best distinction between malignancy and infection because tumors rarely involve the disc space, have different signal characteristics, and typically do not cause as marked edematous changes about the soft-tissue planes. Degenerative changes, such as Modic type I changes, may mimic early infection. However, unlike infection, a degenerative pattern will demonstrate a disc that appears strongly hypointense on T2 due to water loss.

CT scanning has lost some of its value because of the advent of MRI, but remains the best modality for delineation of bony anatomy and extent of osseous involvement. Postmyelography CT can be helpful in evaluating neural compression and/or epidural abscesses. The myelogram also offers an opportunity to obtain cerebrospinal fluid for evaluation and culture. However, the risks of spreading infection with lumbar puncture must be weighed against the benefits of the study.

Definitive diagnosis is best achieved by CT-guided biopsy. If the patient is taking antibiotics, these should be discontinued before obtaining tissue to increase yield. CT-guided biopsy provides an accuracy between 68% and 86%. Tissue from the biopsy specimen should be sent for Gram stain, cultures (including aerobes, anaerobes, mycobacteria, atypical mycobacteria, and fungi), sensitivity, and acid-fast and potassium hydroxide staining. Cultures should be retained to grow out low virulence organisms and mycobacterium. Specimens should also be sent to the pathologist for histologic analysis to rule out a malignancy.

Nonpyogenic Vertebral Osteomyelitis

In developed nations, most spinal infections are caused by pyogenic bacteria. However, in underdeveloped countries and in immunocompromised hosts, a multitude of nonpyogenic infections may be found. With the surge of immunocompromised patients in the last decade, more of these types of infections can be found in the United States. As the number of infected hosts increases, mutation leads to increased virulence and drug resistance. Subsequently, there have been increasing reports of such pathogens in certain groups of immunocompetent hosts.

Granulomatous infections of the spine are uniquely different than pyogenic infections. The most extensively researched pathogen in this category is *Mycobacterium tuberculosis*. It is estimated that 1.7 billion people, or one third of the Earth's population are, or have been, infected with the tuberculosis bacillus. Of all patients with tuberculosis, 10% will have musculoskeletal disease. Half of these patients will have spinal involvement, or Pott's disease (tuberculous spondylitis). Spinal lesions are typically a result of hematogenous seeding from a pulmonary source, although direct extension has been reported, and lymphatic spread from renal involvement has been suggested. Most active cases of spinal tuberculosis in adults are actually reactivations of quiescent lesions produced and disseminated during an earlier infection. Although not fully elucidated, recent studies indicate that the cause of osseous destruction by this disease may be the production of chaperonin 10, a potent stimulator of bone resorption.

Clinical Presentation

There are three subtypes of vertebral tuberculosis: peridiscal, anterior, and central, which are based on patterns of osseous destruction. The peridiscal type, which is the most common and accounts for over half of cases, begins in the metaphyseal region of the vertebra and extends to the adjacent vertebra under the anterior longitudinal ligament. The disc is relatively preserved until late in the disease. The anterior form results in scalloping of the anterior aspects of many adjacent segments because infection remains beneath the anterior longitudinal ligament and periosteum as it tracks cephalad and caudad. The central pattern tends to remain within the body of one vertebra, often mimicking the appearance of malignancy and frequently leading to collapse and deformity.

The disc spaces are somewhat more resistant to invasion by granulomatous infection than they are to pyogenic disease. Therefore, disc involvement, if seen, appears later. The thoracic spine is the most common location for spinal tuberculosis, although lumbar involvement is a close second. Cervical involvement is rare. Multifocal disease ranges from 1% to 24% of patients, seeming to be related to nutritional status and/or immunocompetence. The higher percentages come from studies of patients born in developing countries, although geographic differences in virulence cannot be definitively excluded. Large paraspinal abscesses are more common than with pyogenic infection. Abscess formation in the neck may compress the trachea or esophagus (Figs. 3 through 5). Abscess formation in the thoracic spine may cause pleural adhesions to the diaphragm. Lumbar abscesses may track into the femoral triangle. Sacral lesions may extend into the perineum and perirectal fossa. Skin breakdown and sinus formation may be seen and often lead to superinfection with pyogenic bacteria.

Involvement of the posterior elements with sparing of the vertebral bodies and disc space is exceedingly uncommon, but has been reported. Skip lesions, as well as fully extraosseous spinal involvement, may cause delay in diagnosis unless the clinician is aware of such possibilities. Destructive lesions of the sacrum that are palpable on digital rectal examination may be chordomas or chondrosarcomas, but case reports serve as a reminder that vertebral tuberculosis can occur in this manner.

Although acute onset of symptoms has been reported, the onset of symptoms typically is more insidious than with a pyogenic infection. Most patients have back pain. Rates of neurologic findings in different series vary widely, from 10% to 78%, and are understandably lower in patients with lumbar-level disease. Rates of fever range from 30% to 55% in different series, but patients with tuberculosis seem to have more weight loss and malaise as a result of the chronic nature of the disease and often of the more protracted time to diagnosis than occurs with patients who have pyogenic infection. Deformity at the time of diagnosis is also more common in tuberculosis infection. The diagnosis of skeletal tuberculosis, spine or otherwise, must compel clinicians

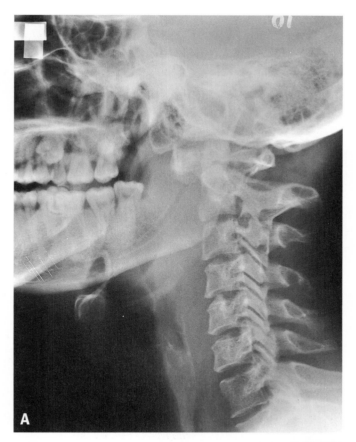

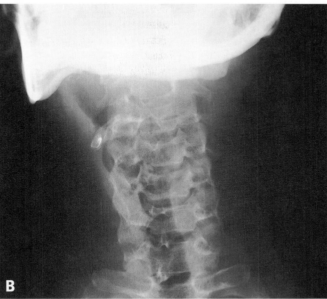

Figure 3 Lateral **(A)** and AP **(B)** radiographs of the cervical spine of a 25-year-old man with a large retropharyngeal tuberculous abscess and atlantoaxial subluxation.

to search for active extraskeletal sites. Almost one third of such evaluations will reveal active disease elsewhere.

Heroin addicts often have a distinct and rapidly progressing syndrome when afflicted with tuberculous

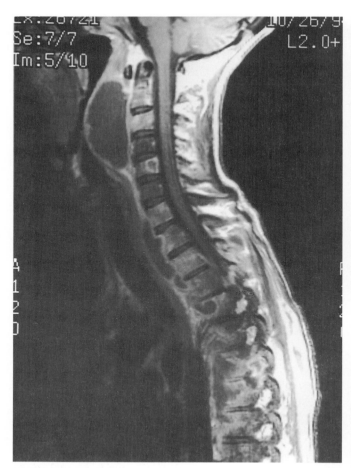

Figure 4 T1-weighted MRI sequence of the same patient noted in Figure 3. A large retropharyngeal abscess is noted and seen to extend from near the base of the skull inferiorly to the level of T9. Although the anterior aspects of the disc spaces are preserved, scalloping of the vertebral bodies anteriorly can be seen.

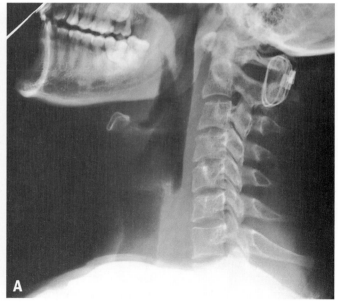

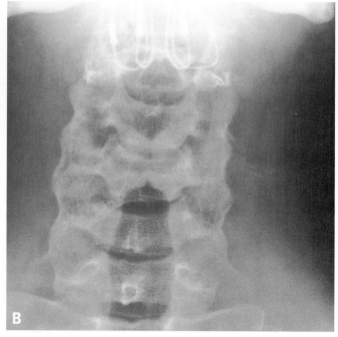

Figure 5 Lateral **(A)** and AP **(B)** views. After débridement of the retropharyngeal abscess; a C1-C2 fusion was performed to stabilize the atlantoaxial subluxation.

spondylitis. They may come to the physician with systemic toxemia, night sweats, weight loss, and rapidly deteriorating neurologic status, and often they have multifocal extravertebral disease.

Epidural granulomata in tuberculous disease is analogous to the epidural abscess in pyogenic infection. Although usually an extension of intraosseous disease, it may be an isolated extraskeletal epidural site of pathology arising from hematogenous seeding. Additional extraskeletal conditions leading to neurologic deficits include tuberculous arachnoiditis, meningitis, and intradural tuberculomas. Extraosseous disease causes paraplegia in about 5% of cases.

Other etiologies of granulomatous infection include fungi, *Candida*, spirochetes, and other mycobacteria. Specifically, chronic granulomatous infections are frequently caused by pathogens of the order *Actinomycetales*. This order includes the families *Mycobacteriaceae* (genus *Mycobacterium*), *Actinomycetaceae* (genera *Actinomyces* and *Arachnia*), and *Nocardiaceae* (genus *Nocardia*).

Aspergillus are ubiquitous saprophytic molds. They often are found in the respiratory tract of healthy adults where the phagocytic functions of macrophages and monocytes keep the organism in check. In immunocompromised hosts, aspergillosis may become an invasive opportunistic infection, especially in patients with hematologic malignancy, tuberculosis, acquired immunodeficiency syndrome, and those on chemotherapeutic agents. Vertebral osteomyelitis has been reported. Patients with chronic obstructive pulmonary disease seem to be at increased risk. Recently, vertebral aspergillosis has been reported in patients with chronic obstructive pulmonary disease who were immunocompetent and received short courses of systemic steroids. Smokers have a much higher rate of pulmonary colonization than do nonsmokers.

Diagnostic Evaluation

As in pyogenic infections, laboratory studies may be helpful, but often are inconclusive. The ESR is typically elevated, but leukocytosis usually is not present. A purified protein derivative is typically positive; however, in the chronically debilitated or immunosuppressed, anergy may lead to false-negative results. Sputum and urine culture and acid-fast staining may be helpful in renal and pulmonary involvement, but culture may take up to 8 to 10 weeks to be diagnostic for mycobacterium. Nuclear imaging modalities are not as reliable as in pyogenic infections. The false-negative rates with technetium Tc 99m and gallium Ga 67 scans approach 40% and 70%, respectively. SPECT scanning may be slightly more useful than planar imaging. MRI remains the best single test for radiographic evaluation. Gadolinium helps demonstrate abscesses; a peripherally enhanced ring of contrast is likely to indicate abscess formation, whereas exuberant enhancement indicates probable granulation tissue. Signal changes are similar to those with pyogenic infection; however, less disc involvement is typically seen.

The definitive diagnosis can best be made by CT-guided biopsy and cultures with staining. The single best diagnostic modality remains polymerase chain reaction (PCR) studies. In recent series, the sensitivity was 95% and the accuracy was 93%. PCR also can help determine resistance before treatment is begun. Although it currently is not used routinely in this clinical setting, the use of PCR clinically is expanding rapidly.

Treatment

The goals of treatment in the face of vertebral infections are (1) eradication of disease, (2) pain relief, (3) preservation or improvement of neurologic function, (4) maintenance or restoration of spinal stability, and (5) prevention of relapse or recurrence. Nonsurgical care is preferred if surgical intervention is not warranted. Indications for surgery include: (1) inability to obtain diagnostic tissue by closed techniques; (2) presence of spinal instability, significant deformity, or fracture; (3) progressive neurologic findings (unless complete paralysis of greater than 72 hours' duration); (4) sepsis (due to the vertebral focus); and (5) failure of medical management.

In all cases, the importance of nutritional repletion

and optimization of medical comorbidities such as coexisting infection or diabetes cannot be overemphasized. The single most important factor in determination of prognosis may very well be the condition of the host. Protein-calorie malnutrition (PCM) is not a problem of only third-world nations. The Ten State Survey in the United States found about 25% of low income children have PCM. In addition, a study of hospitalized surgical patients in large urban hospitals showed over 35% to have PCM. Institutionalized patients, the elderly, and patients with chronic disease are likely to be affected. A weight loss of greater than 10%, serum albumin less than 3g/dL, serum transferrin less than 1.5g/L, anergy, or total lymphocyte count less than 1,200/mm^3 should raise the suspicion of PCM. PCM causes impaired wound healing, impaired cell-mediated immunity, decreased cardiac output and peripheral oxygenation, and impaired integrity of pulmonary immune defenses. The prevention of malnutrition in the hospitalized patient with increased metabolic demands secondary to fever, infection, or surgical insult must be a priority for the health-care team.

Nonsurgical Management

As with any infection, the choice of antibiotics should be made, when possible, based on culture results and the sensitivity of the organism. Unless life-threatening infection is imminent, treatment is best delayed until culture results are obtained. Early initiation of broad-spectrum antibiotics may complicate a second biopsy, if it is necessary. A minimum of 4 weeks of parenteral antibiotic therapy is required to prevent high failure rates in pyogenic infections. Thereafter, the organism, the host, and the patient's response to treatment should guide the decision regarding parenteral versus oral therapy, as well as duration of treatment. The C-reactive protein and/or ESR may help monitor response to therapy.

Immobilization with bed rest and/or orthosis for pain control and deformity prevention are the standard of care. Once the patient is mobilized, a thoracolumbosacral orthosis with a chin extension may be required for upper thoracic lesions. The chin extension is unnecessary in lower thoracic and lumbar lesions, but low lumbar lesions may require a thigh extension for adequate immobilization. Cervical lesions are usually best treated in a halo. Most experts recommend a minimum of 3 months of bracing, but the degree of osseous destruction, location of the lesion, and response to treatment may modulate this time frame. In the preantibiotic era, the mortality rate from pyogenic spondylitis approached 70%. Today, about 75% of patients treated appropriately will have successful cures with nonsurgical management. Patients older than 60 years, those with diabetes, immunocompromised hosts, and the malnourished obviously are overrepresented in the group in whom nonsurgical management fails. Spontaneous fusion of adjacent vertebrae after eradication of infection can be seen in about half of patients and is much more likely in the cervical spine than in the lumbar and thoracic regions.

Tuberculous infections usually are treated with isoniazid, rifampin, and pyrazinamide for 12 months. To prevent relapse and to fully eradicate paucibacillary disease, some experts recommend 18 months of therapy, especially in slow responders. However, many authors and results of some series have shown shorter courses of therapy with a variety of different regimens to be as effective as traditional longer programs. In addition, some studies have shown that nonsteroidal anti-inflammatory drugs (NSAIDs) may decrease osteolysis and deformity by impairing prostaglandin-induced resorption. However, it should be noted that the use of these drugs may greatly complicate surgery or the patient's postoperative course because of platelet inhibition, pseudarthrosis, and the risk of hematoma formation. Perhaps the use of newer COX-2 specific inhibitors will provide the benefits of these drugs without the detrimental effects of traditional NSAIDs. The nonsurgical chemotherapeutic treatment of aspergillosis is by a combination of intravenous amphotericin B, itraconazole, and/or flucytosine. Because of the high incidence of organ toxicity associated with these drugs, these infections should certainly be treated in conjunction with a specialist experienced in their use.

PCR has greatly added to the ability to diagnose and understand tuberculosis. PCR has shown that rifampin resistance is caused by localized mutations in an RNA polymerase (rPOB) gene. Resistance to ciprofloxacin and streptomycin seems due to gyrase A (Gyr A) and ribosomal protein SR (rPSL) mutations. Advanced knowledge of resistance may help to guide appropriate therapy on a patient by patient basis in the near future.

In summary, a team approach to the nonsurgical management of spinal infections is advocated. The value of an infectious disease expert familiar with current trends, local resistance patterns, and management protocols cannot be overemphasized.

Surgical Management

The indications for surgical intervention already have been discussed. The mainstay of surgical treatment is complete and thorough débridement. Almost always this is done through an anterior approach because isolated posterior infections are exceedingly rare. Necrotic bone, disc, soft tissue, and fibrinous exudate should be removed and only viable healthy tissue left at the margins. The spinal canal is almost universally decom-

pressed. Copious irrigation is required. Multiple cultures should be obtained. Most experts advocate that specimens should be sent to pathology to rule out the rare instance of neoplasm or inflammatory conditions presenting as atypical infection. Superinfection of a malignant lesion has been seen.

An adequate débridement and decompression will leave a bony defect that requires reconstruction for stability (Fig. 6). Tricortical iliac crest bone graft (ICBG) can be used to span two or less segments. The autogenous fibula graft provides an alternative for larger defects. Although fusion may be slower with fibula because of a relative lack of cancellous bone, the fibula strut has been shown to be 4.5 times stronger in axial compression than ICBG. Many have advocated the use of the vascularized fibula in special cases of refractory infection or in patients with a high risk of pseudarthrosis. Moreover, the fibula can be osteotomized and folded on itself to provide a double-barrel type graft. If the periosteum and vessels are left intact, the entire graft may remain vascularized, allowing better resistance to infection, less risk of fracture, and more rapid fusion. Obviously the disadvantages of this approach include donor site morbidity and increased time in surgery. The vascularized rib graft does not require anastomosis because it can be rotated on a pedicle. However, despite its occasional value as a vascularized onlay graft, its size, strength, and morphology make it a poor candidate for structural support augmentation.

Some authors have made a strong case for the use of anterior allograft placement following thorough débridement of the spine for tuberculous spondylitis. Fresh frozen allograft has the obvious advantage of avoiding donor site morbidity, and a choice of different sizes and shapes may be available from the bone bank. However, in some series, these grafts have shown increased risks of fracture and infection. Success with allografts in tuberculous spondylitis is encouraging, and reports demonstrate a low incidence of complications when anterior grafting is combined with posterior fusion. However, there are no long-term studies to evaluate the use of allografts in the face of pyogenic infections.

Use of instrumentation raises some concerns because pathogens capable of producing glycocalyx or biofilm may adhere to metallic implants and make eradication difficult. Some have recommended posterior instrumentation following anterior débridement and fusion for tuberculosis. Many surgeons and authors have extended the indications for posterior instrumentation to the management of pyogenic disease. The advantages include more rapid mobilization and deformity correction with decreased requirements for bracing. Many authors have reported good results.

Yilmaz and associates have successfully treated tuber-

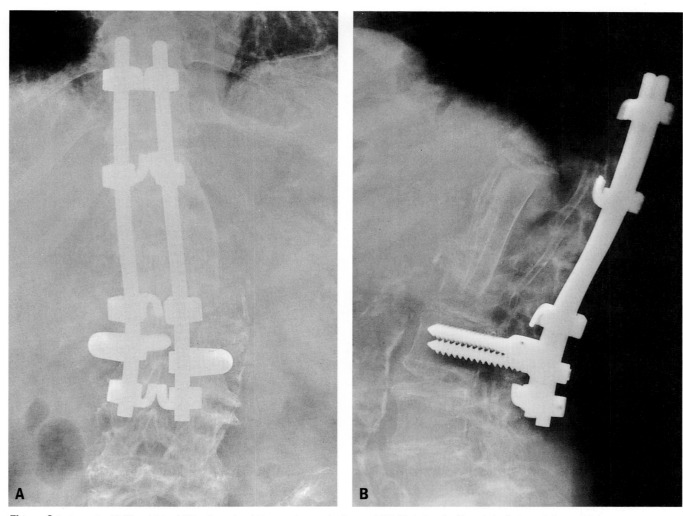

Figure 6 Postoperative AP **(A)** and lateral **(B)** radiographs of L1 corpectomy and subsequent T12-L2 strut graft with posterior instrumentation and fusion.

culous spondylitis with anterior instrumentation, avoiding a second-stage procedure posteriorly. Anterior instrumentation alone is viable only if the posterior column is not involved. Disadvantages of anterior instrumentation include not only direct contact with the infected field, but also reliance on infected and often osteoporotic vertebral bodies for fixation. Often, monosegmental fixation may be feasible posteriorly in the setting of uninvolved pedicles, but may not be feasible anteriorly due to the disease. This situation may lead to increased length of fusion. Also, the removal of anterior hardware poses more serious risks than the extraction of posterior instrumentation. Yilmaz and associates undoubtedly have increased enthusiasm for the anterior instrumentation of tuberculous spondylitis and Rezai and associates have reported good results with anterior instrumentation of the cervical spine in 14 patients with pyogenic infection. Caution should be exercised when applying these techniques until more information is

published. The use of any instrumentation should be scrutinized in the face of pyogenic disease because these patients tend not to have the same degree of deformity as their nonpyogenic counterparts. Additional studies of anterior instrumentation are needed to define its role in all spinal infections.

Iatrogenic Infection

Postoperative infections deserve special mention. These infections may result from inoculation during the index procedure or occur by hematogenous seeding. Prophylaxis for perioperative infection remains controversial. In most series of instrumented fusions there is a reduced rate of infection with the use of prophylaxis. Most authors believe that the dose should be administered for no more than 24 hours, although some argue that drains should be removed before cessation of therapy. The choice of antibiotics depends on many factors including the host, the bacterial flora common in the hospital and region, the type of procedure, the cost, and the side-effect profile. We favor the use of a first-generation cephalosporin, such as cefazolin, for routine prophylaxis in nonallergic patients, but the specific agent should be chosen in conjunction with the institution's infectious disease specialists. With increased concern about resistance, the use of drugs such as vancomycin for prophylaxis has been discouraged. Clindamycin may be a viable alternative in allergic patients. A group from Vanderbilt University, from data intended to elucidate risk factors for postoperative methicillin-resistant *S aureus* wound infections, found that independent risk factors seem to include lymphopenia, recent or current hospitalization, postoperative wound drainage, and alcohol abuse. If vancomycin is to be used for prophylaxis, a selective targeting of high-risk patients seems prudent.

Despite preventive efforts, postoperative infections occur in 2% to 3% of spine procedures. Simple lumbar discectomy has an infection rate of less than 1%, whereas combined fusion and instrumentation are associated with rates between 4% and 8%. Risk factors include increased age, obesity, diabetes, smoking, immunosuppression, length of preoperative hospitalization, spinal dysraphism, myelodysplasia, revision surgery, time in surgery, and use of instrumentation, bone graft, or methylmethacrylate.

Early and decisive treatment should be initiated on diagnosis. As medical management is likely to fail, aggressive surgical intervention typically is suggested for postoperative infections. The débridement should proceed in a systematic fashion. Each layer is débrided and cultured before advancing deeper with the dissection. If subfascial involvement is believed to exist because of subfascial aspiration or gross deep drainage, deep débridement is performed. Although instrumentation is typically left in place in the early postoperative period, all other foreign bodies such as bone wax and absorbable gelatin sponge must be removed. Hardware removal is appropriate if the instrumentation has failed, in refractory infections, or in cases of late hematogenous infection occurring after a fusion has healed. Hematoma should be evacuated thoroughly. Bone graft poses a bit of a dilemma. Many authors will allow it to remain in place, especially if it is adherent. Others recommend removal of loose graft and washing or replacement. Débridement principles are the same as discussed previously. Hemostasis must be meticulous to prevent formation of a hematoma seeded with bacteria. Dead space must be obliterated, and an increasing number of spine surgeons are enlisting the help of plastic surgeons for dead space management when indicated. Primary wound closure over drains, often with retention sutures to prevent dehiscence, is favored when possible. Routine redébridements often are required. Simple wound infections may be packed open and allowed to close by secondary intention. More complex wound infections may require musculocutaneous flaps.

Antibiotic therapy is required for at least 10 to 14 days in the face of soft-tissue and wound infections. Six weeks of parenteral antibiotic treatment is preferred if bony involvement, deep infection, or foreign bodies (metal, graft, and so forth) remain.

Annotated Bibliography

Carragee EJ, Kim D, van der Vlugt T, Vittum D: The clinical use of erythrocyte sedimentation rate in pyogenic vertebral osteomyelitis. *Spine* 1997;22:2089-2093.

   This study helps define the clinical use of the ESR in the diagnosis, treatment, and management of pyogenic osteomyelitis. As a general rule, a falling ESR during the first month of treatment is a good prognostic sign. However, lack of this improvement does not necessarily portend a failure in management because 40% of this latter group will go on to respond to conservative management.

Currier BL, Eismont FJ: Infections of the spine, in Herkowitz HN, Garfin GR, Balderston RA, Eismont FJ, Ball GR, Wiesel SW (eds): *The Spine*. Philadelphia, PA, WB Saunders, 1999, pp 1207-1258.

   This is a current review of spine infections.

Currier BL, Heller JG, Eismont FJ: Cervical spinal infections, in Clark CR, Ducker TB, Dvorak J, et al (eds): *The Cervical Spine*, ed 3. Philadelphia, PA, Lippincott-Raven, 1998, 659-690.

   This is a current review of cervical spine infections.

Dietze D, Fessler G, Jacob R: Primary reconstruction for spinal infections. *J Neurosurg* 1997;86:981-989.

   The authors conclude that primary arthrodesis and instrumentation can be performed in acute spinal infection if aggressive débridement and prolonged parenteral antibiotics are used.

Govender S, Parbhoo AH: Support for the anterior column with allografts in tuberculosis of the spine. *J Bone Joint Surg Br* 1999;81:106-109.

   The authors make a strong argument for the use of fresh frozen allografts anteriorly following thorough débridement of the spine for tuberculous spondylitis. The population studied consisted of children ranging from 2 to 9 years of age.

Krodel A, Kruger A, Lohscheidt K, Pfahler M, Refior HJ: Anterior debridement, fusion, and extrafocal stabilization in the treatment of osteomyelitis of the spine. *J Spinal Disord* 1999;12:17-26.

The use of posterior extrafocal transpedicular stabilization after anterior débridement and fusion for spinal osteomyelitis shortened rehabilitation and offered the advantage of braceless mobilization without adding unpredictable risks.

Levi AD, Dickman CA, Sonntag VK: Management of postoperative infections after spinal instrumentation. *J Neurosurg* 1997;86:975-980.

The authors retrospectively reviewed 452 consecutively treated patients who underwent a spinal instrumentation procedure at a single level to establish which patients and which surgical approaches might be associated with increased risk of deep wound infection. The efficacy of their treatment regimen, which included surgical débridement, antibiotics, and insertion of an antibiotic-containing irrigation system, was examined.

Moon MS: Tuberculosis of the spine: Controversies and a new challenge. *Spine* 1997;22:1791-1797.

The author concludes that tuberculosis of the spine without kyphosis, instability, or neurologic compromise is a medical, rather than a surgical, condition. Surgery should be reserved for advanced cases with unacceptable complications such as paraplegia or deformity.

Pertuiset E, Beaudreuil S, Liote F, et al: Spinal tuberculosis in adults: A study of 103 cases in a developed country, 1980-1994. *Medicine* 1999;78:309-320.

The authors reviewed 103 patients with confirmed spinal tuberculosis, both with and without disc involvement. The study describes diagnostic and radiographic findings and compares both groups. In this series, the atypical form (without disc involvement) was most common in foreign-born subjects in industrialized nations.

Rezai AR, Woo HH, Errico TJ, Cooper PR: Contemporary management of spinal osteomyelitis. *Neurosurgery* 1999;44:1018-1026.

The authors reviewed the results of treatment of a series of patients with spinal osteomyelitis. In their series, early surgical decompression resulted in rapid improvement of neurologic deficits, decreases in kyphotic deformities, and stable bony fusion. Active infection did not preclude the use of internal fixation.

Wimmer C, Gluch H, Franzreb M, Ogon M: Predisposing factors for infection in spine surgery: A survey of 850 spinal procedures. *J Spinal Disord* 1998;11:124-128.

Proven risk factors for infection included extended preoperative hospitalization, high blood loss, prolonged surgical time, diabetes, obesity, smoking, steroid use, alcohol abuse, and revision surgery.

Wuisman PI, Jiya TU, Van Dijk M, Sugihara S, Van Royen BJ, Winters HA: Free vascularized bone graft in spinal surgery: Indications and outcome in eight cases. *Eur Spine J* 1999;8: 296-303.

Vascularized bone graft in spinal surgery facilitates primary mechanical stability and rapid fusion. Vascularized grafts also are more resistant to infection and can be shaped without devascularization. There are situations in which the risk:benefit ratio favors the use of these grafts in spinal surgery.

Yilmaz C, Selek HY, Gurkan I, Erdemli B, Korkusu Z: Anterior instrumentation for the treatment of spinal tuberculosis. *J Bone Joint Surg Am* 1999;81:1261-1267.

The authors demonstrate that anterior instrumentation is more effective than posterior instrumentation for reducing deformity and stabilizing the spine in patients with kyphosis related to spinal tuberculosis. The rate of persistent or recurrent infection was not increased.

Classic Bibliography

An HS, Vacaro AR, Dolinskas CA, Colter JM, Balderston RA, Bauerle WB: Differentiation between spinal tumors and infections with magnetic resonance imaging. *Spine* 1991;16(suppl 8):S334-S338.

Dempsey R, Rapp RP, Young B, Johnston S, Tibbs P: Prophylactic parenteral antibiotics in clean neurosurgical procedures: A review. *J Neurosurg* 1988;69:52-57.

Djukic S, Lang P, Morris J, Hoaglund F, Genant HK: The postoperative spine: Magnetic resonance imaging. *Orthop Clin North Am* 1990;21:603-624.

Eismont FJ, Bohlman HH, Soni PL, Goldberg VM, Freehafer AA: Pyogenic and fungal vertebral osteomyelitis with paralysis. *J Bone Joint Surg Am* 1983;65: 19-29.

Emery SE, Chan DP, Woodward HR: Treatment of hematogenous pyogenic vertebral osteomyelitis with anterior debridement and primary bone grafting. *Spine* 1989;14:284-291.

Guven O, Kumano K, Yalcin S, Karahan M, Tsuji S: A single stage posterior approach and rigid fixation for preventing kyphosis in the treatment of spinal tuberculosis. *Spine* 1994;19:1039-1043.

Horwitz NH, Curtin JA: Prophylactic antibiotics and wound infections following laminectomy for lumbar disc herniation. *J Neurosurg* 1975;43:727-731.

Hsu LC, Cheng CL, Leong JC: Pott's paraplegia of late onset: The cause of compression and results after anterior decompression. *J Bone Joint Surg Br* 1988;70:534-538.

Hsu LC, Leong JC: Tuberculosis of the lower cervical spine (C2 to C7): A report on 40 cases. *J Bone Joint Surg Br* 1984;66:1-5.

Lifeso RM: Pyogenic spinal sepsis in adults. *Spine* 1990; 15:1265-1271.

Lifeso RM, Weaver P, Harder EH: Tuberculous spondylitis in adults. *J Bone Joint Surg Am* 1985;67: 1405-1413.

Massie JB, Heller JG, Abitbol JJ, McPherson D, Garfin SR: Postoperative posterior spinal wound infections. *Clin Orthop* 1992;284:99-108.

Modic MT, Feiglin DH, Piraino DW, et al: Vertebral osteomyelitis: Assessment using MR. *Radiology* 1985; 157:157-166.

Nussbaum ES, Rigamonti D, Standiford H, Numaguchi Y, Wolf AL, Robinson WL: Spinal epidural abscess: A report of 40 cases and review. *Surg Neurol* 1992;38: 225-231.

Oga M, Arizono T, Takasita M, Sugioka Y: Evaluation of the risk of instrumentation as a foreign body in spinal tuberculosis: Clinical and biologic study. *Spine* 1993;18:1890-1894.

Ozuna RM; Delamarter RB: Pyogenic vertebral osteomyelitis and postsurgical disc space infections. *Orthop Clin North Am* 1996;27:87-94.

Rubin G, Michowiz SD, Ashkenasi A, Tadmor R, Rappaport ZH: Spinal epidural abscess in the pediatric age group: Case report and review of literature. *Pediatr Infect Dis J* 1993:12:1007-1011.

Sadato N, Numaguchi Y, Rigamonti D, et al: Spinal epidural abscess with gadolinium-enhanced MRI: Serial follow-up studies and clinical correlations. *Neuroradiology* 1994;36:44-48.

Sapico FL, Montgomerie JZ: Pyogenic vertebral osteomyelitis: Report of nine cases and review of the literature. *Rev Infect Dis* 1979;1:754-776.

Sixth report of the Medical Research Council Working Party on Tuberculosis of the Spine: Five-year assessments of controlled trials of ambulatory treatment, debridement and anterior spinal fusion in the management of tuberculosis of the spine: Studies in Bulawayo (Rhodesia) and in Hong Kong. *J Bone Joint Surg Br* 1978;60:163-177.

Stambough JL, Beringer D: Postoperative wound infections complicating adult spine surgery. *J Spinal Disord* 1992;5:277-285.

Thelander U, Larsson S: Quantitation of C-reactive protein levels and erythrocyte sedimentation rate after spinal surgery. *Spine* 1992;17:400-404.

Chapter 44

Complications of Cervical Surgery

Andrew E. Wakefield, MD

Edward C. Benzel, MD

Infection

The risk of infection after cervical spine surgery, though low, is difficult to determine; a postoperative infection rate of 0 to 6% has been reported. Implantable materials influence the rate of infection. The prevalence of postoperative infections varies with the type of surgery performed, duration of the procedure, and the preoperative condition of the patient. Patient-specific risk factors for infection are related predominantly to the general medical condition of the patient, including malnutrition, obesity, diabetes mellitus, steroid therapy, immunosuppression, age, shock, and prolonged hospital stay. For example, a recent weight loss of 10 lbs, a serum albumin of less than 3.4 g/dL, or a total lymphocyte count of less than 15,000 cells/mL, should alert the surgeon to the possibility of inadequate nutrition. If on further testing, the transferrin level is less than 150 mg/dL and/or the patient is anergic to skin testing, elective surgery should be postponed and the nutritional status improved. If these secondary tests are within the normal range, the surgery can proceed with attention paid to the postoperative nutritional status of the patient.

Obesity is also a risk factor for postoperative infection. The surgeon should be mindful that adipose tissue is poorly vascularized. During closure of the wound, care should be taken to irrigate the wound thoroughly and to minimize dead space. When possible, the patient should be counseled on weight loss before surgery. Risk of infection is not greater in patients with well-controlled diabetes, but is greater in patients with uncontrolled diabetes, especially those in ketoacidosis.

Immunosuppression is associated with a variety of problems including acquired immune deficiency syndrome, hematopoietic tumors, malnutrition, organ transplantion, steroid therapy, and chemotherapy. When possible, steroid medications should be tapered; however, if this cannot be done, steroids may be required during the perioperative period. Infection distant to the surgical site should be identified and treated. Urinary tract and respiratory infections are common sources for spread to surgical wounds. Patients with prolonged hospitalization are also at increased risk of infection.

Adherence to sound surgical technique is an important aspect of preventing wound infections. There is a direct correlation between the duration of the surgery and the infection rate. Tissue should be handled gently, and self-retaining retractors should be released periodically. Hemostasis should be meticulous, although extensive use of electrocautery can actually increase infection rates. A closed suction drain may be used; however, some believe that drains may increase the infection rate. If a drain is used, it should be discontinued within 24 hours, whenever possible.

Prophylactic antibiotics are used to prevent naturally occurring organisms from proliferating, organisms contaminating a normally sterile site from producing disease, and infection by exogenous organisms. Clinical studies have shown infection rates reduced from 9% to 1% for lumbar laminectomy with the use of prophylactic antibiotics. Cephalosporins are used most commonly. They provide excellent coverage for gram-positive organisms, namely *Staphylococcus aureus*. For patients who are hospitalized for more than 1 week or who are immunosuppressed, broad-spectrum or two-agent coverage should be used. The surgeon must be aware of institutional variation in bacterial susceptibility and adjust antibiotic coverage accordingly. The penetration of antibiotics within the disc space and the timing thereof are poorly defined; however, it is generally believed that antibiotics should be administered 1 to 2 hours before surgery, allowing time for the drug to reach the poorly vascularized tissue in the disc space.

In the initial postoperative period, the patient with an incipient wound infection may not show remarkable signs. Fever in the immediate postoperative period may be due to microatelectasis, thrombophlebitis, urinary tract infection, or wound infection. A superficial infection may appear benign for the first 3 to 4 days, but the patient will usually report that the wound is becoming more painful rather than less. Fever is often low grade and white blood cell (WBC) counts and erythrocyte sedimentation rate (ESR) may be mildly elevated. The patient with a deep wound infection typically seeks care 7 to 14 days after surgery. Common complaints include increased surgery site pain, general malaise, fever, and fullness of the neck. If a ventral approach was used, an esophageal injury must be considered. A plain radiograph may show subcutaneous emphysema, and esophagoscopy may confirm the diagnosis. If the wound requires reexploration, the surgeon must inspect the esophagus and be prepared to repair it if needed. With either superficial or deep wound infections, the discharge should be cultured and appropriate antibiotic treatment begun. When the culture is completed and sensitivity determined, the antibiotic coverage may be adjusted.

Discitis occurs infrequently and is not completely avoidable. The prevalence in large series ranges from 0 to 1%. The incidence of discitis increases with the complexity of the procedure and the use of metallic implants. The typical history includes increasing neck pain and paravertebral muscle spasm, with an onset from days to weeks and even months after surgery. Vital signs and the WBC count are typically normal, but the ESR usually is elevated. The study of choice is MRI, with and without gadolinium. T1-weighted images show decreased signal intensity in the marrow cavity adjacent to the involved disc and the normal definition between the disc space and vertebral body is lost. On T2-weighted images, signal intensity in the disc space is increased. The use of gadolinium helps exclude other postoperative conditions with similar appearances, such as epidural abscess or recurrent disc herniation. The most common organism causing discitis is *S aureus*, but *S epidermidis*, *Escherichia coli*, and diptheroids also occur. Antibiotic coverage should be dictated accordingly and continued for 6 weeks or until the ESR returns to normal.

Epidural abscess after cervical spine surgery is rare. The cumulative prevalence is 0.06%. Despite its rarity, the appearance is typical. All patients report severe neck pain, are febrile, and have an elevated WBC count. The patient may exhibit radicular symptoms and/or be myelopathic with varying degrees of quadraparesis or paraparesis. The preferred study is an MRI with gadolinium. The treatment usually involves emergency surgery. The approach is dictated by the location of the epidural abscess.

Dural Injury and Cerebrospinal Fluid Leaks

The exact prevalence of cerebrospinal fluid (CSF) leaks is difficult to determine. Current reports suggest an incidence of dural tear and CSF leak in the range of 0.8% to 1.8%. The one entity that carries a higher incidence of dural mishap is ossification of the posterior longitudinal ligament. The calcified posterior longitudinal ligament can be adherent to the underlying dura mater or the dura may be absent. Reexploration of a surgery site carries an increased risk of dural injury. Dural laceration is related most commonly to the use of a high-speed drill.

The presence of a CSF leak can be detected at the time of surgery or afterward. Clear drainage should always raise the suspicion of a CSF leak. In addition, a palpable mass at the incision site may represent a CSF collection and can lead to an external fistula. The patient usually complains of headache that is continuous, but worsens when the head is elevated. An MRI may demonstrate fluid or a dural defect. If the patient cannot undergo an MRI or if no leak is identified, a myelogram and postmyelogram CT may reveal the problem.

If a CSF leak is detected at surgery, primary closure should be attempted aggressively. If the edges of the deficit cannot be reapproximated, a patch graft can be placed. When possible, autologous tissue should be used. Muscle and fascia may be harvested from the incision or fascia lata may be harvested from a second incision. Cadaveric tissues can be a source of disease transmission. Creutzfeldt-Jakob disease transmission has been reported with cadaveric dura. The use of commercially prepared tissues may be an alternative to autologous material, but long-term studies are not available. Even with a watertight closure, a lumbar subarachnoid drain may be used.

If a CSF leak is detected in the postoperative period, a lumbar drain may be used for management of this complication. The basic protocol for the management of the lumbar drain is the same as if it was placed at the time of surgery or postoperatively. The patient is kept at bed rest. The lumbar drainage of 200 to 300 cc per 24 hr usually occurs. This is drained for 72 to 96 hr, then the drain is pulled and the patient allowed to ambulate. This strategy of bed rest and lumbar drainage works in most patients. Patients that fail conservative treatment will require surgery.

Neural Injury

Injury to the recurrent laryngeal nerve or the vagus nerve can result in vocal cord paralysis. Postoperative voice changes following ventral cervical spine surgery occur in approximately 7% of patients. However, most changes are temporary (hoarseness). The recurrent laryngeal nerve on the right side exits the carotid sheath medially, at a variable level, to course in the tracheoesophageal groove. On the left side the recurrent laryngeal nerve has a more predictable and protected course in the tracheoesophageal groove. Staying within fascial planes and avoiding sharp dissection helps avert injury. Care should be taken during placement of retractors. A stretch injury can occur with overdistraction of the recurrent laryngeal nerve.

Horner's syndrome will occur if the sympathetic nerve fibers are irritated or damaged in their course over the longus capitis muscles and the transverse processes. This problem may be avoided if these muscles are not disturbed or if they are retracted only slightly and subperiosteally from the midline.

Injuries to nerve roots have been reported with both ventral and dorsal approaches. Fortunately, most of these injuries are transient. The risk of neural element injury is ever present. This risk is increased in patients with myelopathy. Often the spinal cord's physiologic reserve has been compromised partially, leaving the cord highly susceptible to injury, even with minor indirect trauma or vascular compromise. A patient with cervical disc disease or spondylosis associated with myelopathy has a greater than 10% risk of deterioration of neurologic status when approached dorsally.

Vascular Complications

Vascular injuries to the vertebral and carotid arteries and jugular vein are rare. The use of high-speed drills, misdirected drill bits, screws, or instruments wandering out of fascial planes, and misplaced retractors have all been implicated as causes of injury. Other vascular structures at risk of injury are the anterior spinal artery, superior thyroid artery, and thoracic duct (left-sided approach).

Hematomas can be present as localized swelling at the incision site or be deeper and cause compression of the trachea and neural structures. These are rare occurrences, but can constitute a surgical emergency.

In the case of expanding hematomas, the incision may need to be opened at the bedside to relieve pressure on the airway and/or the spinal cord. However, careful postoperative monitoring can identify these patients and allow their return to the operating room for proper reexploration and control of the bleeding source.

Complications of Cervical Spine Bracing

Devices for cervical bracing range from a soft cervical collar to the halo and Minerva braces. Several complications, such as skin and soft-tissue injuries, muscle atrophy, and compliance, are common to all braces. Miscellaneous complications, such as dysphagia and cardiopulmonary and gastrointestinal dysfunction, also have been reported. Ineffective spinal stabilization is a detriment common to all spinal bracing to varying degrees. It is beyond the scope of this chapter to review bracing biomechanics. However, complications of halo and Minerva bracing are discussed.

For an orthosis to be effective, it must have skin contact; therefore, skin breakdown can result. The incidence of integument injury with bracing is not known; however, the physiologic conditions and the stages of breakdown are known. Important factors for the development of pressure sores include the magnitude and duration of contact, associated shear and friction of the skin, tissue hydration, and general nutrition of the patient. Pressure sores are preventable complications. Patients, families, and caregivers should be educated regarding the early warning signs of skin ulceration and should play active roles in prevention. Prevention is particularly important in comatose patients and patients with anesthetic skin. Nutritionally depleted patients have altered wound-healing capabilities, tissue and skin turgor, and an increased risk of infection. Muscle atrophy can occur even with short-term bracing. If profound muscle weakness results from prolonged use of a brace, active rehabilitation may be required when arthrodesis is achieved and the brace is discontinued. Contractures can occur with long-term bracing. Up to 80% residual neck pain and stiffness has been reported after halo bracing.

Halo fixation devices have unique complications, most of which are related to the halo pins. The incidence of pin loosening can range from 4.5% to 60%. The pin-site infection rate is around 20%. Supraorbital nerve injury has been reported (2% incidence), and penetration of the cranial vault by a halo pin has a reported incidence of 1%. To minimize complications, pins should be placed ventrolaterally and dorsolaterally, and below the equator of the skull. Ventral pins should be placed 1 cm above and lateral to mideyebrow. The surgeon must be careful not to place the pin in the area of the supraorbital nerve medially or the temporalis muscle laterally. The pins should be inserted perpendicular to the bone and torqued to 6 to 8 in/lb. They should be tightened again at 24 hr to 6 to 8 in/lb.

Usually four pins are all that is required in the adult. However, additional pins (8 to 10) are needed in adolescents and children due to thinner bone or in patients with poor bone quality.

If a pin becomes loose, it can be torqued to 6 to 8 in/lb. However, if the pin requires more than two turns to become secure, it should be removed and a new pin inserted at a new site. The pin sites should be cleaned daily with hydrogen peroxide.

Bone Graft Complications

The iliac crest is a common bone graft harvest site, with a reported complication rate of about 20%, including both major and minor complications. In general, complications include injury to adjacent structures (vascular, neural, and visceral), hernias, fractures, and infections. Hematomas and infections are the most common complications reported. Injuries to neural structures are also common, with a reported rate of 8%. The lateral femoral cutaneous nerve is at risk during ventral crest exposure, but injuries to the femoral, genitofemoral, and ilioinguinal nerves have been reported. The incision should be made approximately 3 to 4 cm lateral to the anterior superior iliac spine. This protects the inguinal ligament, lateral femoral cutaneous nerve, and the attachments of the sartorius muscle. Superior cluneal nerve injury is the most common injury related to harvest of dorsal iliac crest grafts.

The dorsal iliac crest can be harvested by palpating the crest and making a skin incision that begins approximately 6 to 8 cm lateral to the midline and parallel to the crest. The fascial incision also is made 6 to 8 cm lateral to the midline. If the fascial incision is made too far laterally, injury to the superior cluneal nerve can occur. Injury to the superior gluteal artery as it exits the sciatic notch also can occur with the dorsal approach. This injury can be discovered late with formation of a pseudoaneurysm. The most common vascular-related complication is hematoma with an incidence of 6% to 21%. Herniation of abdominal contents is rare but can occur in both ventral and dorsal exposures. It usually is related to full-thickness grafts, but inadequate fascial closure also has been implicated. If a hernia does occur, reduction of the hernia and repair of the defect are required.

Fractures rarely occur following graft harvesting. However, with the ventral approach, it is important to leave adequate bone lateral to the anterior iliac spine to prevent avulsion fracture by the sartorius muscle. With the dorsal approach, the sacroiliac joint must not be violated lest pelvic instability or pain results. Infection of the harvest site can be deep (2.5%) or superficial (20.6%). Osteomyelitis is rare. Incidence of chronic pain at the donor site ranges from 1.6% to 39%.

If fibula is used for autologous bone graft, the common peroneal nerve is at risk of injury, as well as the vascular structures adjacent to the fibula. Subperiosteal dissection helps avoid these structures. In harvesting the graft, the surgeon must stay at least 6 cm above the lateral malleolus to prevent instability of the ankle.

Extrusion of bone graft from interbody fusions has been reported for single-level fusion in 0 to 1.2% of patients, and for multilevel fusion in as high as 11%.

These rates are lower for instrumented fusion. The use of spinal instrumentation has increased over the past 10 years. Even with instrumentation, there can be dorsal displacement of the bone graft. With displacement of the bone graft, the patient may be asymptomatic or can have dysphagia, neural compression, and/or instability. Displacement or failure of spinal instrumentation can cause similar complications. Patients who do not exhibit dysphagia, pain, or loss of alignment may be followed clinically with serial radiographs. Others will require surgical correction.

Both autograft and allograft bone can be used for fusion. Pseudarthrosis can occur with either, but the rate is generally higher for allograft, especially for multilevel discectomy and corpectomies. Spinal instrumentation has increased the fusion rates with both autograft and allograft. Instrumentation that allows stress sharing between the graft and the plate and screws is ideal. The bone graft is not a static structure; it will remodel, and subsidence can occur. Subsidence increases the stresses placed on the plate and screw and thus will reduce the load on the graft. The off-loading of the graft may increase the risk of pseudarthrosis because of stress shielding. Increased stress on the plate and screw can cause plate and screw displacement or breakage. A system that allows settling over time and the use of intermediate points of fixation may reduce the incidence of failure.

Dorsal instrumentation techniques have advanced over the past 10 years. The complications associated with lateral mass or pedicle screws are predominantly injury to neural and vascular structures. Breakage or dislodgment of plates and screws are known complications. Dorsal wiring remains a viable option for spinal stabilization, but like other instrumentation systems, it can break or pull out.

Transoral Approach

The most common problems encountered with the transoral approach are wound closure, infection, and complications related to inadequate exposure. Various retractor systems are available. They all have an upper blade that engages the teeth and a lower tongue blade. The upper lip must be clear of the retractor. The application of steroid cream to the lips and gums may help prevent postoperative swelling. In addition, the tongue blade should be relaxed periodically during the operation to minimize lingual edema. The surgical corridor makes the risk of postoperative infection relatively high; therefore, preoperative antibiotics with a broad coverage, and postoperative antibiotics for 72 hours, often are used. To limit wound dehiscence, a tension-free layered closure should be used.

Ventral Approach to the Midcervical Spine

There are a number of complications associated with this approach. However, the overall complication rate is approximately 4%. Infection, hematoma, vascular and esophageal injury, tracheal perforation, dysphagia, vocal cord paralysis, neural injury, implant complications, dislodgment of the bone graft, and pseudarthrosis have all been reported.

Ventral Approach to the Lower Cervical Spine

All the complications listed above for the midcervical region have been reported for this approach. In addition, the pleura should be inspected for injury when exposed, and postoperative chest radiographs are required to role out a pneumothorax. With a left-sided approach, injury to the thoracic duct is possible.

The thoracic duct ascends behind the esophagus to join the left jugular and subclavian veins. This anatomy can be variable, and branching and right-sided confluence are not uncommon. If the thoracic duct is injured during surgery, it should be ligated if possible, the area tightly oversewn, and the patient placed on a low-fat diet. If the injury goes unnoticed at the time of surgery it may manifest itself as a chylous effusion from the wound or as a collection within the chest. Most thoracic duct injuries resolve with time but can result in a significant caloric loss. If reexploration is required, the thoracic duct is difficult to locate at best. If the duct can be found it should be ligated; if not, the approximate area of the leak should be oversewn in a multilayered fashion. The patient also should be placed on a low-fat diet and followed with chest radiographs in the postoperative period.

Injury to the phrenic nerve and paralysis of the diaphragm also can occur. The innominate vessels may be injured with a low midline exposure.

Dorsal Occipitocervical Approach

The occipitocervical junction is often decompressed before stabilization and fusion. The placement of burr holes in the occipital bone can result in injury to the dura mater and to the underlying cerebellum.

If a dural injury is caused and a CSF leak results, a primary closure may be difficult. Placing gelfoam within the burr hole and closing the wound in a watertight fashion are all that usually is required. However, if bleeding is encountered meticulous homeostasis is needed. The rare development of a posterior fossa subdural hematoma can have dire consequences and can be manifested acutely or in a delayed fashion in the postoperative period. If the source of the blood can be seen then a bipolar cautery may be used. If homeostasis is not obtained or the source of bleeding not seen, then gelfoam and/or oxycellulose can be placed within the burr hole and held in place with a cottonoid patty. This patty should be left in place for several minutes and irrigated with warm saline until the fluid is clear. If this step does not obtain homeostasis, the gelfoam and oxycellulose can be removed and replaced as described above. If this second attempt does not control the bleeding, the burr hole may need to be enlarged to find the source. The surgeon should not attempt this potential exploration of the posterior fossa unless he or she is familiar with the anatomy and techniques of intracranial surgery. The assistance of a neurosurgeon may be warranted. Even with homeostasis, this site should be inspected at the end of the case for the presence of a hematoma. Care also should be taken to close the wound in a watertight fashion.

The passage of wires under the lamina can traumatize the spinal cord or dura. Once the wires are passed, they should be kept under tension to prevent migration into the spinal canal and injury to underlying structures. The vertebral artery and the venous plexus may be damaged during decompression or the placement of a transarticular screw. The implant is secured to the occiput with wires, screws, or occipital buttons. These can pull out either at surgery or postoperatively.

Dorsal Approach to the Lower Cervical Spine

Complications in this region are similar to those at the occipitocervical junction. They include vascular and neural injury, instrumentation complications, and/or pseudarthrosis. When drilling holes and passing wires through the spinous processes the surgeon must be careful to prevent injury to the dura or spinal cord. Lateral mass screws, if misplaced, can injure the vertebral artery or nerve roots. If a laminectomy is done, injury to underlying neural and vascular structures is possible.

Annotated Bibliography

Benzel EC (ed): *Spine Surgery: Techniques, Complication Avoidance, and Management.* New York, NY, Churchill Livingstone, 1999, pp 879-881.

The author discusses bone graft choice and harvesting techniques and complications.

Benzel EC (ed): *Spine Surgery: Techniques, Complication Avoidance, and Management.* New York, NY, Churchill Livingstone, 1999, pp 1372-1376.

The author discusses the complications of cervical bracing.

Geer CP, Papadopoulos SM: The argument for single-level anterior cervical discectomy and fusion with anterior plate fixation. *Clin Neurosurg* 1999;45:25-29.

The authors make the case for plating single-level anterior discectomy and fusions.

Hart BL, Benzel EC, Ford CC (eds): *Fundamentals of Neuroimaging*. Philadelphia, PA, WB Saunders, 1997, pp 167-171.

This short book describes the fundamentals of neuroimaging. Imaging of the spine is approached from a practical perspective.

Kameyama O, Ogawa K, Suga T, Nakamura T: Asymptomatic brain abscess as a complication of halo orthosis: Report of a case and review of the literature. *J Orthop Sci* 1999;4:39-41.

Brain abscess, a known complication of the halo, is illustrated nicely in this manuscript.

Manski TJ, Wood MD, Dunsker SB: Bilateral vocal cord paralysis following anterior cervical discectomy and fusion: Case report. *J Neurosurg* 1998;89:839-843.

Vocal cord paralysis is uncommon following anterior cervical surgery. The authors present a case of bilateral injury and discuss the etiology and treatment.

Sampath P, Rigamonti D: Spinal epidural abscess: A review of epidemiology, diagnosis, and treatment. *J Spinal Disord* 1999;12:89-93.

This is a comprehensive review of spinal epidural abscess.

Classic Bibliography

Agrillo U, Simonetti G, Martino V: Postoperative CSF problems after spinal and lumbar surgery: General Review. *J Neurosurg Sci* 1991;35:93-95.

Botte MJ, Byrne TP, Abrams RA, Garfin SR: The halo skeletal fixator: Current concepts of application and maintenance. *Orthopedics* 1995;18:463-471.

Cruse PJ, Foord R: A five-year prospective study of 23,649 surgical wounds. *Arch Surg* 1973;107:206-210.

Fowler BL, Dall BE, Rowe DE: Complications associated with harvesting autogenous iliac bone graft. *Am J Orthop* 1995;24:895-903.

Heller JG, Silcox DH III, Sutterlin CE III: Complications of posterior cervical plating. *Spine* 1995;20:2442-2448.

Horwitz NH, Curtin JA: Prophylactic antibiotics and wound infections following laminectomy for lumbar disc herniation. *J Neurosurg* 1975;43:727-731.

Iversen E, Nielsen VA, Hansen LG: Prognosis in postoperative discitis: A retrospective study of 111 cases. *Acta Orthop Scand* 1992;63:305-309.

Jensen JE, Jensen TG, Smith TK, Johnston DA, Dudrick SJ: Nutrition in orthopaedic surgery. *J Bone Joint Surg Am* 1982;64:1263-1272.

Lind B, Sihlbom H, Nordwall A: Halo-vest treatment of unstable traumatic cervical spine injuries. *Spine* 1988;13:425-432.

Smith MD, Bolesta MJ, Leventhal M, Bohlman HH: Postoperative cerebrospinal-fluid fistula associated with erosion of the dura: Findings after anterior resection of ossification of the posterior longitudinal ligament in the cervical spine. *J Bone Joint Surg Am* 1992;74:270-277.

Smith TK: Nutrition: Its relationship to orthopedic infections. *Orthop Clin North Am* 1991;22:373-377.

Yamada S, Aiba T, Endo Y, Hara M, Kitamoto T, Tateishi J: Creutzfeldt-Jakob disease transmitted by a cadaveric dura mater graft. *Neurosurgery* 1994;34:740-744.

Zeidman SM, Ducker TB: Posterior cervical lamino-foraminotomy for radiculopathy: Review of 172 cases. *Neurosurgery* 1993;33:356-362.

Chapter 45

Complications of Adult Thoracolumbar Surgery

Brett A. Taylor, MD, Major, USAF

Todd J. Albert, MD

Pedicle Screw Placement

Recent studies of complications related to posterior thoracolumbar surgery focus on instrumentation. Pedicle screw placement increases the length of surgery, infection rate, and general morbidity. Inaccurate pedicle screw placement risks nerve root injury, especially at the medioinferior aspect of the pedicle. Nerve damage can result from eccentric screw placement or improper sizing of the pedicle. Nerve impingement occurs from pedicle fracture fragments or pedicle screw contact. In a study of 30 patients with 131 screws placed under fluoroscopic control by experienced spine surgeons, CT images indicated cortical penetration in 40% and medial wall penetration in 29% of screws. Deviation on CT of more than 6 mm indicated a high risk of nerve root injury. Other authors have indicated similar findings. Minimal penetration poses little risk to the neural elements. In a review of 50 patients (244 pedicle screws), CT after routine hardware removal revealed a 59% accuracy rate in pedicle screw placement. In 20.9% of screws, less than 2 mm of medial pedicle breech was noted. In this study only one patient (0.5%) showed signs of nerve root impingement. The authors recommend meticulous preoperative planning, including measurements of pedicle angle, diameter, and length. A 5-

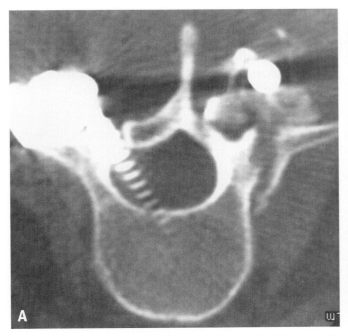
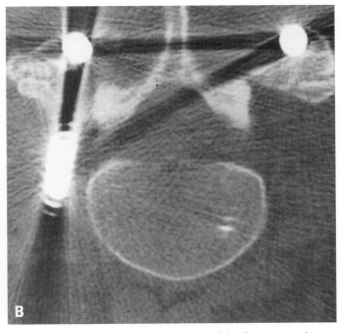

Figure 1 CT scan of inaccurate pedicle screw placement. **A,** Pedicle screw medial to pedicle in neural canal. **B,** Pedicle screw lateral to pedicle adjacent to neural foramen.

One or more of the authors or the departments with which they are affiliated have received something of value from a commercial or other party related directly or indirectly to the subject of this chapter.

mm-diameter screw may safely be placed in pedicles smaller than 8 mm, a 6-mm screw in pedicles of 8 to 9.5 mm, and a 7-mm screw in pedicles larger than 9.5 mm. In this study eccentric pedicle screws occur more often than the incidence of postoperative radiculopathy (Fig. 1).

In the elderly patient, pedicle screws can be used in arthrodesis with clinical success. A retrospective review of 38 patients age 60 years and older showed outcomes similar to younger populations. The mean number of comorbidities in this patient pool was 1.7, with no deaths reported at 2-year follow-up. Complications in this study group included dural lacerations, myocardial infarction, and inability to place screws due to osteoporotic bone. Female patients suffered more complications, but had comparable functional outcomes. These results imply that age alone is not a contraindication to extensive spinal surgery.

Postoperative radicular complaints are best evaluated by myelogram and CT. Numerous studies indicate that CT provides reliable documentation of pedicle screw placement. These studies have been verified with in vitro macroscopic anatomic dissection. Evidence of direct nerve root impingement requires screw removal and/or redirection. Less frequently reported complications of pedicle screws include a report of fatal cardiac tamponade after placement of a thoracic pedicle screw. The patient died from a coronary artery injury caused, presumably, by an intraoperative wire pedicle marker.

Intraoperative electromyographic (EMG) monitoring has been shown to be an effective method of improving pedicle screw placement. In one study of 90 patients with 512 pedicle screws, intraoperative pulsed current stimulation of the screw proved an excellent technique to improve placement accuracy. In 9% of patients EMG data detected screw malposition when intraoperative radiographs appeared satisfactory. The authors report that a stimulation threshold greater than 15 mA provides a 98% confidence that the screw was well positioned. A threshold between 10 and 15 mA provides an 87% confidence; however, exploration is suggested to rule out cortical breach. With this technology, 3% of screws were determined to be outside of the pedicle on CT imaging. In another study of 35 patients a constant current threshold of 6 mA or less indicated a pedicle wall breach. This study found EMG to be 93% sensitive to cortical penetration. Electrophysiologic monitoring is an effective adjunct to prevention of neurologic injury during pedicle screw placement. This technology provides intraoperative warning of altered neurologic function, allowing the surgeon to intervene.

Hardware fracture occurs as a late complication frequently associated with pseudarthrosis. Pedicle screw fracture occurs more frequently with small, minor-diameter screws. Increasing the minor diameter decreases screw fracture rates but also decreases pullout resistance because of smaller thread depth. Construct rigidity may also affect pedicle screw fracture risk. The addition of cross-links to a pedicle screw construct significantly increased rotational and lateral bending stiffness in in vitro studies. Thus, the surgeon can modify construct stiffness by altering the number of cross-links. Hardware fracture does not always require surgical management; however, a thorough assessment of fusion status is indicated in the presence of hardware fracture.

A complication of screw removal includes potential large vessel injury. In a case report, a screw removal instrument resulted in the screw fragment migrating into the retroperitoneal cavity. This required CT evaluation and anterior surgical removal. With screw failure rates reported as high as 20%, routine removal of pedicle screws is not warranted and may result in nontrivial complications.

Anterior Thoracolumbar Surgery

Among the most serious exposure-related complications of anterior surgery is vascular injury. Vascular complications include hemorrhage, hematoma, and thromboembolism. The risk of thromboembolism is not known; however, careful vessel manipulation and the use of sequential compression devices and elastic stockings may decrease this complication.

Neurologic damage can result from exposures that damage the lumbar sympathetic plexus, resulting in retrograde ejaculation in male patients or sympathectomy symptoms in the lower extremities. Retrograde ejaculation is an underreported complication, with published rates of 0 to 2%. Avoidance of monopolar electrocautery and use of blunt dissection anterior to the L5-S1 disc may reduce risk of this complication. Lower extremity sympathectomy can occur in up to 10% of patients; it usually is transient.

Horner's syndrome is associated with high thoracotomy if dissection is proximal to T1 or T2. Identification of the stellate ganglion and avoidance of electrocautery in this region may decrease the risk of this complication. Lumbar plexus injury also is associated with dissection lateral to the psoas muscle. Avoidance of dissection lateral to the pedicle is suggested in anterior spinal exposure.

Another exposure-related complication is visceral injury. The ureter is at increased risk in patients who have had prior surgery and in obese patients because of elevation by periureteral fat. Delayed detection of ureteral injury may lead to obstruction with acute signs and symptoms or extravasation of urine, which was described in a case report of a subtle presentation that included ileus, nausea, vomiting, and anorexia. The urinoma later resulted in hydronephrosis, fever, and leukocytosis. Final diagnosis required CT and aspiration of the fluid collection. An intraoperative finding of clear fluid on exposure should prompt investigation to rule out cerebrospinal fluid (CSF) leakage, thoracic duct injury, or ureteral injury. If possible, exposures should be on the opposite side of previous surgical fields.

The risk of paraplegia from vessel ligation during anterior thoracolumbar spine exposures was reviewed in 1,197 cases. No paralyses were noted. The authors suggest unilateral vessel ligation at the midvertebral body level and the avoidance of hypotensive anesthesia.

Wound complications in anterior surgery include infection, dehiscence, hernia, and seroma formation. Frequently, wound complications can be treated without additional surgical interventions.

In a large review of perioperative complications in 1,223 thoracolumbar anterior fusions, risk was associated with age older than 60 years. The direct complication rate of anterior surgery was 11.5% with rare serious complications.

Fixation-related complications include graft displacement, collapse, resorption, fracture, and nonunion. The popularity of interbody fusion cage technology has led to an increase in anterior lumbar fusion procedures. Incidence of vascular injury related to cage placement ranges from 1% to 6% in most studies. Neurologic injury is also possible during cage placement. Malpositioning of interbody devices can result if the midline position is inaccurately assessed. Excessive lateral cage placement can result in nerve root impingement and postoperative radicular symptoms. Evaluations of postoperative radiculopathy include myelogram and/or CT. In a case report, iatrogenic spinal stenois resulted after retropulsion of an interbody cage device.

Anterior instrumentation complications related to technique include those resulting from inaccurate incision placement, poor patient positioning, and failure to contour the plate to provide compression at the graft-host interface. In the thoracic spine, exposure generally requires excision of a rib two levels above the desired level. A retroperitoneal approach will allow plate application as high as L2 and as caudal as L4. Plate application at L5 requires extensive psoas muscle retraction and iliac crest removal. For these reasons, instrumentation into the lateral body of L5 is not recommended. Plate application above L2 requires a twelfth rib approach. During the procedure, the surgeon must maintain the patient in a true lateral orientation. The risk of canal penetration is increased if the patient inadvertently falls forward or backward during the procedure. If the operating table has been flexed to aid exposure, the table

must be neutralized before instrumentation to avoid deformity.

Device-related complications include erosion of hardware through vascular structures, hardware fracture, or loss of fixation. The force required for screw pullout in thoracolumbar plating is increased with bicortical placement. Careful preoperative planning is helpful in determining adequate screw length. Polymethylmethacrylate can be added to screw holes to improve purchase in cases of severe osteoporosis. Structural graft used in conjunction with thoracolumbar plating can be applied with compression to the cartilage-free end plates. The graft should be placed on the side of the spine contralateral to the plate. Screws should not be placed into the graft because this placement weakens graft stability.

In a series of 12 patients, the Z plate was successfully applied after anterior decompression for burst fractures without complication. A review of 150 burst fractures treated with the Kaneda device found a 93% fusion rate and marked reduction in canal compromise, from a mean of 47% to a postoperative mean of 2%. Nine patients suffered hardware fracture; however, none required implant removal. Seven patients had pseudarthroses without neurologic deterioration, which resolved after posterior spinal instrumentation.

Minimally Invasive Surgery

Minimal incision surgery offers the advantage of faster recovery. Endoscopic surgery introduces complications unique to the procedure. A steep learning curve is associated with the application of endoscopic technology (5 to 10 cases).

Thoracoscopic surgery has been used successfully to treat a number of thoracic pathologies including disc herniation, disc abscess, tumors, and deformity. Anesthesia by dual lumen intubation is required. Broncoscopy is useful in determining the tube position for allowing sufficient lung collapse. Complications include effusions, atelectasis, diaphragm injury, lung injury, mediastinal shift, emphysema, and intercostal paresthesias. Intercostal neuralgia is reported in up to 28% of patients undergoing thoracoscopy. This complication is limited if dissection is maintained at the superior aspect of the caudal rib. Dural injury is infrequently amenable to endoscopic repair; it usually requires open conversion. As with all minimally invasive procedures, emergency equipment must always be available in the event that open conversion is required. Complications related to instrument breakage frequently can be corrected endoscopically.

Unlike thoracoscopic procedures, laparoscopic surgery requires the use of CO_2 insufflation and positioning to distend the abdomen. Impaired visualization results when an inadequate seal is present. Trendelenburg positioning allows cephalad displacement of visceral structures. Laparoscopic technique has successfully allowed cage placement at the L4-5 interspace as well as the L5-S1 interspace as documented by numerous studies. Complications of this technique because of inadequate exposure include expansion injury to viscera or vessels. In addition, these structures can be damaged during instrument placement in the abdomen. Use of electrocautery with inadequate visualization can result in thermal injury.

In one comparison of laparoscopic and open threaded interbody cage placement, complication rates were comparable, with 4.2% occurring in the open procedures and 4.9% in the laparoscopic. However, the device-related reoperation rate was 4.7% in the laparoscopic group and 2.3% in the open group. In addition, 10% of the intended laparoscopic cases were converted to open placement. Complications include iliac vein lacerations, broken or dislodged hardware, and intraoperative disc herniation, with the latter complication associated with lateral cage placement. Monopolar electrocautery usage probably increases the rate of retrograde ejaculation. The transabdominal retroperitoneal approach is believed to have the lowest risk of autonomic dysfunction and should be considered in young male patients planning a family.

The following guidelines are suggested for cage placement. A history of multiple abdominal surgeries or intra-abdominal disease indicating a risk of scarring is a contraindication to laparoscopic cage procedures. A general surgeon trained in use of laparoscopic procedures should be available for the exposure. Only the initial blunt trochar is placed blindly, with all other trochar insertions under direct vision. The initial trochar is placed in a caudal direction to limit risk to bowel and vessels. Insufflation flattens the iliac veins and inferior vena cava, mandating clear observation of these structures at all times. Biplanar fluoroscopy is essential to accurate cage placement. Disc material must be removed to prevent herniation. Hemostasis must be assured at reduced insufflation to avoid postoperative bleeding. Incisional hernia results if trochar sites larger than 11 mm are left unsutured.

Circumferential Fusion

Anterior and posterior (A/P) fusion is the procedure of choice for many adult spinal pathologies, including pseudarthrosis, complex deformity, and correction of flatback syndrome. In a comparison of one-stage versus two-stage A/P spinal reconstructions, fewer infectious complications occurred in one-stage procedures. Both treatment groups had a high incidence of postoperative malnutrition (64% to 76%). All infections occurred in malnourished patients. Blood loss, transfusion requirements, and time in surgery were similar in the two groups. Hospital stay was an average of 7 days less in the single-stage group. Patients polled postoperatively preferred a one-stage procedure.

A history of prior surgery does not affect the short-term complication rate in adult patients undergoing A/P spinal fusion for deformity. Total surgery time and hospital costs were similar, with blood loss slightly higher in the primary group. Complications included prolonged ileus, deep venous thrombosis (DVT), deep wound infections, hardware failure, and neurologic deficit. Complications were similar in the two groups. In the revision group there was a greater use of total parenteral nutrition (TPN). It is possible that the use of TPN may have affected morbidity, in particular reducing the risk of deep wound infection.

Pseudarthrosis management in the lumbar spine with A/P fusion results in a high fusion rate. However, improved fusion status resulted in minimal change in functional status. Satisfactory outcome was 50% in one study with only a 53% return-to-work rate. Complications included wound dehiscence, pneumonia, and painful instrumentation. In a similar study of 37 patients, a 31% functional failure rate was found after A/P fusion for lumbar pseudarthrosis. Significant risk factors for failure were preoperative use of narcotics and abnormal neurologic findings. Patients with degenerative disc disease and pseudarthrosis are radiographically improved by A/P fusion surgery with less predictable functional improvement.

Flatback deformity results from reduction of normal lumbar lordosis. The resulting sagittal imbalance leads to muscle fatigue and pain. Patients treated with Harrington distraction instrumentation for adolescent scoliosis often become symptomatic 20 to 30 years postoperatively. Surgical treatment options include posterior osteotomy with or without anterior fusion, pedicle subtraction osteotomy, and combined A/P osteotomies. A review of 28 patients surgically treated for flatback deformity found poor patient satisfaction related to insufficient sagittal correction, pseudarthrosis, coronal imbalance, and four or more medical comorbidities. Avoiding these complications can result in significant pain reduction.

Vertebroplasty

Developed in Europe in the 1980s, vertebroplasty is a percutaneous technique that places polymethylmethacrylate (PMMA) into neoplastic and osteoporotic compression fractures. A paravertebral transpedicular approach under CT or fluoroscopic guidance has proven effective in the application of vertebroplasty. Preprocedure CT is valuable in determining both pedicular size and fracture extension. During injection, attention is paid to avoid entrance of PMMA into the epidural space, spinal canal, or perivertebral veins. Possible complications include thermal injury, nondisplaced rib fractures, PMMA embolization to the lungs, PMMA extravasation into the disc, cement displacement of nerve roots resulting in radiculopathy, and PMMA injection into the venous plexus resulting in thecal sac flattening. In a review of 29 patients, 90% reported pain relief within 24 h. A review of 38 patients found a minor complication rate of 6%. In this study there was complete or marked pain relief in 95% of osteoporotic compression fracture patients. Patients treated for neoplasm did not have consistent pain relief.

Nutritional Deficiency

Numerous studies indicate nutritional deficiencies lead to increased postoperative complications and morbidity. Standard nutritional assessment includes measurements of serum albumin (< 3.5g/dL is abnormal) and total lymphocyte count (< 1,500 to 2,000 cells/mm^3 is abnormal). Nutritionally at-risk patients include those with spinal cord injury and vertebral osteomyelitis. In one study, postoperative complications were found predominately in malnourished patients in these groups. The risk of postoperative wound infection was 15 times greater in malnourished patients. In elective adult lumbar spinal surgery 25% to 42% of patients are inadequately nourished at surgery. Patients found with inadequate parameters should be replenished before elective procedures. In patients requiring complex spinal procedures (A/P surgery) use of TPN results in less nutritional depletion. It is presumed that improving nutritional status with TPN will decrease postoperative complications. In a prospective study of 40 adult spinal patients, TPN use improved nutritional parameters without additional TPN-related complications.

Wound Infection

Wound infections occur in 1% to 6% of spinal surgeries. Instrumented fusion is associated with a higher rate of infection than noninstrumented fusion. Infected instrumented wounds are managed with serial irrigation and débridement and extended antibiotic treatment. In a study of 19 deep wound infections, antibiotic-impregnated beads and serial irrigation and débridement were used to control deep infections without hardware removal. At 1-year follow-up no recurrence of infection was detected.

Dural Tears

Acute tears encountered intraoperatively can be posttraumatic or iatrogenic. Posttraumatic dural injury associated with lamina fractures requires surgical exploration to assess for neural element interposition. The major risk of posttraumatic dural tear is neurologic injury, not persistent leakage of CSF. Iatrogenic dural tears noted intraoperatively require closure by primary repair when possible. In a retrospective review, patients with repaired incidental durotomies were allowed to ambulate without restriction. This early postoperative ambulation was effective in 75% of patients; 20% reported headache, nausea, or other symptoms. Reoperation was required in 5% for stitch loosening. The authors of this review support dural repair and fibrin glue as adequate treatment without mandatory bed rest. Intraoperative repairs should be tested with reverse Trendelenburg positioning and Valsalva maneuver.

Dural injury and CSF leakage noted postoperatively pose different challenges. Beta-2-transferrin can be tested in wound drainage to determine the presence of CSF. Other diagnostic tools include myelography and MRI. Subarachnoid drains have been successful in eliminating CSF leakage in this circumstance. Drainage rates of 50 to 100 cc every 8 h for up to 4 to 6 days are well

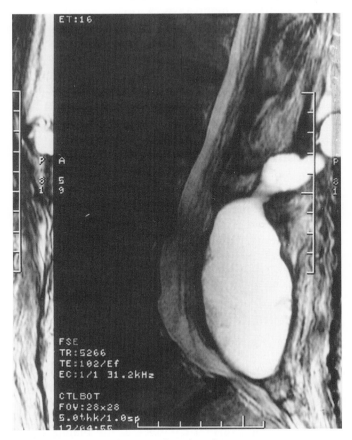

Figure 2 Sagittal MRI of large pseudomeningocele.

tolerated without side effects. The drain fluid should be closely monitored for white blood cells to prevent infections. The epidural blood patch is another treatment modality for postoperative CSF leaks. The combination of spinal drainage and a blood patch has successfully treated both CSF fistulas and pseudomeningoceles. In some cases reoperation is required when nonsurgical measures fail (Fig. 2).

Bone Graft Harvest

The use of autogenous bone graft from the ilium is common in spinal surgery. Knowledge of the reported complications and meticulous surgical technique can avoid major complications and reduce the occurrence of minor complications. Bone graft complications include pain, nerve injury, hemorrhage, arterial injury, deformity, infection, stress fracture, gait abnormalities, peritoneal perforation, pelvic instability, visceral injury, and herniation of abdominal contents. Superior gluteal artery injury with uncontrolled hemorrhage has been managed with pressure application, enlargement of the sciatic notch, emergent anterior approach, and embolization. An additional technique includes detachment of the origin and reflection of the gluteus maximus, providing adequate exposure of the superior gluteal artery for hemostasis. A review of 261 operations by one surgeon revealed a 39% incidence of minor complications. Risk factors for complication included female sex, separate incision harvest, and age younger than 20 years, with the latter being attributed to poor patient acceptance of scarring. Meticulous closure technique with minimal tension on the skin closure may improve results.

Thromboembolism

The literature on thromboemboli after spinal surgery is limited. A prospective review of 116 adult spinal surgery patients found a 0.9% incidence of asymptomatic DVT diagnosed by screening duplex scan. The symptomatic pulmonary embolism (PE) rate was 2.6% of all patients (posterior only and A/P procedures), with all occurring in combined A/P procedures. This represented a 6% rate of symptomatic PE in combined A/P procedures. All patients in this study were treated prophylactically with thigh-length compression hose and pneumatic compression leggings. The authors believed that screening duplex scans were not helpful in detecting subclinical DVT. In addition, patients undergoing A/P fusion with manipulation of the great vessels are at increased risk of DVT and PE. Routine mechanical prophylaxis may be inadequate in this patient population.

Heparinization further complicates the management of spinal surgery patients with PE. The use of heparin

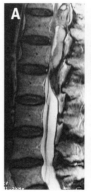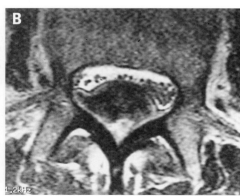

Figure 3 A, Sagittal MRI of an epidural hematoma resulting from postoperative anticoagulation. **B,** Axial MRI of hematoma compressing thecal sac.

for nonfatal PE in postoperative spinal surgery patients is associated with a 67% complication rate. These complications include wound hematoma, infection, gastrointestinal bleeding, and epidural hematoma resulting in cauda equina syndrome and paraplegia (Fig. 3). The high wound complication rate is thought to be related to the decortication effect and dead space created in spinal surgery. In comparison, the complication rate of filter placement is 1% to 10%. Inferior vena cava filter placement is favored for patients with nonfatal PE after spinal surgery.

Visual Function

Ophthalmic complications are serious but rare in spinal surgery. In a series of 3,450 spinal procedures 0.20% were complicated by loss of vision. Classically, these complications are attributed to undue pressure on the prone orbit. However, hypertension and peripheral vascular disease may also contribute to these complications. Etiologies of postoperative visual loss include posterior optic nerve ischemia, occipital lobe infarcts, retinal artery occlusion, and central retinal vein thrombosis. Chronic hypertension, diabetes, smoking, intraoperative hypotension, and low flow states may contribute to the ischemia-related complications. Ischemic optic neuritis may be reversible in its early course; therefore, prompt ophthalmology consultation is indicated in patients with changes in postoperative visual function. In a review of 37 visual loss cases, the complication was associated with complex instrumented fusion. In most cases the deficit was permanent. The authors concluded the visual complication rate might be as high as one case per 100 spine surgeons per year. They suggest vigilance in eye protection during positioning, as well as establishing a minimum systolic blood pressure preoperatively to prevent excessive hypotension.

Annotated Bibliography

Albert TJ, Pinto M, Denis F: Management of symptomatic lumbar pseudarthrosis with anteroposterior fusion: A functional and radiographic outcome study. *Spine* 2000;25:123-130.

The authors provide a retrospective review of 39 patients with lumbar pseudarthrosis to assess functional and radiographic results of A/P revision surgery. Radiographically there was a 10% pseudarthrosis rate and 31% functional failure rate. Preoperative narcotic usage and abnormal neurologic findings were associated with poor functional outcome.

Barr JD, Barr MS, Lemley TJ, McCann RM: Percutaneous vertebroplasty for pain relief and spinal stabilization. *Spine* 2000;25:923-928.

This is a retrospective review of 47 patients treated with percutaneous vertebroplasty for osteoporotic fractures and spinal neoplasm. Among the 38 patients treated for osteoporotic fractures, 63% had marked relief of pain and 32% moderate relief of pain. There was a 6% minor complication rate.

Booth KC, Bridwell KH, Lenke LG, Baldus CR, Blanke KM: Complications and predictive factors for the successful treatment of flatback deformity (fixed sagittal imbalance). *Spine* 1999;24:1712-1720.

This review of 28 patients treated with spinal osteotomy to correct flatback deformity provides a detailed review of the anatomy, diagnosis, and treatment options for this pathology. Poor patient satisfaction is associated with inadequate sagittal correction, pseudarthrosis, and four or more major medical comorbidities.

Castro WH, Halm H, Jerosch J, Malms J, Steinbeck J, Blasius S: Accuracy of pedicle screw placement in lumbar vertebrae. *Spine* 1996;21:1320-1324.

The authors studied pedicle screws placed in 30 patients, with CT images obtained to verify accuracy. In the clinical group 40% of all screws were improperly placed and 29% had medial wall pedicle breech. Medial deviation greater than 6 mm placed the nerve root at high risk for injury.

Dearborn JT, Hu SS, Tribus CB, Bradford DS: Thromboembolic complications after major thoracolumbar spine surgery. *Spine* 1999;24:1471-1476.

This prospective study was undertaken to determine the incidence of subclinical DVT in spinal surgery. Screening duplex ultrasound was unable to detect clots prior to embolization. In addition patients undergoing A/P spinal fusion may not receive adequate prophylaxis by simple mechanical means.

Faciszewski T, Winter RB, Lonstein JE, Denis F, Johnson L: The surgical and medical perioperative complications of anterior spinal fusion surgery in the thoracic and lumbar spine in adults: A review of 1223 procedures. *Spine* 1995;20:1592-1599.

This retrospective review of 1,223 anterior thoracolumbar fusions reported a 0.3% death rate and a 0.2% paraplegia rate. The complication rate attributable to the anterior procedure was 11.5%.

Gertzbein SD, Hollopeter MR, Hall S: Pseudarthrosis of the lumbar spine: Outcome after circumferential fusion. *Spine* 1998;23:2352-2357.

This is a retrospective review of 25 patients with pseudarthrosis after failed lumbar fusions for degenerative disc disease. Revision A/P fusion resulted in a 100% fusion rate without an appreciable improvement in patient outcome. Postoperatively 41% were on narcotics, and only 53% had returned to work. Revision fusion surgery offers questionable benefit to patients with degenerative disc disease.

Ghanayem AJ, Zdeblick TA: Anterior instrumentation in the management of thoracolumbar burst fractures. *Clin Orthop* 1997;335:89-100.

This excellent review of anterior plate fixation indications, surgical technique, and complications includes the clinical results from 12 patients treated successfully with anterior decompression and instrumentation after burst fractures.

Glassman SD, Dimar JR, Puno RM, Johnson JR, Shields CB, Linden RD: A prospective analysis of intraoperative electromyographic monitoring of pedicle screw placement with computed tomographic scan confirmation. *Spine* 1995;20:1375-1379.

This large prospective clinical study showed that intraoperative pedicle screw EMG monitoring is a valuable adjunct to spinal instrumentation. A stimulation threshold more than 15 mA provides a 98% confidence of accurate pedicle screw placement.

Klein JD, Hey LA, Yu CS, et al: Perioperative nutrition and postoperative complications in patients undergoing spinal surgery. *Spine* 1996;21:2676-2682.

In this three-part study on nutritional status of patients with vertebral osteomyelitis, spinal cord injury, and elective spinal surgery, preoperative nutritional status was an independent predictor of postoperative complications. In elective surgery 25% to 42% of patients were found to be inadequately nourished.

Regan JJ, Yuan H, McAfee PC: Laparoscopic fusion of the lumbar spine: Minimally invasive spine surgery: A prospective multicenter study evaluating open and laparoscopic lumbar fusion. *Spine* 1999;24:402-411.

This excellent prospective multicenter study investigated the safety of laparoscopic cage placement. The laparoscopic group had shorter length of hospital stay and increased surgery times. The device-related complications were higher in the laparoscopic group.

Schulze CJ, Munzinger E, Weber U: Clinical relevance of accuracy of pedicle screw placement: A computed tomographic-supported analysis. *Spine* 1998;23:2215-2221.

Fifty patients underwent routine removal of 244 pedicle screws and postoperative CT scanning. The images were reviewed to assess pedicle anatomy without the artifact of hardware. Fifty-nine percent of screws were placed centrally and only 20% showed medial pedicle violation (none greater than 2 mm). There was only one case of neurologic damage with nerve root irritation. There is a safety zone between the medial pedicle wall and the nerve root, resulting in a minimal incidence of neurologic complication.

Classic Bibliography

Banwart JC, Asher MA, Hassanein RS: Iliac crest bone graft harvest donor site morbidity: A statistical evaluation. *Spine* 1995;20:1055-1060.

Cain JE Jr, Major MR, Lauerman WC, West JL, Wood KB, Fueredi GA: The morbidity of heparin therapy after development of pulmonary embolus in patients undergoing thoracolumbar or lumbar spinal fusion. *Spine* 1995;20:1600-1603.

Dick J, Boachie-Adjei O, Wilson M: One-stage versus two-stage anterior and posterior spinal reconstruction in adults: Comparison of outcomes including nutritional status, complication rates, hospital costs, and other factors. *Spine* 1992;17(suppl 8):S310-S316.

Glassman SD, Dimar JR, Puno RM, Johnson JR: Salvage of instrumental lumbar fusions complicated by surgical wound infection. *Spine* 1996;21:2163-2169.

Grimes PF, Vaccaro AR, Garfin SR: Treatment complications of thoracolumbar spine trauma. *Semin Spine Surg* 1995;7:141-151.

Isiklar ZU, Lindsey RW, Coburn M: Ureteral injury after anterior lumbar interbody fusion: A case report. *Spine* 1996;21:2379-2382.

Kaneda K, Taneichi H, Abumi K, Hashimoto T, Satoh S, Fujiya M: Anterior decompression and stabilization with the Kaneda device for thoracolumbar burst fractures associated with neurological deficits. *J Bone Joint Surg Am* 1997;79:69-83.

Lynn G, Mukherjee DP, Kruse RN, Sadasivan KK, Albright JA: Mechanical stability of thoracolumbar pedicle screw fixation: The effect of crosslinks. *Spine* 1997;22:1568-1573.

Maguire J, Wallace S, Madiga R, Leppanen R, Draper V: Evaluation of intrapedicular screw position using intraoperative evoked electromyography. *Spine* 1995;20:1068-1074.

Myers MA, Hamilton SR, Bogosian AJ, Smith CH, Wagner TA: Visual loss as a complication of spine surgery: A review of 37 cases. *Spine* 1997;22:1325-1329.

Shin AY, Moran ME, Wenger DR: Superior gluteal artery injury secondary to posterior iliac crest bone graft harvesting: A surgical technique to control hemorrhage. *Spine* 1996;21:1371-1374.

Stevens WR, Glazer PA, Kelley SD, Lietman TM, Bradford DS: Opthalmic complications after spinal surgery. *Spine* 1997;22:1319-1324.

Vanichkachorn JS, Vaccaro AR, Cohen MJ, Cotler JM: Potential large vessel injury during thoracolumbar pedicle screw removal: A case report. *Spine* 1997;22:110-113.

Winter RB, Lonstein JE, Denis F, Leonard AS, Garamella JJ: Paraplegia resulting from vessel ligation. *Spine* 1996;21:1232-1234.

Section 4

New and Future Developments

Section Editor:
Scott D. Boden, MD

Chapter 46

Biologic Enhancement of Spinal Arthrodesis: Past, Present, and Future

K. Craig Boatright, MD

Scott D. Boden, MD

Previously, the goals for bone-graft substitutes were to match fusion rates with autologous bone-grafting techniques while avoiding the morbidity of bone-graft harvest and extending the quantity of available graft material. As bone-graft substitutes and growth factors become clinical realities, new standards will be defined.

An ideal bone-generating combination is now the goal. It will integrate an osteoconductive matrix with growth factors delivered in a localized environment and, over the appropriate time course, attract and sustain osteoprogenitor cells as they differentiate into osteogenic cells. The osteoinductive growth factors will be the product of cells genetically engineered to synthesize these substances under specific conditions controlled by the physician. Finally, the ideal graft substitute will provide structural support as necessary, but as the graft matures, the graft matrix will allow transition of functional weight bearing to the new host bone.

Biology of Spine Fusion

The first step in the search for a superior bone generator is understanding the biology of spinal fusion. The fracture-healing of long bones and the healing of segmental defects in long bones both differ greatly from the incorporation of bone graft that occurs at the site of a spinal fusion mass. The biologic environment differs even between the various types of fusions used in spine surgery. The compressive environment of an interbody fusion is different from that found in posterolateral intertransverse-process fusions, the most common type of spinal arthrodesis performed in clinical practice. Compressive forces are much less significant in the early

healing of intertransverse fusion because consolidation is necessary before a newly formed posterolateral bone mass is subjected to any weight bearing.

With the utilization of autogenous bone graft, a characteristic set of events must occur for a fusion mass to form. First, osteoprogenitor cells must enter the fusion area by decortication of the host bone. This allows cells to escape from the bone marrow into the fusion environment. These progenitor cells then differentiate into osteoblasts that deposit new bone matrix on the structural component of the transplanted bone graft. Finally, remodeling of the initial fusion mass occurs according to Wolff's law; this results in a mature fusion mass that is able to provide long-term, durable stability to the spine.

The development of appropriate animal models has greatly facilitated the study of this process. With animal models, causal factors can be isolated and the end point of fusion determined with certainty by a variety of methods. Fusion masses resulting from decortication and autogenous bone grafting have been characterized using biomechanical analysis, histomorphometric techniques, and radiographic evaluation (Figs. 1 through 3).

Advances in molecular biology have been used to investigate the characteristic sequence of temporal and spatial gene expression that leads to the formation of a fusion mass in posterolateral intertransverse spinal fusion. Both membranous and enchondral bone formation are seen to occur at specific, predictable times and locations within a fusion mass. These events are orchestrated by a similarly reproducible pattern of osteoinductive growth factors that include several bone morphogenetic proteins (BMPs). These studies provide a basic level of understanding that can systematically direct further research efforts (Fig. 4).

Interventions such as internal fixation to improve control of the local biomechanical environment have improved the success rate of spinal arthrodesis. Still, a nonunion rate of 10% to 15% exists. Characterization of histologic and corresponding molecular events surround-

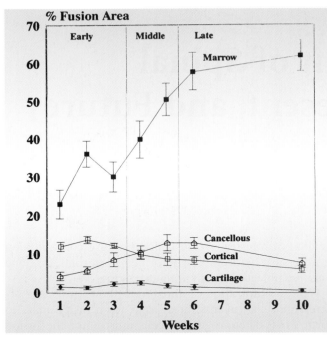

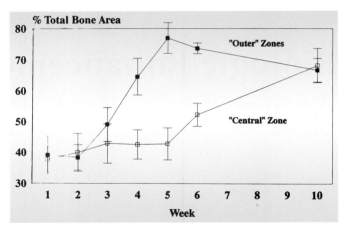

Figure 1 Quantitative histologic healing sequence of rabbit spine fusions depicted graphically. Note the continuous increase in bone marrow content of the fusion mass beginning in the early phase and continuing through the late phase of healing. During the middle phase of healing, a reversal of the cortical:cancellous bone ratio is seen as well as a small peak in the relative percentage of cartilage corresponding to the central region endochondral ossification. *(Reproduced with permission from Boden SD, Schimandle JH, Hutton WC, Chen MI: The use of an osteoinductive growth factor for lumbar spinal fusion: Part I. Biology of spinal fusion. Spine 1995;20:2626-2632.)*

Figure 2 Histologic fusion maturation in rabbit depicted graphically with measurement of cancellous bone area (mean ± SEM). Note the temporally more advanced fusion maturation in the "outer" zones (near the transverse processes) compared with the less mature fusion in the "central" zone. A similar temporal sequence of maturation occurred in the central zone but was delayed in time–the "lag effect." By 10 weeks, fusion maturation (as measured by cancellous bone area) was similar in both zones. *(Reproduced with permission from Boden SD, Schimandle JH, Hutton WC, Chen MI: The use of an osteoinductive growth factor for lumbar spinal fusion: Part I. Biology of spinal fusion. Spine 1995;20:2626-2632.)*

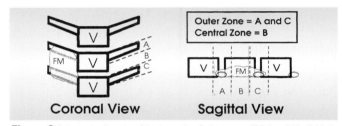

Figure 3 Schematic diagram of lumbar spine fusion mass (FM) in rabbit divided into thirds in the coronal and sagittal views and their relationship to the vertebral bodies (V). The two outer zones (A and C) are distinguished from the central zone (B). *(Reproduced with permission from Morone MA, Boden SD, Hair G, et al: Gene expression during autograft lumbar spine fusion and the effect of bone morphogenetic protein 2. Clin Orthop 1998;351:252-265.)*

ing posterolateral fusion has led to exciting advances in the understanding of this process. In the future, this knowledge will be applied to the quest for a superior bone generator to replace autogenous bone graft. Attention now is focused on the biology of spine fusion to further enhance the rate of successful arthrodesis.

Classifying Bone-Generating Substances

A superior bone generator will need to meet many requirements. As an osteoconductive substance, it will provide the scaffolding that the cells of bone metabolism require. At least one component of the substance must provide osteoinduction. This is accomplished by inducing progenitor cells to differentiate into bone-forming cells. Growth factors such as BMPs function to effect osteoinduction. Through osteoinduction, the bone-forming environment becomes osteogenic.

Osteogenesis requires the presence of cells capable of forming bone. Autogenous bone graft is osteogenic under circumstances in which osteoblasts remain viable after harvesting and implantation. Only autogenous bone graft and bone marrow contain bone-forming cells initially; all other substances must rely on osteoinduction to establish an osteogenic environment.

Available bone-graft substitutes can be broadly classified under three major headings: bone-graft extender, bone-graft enhancer, or bone-graft substitute. The terms extender, enhancer, and substitute all inherently reference the current gold standard, autogenous bone graft. One of the major shortcomings of autograft bone is the finite supply available in each patient. As the term implies, an extender is used to add to available autograft to expand the coverage or decrease the required volume of autograft. By definition, rates of fusion in a successful bone-graft extender–autograft combination are at best equal to those of autograft alone. In contrast, a bone-graft enhancer is a substance that, when used in conjunction with autograft, will increase the successful rate of fusion above that reported for autograft alone (70% to 90%) under the specific clinical circumstance. Finally, a bone-graft substitute is unique in that it can replace autogenous bone graft, achieving equal or

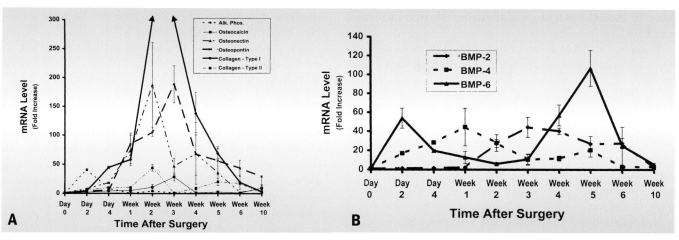

Figure 4 **A,** Graph of the sequential osteoblast-related gene expression in the central zone of rabbit posterolateral spine fusion masses (n = 3 per time point) with autogenous bone graft. The values were determined by semiquantitative reverse transcriptase–polymerase chain reaction (RT-PCR) and expressed as fold increases over the level present in iliac crest bone (day 0). A reproducible and orderly sequence of gene expression was seen that was paralleled in the central zone (not shown) but delayed by 1 to 3 weeks. **B,** BMP gene expression determined by RT-PCR in the outer zone of the spine fusion mass at specific times after surgery. The values of messenger RNA (mRNA) levels are given as fold increases over the level present in iliac crest bone (day 0). A reproducible sequence of gene expression was seen with BMP-6 mRNA peaking earliest on day 2, followed by BMP-4 mRNA, BMP-2 mRNA, and a second peak of BMP-6 mRNA. These results suggest that different BMPs have unique temporal patterns of expression during the spine fusion healing process. *(Reproduced with permission from Morone MA, Boden SD, Hair G, et al: Gene expression during autograft lumbar spine fusion and the effect of bone morphogenetic protein 2. Clin Orthop 1998;351:252-265.)*

better rates of fusion and thereby obviating the need for autogenous bone-graft harvest and avoiding its concomitant morbidity. The next generation of stand-alone bone-graft substitutes, which likely will be made up of an optimum combination of the substances reviewed here, can realistically be expected to have an enhanced rate of fusion compared with that of autograft.

Clinical data exist to classify many of the available materials into one of these three categories for various grafting scenarios. Performance results reported for spinal fusion with each substitute or combination of substitutes are reviewed below.

Current Options

Autogenous Bone Graft in Spinal Fusion

During the 1990s, spinal fusion surgery became the most common reason for autologous bone grafting. Despite the fact that autograft bone is osteoconductive, osteoinductive, and osteogenic, it has major shortcomings as an ideal bone generator. The rate of nonunion after spinal arthrodesis is reported to range from 5% to 35%. As noted earlier, the addition of internal fixation has lowered the nonunion rate, but pseudarthrosis still can be expected in 10% to 15% of instrumented cases when posterolateral lumbar fusion is attempted.

Aside from the significant nonunion rate, bone-graft harvest is associated with well-known complications in up to 25% of cases; these include infection, fracture of the ilium, abdominal herniations, increased blood loss, increased hospital stay, and increased postoperative

pain. In addition, autograft is available in a limited supply that can be inadequate for revisions or multilevel procedures. The clinical track record of autogenous bone graft makes it the present gold standard for spinal arthrodesis.

Allogenic Bone Graft in Spinal Fusion

The performance of allograft bone in spinal fusion varies greatly with each specific clinical scenario. With a few notable exceptions, it has functioned well for anterior structural grafts and poorly when used alone for posterior spinal fusion. It remains the most commonly used bone-graft extender.

Methods of sterilization and preservation kill the cells within allograft and damage other soft-tissue components, including proteins. For this reason, allograft does not function as an osteogenic substance and has only weak osteoinductive potential. Allograft is the quintessential example of osteoconductivity, which varies directly with a substance's structural similarity to natural bone.

Cortical allografts have been used with success in anterior cervical surgery as structural interbody implants. Fusion rates are reported to be equal to those of autograft for single-level anterior cervical discectomy and fusion, with successful arthrodesis rates of 95%. The use of allogenic strut grafts for anterior column support after complete or partial corpectomy is common throughout the spine. In this setting, morcellized autograft is placed at the site of the construct by most surgeons, and although the allograft strut may take up to a year to incorporate, clinical sequelae of pseudarthrosis are rare.

With one notable exception, allograft bone as a bone-graft substitute has functioned poorly in posterior spinal surgery. The exception has been reported in adolescent idiopathic scoliosis, in which small amounts of local autogenous bone were mixed with allograft chips and found to have a fusion rate equal to that of an iliac crest autograft–local autograft combination. Although this does not represent use as a true stand-alone bone-graft substitute (local autograft was added), secondary donor site morbidity was avoided, and this was reflected in patient outcome.

Allograft bone functions well for structural support of the anterior column and as a bone-graft extender when sufficient autograft is not available. At this time, data do not support its use as a stand-alone bone-graft substitute in posterior spinal surgery.

Osteoconductive Bone-Graft Substitutes

The basic science of osteoconductive materials has centered on the analysis of the porous physical structure of compounds that have demonstrated efficacy as bone-graft substitutes. Porosity allows vascularization and provides surface area for the adherence of osteogenic cells, including osteoblasts and osteoclasts. The optimal pore size for bony ingrowth has been studied in detail and appears to be between 100 and 500 μm, with a total porous volume of 75% to 80%. The topographic structure of the channels appears to be most successful when it closely resembles that of natural bone. Also critical for the ultimate goal of bony union followed by physiologic remodeling is the ability of a material to be reabsorbed over a time course that encourages bony replacement.

Calcium Sulfate

Reported in 1892 by Dresmann, plaster of Paris was the first substance used to fill bony defects in patients. Dresmann noted that bony voids filled with this calcium sulfate compound showed evidence of bone ingrowth. Since that time, multiple preparations of calcium-containing compounds have been used with varying success as bone-graft extenders or substitutes.

Calcium sulfate, the primary ingredient in plaster of Paris, continues to be available for clinical use, albeit in a different form from that used by Dresmann in 1892. Compounds of calcium sulfate generate very little foreign-body reaction, and osteoclasts actively reabsorb calcium sulfate in a manner similar to physiologic bone remodeling. Despite these desirable traits, previous heterogenous compounds were unreliable and dissolved quickly, so that fibrous tissue formed instead of bone. Recently, a more crystalline form of calcium sulfate that dissolves at a more predictable rate has become available. This substance, OsteoSet (Wright Medical Technology, Arlington, TN), has shown promising results in several animal models. It is marketed for clinical use as "bone void filler."

Coralline Substitutes

Similarity between the exoskeletons of certain naturally occurring marine corals and bone was first recognized in the 1970s. This similarity has been exploited as naturally occurring corals have served as templates for the generation of various implants for bone grafting. The term coralline was coined to classify this subset of bone-graft substitutes.

Either of two general processes is used to prepare marine corals for implantation. The first uses the calcium carbonate exoskeleton directly after it has undergone a detergent-based process to remove the organic phase of the coral organism; this results in the product whose trade name is Biocoral (Inoteb, Saint Gonnery, France). The second general process converts the calcium carbonate to hydroxyapatite by a hydrothermal exchange reaction known as replamineform. Products produced by this process are Pro Osteon and Interpore porous hydroxyapatite (Interpore Cross International, Irvine, CA).

Multiple animal studies have demonstrated the biocompatibility as well as the bioactivity of coralline implants because osteoblasts and vascular tissues readily migrate into their matrix. Remodeling also occurs as the implants are resorbed and replaced by host bone. This process is described by Wolff's law and is accomplished through osteoclastic activity similar to physiologic bone remodeling. Many of these data have been accumulated using long-bone defect models; however, despite encouraging results, these products have not proved to be stand-alone bone-graft substitutes, especially in the challenging environment of posterolateral spinal fusion.

Ceramics

Ceramic forms of calcium phosphates are formed by heating and pressurizing these nonmetallic materials. Although the biocompatibility of these substances has been excellent as a group, bioresorbability has varied among the ceramics. In fact, several ceramic substances have been abandoned because the rate of resorption is too slow. The retained implant creates a stress riser within the fusion mass and thus compromises it mechanically.

An example of poor resorbability is ceramic hydroxyapatite. At the other extreme of resorbability are some calcium sulfate compounds, such as those mentioned earlier, that can dissolve so quickly that fibrous tissue ingrowth occurs instead of bone formation. In the intermediate range are the tricalcium phosphate implants that dissolve within 6 weeks, a time course that is still quite short for posterolateral fusion in primates. One strategy used to deal with these shortcomings is to integrate two substances into one composite, thus providing a more favorable timeline of dissolution.

Collagen

The use of collagen as a bone-graft substitute was suggested by its role in normal bone physiology. Type I collagen catalyzes the events surrounding bone formation, acting in both a structural and biochemical manner. The use of collagen as a stand-alone bone-graft substitute has been unsuccessful, but it greatly potientiates the effects of other osteoinductive and osteoconductive substances, including bone marrow and composites of hydroxyapatite and tricalcium phosphate. Although collagen has been a successful bone-graft extender, its primary future role will likely be as an ingredient in stand-alone bone-graft substitute composites because it appears to contribute significantly to an ideal environment for new bone formation.

The role of osteoconductive bone-graft substitutes has changed considerably as more data have become available and as bone-grafting strategies have developed. At this time, the use of osteoinductive implants has moved from their use alone as bone-graft substitutes. Despite this, interest in and the development of these substances has intensified. The goal now is to integrate an ideal osteoconductive substance with a potent osteoinductive substance to create a superior bone generator.

Demineralized Bone Matrix

Demineralized bone matrix (DBM) became available for clinical use in 1991. Its use since then has increased; in 1999 in the United States, more than 500,000 mL of DBM was estimated to have been implanted. The seminal work of Urist, first reported in 1965, proved the osteoinductive capacity of DBM, which is prepared from allograft by decalcification of cortical bone. This process leaves the extracellular matrix, which contains type I collagen and nonstructural proteins, including small amounts of growth factors. Among the growth factors are the BMPs that make up approximately 0.1% of the total weight of all proteins in bone and are responsible for the osteoinductive capacity of DBM. Although DBM provides no structural integrity and is meant to be used in a mechanically stable environment, nevertheless it has variable osteoconductive potential because of the presence of collagen.

Despite the widespread clinical use of DBM, prospective clinical data are very limited. Many of the data have been generated in small-animal models in which DBM has been shown to have variable osteoinductive potency depending on the details of preparation, composite

form, and the healing environment being tested. Data from animal studies comprise the greatest source of information on DBM in spinal fusion, where it has been tested as a bone-graft substitute and as an autogenous bone-graft extender. DBM consistently performs better than mineralized allograft bone but not as well as autogenous bone in small-animal models.

Studies in human subjects are limited; however, equivalent fusion rates have been reported in comparing DBM (Grafton, Osteotech, Eatontown, NJ) and autograft composite with autograft alone in posterolateral fusion.

As noted, DBM has shown promising results as a bone-graft extender and even as a substitute in small-animal models. Care must be taken, however, in extrapolating results from small-animal models to humans because of the increased difficulty of initiating osteoinduction in primates. In evaluating the presently available DBM compounds, the prevailing clinical attitude is that DBM compounds function as bone-graft extenders, not as substitutes.

Future Options

After initially identifying DBM and its osteoinductive ability, Urist proceeded to fractionate the osteoinductive portion of the DBM. From this portion, he eventually reported on a series of soluble, low-molecular-weight glycoproteins responsible for inducing bone formation. These became known as BMPS and are the most widely investigated group of growth factors that result in bone formation. By the early 1990s, nine specific molecules, designated BMP-1 through BMP-9, had been isolated and cloned using the molecular techniques of genetic engineering. Through these processes, recombinant human BMPs (rhBMPs) can be generated in standard potencies and unlimited quantities, making the study of these compounds easier. As a result, these cloned growth factors are being applied to many models of bone healing with exciting results.

Extracted BMPs: Bovine-Derived Bone Protein Extract

Bovine-derived bone protein extract, commercially known as Ne-Osteo (Sulzer Orthopedics Biologics, Denver, CO), is the product of improved techniques of extraction and purification and results in a concentrated mixture of BMPs. This osteoinductive cocktail has been investigated in both rabbit and nonhuman primate models for variables such as time to fusion, biomechanical properties, and the histology of the resulting fusion mass. Results have shown that Ne-Osteo functions successfully for fusion when delivered in autograft, DBM, natural coral, or coralline hydroxyapatite.

The systematic investigation of this compound serves

as a model for methodology in the search for the ideal bone generator. Various delivery systems in appropriate animal models have demonstrated an effective method to investigate the optimization of new growth factor–bone graft substitute combinations.

Recombinant BMPs

Recombinant Human Bone Morphogenetic Protein-2

At this time, rhBMP-2 (Genetics Institute, Cambridge, MA) has been investigated in more detail than have other BMPs. In 1990, this particular glycoprotein molecule was found to induce ectopic bone formation in rats. Since then, rhBMP-2 has been effective for bone generation in many spinal fusion models, including in rabbits, dogs, sheep, goats, and rhesus monkeys. Recent results reported in nonhuman primates and in pilot human clinical trials have been very encouraging.

To date, published primate research using rhBMP-2 has focused on use of the growth factor in the interbody fusion environment. In a rhesus monkey anterior interbody fusion model that compared freeze-dried allograft bone dowels filled with either autograft or rhBMP-2–soaked collagen sponges, the rhBMP-2–soaked collagen sponges had superior results. Specifically, the rhBMP-2–collagen sponge fusion sites demonstrated 100% fusion at 6 months and extensive replacement of allograft with new host bone. The autograft-filled dowel sites showed no similar remodeling of initial allograft dowels. Similar successful results in adult rhesus monkeys have been reported by a separate group of investigators who also used the lumbar interbody environment. In this experiment, titanium cages were implanted with various doses of rhBMP-2–soaked collagen sponges in five animals; two control animals were implanted with cages containing collagen sponge without rhBMP-2. All animals receiving cages with rhBMP-2 showed solid fusion through the cages, whereas neither of the control animals fused (Fig. 5).

These data set the stage for a recently published pilot study of single-level anterior lumbar interbody fusions in humans that has shown definitive evidence of osteoinduction by rhBMP-2 in humans. Fourteen patients with single-level lumbar degenerative disc disease were prospectively randomized to receive tapered cylindrical threaded fusion cages filled with either rhBMP-2–soaked collagen sponges or autogenous iliac crest autograft. All 11 patients randomized to the rhBMP group were fused at 6 months postoperatively, whereas one of the three patients randomized to the control group receiving autograft in their cages was deemed a nonunion at 1 year. These studies have provided the data necessary to justify further human trials. Human trials investigating rhBMP in the human pos-

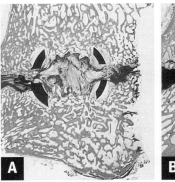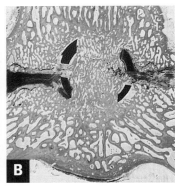

Figure 5 A, Coronal section of a rhesus monkey lumbosacral spine 24 weeks after interbody arthrodesis using hollow titanium threaded fusion cage (methylene blue/basic fuchsin, ×1). In this monkey, the cage was filled with collagen sponge carrier without any bone growth factor to serve as a control. The cage is filled with fibrous tissue rather than new bone. **B,** Coronal section of a rhesus monkey lumbosacral spine 24 weeks after interbody arthrodesis using hollow titanium threaded fusion cage (methylene blue/basic fuchsin, ×1). In this monkey, the cage was filled with collagen sponge carrier soaked with rhBMP-2 (1.5 mg/mL). The cage is filled with new bone that connects the two vertebral bodies through the opening in the upper and lower margin of the cage. *(Reproduced with permission from Boden SD, Martin GJ Jr, Horton WC, Truss TL, Sandhu HS: Laparoscopic anterior spinal arthrodesis with rhBMP-2 in a titanium interbody threaded cage. J Spinal Disord 1998;11:95-101.)*

terolateral intertransverse fusion environment are presently under way.

The administration of rhBMP-2 is being explored in an attempt to generate the optimum regimen to achieve fusion. It is evident that each fusion environment is unique as characterized by the species of animal, the location of the fusion within the animal, and the maturity of the animal. Much of this research centers on the dosing of growth factor for each situation. Dosing thresholds for osteoinduction have been shown to differ by several orders of magnitude between successful cell response in in vitro experiments and that necessary for in vivo bone induction. Evidence suggests that fusion in larger animals such as primates is more difficult to achieve than in the smaller animals used for many fusion models. This difficulty has been directly related to dosing.

Other avenues presently being explored involve the interaction of rhBMP-2 with its carrier. Collagen has proved to be a successful carrier. Binding of BMPs to collagen results in gradual-release kinetics for the growth factor. Some synthetic polymers also offer steady time release that gives a more desirable dosing profile, especially in animals that require longer times to fusion, such as primates. In fact, the excitement for polymers as a delivery substance is because of the ability to change release kinetics by altering the production procedure or component ratio of some polymers.

Under the paradigm of dosing through release kinetics, controlled release will be necessary for the longer time course of spinal fusion in humans. New approaches such as gene therapy for de novo production of growth factor at the fusion site are presently being explored in an attempt to provide growth factor within the fusion environment at the ideal concentration and with the right timing.

Recombinant Human Osteogenic Protein-1

Recombinant human osteogenic protein-1 (rhOP-1), also known as rhBMP-7 (Genetics Institute, Cambridge, MA), has been investigated in detail in long-bone defect and fracture models. In these environments, rhOP-1 has functioned to promote filling of bone defects and to speed healing. Results in spinal fusion have been reported for both an anterior thoracic interbody sheep model and a posterior dog model. In both anterior interbody and posterior spinal fusion models, rhOP-1 has been shown to act as a bone-graft substitute, achieving biomechanically stable fusions in much shorter times compared with autograft under similar conditions.

Human trials with mixed results have been reported from northern Europe. Successful long-bone healing has been reported for high tibial osteotomy fibular defects in comparing rhOP-1 delivered on collagen sponge with controls of collagen sponge alone. Reports of use in human spinal surgery have been disappointing. Injection of rhOP-1 into unstable single-level thoracolumbar fractures in five patients had disappointing results, with failure of posterior fixation before healing of fractures in all five patients. The use of rhOP-1 delivered on a collagen carrier for four attempted C1-2 fusions in rheumatoid patients resulted in three of four nonunions at 6 months. The use of rhOP-1 for controlled human trials in spinal fusion has not been reported.

Innovative Approaches to Bone Formation

As described earlier, the ideal bone generator for clinical use in spinal surgery will function to induce the migration of cells capable of becoming bone-forming cells and then activate the system of signals necessary to cause these cells to differentiate into osteoblasts. This bone generator also must supply the proper spatial environment for these bone-forming cells to function; this requires that neovascularization occur in proximity to surface areas that provide physiologically resorbable scaffolding to act as a template for the various cells involved in bony remodeling. In this manner, the grafted material can be replaced by functional bone that can be maintained physiologically during the patient's lifetime.

As the necessary ingredients for this ideal bone generator are better understood, it becomes clearer why no single substitute has been able to supplant autograft. It is also easier to explain why even autograft is not uniformly successful because at times it fails to provide a sufficient quantity of osteoinductive substances over an appropriate time course once it has been devitalized by the grafting process. Focus has now shifted to synthesis of a composite that maximizes the potential of each ingredient.

Growth factors and an adequate supply of progenitor cells are the key to osteoinductivity. As discussed earlier, the glycoprotein molecules of the BMP family are effective bone-generating growth factors. The challenge now lies in delivering a potent growth factor over the appropriate time course for each specific clinical need. The time course for many spinal fusion models appears to be several months, especially in larger animal models. The normal physiologic half-life of glycoprotein molecules in the cellular environment is measured in hours and days, not the weeks or months necessary for spinal fusion in primates.

In addition, it is necessary to find a "growth factor" that works early enough in the cascade of events leading to bone formation so that all of the conditions for bone formation will be in place at a clinical site with appropriate physiologic timing. The ideal factor will initiate bone formation by triggering the construction of the biochemical bone-forming environment, attracting and effecting differentiation of osteoprogenitor cells, and then potentiating the activity of those cells involved in physiologic bone formation and remodeling.

As more physiologic environments are characterized, the complexity of each has become increasingly evident. It is likely that bone generation requires a molecular milieu that is provided at specific phases of the wound-healing process. During each phase, a different milieu of permissive factors is available. These factors are substances such as transforming growth factor-beta, fibroblast growth factor, glucocorticoids, and vitamin D. It is important that these permissive and/or potentiating factors be present within the bone-forming environment at the appropriate concentrations for factors such as the BMPs to be maximally effective.

Delivery of Growth Factors

Current data on rhBMPs indicate that these substances can lead to bone formation within the spinal fusion environment. These growth factors must be delivered appropriately in both a spatial and temporal sense. As discussed earlier, strategies for accomplishing this have included the utilization of differing doses and/or carriers with different breakdown rates in the hope that some of the growth factor will be available at the appropriate times. Recent pilot studies have proved that it is possible for BMP to induce bone consistently in humans, but both Ne-Osteo bovine bone protein extract and rhBMP-2 require higher dosing and take longer for

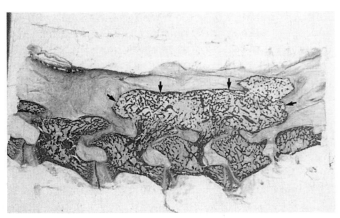

Figure 6 Low-power sagittal view (×1) photomicrograph through a rat lumbar spine that received devitalized bone matrix with bone marrow cells transfected with active LMP-1 cDNA. A continuous solid bridge of cancellous bone (*arrowheads*) attached to the sinuous processes and laminae was seen. (*Reproduced with permission from Boden SD, Titus L, Hair G, et al: Lumbar spine fusion by local gene therapy with a cDNA encoding a novel osteoinductive protein [LMP-1]. Spine 1998;23:2486-2492.*)

osteoinduction in primates than in smaller animals. These substances can be effective in primates, but the high doses necessary and the length of time to fusion demonstrate the need to refine these systems before they will be clinically practical.

One major strategy is to develop a better delivery system for growth factor. Multiple alternatives have been explored that use the various available osteoconductive substances soaked with growth factors. These synthetic bone-graft substitute materials integrated with rhBMP have been explored in several posterolateral canine fusion models in which rhBMP-2 in a biodegradable polymer was superior or equal to autogenous iliac crest bone graft for inducing transverse-process arthrodesis and strength of fusion mass.

Gene Therapy

Gene therapy is a more sophisticated delivery system for growth factors. Utilizing various molecular strategies, genes encoding for factors of the bone-formation cascade are inserted into the patient's own cells that exist at the site for fusion (in vivo) or that have been removed and will be reimplanted at the site of fusion (ex vivo). Once these cells are in place, they will produce a protein product from the transfected gene that leads to bone formation. In this manner, the half-life of the cell or the gene within the cell, not the actual glycoprotein, is the limiting temporal factor for the presence of a specific growth factor at the fusion site.

This strategy has been used in a rat posterolateral spine fusion model with excellent results. A novel protein was recently reported that appears to function very

early in the cascade of events leading to bone formation. The protein is an intracellular signaling protein, named LIM mineralization protein-1 (LMP-1). It was isolated by molecular techniques and its gene was identified. By the use of an ex vivo methodology, this gene was transfected into harvested bone marrow cells of rats and then reimplanted at sites for posterolateral spine fusion. Sites implanted with cells containing the LMP-1 gene fused solidly, whereas control sites implanted with control cells had no fusion (Fig. 6). This study validates the feasibility of local gene therapy to induce bone formation and spinal fusion in a mammal.

An in vivo strategy for gene therapy in a rodent model also has been reported. An adenovirus vector containing the growth factor rhBMP-9 was injected directly into the paraspinal musculature of rodents. These injections resulted in solid posterior arthrodesis at all experimental sites, thus demonstrating success in a rodent model with another strategy for gene therapy and a different growth factor.

Optimizing gene therapy introduces even more challenges to the search for an ideal bone generator. Vectors for the delivery of genes into cells, the types of cells transfected, and the control of gene expression are all areas to be explored. As knowledge of each growth factor and its mechanism of action is elucidated, the most potent factor can be identified and exploited. As knowledge of spinal fusion expands on a molecular level, the search for a complete bone-graft substitute will proceed in a more logical, systematic fashion and rely less on empirical trial and error.

Annotated Bibliography

Biology of Spine Fusion

Boden SD, Schimandle JH, Hutton WC, Chen MI: The use of an osteoinductive growth factor for lumbar spinal fusion: Part I. Biology of spinal fusion. *Spine* 1995;20: 2626-2632.

This investigation in a rabbit model characterizes the posterior intertransverse fusion environment using quantitative histology. Both geographic and temporal events of fusion are described. Three phases and a reproducible pattern of healing are identified.

Boden SD, Schimandle JH, Hutton WC: The use of an osteoinductive growth factor for lumbar spinal fusion: Part II. Study of dose, carrier, and species. *Spine* 1995;20: 2633-2644.

The threshold dose of bovine bone-derived osteoinductive protein extract (Ne-Osteo) necessary for fusion was found to be 8 to 10 times higher in monkeys versus rabbits. DBM, autograft carrier, and coral were found to be acceptable carriers for Ne-Osteo in these models.

Boden SD, Schimandle JH, Hutton WC: Lumbar inter-transverse-process spinal arthrodesis with use of a bovine bone-derived osteoinductive protein: A preliminary report. *J Bone Joint Surg Am* 1995;77:1404-1417.

Using a rabbit model for posterolateral intertransverse spinal fusion, bovine bone-derived osteoinductive protein extract (Ne-Osteo) delivered on DBM was compared with autograft. The Ne-Osteo–DBM combination had a higher fusion rate (100% versus 62%), and biomechanical testing revealed a stronger, stiffer fusion mass.

Morone MA, Boden SD, Hair G, et al: Gene expression during autograft lumbar spine fusion and the effect of bone morphogenetic protein 2. *Clin Orthop* 1998;351:252-265.

Messenger RNA expression within fusion masses of a rabbit posterolateral intertransverse fusion model revealed a reproducible geographic and temporal pattern of osteoblast-related gene expression. The pattern of expression for various BMPs was altered by the addition of exogenous rhBMP-2.

Demineralized Bone Matrix

Cook SD, Dalton JE, Prewett AB, Whitecloud TS III: In vivo evaluation of demineralized bone matrix as a bone graft substitute for posterior spinal fusion. *Spine* 1995;20:877-886.

In an adult dog posterior spine fusion model, allograft and autograft were compared with DBM and a DBM-autograft mix. DBM with or without allograft was inadequate for fusion.

Morone MA, Boden SD: Experimental posterolateral lumbar spinal fusion with a demineralized bone matrix gel. *Spine* 1998;23:159-167.

Grafton DBM functioned as a bone-graft extender, showing equal effectiveness with autograft in a 1:1 or 3:1 dosing ratio in a rabbit posterolateral intertransverse fusion model. However, it did not function as a graft enhancer because it did not increase the fusion rate above the usual 70%.

Bone Morphogenetic Protein-2

Boden SD, Martin GJ, Horton WC, Truss TL, Sandhu HS: Laparoscopic anterior spinal arthrodesis with rhBMP-2 in a titanium interbody threaded cage. *J Spinal Disord* 1998;11:95-101.

A titanium interbody fusion model was used to demonstrate the efficacy of rhBMP-2 as a bone graft substitute in nonhuman primates. Histologic and radiographic analysis demonstrated fusion in five adult rhesus monkeys implanted with rhBMP-2 while no fusion occurred in two control monkeys.

Boden SD, Zdeblick TA, Sandhu HS, Heim SE: The use of rhBMP-2 in interbody fusion cages: Definitive evidence of osteoinduction in humans. A preliminary report. *Spine* 2000;25:376-381.

This pilot human clinical trial demonstrated the successful use of rhBMP-2 in the lumbar interbody fusion environment. Five independent reviewers using CT and radiographs found that 11 of 11 patients treated with rhBMP-2 delivered on collagen sponge within a titanium cage fused.

Hecht BP, Fischgrund JS, Herkowitz HN, Penman L, Toth JM, Shirkhoda A: The use of recombinant human bone morphogenetic protein 2 (rhBMP-2) to promote spinal fusion in a nonhuman primate anterior interbody fusion model. *Spine* 1999;24:629-636.

A rhesus monkey model of L7-S1 anterior lumbar interbody fusions using freeze-dried cortical bone dowels filled with either rhBMP-2–soaked collagen sponges or autograft showed three of three fusions in the rhBMP-2 group versus one of three in the autograft group. In comparison, the sites treated with rhBMP-2 had earlier fusion and extensive remodeling of allograft bone dowels.

Osteogenic Protein (OP-1)

Cook SD, Dalton JE, Tan EH, Whitecloud TS III, Rueger DC: In vivo evaluation of recombinant human osteogenic protein (rhOP-1) implants as a bone graft substitute for spinal fusions. *Spine* 1994;19:1655-1663.

In a canine posterior spine fusion model, rhOP-1 (rhBMP-7) delivered on collagen demonstrated a 100% fusion rate over a significantly faster time course compared with allograft (6 to 12 weeks versus 26 weeks).

Cunningham BW, Kanayama M, Parker LM, et al: Osteogenic protein versus autologous interbody arthrodesis in the sheep thoracic spine: A comparative endoscopic study using the Bagby and Kuslich interbody fusion device. *Spine* 1999;24:509-518.

In a sheep thoracic interbody fusion model, rhOP-1 and autograft delivered in titanium cages were compared. rhOP-1 demonstrated equivalent efficacy to autograft in this environment for fusion rate and biomechanical and histologic testing of the fusion mass.

Geesink RG, Hoefnagels NH, Bulstra SK: Osteogenic activity of OP-1 bone morphogenetic protein (BMP-7) in a human fibular defect. *J Bone Joint Surg Br* 1999;81:710-718.

This prospective, randomized, double-blind human study demonstrated the osteogenic activity of rhOP-1 in a long-bone defect model. In high tibial osteotomy fibular defects, patients received either rhOP-1 in a collagen carrier or collagen carrier alone. New bone formation was seen in the rhOP-1 group only.

Gene Therapy

Boden SD, Titus L, Hair G, et al: Lumbar spine fusion by local gene therapy with a cDNA encoding a novel osteoinductive protein (LMP-1). *Spine* 1998;23: 2486-2492.

The gene of osteoinductive protein LMP-1 was used to transfect bone marrow cells from athymic rats in an ex vivo gene therapy model. Successful gene therapy was demonstrated as the cells were reimplanted and subsequently led to successful posterior spinal fusions.

Helm GA, Alden TD, Beres EJ, et al: Use of bone morphogenetic protein-9 gene therapy to induce spinal arthrodesis in the rodent. *J Neurosurg* 2000:92(suppl 2):191-196.

An in vivo gene therapy strategy was used to induce posterior spine fusion in a rodent model. An adenovirus vector containing rhBMP-9 was directly injected into the paraspinal musculature of rats. This resulted in robust bone formation and a 100% fusion rate.

Scaduto AA, Lieberman JR: Gene therapy for osteoinduction. *Orthop Clin North Am* 1999;30:625-633.

The authors present a basic description of the various molecular techniques and strategies of gene therapy presently being investigated.

Classic Bibliography

Albee FH: Transplantation of a portion of the tibia into the spine for Pott's disease: A preliminary report. *JAMA* 1911;57:885-886.

Chiroff RT, White EW, Weber KN, Roy DM: Tissue ingrowth of replamineform implants. *J Biomed Mater Res* 1975;9:29-45.

Dubuc FL, Urist MR: The accessibility of the bone induction principle in surface-decalcified bone implants. *Clin Orthop* 1967;55:217-223.

Hibbs RA: An operation for progressive spinal deformities: A preliminary report of three cases from the service of the Orthopaedic Hospital. *NY Med J* 1911;93: 1013-1016.

Peltier LF: The use of plaster of paris to fill large defects in bone: A preliminary report. *Am J Surg* 1959;97: 311-315.

Urist MR: Bone: Formation by autoinduction. *Science* 1965;150:893-899.

Wang EA, Rosen V, D'Alessandro JS, et al: Recombinant human bone morphogenetic protein induces bone formation. *Proc Natl Acad Sci USA* 1990;87:2220-2224.

Wozney JM: The bone morphogenetic protein family and osteogenesis. *Mol Reprod Dev* 1992;32:160-167.

Chapter 47

Minimally Invasive Spinal Surgery

Isador H. Lieberman, BSc, MD, FRCS

Introduction

Endoscopic surgery dates to 1853, when urologists used crude tubes with mirrored light sources to perform cystoscopies. In the early 1900s, thoracic and general surgeons performed thoracoscopies and laparoscopies in a similar fashion. These techniques were exclusively diagnostic and it was not until the 1970s and 1980s that gynecologists and general surgeons ushered in the therapeutic advances of endoscopic surgical techniques.

Orthopaedics has witnessed a revolution in endoscopic techniques with the advent and acceptance of knee arthroscopy. Takagi was the first to describe and Watanabe the first to advance diagnostic knee arthroscopy in 1939 and 1957, respectively. Casscells in 1971 and Jackson in 1972 are credited with promoting the Japanese methods in North America. Their efforts led to important therapeutic advances in knee, shoulder, wrist, elbow, and ankle arthroscopy. Today, in essentially every surgical specialty, the benefits of minimally invasive surgery are being realized. Spinal surgery is catching up with this revolution.

Endoscopy refers to the use of a scope and light source for visualization and magnification through small percutaneous portals. The term minimally invasive surgery has become synonymous with any surgical procedure that involves endoscopic access to a body cavity or joint. This terminology emphasizes the philosophy of targeting the pathology and applying the therapeutic intervention with little or no damage to surrounding nonpathologic tissues. The advantages of this philosophy have now been realized as less postoperative pain, thereby alleviating the physiologic concerns of healing associated with large incisions into the thoracic, peri-

toneal, or retroperitoneal cavities; improved visualization of the target tissues; improved cosmetic result because of smaller incisions; and reduced recovery time and hospital stay. Disadvantages include a steep learning curve, limitations in tactile feedback, two-dimensional video visualization that results in limited depth perception, the necessity for specialized instruments, and the ability to deal with certain complications. As the surgeon gains experience, however, these disadvantages become much less limiting.

In spinal surgery, the term minimally invasive has come to mean much more than the endoscopic techniques described above. Minimally invasive spinal therapy encompasses everything from traditional injection techniques (epidural injections, discography, facet and nerve root blocks) to percutaneous therapeutic modalities (intradiscal electrothermal therapy, vertebroplasty, kyphoplasty) to true endoscopic procedures (endoscopic discectomies, endoscopic lumbar fusions, endoscopic transthoracic procedures). A more formal definition of minimally invasive spinal therapy could become even more elusive as new advances in technology (image-guided surgery), in biology (bone substitutes and enhancers, nuclear regeneration), and in diagnostic techniques are developed and affect spinal treatment modalities. However, although a clear trend shows that technologic advances will improve what can be done surgically to the spine, a reciprocal trend shows that biologic advances will limit what has to be done to the spine.

Discectomies for Symptomatic Herniated Discs With Radiculopathy

The treatment of symptomatic lumbar disc herniations with radiculopathy has evolved from extensive open laminectomies to lesser laminotomies to percutaneous chemonucleolysis to percutaneous/arthroscopic mechanical central disc evacuations and then back to the cur-

The author or the departments with which he is affiliated have received something of value from a commercial or other party related directly or indirectly to the subject of this chapter.

rent gold standard, microdiscectomy. To date, not one of the newer techniques has been able to equal or improve on the excellent outcome of microdiscectomy. Microdiscectomy is in the purest sense a minimally invasive procedure because of the limited exposure, minimal (if any) bone resection, and minimal manipulation of the epidural contents. The newer techniques have promise but will play roles in future treatment protocols only when the technology improves to allow for outcomes better than current results.

Symptomatic thoracic disc herniations might be amenable to endoscopic transthoracic decompressions. The technical details are similar to those described below for endoscopic transthoracic releases and osteotomies for deformity. Only a few centers employ endoscopic techniques to decompress thoracic disc herniations, and only a few clinical reports have been published. The critical issue in this clinical scenario is patient selection. In practice, thoracic disc herniations with true radicular or myelopathic symptoms are rare. The more common scenario is diffuse midthoracic back pain, with imaging showing multiple degenerative segments with or without herniations. These patients typically are not ideal candidates for discectomy of any form, either open or endoscopic.

Minimally Invasive Lumbar Fusions

Exposure for spinal fusion has evolved in an attempt to minimize the soft-tissue surgical trauma. A number of percutaneous or minimally open posterior techniques have been reported but have not been readily accepted. These techniques involve a combination of posterolateral percutaneous endoscopic or arthroscopic disc evacuation and bone graft or cage application, followed by some form of percutaneous transpedicular fixation. All attempts undertaken so far with existing equipment have been cumbersome and technically challenging.

Anterior lumbar spine exposure also has evolved from the traditional open transperitoneal approach to open retroperitoneal to muscle-sparing retroperitoneal to endoscopic retroperitoneal to a laparoscopic transperitoneal approach. A variety of devices (threaded cylinders, disc spacers, allograft rings) has been used to stabilize the disc space and restore it to its native height and to facilitate fusion. Compared with the formal open techniques, the minimally invasive techniques have shown advantages in pain relief, recovery time, and cosmetic appearance of the scars without a significant sacrifice in access or a significant increase in complications. In keeping with a minimally invasive philosophy, some cases (depending on the implant) might be done as a standalone anterior procedure, avoiding the necessity of a combined anterior-posterior exposure. Currently the

most utilized is either a "miniopen" retroperitoneal-transperitoneal approach or a transperitoneal laparoscopic approach.

The miniopen retroperitoneal-transperitoneal approach recently has been repopularized with the advent of corridor-type retractor frames and the widespread use of magnification and illumination. To access the L2 to L5 levels, a retroperitoneal approach seems most convenient. To access the L5-S1 level, a transperitoneal approach technically is easier. For two-level cases, depending on the patient's body habitus and the way the patient is positioned at the time of surgery, the surgeon can choose either retroperitoneal or transperitoneal lumbar spine exposure. The retroperitoneal approach to L5-S1, with the patient in the lateral position, is technically a little more demanding, yet it is preferred for the L4-5 level. The transperitoneal approach to L4-5, with the patient in the supine position, is likewise technically more demanding, requiring mobilization of the great vessels and more manipulation of the abdominal contents; yet it is the preferred approach to L5-S1. The blood loss for either approach is minimal and the surgical time, acceptable. Hospital length of stay does not seem to depend on approach.

The laparoscopic lumbar spine exposure also has recently gained popularity because of the growing use of threaded cylindrical cages and the adoption of laparoscopic techniques in general surgery. This exposure is accomplished through the standard five-portal laparoscopic approach to the abdominal cavity. In a recently published series, no significant complications and only one conversion to open surgery occurred. The blood loss, surgical time, hospital stay, and complications were comparable with those of any published series of open exposures.

Each of these exposure techniques has its own advantages and disadvantages. The laparoscopic approach requires an experienced laparoscopic surgeon and is equipment dependent. It is advantageous in select patients with intact posterior elements when threaded cylindrical cages are used because the procedure can be done as a stand-alone anterior procedure. It is particularly suitable for the isolated L5-S1 fusion. The disadvantage of the laparoscopic approach is the difficulty in mobilizing the vessels over the L4-5 level. The miniopen retroperitoneal technique is more familiar to most spinal surgeons and is more versatile for gaining exposure from the L2 to L4 levels. On the other hand, exposing the lumbosacral junction through this approach can be problematic in certain patients, especially the obese and men with a low-lying L5-S1 segment and a narrow pelvis. The most difficult scenario typically encountered is the two-level L4-5 and L5-S1 case. The exposure decision must be based on the patient's morphology, the condition of the posterior elements, the implants to be used, and the surgeon's familiarity with the exposure.

Transthoracic Releases and Osteotomies for Deformity

During traditional thoracotomy or thoracophrenicolumbotomy, the chest and/or retroperitoneal structures are exposed and manipulated and can become desiccated. As a consequence of these exposures, patients develop a measurable reduction in pulmonary and shoulder girdle function. In considering these exposures, distinct issues related to pain, cosmesis, and morbidity should be weighed. Endoscopic transthoracic exposures might minimize or eliminate these issues because of improved visualization (illumination and magnification of the surgical site by the video system), less postoperative incisional pain (less muscle dissection and no rib spreading), and more cosmetically acceptable scars. Other potential advantages include the opportunities to perform simultaneous procedures, reduce blood loss, reduce the risk of infection, eliminate compromise of respiratory and shoulder mechanics, and reduce the length of intensive care stays and hospitalization. The disadvantages include a steep learning curve (because of the loss of depth perception associated with the change from binocular vision to monocular, video-assisted vision and the loss of tactile feedback associated with long-handled instruments) and the theoretic technical limitations in treating intraoperative complications. Other potential disadvantages include the anesthetic demands of double-lumen intubation and single-lung ventilation and the currently limited ability to place structural bone graft or bone substitutes or to apply implants to the spine.

Endoscopic surgery can directly or indirectly address the goals of deformity surgery: arresting progression, achieving and maintaining correction, achieving a solid fusion, and decompressing and protecting the neural elements. The indications for endoscopic techniques are the same as those for thoracotomy: release of a rigid curve to rebalance the sagittal and coronal contours and to minimize the risk of pseudarthrosis by bone grafting to achieve an interbody fusion. In the patient with preexisting compromised pulmonary mechanics caused by the spinal deformity or associated neurologic syndromes (eg, polio), endoscopic techniques might be indicated to minimize any thoracotomy-related pulmonary compromise.

Before undertaking an endoscopic exposure, the surgeon must be familiar with open anterior spinal anatomy and surgical techniques. The surgical procedures are the same but the methods are different enough to challenge even experienced spinal surgeons. Although the loss of depth perception and the necessity

for triangulation might be familiar to a small-joint arthroscopist, the change in working distance and instrument excursion from 4 to 30 cm demands its own learning curve.

Absolute patient contraindications to an endoscopic transthoracic approach include previous open thoracotomy, empyema, pleurodesis, bullous lung pathology, and inability to tolerate single-lung ventilation. A further relative contraindication is a narrow anterior-posterior chest diameter and/or significant vertebral rotation at the apex. These anatomic variants limit the working space in the chest cavity; the rotation in particular might cause the mediastinal organs to obstruct exposure. These variables can be overcome by adding more working portals, but under such circumstances, a formal open thoracotomy might be prudent.

In preparation for the procedure, patients undergo selective double-lumen endotracheal intubation, depending on which chest cavity is to be exposed. Patients are usually positioned in a lateral decubitus position with the appropriate chest up. Patients also might be positioned prone if the simultaneous approach is to be used. The lateral position affords the surgeon a more familiar anatomic alignment and approach. The prone position allows the mediastinal organs to fall away from the spine, obviating the need for retraction.

After positioning, the appropriate lung is deflated by clamping the lumen of the double-lumen tube. With the lateral position, the skin over the chest, back, and iliac crest is prepared and draped widely, as for a thoracotomy. With the prone position, the chest and back are prepared and draped to the anterior axillary lines bilaterally. The function of the double-lumen tube must be monitored continuously throughout the case.

For kyphosis correction, the spine can be approached from either chest at the surgeon's discretion. A theoretical risk exists, depending on which approach is selected. The aorta is a thick, resilient structure, less prone to injury. On the other hand, in the right chest, the azygous system with large, friable, tortuous veins might prove to be more problematic.

For scoliosis correction, the spine can be exposed on the convexity or the concavity, depending on the clinical circumstances and surgeon's preference. Release on the convexity might require more portals so as to gain parallel access to each disc space; to release the structural tether in some curves, gaining access to the posterolateral corner on the concavity at the proximal and distal levels might be difficult. However, if thoracoplasty is indicated, then only the convex approach is applicable. On the other hand, working on the concavity allows for fewer portals and provides direct access to the structural tether (posterolateral corner and costotransverse ligaments) over the entire curve. This concave approach, however, does require more meticulous dissection of the aorta, which unfolds into the concavity of the curve.

The first portal is inserted into the chest through a skin incision opposite the apex of the deformity in the anterior axillary line. This becomes the main working portal and is the only portal inserted blindly. It should be inserted after blunt dissection with a Kelly forceps just over the top of the rib to avoid damage to the neurovascular bundle or deep structures. The endoscope is then inserted into the chest, and the chest cavity is inspected. Any minor lung adhesions are released and the spinal levels are identified. The remaining portals are inserted under direct view with the lung protected. The pattern of portal placement can be either an L or V shape, depending on the chest wall morphology and the level of the spine to be approached.

With the patient in the lateral position, the lung might require retraction with an endoscopic fan retractor or strategically placed sponges. The levels of interest are identified by counting ribs and then are verified with a radiograph. Once identified, the pleura can be incised with cautery over the appropriate levels either longitudinally, parallel to the spine, or transversely, parallel to each disc space. If the segmental vessels are to be preserved, smaller pleural incisions are created parallel to the disc space. The parietal pleura is then bluntly dissected proximally, distally, and anteriorly to expose as much of the vertebral margins as is necessary. The anulus is then incised with cautery over a 1- to 2-cm segment, and the nucleus and cartilage end plates are evacuated to subchondral bleeding bone with pituitary rongeurs, Cobb elevators, and curettes. The evacuation is completed to the posterior longitudinal ligament. Once completed, the remaining anulus is then incised. For kyphosis correction, the anterior longitudinal ligament and the anulus on the opposite side must be incised. For scoliosis, if working on the convexity, the concave posterolateral corner must be released to achieve a complete release. If working on the concavity, the posterolateral corner and costotransverse junction are released under direct view, and the convex lateral anulus is left intact to act as a tether to prevent overdistraction and as a pivot point during the posterior correction.

Once all levels are released, the disc spaces are bone-grafted with either morcellized cancellous iliac crest graft delivered by a funnel or, especially in kyphosis, a structural tricortical crest graft or femoral allograft ring. The chest cavity is then irrigated to remove any disc debris, a chest tube is inserted through one portal, and the remaining portals are closed.

Internal thoracoplasty also might be performed endoscopically, either at the same time as the release or as an independent procedure. The patient is positioned in the lateral decubitus position with the convexity up. The operating room table is tilted 15° to 20° toward the prone to help with lung retraction. The rib resections are planned as an ellipse to ensure that the chest contours are smooth. The ribs are resected using a combination of periosteal stripping and high-speed burrs to create the osteotomies. It is advisable to drape the arm free to allow intraoperative scapula mobilization to ensure the expected clinical and functional results. The bone from the rib resections can be used for the interbody or posterior grafting, as necessary.

Vertebral corpectomies or osteotomies also can be completed using similar endoscopic techniques. The patients are positioned either laterally or prone, depending on the necessity for subsequent procedures. The spine is exposed by bluntly dissecting the pleura and ligating only those segmental vessels in the surgical field. Combinations of pituitary rongeurs, curettes, Cobb elevators, and high-speed burrs are used in the same fashion as would be done with the chest open. The corpectomy reconstruction can be completed by negotiating allograft struts, or mesh cages, into the defect after inserting them into the chest through one of the portals.

During endoscopic surgery, the camera assistant must maintain the camera orientation, keep the surgical field centered in view, and have a steady hand. It is vital to keep the camera and instruments in the same 180° arc to avoid the difficulties associated with working in a mirror image. The camera assistant and the operating surgeon must work in unison with small serial movements always under direct view. In the many recently published reports of transthoracic endoscopic techniques, results overall have been predictable and satisfying for both the surgeons and patients. The reported complication rate seems to be equivalent to that of similar traditional open procedures. The advantages of the endoscopic techniques in postoperative pain relief and preservation of pulmonary function have been realized. The surgical time associated with the endoscopic procedure, initially reported as lengthy, has improved considerably as surgeons have gained experience. It now takes experienced endoscopic spinal surgeons approximately 20 min to place portals and expose the spine, and 10 to 15 min to release and bone graft each disc space. Comparisons with the extent of spinal correction in adult deformity to historical cohorts match or exceed the published curve corrections, and two recently published animal studies conclude that the extent of discectomy and quality of release is comparable to open techniques.

The next major step in endoscopic transthoracic spinal surgery is the development and application of spinal implants capable of stabilization and correction. The use of threaded cylindrical interbody fusion cages has become widespread in the lumbar spine, and this experience has been extended to the thoracic spine. The cages are being applied in the coronal or oblique plane. Their application in the thoracic spine might be technically less demanding, but the risks of malposition are clearly more significant. The fusion rates of single cages in the thoracic spine still must be evaluated.

A number of centers are now using existing posterior or anterior rod-and-screw implant systems in an endoscopic fashion. Recently published animal studies reveal that the spine can be instrumented and deformed or straightened using an endoscopic percutaneous technique. From a clinical standpoint, there are major concerns with the existing systems. The scoliotic spine is a three-dimensional deformity, and these implants and application techniques assume a two-dimensional correction. The thoracic cage limits access to the implants, thus requiring extensions beyond the chest wall to manipulate the implants. These extensions will be limited in their excursion and correction ability by the chest wall. Also, by using these extensions, an exaggerated lever arm will be applied to the implant-bone interface and might jeopardize screw purchase and cause premature implant loosening, resulting in pseudarthrosis or loss of correction. Under select circumstances, these approaches to endoscopic instrumentation might be worthwhile, but this area deserves further biomechanical and clinical scrutiny.

Vertebral Body Augmentation for Osteoporotic or Lytic Compression Fractures

An estimated 700,000 pathologic vertebral body compression fractures occur in the United States each year, of which more than one third become chronically painful. The majority of these fractures (about 85%) are the result of primary osteoporosis; the remainder are caused by secondary osteoporosis or lytic spinal metastases. These compression fractures lead to progressive deformity and changes in spinal biomechanics and are believed to contribute to increased risk of further fracture. Whether the fracture is painful or not, the spinal deformity caused by two or more fractures dramatically affects health, activities of daily living, and medical costs through loss of lung capacity, reduced mobility, chronic pain, loss of appetite, and/or clinical depression. With each osteoporotic vertebral compression fracture, a 15% age-adjusted increase in mortality and a 9% loss in predicted forced vital capacity have been shown to occur.

Traditionally, vertebral body compression fractures were treated with medical and rarely with surgical modalities. Unfortunately, the medical management of painful fractures (bed rest, hospitalization, narcotic analgesics, and bracing) does nothing to restore spinal alignment and might compound the problem. Because

of its inherent risks and invasive nature and the poor quality of osteoporotic bone, surgical treatment of vertebral body compression fractures has been limited to patients with concurrent spinal instability or neurologic deficit.

In response to the limited results of medical and surgical modalities, to stabilize and strengthen the collapsed vertebral bodies, interventional neuroradiologists, first in France and now in the United States, have begun bilateral transpedicular percutaneous bone cement injections. Direct cement injection, or vertebroplasty, has been shown to reduce or eliminate fracture pain and prevent further collapse. This is of significant benefit because it allows a rapid return to mobility, preventing the known bone loss caused by bed rest. In addition, no cement failures have been reported, and only two cases of fracture progression in the treated vertebral bodies (caused by inadequate cement fill) have been reported. The longest reported follow-up is 3 years, although the first article on vertebroplasty was published in 1986. The most recent report in the United States involves 47 patients with an average follow-up of 18 months. Marked to complete pain relief was reported in 63% of patients with osteoporosis vertebral compression fractures. Results of vertebroplasty in osteolytic metastatic vertebral collapse in eight patients revealed that only four patients experienced any pain relief. In this group of patients, there was a 6% complication rate, which in 4% of patients was unrelated to the vertebroplasty.

Although vertebroplasty can reduce or eliminate fracture pain, it does not address the spinal deformity. Also, this technique requires a high-pressure cement injection using low-viscosity cement, thus increasing the risk of cement leaks. In four recent studies, cement leaks were observed in 30% to 80% of procedures. Most of these leaks had no clinical consequences; however, there have been a number of significant complications.

Kyphoplasty is a technique with a number of potential advantages. Kyphoplasty involves the extrapedicular or transpedicular cannulation of the vertebral body, under fluoroscopic guidance, followed by insertion of an inflatable bone tamp. Once inflated, the tamp restores the vertebral body back toward its original height while creating a cavity to be filled with bone cement. The cement injection is done under relatively low pressure in an attempt to reduce the risk of extravasation.

In a phase 1 institutional review board-approved study just recently completed, 59 consecutive kyphoplasty procedures were performed in 25 patients during 31 sessions. The mean age was 68.6 years (range, 48 to 86 years). The indications included 17 painful primary or 3 secondary osteoporotic vertebral compression fractures in 20 patients unresponsive to nonsurgical modalities. Another five patients presented with painful compression fractures resulting from multiple myeloma. The mean duration of symptoms was 3.5 months (range, 0.5 to 12 months). Symptomatic levels were identified by correlating the clinical data with MRI findings of marrow signal changes consistent with compression fractures. Outcome data were obtained by comparing patient preoperative and latest postoperative data using the Medical Outcomes Study 36-Item Short Form Health Survey (SF-36).

In this study, all 25 patients tolerated the procedure well, and improvement in pain and mobility was seen early. Virtually all patients subjectively reported immediate relief of their typical fracture pain, and no patient complained of worse pain at the treated levels. The levels treated ranged from T6 to L5, with the majority at the thoracolumbar junction (T11 = 7, T12 = 14, L1 = 9). Radiologic height measurement of all 59 levels treated (regardless of fracture age) demonstrated that the mean percentage of height lost that was restored by the procedure was 38% (range, 0 to 100%). SF-36 scores for bodily pain, physical function, and role physical subscales all showed statistically significant improvement. At final follow-up, no major complications related directly to the use of this technique or the inflatable bone tamp were reported. The results of this initial series show that kyphoplasty is a well-tolerated procedure indicated for the treatment of painful osteoporotic or osteolytic vertebral compression fractures. Kyphoplasty is associated with early clinical improvement of pain and function as well as with restoration of vertebral body height. The long-term benefits of kyphoplasty are currently being studied in a multicenter phase 2 randomized controlled trial.

Intradiscal Modalities for Symptomatic Degenerative Disease

Discogenic low back pain is difficult to diagnose and treat. Traditional treatment involves nonsurgical modalities such as anti-inflammatory medications, epidural steroid injections, spinal manipulation, and back-specific exercise rehabilitation. In patients unresponsive to the nonsurgical modalities, surgical intervention in the form of a lumbar fusion is typically recommended. The outcome of lumbar fusion in this group of patients is unpredictable, with fusion rates varying depending on the technique. Because of this, a more predictable and less invasive method to treat discogenic low-back pain would be desirable.

Targeted thermal energy is currently being used in select applications (joint instability, capsular shrinking,

ligament shortening) to shrink collagen fibrils. Basic science studies verify that the thermal energy does in fact reorganize the collagen structure; however, other studies have demonstrated that the structural strength of these treated tissues is compromised. In the lumbar spine, this technology is being applied to the disc/anulus complex as a potential tool to shrink disrupted annular fibers, to cauterize inflammatory granulation tissue, and to ablate nociceptive nerve endings. Intradiscal electrothermal anuloplasty is performed through a percutaneous fluoroscopic-assisted approach with a navigable catheter and thermal probe. The catheter probe complex is steered to the length of the posterior annular wall, where the tissues are heated to 65°C for a 17-min period. The reported advantage of this probe over radiofrequency or laser modalities is a more controlled, broader application of thermal energy to the posterior anulus.

In a recently published preliminary report of 25 consecutive patients with an average follow-up of 7 months, the authors reported that 80% of the patients realized a two-point difference in pain reduction as measured with a visual analog pain scale. The authors also noted a statistically significant improvement in the SF-36 physical function and bodily pain subscales in 72% of patients. The authors did not detect any deterioration in these results over the short term follow-up and reported that no patients experienced any neurologic or catheter-related complications. The short-term results in this group of patients with chronic discogenic back pain symptoms is promising. The long-term consequences of intradiscal thermal treatment are not yet defined. This modality deserves further clinical study.

Conclusion

Minimally invasive spinal surgery is an important tool in the spine surgeon's armamentarium to gain access to and/or expose the spine, with little or no damage to the surrounding nonpathologic tissues. As technologic and biologic advances develop, the combination of minimally invasive techniques will become more refined and specific to the treatment of various spinal pathologies. Spinal surgeons, however, must be vigilant in not converting excellent, open, traditional surgical techniques to mediocre minimally invasive or minimally beneficial techniques. Although the indications for any surgical intervention remain unchanged, with the anticipated advances in technology, robotics, biology, and physiology, the indications could be refined to address specific pathologic spinal entities.

Annotated Bibliography

Discectomies for Symptomatic Herniated Discs With Radiculopathy

Ditsworth DA: Endoscopic transforaminal lumbar diskectomy and reconfiguration: A postero-lateral approach into the spinal canal. *Surg Neurol* 1998;49:588-597.

The author presents his initial experience in 110 patients, evaluated independently, at a minimum of 2 years after a transforaminal endoscopic discectomy. He concludes that the endoscopic transforaminal approach can be safe and effective and has a 91% success rate.

Hermantin FU, Peters T, Quartararo L, Kambin P: A prospective, randomized study comparing the results of open discectomy, with those of video-assisted arthroscopic microdiscectomy. *J Bone Joint Surg Am* 1999;81:958-965.

The authors report a randomized trial of 60 patients with lumbar radiculopathy treated by either open discectomy or video-assisted arthroscopic discectomy. Their findings suggest that arthroscopic microdiscectomy might be useful for the treatment of specific symptoms in properly selected patients.

Rosenthal D, Dickman CA: Thoracoscopic microsurgical excision of herniated thoracic discs. *J Neurosurg* 1998;89:224-235.

The authors describe their experience, using endoscopic modalities, in their first 55 patients with thoracic disc herniations who presented with myelopathy or radiculopathy. They report shorter surgical times, less blood loss, and shorter hospitalizations compared with a similar patient group that underwent costotransversectomy. They report excellent clinical and neurologic results and conclude that endoscopic techniques are safe and reliable.

Minimally Invasive Lumbar Fusions

Lieberman IH, Willsher PC, Litwin DE, Salo PT, Kraetschmer BG: Transperitoneal laparoscopic exposure for lumbar interbody fusion. *Spine* 2000;25:509-515.

In a prospective clinical trial to determine the safety and effectiveness of a transperitoneal laparoscopic exposure for lumbar interbody fusion, the authors concluded that laparoscopic exposure for single- or multiple-level anterior lumbar interbody fusion can be performed with acceptable perioperative risk.

Mayer HM: A new microsurgical technique for minimally invasive anterior lumbar interbody fusion. *Spine* 1997;22:691-700.

The author presents his series of 25 patients who underwent anterior lumbar interbody fusion with a microsurgical modification to the standard open retroperitoneal approach to L2-4 and transperitoneal approach to L5-S1. All patients also underwent posterior stabilization. The author encountered no significant complications with the miniopen anterior exposure.

Transthoracic Releases and Osteotomies for Deformity

Ebara S, Kamimura M, Itoh H, et al: A new system for the anterior restoration and fixation of thoracic spinal deformities using an endoscopic approach. *Spine* 2000;25:876-883.

This article reports the results of animal experiments in which a new endoscopic spinal fixation system allows for correction and stabilization of the scoliotic spine. In the animal, the authors were able to alter the Cobb angle using an outrigger system extending beyond the chest wall.

Lieberman IH, Salo PT, Orr RD, Kraetschmer B: Prone position endoscopic transthoracic release with simultaneous posterior instrumentation for spinal deformity: A description of the technique. *Spine* 2000;25:2251-2257.

The authors describe the technique and clinical results of endoscopic transthoracic anterior release performed for the correction of adult spinal deformity with the patient prone, on the concave side for scoliosis or on either side for kyphosis, with simultaneous posterior instrumentation and correction. They claim this technique offers a minimally invasive method of accessing the anterior spinal column, with the benefits of excellent visualization, minimal soft-tissue disruption, and an improved cosmetic result. This simultaneous technique obviates the need for staged or subsequent procedures.

McAfee PC, Regan JR, Zdeblick T, et al: The incidence of complications in endoscopic anterior thoracolumbar spinal reconstructive surgery: A prospective multicenter study comprising the first 100 consecutive cases. *Spine* 1995;20:1624-1632.

This is a report on a prospective multicenter study of 100 consecutive endoscopic spinal procedures. The series included both thoracoscopic and laparoscopic procedures. In this series, no permanent iatrogenic neurologic injuries occurred. The authors concluded that the endoscopic techniques were safe.

Mehlman CT, Crawford AH, Wolf RK: Video-assisted thoracoscopic surgery (VATS): Endoscopic thoracoplasty technique. *Spine* 1997;22:2178-2182.

The authors describe their initial experience and the technique of endoscopic rib resection for cosmetic correction of the scoliotic rib hump.

Newton PO, Cardelia JM, Farnsworth CL, Baker KJ, Bronson DG: A biomechanical comparison of open and thoracoscopic anterior spinal release in a goat model. Spine 1998;23:530-536.

This article compares the relative efficacy of anterior release in achieving spinal mobility for deformity correction through either an endoscopic or open approach. No detectable difference between the two techniques was noted.

Newton PO, Wenger DR, Mubarak SJ, Meyer RS: Anterior release and fusion in pediatric spinal deformity: A comparison of early outcome and cost of thoracoscopic and open thoracotomy approaches. *Spine* 1997;22:1398-1406.

The authors report on the outcome and economics of thoracoscopic versus conventional thoracotomy in the treatment of pediatric spinal deformity. They concluded that the open technique was 29% less expensive, although they implied that the thoracoscopic technique was better for the patients.

Wall EJ, Bylski-Austrow DI, Shelton FS, Crawford AH, Kolata RJ, Baum DS: Endoscopic discectomy increases thoracic spine flexibility as effectively as open discectomy: A mechanical study in a porcine model. *Spine* 1998;23:9-16.

The authors set out to biomechanically compare two surgical techniques for anterior discectomy in a porcine model. They concluded that the open and endoscopic techniques were equally effective in increasing spine flexibility.

Vertebral Body Augmentation for Osteoporotic or Lytic Compression Fractures

Barr JD, Barr MS, Lemley TJ, McCann RM: Percutaneous vertebroplasty for pain relief and spinal stabilization. *Spine* 2000;25;923-928.

This is a retrospective review of the authors' initial experience with vertebral body cement augmentation in 47 patients with osteoporotic compression fractures and metastatic dis-

ease. Ninety-five percent of their patients at average follow-up of 18 months reported pain relief. The authors report a 6% rate of minor complications.

Lieberman IH, Dudney MS, Reinhardt MK, Bell G: Initial outcome & efficacy of kyphoplasty in the treatment of painful osteoporotic vertebral compression fractures. *Spine*, in press.

The authors report their phase 1 efficacy study of inflatable bone tamp usage in the treatment of symptomatic osteoporotic compression fractures in 30 consecutive patients. Kyphoplasty was associated with early statistically significant clinical improvement in pain and function as well as restoration of vertebral body height and low risk of cement extravasation.

Intradiscal Modalities for Symptomatic Degenerative Disease

Saal JS, Saal JA: Management of chronic discogenic low back pain with a thermal intradiscal catheter: A preliminary report. *Spine* 2000;25:382-388.

This article presents the preliminary results of managing back pain using a thermal intradiscal catheter. At mean follow-up of 7 months, the authors noted that 20 of 25 patients reported at least a 2-point improvement on the visual analog pain scale.

Classic Bibliography

Casscells SW: Arthroscopy of the knee joint: A review of 150 cases. *J Bone Joint Surg Am* 1971;53:287-298.

Jackson RW, Abe I: The role of arthroscopy in the management of disorders of the knee: An analysis of 200 consecutive examinations. *J Bone Joint Surg Br* 1972;54:310-322.

Takagi K: The classic: Arthroscope. *J Jpn Orthop Assoc* 1939. *Clin Orthop* 1982;167:6-8.

Watanabe M, Takeda S: The number 21 arthroscope. *J Jpn Orthop Assoc* 1960;34:1041.

Chapter 48

Disc Replacement Prosthetics

Qi-Bin Bao, PhD

Hansen A. Yuan, MD

Introduction

Among the many evolutions of spine surgery, the development of a prosthetic disc or nucleus has accelerated in the last decade. In 1989, the First International Symposium on The Artificial Disc was held in Berlin. Since then, the artificial disc has been a topic of interest at many spinal meetings, symposia, and summits, and it has been the subject of several books, book chapters, and review articles.

Theoretically, the ultimate treatment for symptomatic disc degeneration should be disc arthroplasty instead of arthrodesis. Such a step is similar to what has transpired for the treatment of hip and knee joint disease, although a patient's function is not as greatly impaired by a single-level disc fusion as by fusion of the hip or knee. Currently, however, spinal surgeries alter the normal disc structure and function and too often result in complications associated with these changes. The primary goal of disc arthroplasty, therefore, is to maintain or restore the disc's normal anatomy and functions while successfully treating the patient's pain.

Because of the multicomponent structure of a disc, attempts to achieve the goals of disc arthroplasty have involved either replacement of the entire disc or replacement of that part of the disc most directly related to the pathology.

Total Disc Replacement

An artificial total disc is designed to replace the entire disc. Because the entire original disc is removed, the condition of specific components causing the symptoms is less significant. Therefore, the procedure can be used for patients at any stage of disc degeneration as long as the integrity of the adjacent tissues is maintained. Although the stiffness and strength of discs in compression, flexion, extension, and torsion have been fairly well documented, it has not been possible thus far to design an artificial disc that mimics all the mechanical properties of a natural disc and has the necessary endurance. For such a disc, a multicomponent design made of several materials of very different mechanical properties would be required, and researchers would have to consider issues such as interfacial bonding and wear.

Artificial discs often are designed to have a size close to the cross-sectional area of the vertebrae so that the load can spread over a large surface area, thereby minimizing contact stress. Although this design makes perfect mechanical sense, it makes surgical insertion more difficult, usually requiring an open anterior approach and lengthy surgery. Hard or rigid materials for superior and inferior surfaces further increase the bulkiness of the implant. To prevent migration, the implant must be fixed firmly to the vertebrae. Fixation failure of a bulky implant with hard and rigid surfaces could result in catastrophic complications.

For any new technology, acceptance depends on the benefit-to-cost and benefit-to-risk ratios. Although artificial discs promise some benefits over discectomy and fusion, risks and costs should be comparable to those of current surgical treatment, especially in the beginning, before the clinical benefits have been demonstrated.

In 1990, four prosthetic disc concepts, three total disc prostheses and one nucleus prosthesis, were presented at the fifth annual meeting of the North American Spine Society (NASS). The three disc prostheses—the all-metal design of Kostuik, the all elastomer design of Lee, and the metal-elastomer-metal sandwich of Steffee— had undergone significant preclinical testing of their function, fatigue, and wear properties. From October 1988 to October 1989, Steffee even had the opportunity to implant disc prostheses in six of his patients with approval from the hospital Institutional Review Board. Estimating the time line for clinical studies and approval process required by the US Food and Drug Administration (FDA), it was believed at that time that some artificial disc prostheses should be commercially available by the year 2000.

Now, over a decade later, no disc prosthesis is commercially available in the United States. For several reasons, we believe it will take at least another 4 to 5 years for any disc prostheses to be commercially available. First, there is considerable challenge involved in designing a prosthesis that mimics disc structure and function without being too complicated to manufacture and too bulky to implant. Second, the potential risk of surgery and implant dislodgement for any of the current artificial disc designs is perceived to be high, and because the prosthetic disc is not a life-saving device, its risk must be low relative to clinical benefits. Third, the tight regulatory and litigious environments in the United State significantly affect clinical testing of artificial discs.

Medical device regulations exist to protect the safety of patients. While adequate preclinical testing is required to demonstrate the safety and efficacy of a medical device, it is not sufficient in itself. The ultimate efficacy of the device and its ultimate safety can be determined only in clinical studies. Often, clinical studies allow researchers to identify and correct occult problems that are difficult to find in the laboratory.

The tight regulations and litigious environment of the United States make clinical studies more costly and more difficult to fund. Thus, regulations designed to protect patients from harm sometimes retard the development of technology that could relieve the suffering of many. This problem is particularly apparent in the case of disc replacement.

For those who have gained Investigational Device Exemption (IDE) approval for a pilot study, delays occur in expanding the trials. Such delays have been larger in the United States than in Europe. The SB Charite disc prosthesis of Buttner-Janz and Schellnack in Germany and the Steffee disc prosthesis in the United States both were developed in the mid 1980s and began pilot clinical studies in the late 1980s. Both prostheses were found to contain some design defects in the early clinical series. Although the SB Charite disc was modified quickly from generation I to generation III with continued clinical use in Europe, it took almost 5 years to gain IDE approval to start a pilot study in 1993 for a second-generation Steffee disc, and further modifications are currently awaiting FDA approval for clinical trial. At this writing, over 2,000 SB Charite devices of all three generations have been implanted in Europe; this far exceeds the American experience.

Many questions related to indications for and justifi-cations of using a disc prosthesis are yet to be answered. The lack of thorough understanding of pain mechanisms and precise methods of diagnosing pain generators cloud these issues. In general, the indications and contraindications for use of an artificial disc should be the same as those for use of an interbody fusion device. If a disc prosthesis can be shown to produce the same clinical outcome as an interbody fusion device without significantly increasing the complication rate and risk, it should be easy to justify the use of the disc prosthesis. If clear benefits and acceptable risks are proven for such patients, it would be possible to consider use of a disc prosthesis for patients with moderate disc degeneration or disc herniation who would otherwise be treated by discectomy, but with some concern of instability. Conceptually, a disc prosthesis could be an ideal adjunctive device next to a fusion for patients with multiple disc degeneration; however, the device must pass more vigorous testing for shear fatigue strength because of the added shear stress at the junctional disc.

Nucleus Replacement

Replacement of part of a disc could be achieved by replacing either the nucleus or the anulus. Surgical treatment of disc herniation has been focused on removing part or all of the nucleus material. Likewise, when considering disc arthroplasty by partial disc replacement, almost all attention has been focused on replacing the nucleus with a nucleus prosthesis.

There are several obvious advantages of a nucleus prosthesis as opposed to total disc replacement. Replacing only the nucleus preserves the anulus and end plates and their functions. Because the nucleus has much simpler structure and function than the anulus and end plate, design of a nucleus prosthesis is less demanding. A nucleus prosthesis could potentially be implanted by minimally invasive surgery; possibly, an arthroscopic technique could be used with only a small incision in the anulus and a surgery time comparable to that of discectomy.

The risk associated with a nucleus prosthesis should be lower than that associated with a total disc prosthesis. Although implant extrusion is a significant concern with a nucleus implant, there is less risk of permanent injury to neural structures because of its relatively smaller size and soft nature. In case of failure, a nucleus prosthesis can be converted to a primary fusion or a total disc replacement.

The primary objectives of a nucleus prosthesis are to reinflate the disc space and to share a significant portion of the compressive load. Because the nucleus is significantly stiffened by the constraint from the anulus, a wide range of materials with modulus differences of several orders of magnitude could achieve the above objectives. Also, the shape of the nucleus implant affects stress distribution; implants with better conformity with the end plates and anulus likely provide better stress distribution.

The first major clinical use of any type of disc prosthesis was a nucleus prosthesis developed by Ferstrom in 1964, but most attention since then has been on the total disc prosthesis. At the 5th NASS meeting in 1990, only one nucleus prosthesis concept was presented. Ray suggested using a paired sausage-shaped implant with a flexible outer shell made from two different kinds of filaments, one biodegradable for tissue ingrowth and one nondegradable for mechanical strength. The membrane of the sausage would be semipermeable and filled with hyaluronic acid solution so that water could diffuse through during cyclic loading.

Bao and associates developed the concept of using hydrogel material for a nucleus prosthesis. Their rational for using a hydrogel material for a nucleus prosthesis was that its properties are similar to those of the natural nucleus pulposus and it is capable of restoring the biologic function of the nucleus. They demonstrated in the laboratory that the hydrogel nucleus prosthesis could restore disc height and normal mechanical function and that it could mimic the water imbibe-and-release capability of nucleus tissue under cyclic loading. Their animal study, using a baboon model, showed no adverse tissue reactions with the hydrogel and that the implant tended to delay disc degeneration compared to a sham-operated disc.

Ray changed his original material to a hydrogel and the geometry of his device from cylindrical to pillow-shape. Since 1996, over 150 patients have received this nucleus prosthesis. The procedure has been reported to afford good pain relief and functional improvement to the patients with the implant staying in place. However, there were 17 implant extrusions in the first 101 patients. The relatively large annular excision required to insert the implant is believed to be the major cause for this high implant extrusion rate. The device received its CE mark approval in Europe in 1998 and is currently under a pilot IDE study in the United States.

One way to address the problem of nuclear implant extrusion is to have a nucleus prosthesis that can be inserted through a small annular incision. Using in situ curable polymer, which can be injected through a small annular opening and cured in the disc space, could reduce the risk of implant extrusion. An in situ cured nucleus prosthesis could also have the advantage of better conformity between the implant and nucleus cavity. Because the size and shape of the cavity depend on surgical technique and the patient's anatomy and are highly variable from patient to patient, it is very diffi-cult to match the size and shape of a preformed prosthesis with the cavity. Oversized implants make implantation more difficult and increase the chance of implant extrusion, while undersized implants are not as effective in restoring the mechanical properties of the disc. An unmatched geometry will cause uneven stress distribution on the end plates and anulus.

Indications and justifications for using a nucleus prosthesis are at least as complicated as those for total disc replacement. Ideally, nucleus replacement should be used with most discectomy procedures if the anulus is not grossly damaged, so that disc height and stability are maintained. However, because short-term clinical results of discectomy in relieving sciatic pain are so good, it might be difficult to justify the added cost and potential risk of a nucleus prosthesis. A nucleus prosthesis might be more suitable for patients with discogenic pain because discectomy has not been very effective for these patients, and, currently, most of these patients are treated with fusion that might be excessive. If the nucleus prosthesis shows the same or better clinical outcome for this group of patients, it would definitely be a better choice than fusion.

Anulus Replacement/Repair

Almost all patients with symptomatic degenerative disc disease have a weakened and damaged anulus. When a degenerated nucleus is contained by an intact anulus, the diseased or degenerated nucleus itself should not cause pain. It is in conjunction with a weakened or damaged anulus that the nucleus can cause pain by chemical irritation or mechanical compression of nerve roots. In spite of these observations, very little effort has been made to effect disc arthroplasty by replacing or repairing the anulus. Many animal studies have shown that the anulus, once damaged, heals poorly. Limited attempts to repair the anulus have not been successful.

Advancements in tissue engineering might offer some means to repair or replace an annular defect, whether it is preexisting or created during a discectomy. Then annuloplasty might prevent disc reherniation and pain caused by nuclear fluid leakage. Because unrepaired annular defects have been found to be associated closely with disc degeneration in both humans and animals, an additional benefit of annuloplasty could be prevention of further disc degeneration after a discectomy. Furthermore, because many nucleus prostheses rely on a competent anulus, annular repair should enhance the effectiveness of a prosthetic nucleus implant. Indications for an annular repair device should be the same as those for discectomy. Outcome assessment should include radiographic examination, reherniation rate, and reduction of pain.

Conclusion

Compared with arthroplasty of knee and hip joints, progress has been slow for disc arthroplasty. Significant research has been conducted and knowledge and experience accumulated in the last 35 years, especially in the last 10 years. Several designs have had initial clinical testing with promising results, and many others are close to being tested clinically. Most importantly, the demand, from both physicians and patients, for a better solution for back pain has never been stronger. Although fusion cages and other advances in fixation and fusion biology have made fusion easier with higher fusion rates, these devices do not address the fundamental pitfalls of fusion itself. Recent advances in minimally invasive techniques should reduce the risks and broaden the applicability of replacement of disc components. There is much to be done but the need is compelling, and the potential of these new technologies is great.

Annotated Bibliography

Ahlgren BD, Vasavada A, Brower RS, Lydon C, Herkowitz HN, Panjabi MM: Anular incision technique on the strength and multidirectional flexibility of the healing intervertebral disc. *Spine* 1994;19:948-954.

Ahlgren BD, Lui W, Herkowitz HN, Panjabi MM, Guiboux JB: Effect of anular repair on the healing strength of the intervertebral disc: A sheep model. *Spine* 2000;25:2165-2170.

The authors report on two different annular incisions made in sheep discs. It was found that the big (box) incision causes disc instability and leads to a slower healing process than the small incision. Suturing and fascial plugs did not effect annular healing.

Allen MJ, Schoonmaker JE, Ordway NR, et al: Preclinical testing of a poly(vinyl alcohol) hydrogel nucleus in baboons. *Proceedings of the 15th Annual Meeting of the North American Spine Society*. Rosemont, IL, North American Spine Society, 2000, p 1.

The histologic and radiographic examination showed that the poly(vinyl alcohol) hydrogel nucleus has no adverse local and systemic reaction and delays the degenerative change of an implanted disc in a baboon model.

Enker P, Steffee A, McMillin C, Keppler L, Biscup R, Miller S: Artificial disc replacement: Preliminary report with a 3-year minimum follow-up. *Spine* 1993;18:1061-1070.

A preliminary clinical study of the Acroflex disc on six patients with minimum follow-up of 3 years showed four patients with satisfactory results (one excellent, two good, and one fair) and two with failure due to a fracture through the rubber core (one) and unresolved pain (one).

Langrana NA, Parsons JR, Lee CK, Vuono-Hawkins M, Yang SW, Alexander H: Materials and design concepts for an intervertebral disc spacer: I. Fiber-reinforced composite design. *J Appl Biomater* 1994;5:125-132.

Vuono-Hawkins M, Langrana NA, Parsons JR, Lee CK, Zimmerman MC: Materials and design concepts for an intervertebral disc spacer: II. Multidurometer composite design. *J Appl Biomater* 1995;6:117-123.

These articles present a disc prosthesis of a composite design, using biocompatible thermoplastic elastomers of various stiffnesses with and without fiber reinforcements, which can achieve a range of compressive and torsional properties similar to that of a natural lumbar disc.

Ordway NR, Zheng YG, McCullen GL, et al: Biomechanical evaluation of the functional spine unit with a hydrogel implant. *Proceedings of the 11th Annual Meeting of the North American Spine Society*. Rosemont, IL, North American Spine Society, 1996, p 164.

A cadaver study using a hydrogel nucleus prosthesis demonstrated the restoration of disc height and function under physiologic loading and no implant extrusion under the failure load.

Ray CD: Prosthetic disc nucleus implant: Update. *Proceedings of the 13th Annual Meeting of the North American Spine Society*. Rosemont, IL, North American Spine Society, 1998, p 252.

An update on this nucleus prosthesis showed that the modified design has favorable laboratory results, improvement in disc height and flexibility, and reduction in discogenic pain in 83% of the 42 patients in this study.

Classic Bibliography

Ahrens JE, Shelokov AP, Carver JL: Normal joint mobility is maintained with an artificial disc prosthesis. *Proceedings of the 12th Annual Meeting of the North American Spine Society*. Rosemont, IL, North American Spine Society, 1997, pp 110-111.

Bao QB, McCullen GM, Higham PA, Dumbleton JH, Yuan HA: The artificial disc: Theory, design and materials. *Biomaterials* 1996;17:1157-1167.

Brock M, Mayer HM, Weigel K (eds): *The Artificial Disc*. Berlin, Germany, Springer-Verlag; 1991.

Ethier DB, Cain JE, Yaszemski MJ, et al: The influence of anulotomy selection on disc competence: A radiographic, biomechanical, and histological analysis. *Spine* 1994;19:2071-2076.

Griffith SL, Shelokov AP, Buttner-Janz K, LeMaire JP, Zeegers WS: A multicenter retrospective study of the clinical results of the LINK SB Charité intervertebral prosthesis: The initial European experience. *Spine* 1994;19:1842-1949.

Hedman TP, Kostuik JP, Fernie GR, Hellier WG: Design of an intervertebral disc prosthesis. *Spine* 1991;16(suppl 6):S256-S260.

Herron L: Recurrent lumbar disc herniation: Results of repeat laminectomy and discectomy. *J Spinal Disord* 1994;7:161-166.

Kostuik JP: Intervertebral disc replacement: Experimental study. *Clin Orthop* 1997;337:27-41.

Lemaire JP, Skalli W, Lavaste F, et al: Intervertebral disc prosthesis: Results and prospects for the year 2000. *Clin Orthop* 1997;337:64-76.

McKenzie AH: Ferstrom intervertebral disc arthroplasty: A long-term evaluation. *Orthopaedics Int Ed* 1995;3:313-324.

Osti OL, Vernon-Roberts B, Fraser RD: Anulus tears and intervertebral disc degeneration: An experimental study using an animal model. *Spine* 1990;15:762-767.

Osti OL, Vernon-Roberts B, Fraser RD: Annular tears and disc degeneration in the lumbar spine: A post-mortem study of 135 discs. *J Bone Joint Surg Br* 1992;74:678-682.

Chapter 49

Restoration of Spinal Cord Function

Michael G. Fehlings, MD PhD, FRCSC

Lali H.S. Sekhon, MB, BS, PhD, FRACS

Introduction

Spinal cord injury occurs through various countries throughout the world with an annual incidence of 15 to 40 cases per million. Despite much work, no treatment has been shown to reliably clinically ameliorate neurologic dysfunction that occurs at or below the level of neurologic injury. Understanding both the primary and secondary mechanisms of injury indicates that functional secondary gains begin with limitation of the primary injury effects and the subsequent deleterious cascade of events. Once the injury has been sustained, the repair of the chronic injury and the modification of fiber tracts are key targets in the restoration of function.

Neural Protection

Limitation of Acute Injury

Acute spinal cord injury is a two-step process involving primary and secondary mechanisms. The primary or initial mechanical injury occurs as a result of local deformation and energy transformation. The secondary mechanisms encompass a cascade of biochemical and cellular processes that are initiated by the primary process and may cause ongoing cellular damage and even cell death. Although lipid peroxidation and vascular disruptions were initially thought to be key mediators, the increasing contribution of glutaminergic pathways, sodium- and calcium-mediated mechanisms, and programmed cell death also play a part. Limitation of the acute injury focuses on the prevention of further mechanical injury by stabilizing the spinal column, both in the field and in the hospital setting, and by limiting exposure to possibly avoidable secondary mechanisms, coupled with adequate systemic resuscitation. The maintenance of adequate spinal cord perfusion, with the avoidance of hypotension and hypoxia is paramount, particularly as neurogenic shock and loss of autoregulation leave the spinal cord vulnerable to further injury that is potentially avoidable.

Surgery and Pharmacotherapy

There recently has been an increased focus on the roles of pharmacotherapy and emergent surgical decompression in the amelioration of the effects of spinal cord injury.

Methylprednisolone

Recent studies of the use of methylprednisolone, as recommended on the basis of the National Acute Spinal Cord Injury Studies (NASCIS-2 and NASCIS-3), have shown improved recovery in patients with spinal cord injury. Unfortunately, the improved neurologic recovery observed to date has been modest and primarily root related, with only slight improvement in the functional status.

Methylprednisolone has a number of neuroprotective effects, including inhibition of oxidative cell injury from reactive free radical species, inhibition of lipid peroxidation, attenuation of excitatory amino acid release, reduction of intracellular calcium influx, and augmentation of posttraumatic spinal cord blood flow. The three major studies evaluating the effects of intravenous methylprednisolone on recovery from acute spinal cord injury are summarized here. NASCIS-1 in 1984 compared the efficacy of 1,000 mg/day with that of 100 mg/day of intravenous methylprednisolone semisuccinate (MPSS). Both doses were administered for 10 days in patients with an acute spinal cord injury, starting within 48 hours of trauma. No placebo group was included. The results showed no difference between the two treatment arms. Consequently, the use of steroids for acute spinal cord injury fell out of favor. NASCIS-2, in 1990, addressed the shortcomings of NASCIS-1. In this study, 487 patients were placed into one of three treatment groups: (1) high-dose MPSS (30 mg/kg bolus followed by 5.4 mg/kg/h for 23 h); (2) naloxone (5.4 mg/kg bolus followed by 4.0 mg/kg/h for 23 h); or (3) placebo. It was found that in patients treated within 8 h of injury, MPSS therapy led to improved motor and sensory recovery at

6 weeks, 6 months, and 1 year, compared with naloxone or placebo. This group did, however, have a higher wound infection rate (7.1%) than the other groups. Despite criticisms, this study established the neuroprotective role of steroids in acute spinal cord injury.

NASCIS-3, in 1997, assessed the hypotheses that (1) ultra-early (within 3 h) MPSS therapy was more effective than standard therapy, (2) prolonged infusion of MPSS for 48 h improved functional recovery, and (3) therapy with tirilazad, a 21-aminosteroid with potent effects on lipid peroxidation and few corticosteroid effects would be more effective than MPSS therapy. Patients received either a 24-h infusion of MPSS (5.4 mg/kg/h), a 48-h infusion of MPSS (5.4 mg/kg/h), or tirilazad mesylate (2.5 mg/kg every 6 h for 48 h). The results showed that those patients in all three treatment arms who received drug treatment within 3 h after spinal cord injury had similar neurologic recovery. In contrast, patients who received treatment within 3 to 8 h showed improved motor and functional independence. Tirilazad provided similar effects in terms of functional outcome to 24-h infusion of MPSS. However, the 48-h MPSS regimen was associated with a higher rate of severe sepsis (2.6%) and pneumonia (5.8%). On the basis of NASCIS-2 and NASCIS-3 data, the current recommendation is for all adult patients with acute, nonpenetrating spinal cord injury to receive MPSS within 8 h, and preferably within 3 h, of trauma. Those receiving the initial bolus of MPSS between 3 and 8 h should receive a 48-h infusion of MPSS rather than the standard 24-h regimen. MPSS is not indicated in patients who are first seen more than 8 h after spinal cord injury.

Ganglioside

The gangliosides are a group of sialic acid-containing glycosphingolipids found in high concentration in the outer cell membranes of central nervous system (CNS) tissue. Monosialotetrahexosylganglioside (GM-1) ganglioside has been shown to have some neuroprotective effect in animal models of spinal cord injury. GM-1 ganglioside works by an unknown mechanism of action, but it may exert a neurotrophic effect. GM-1 ganglioside inhibits the neuroprotective effect of MPSS, probably via its effect on lipocortin, and infusion of GM-1 ganglioside typically is delayed until MPSS infusion is completed. Early clinical studies are encouraging, with suggestions that some improvement in functional outcome after spinal cord injury can be achieved. A large randomized trial evaluating GM-1 ganglioside has recently been completed by Geisler and associates. The results of this trial, which to date have not been published, suggest that GM-1 ganglioside may promote earlier recovery of function.

Surgical Intervention

Recent advances in the safety and efficacy of surgical decompression of the spinal cord offer significant potential for repairing some of the neurologic damage caused by spinal cord injuries. Despite the widespread use of surgery in patients with acute spinal cord injury in North America, the role of this intervention in improving neurologic recovery remains controversial because of the lack of well-designed and executed randomized controlled trials.

There is strong experimental evidence from animal models that decompression of the spinal cord improves recovery after spinal cord injury. However, it is difficult to determine a time window for the effective application of decompression in the clinical setting from these animal models. Studies of secondary injury mechanisms suggest that early intervention, within hours after spinal cord injury, is critical to attain a neuroprotective effect. Whether the same time window applies to surgical treatment is unclear. The clinical studies in which the role of surgical decompression in spinal cord injury have been examined are limited. Surgery remains a valid practice option, although there are no conclusive data showing a benefit over nonsurgical management approaches. There is limited evidence suggesting that either early (< 25 h) or delayed (> 200 h) surgical intervention is safe and equally effective. To better define the role of surgery in the management of acute spinal cord injury, randomized, controlled prospective trials are required.

Limitation of Programmed Cell Death

Apoptosis is a form of programmed cell death that occurs in a wide variety of disease states in eukaryotic cells. Unlike necrosis, apoptosis is an active process, which is characterized by cell shrinkage, chromatin aggregation, and nuclear pyknosis. Apoptosis is a tightly regulated process with a sequence of activation steps that require energy and specific macromolecular synthesis such as de novo gene transcription. Apoptosis occurs during development, and now is also believed to play a role in many postdevelopmental disorders of the CNS, including ischemia, trauma, inflammation, and neurodegenerative states. A family of cystein proteins, the caspases, are believed to play an important role in apoptosis. Caspase-3 activation in vitro can be triggered by upstream events, leading to the release of cytochrome *c* from the mitochondria and the subsequent transactivation of procaspase-9 by Apaf-1. These upstream and downstream components of the caspase-3 apoptotic pathway are activated after traumatic spinal cord injury in rats; they may occur early in neurons in the injury site and hours to days later in oligodendroglia adjacent to and distant from the injury site. Oligodendrocytes appear to be the major cell type that undergo apoptosis after spinal cord injury. The mechanism behind this is unclear, but it may occur either as a result of adverse changes in the cellular environment resulting in axonal demyelination, as a result of wallerian degeneration, or by a combination of both these processes. It also has been suggested, that this death of oligodendrocytes may be as a consequence of microglial activation, and peaks at 8 days after injury. Apoptosis occurs around the lesion epicenter as well as within areas of wallerian degeneration in both ascending and descending white-matter tracts. Targeting the upstream events of the caspase cascade to protect neurons and oligodendrocytes from undergoing apoptotic death may have therapeutic potential in the treatment of acute spinal cord injury. Agents such as the oncogene Bcl-2 have been shown to limit the degree of histologic injury in acute experimental spinal cord injury in rats, possibly by regulating an antioxidant pathway that limits free radical generation.

Repair of Chronic Injury

Regeneration

Regeneration occurs more easily in the peripheral nervous system; the CNS does not undergo meaningful spontaneous regeneration. The reasons for this disparity are in part related to myelin-associated proteins in CNS white matter that act as strong inhibitors of the growth of nerve fibers. Neutralization of these proteins by monoclonal antibodies such as IN-1 can lead to pronounced regeneration in the adult rat spinal cords.

The process of regeneration, if initiated, is complex. In order for transected neurons to regenerate, assuming survival after the initial injury, a series of specific events must occur. These include regrowth (spontaneous sprouting) of the damaged axon, passage through the lesion site, elongation in the correct direction, topographic reinnervation of the normal target, and restoration of former electrophysiologic properties.

Attempts to manipulate the regrowth response of lesioned neurons have centered on two primary strategies: (1) the modification of the nonpermissive environment in the lesioned CNS tissue by the implantation of acellular guiding prostheses, fetal neural tissue, and glial cells, or the neutralization of growth inhibitory molecules and the permiabilization of the lesion scar, respectively; (2) the activation of intrinsic neuronal capacities by overexpression of regeneration-promoting genes (*GAP-43*, *Bcl-2*, *c-Jun*), or via the delivery of neurotrophic substances (nerve growth factor [NGF], brain-derived neurotrophic factor [BDNF], neurotrophin

[NT]-3, NT-4/5, platelet-derived growth factor, fibroblast growth factor [FGF], transforming growth factor, insulin-like growth factor, and others) in the vicinity of lesioned axons or perikarya of injured neurons. This gene therapy may provide a new strategy for the treatment of traumatic injury.

Problems such as the relative impermeance of the blood-brain barrier to neurotrophic substances are being addressed by strategies such as slow-releasing intracerebral implants containing the active protein in a biodegradable polymer matrix. In vivo viral vector-mediated gene transfer can also be used. Finally, the stimulation of synthesis, release, and activity of endogenous growth factors may address delivery issues.

Peripheral Nerve Grafts and Other Bridges

The use of peripheral nerves transplanted into a damaged CNS provides direct evidence that adult axons have the capacity to regenerate over long distances. In general, the growth stops close to the distal end of the transplanted nerve, with these axons seldom penetrating far into the CNS. Functional regeneration has been demonstrated in the completely transected spinal cord by using several peripheral nerves stabilized by FGF-impregnated fibrin glue to bridge individual spinal axon bundles to the gray matter of the distal stump. The presence of viable Schwann cells in the graft may be a prerequisite. These cells are believed to provide not only scaffolding and guidance tubes for regenerating peripheral axons, but also may synthesize a number of neurotrophic factors (for example, NGF and BDNF). Schwann cell suspensions have also been used, and the neurotrophic factors secreted by the Schwann cells could play a more important role than previously was realized.

Acellular bridges as well as glial implants have been used, and more recently, embryonic stem cells have been used (see section on stem cells). The implants not only may act as facilitators of neuronal bridges across scar tissue, they also may be a source for trophic factors. Acellular bridges orient paths of low-resistance to guide regrowing axons and provide support frames for glial and vascular reorganization in lesioned CNS tissue. Collagens, hydrogels, omentum, nitrocellulose membranes, glass and carbon filaments, gelfoam, and other materials have all been used with variable success. In general, limited axon growth may occur, but reentry into spinal cord tissue does not occur.

Growth Factors

Most of the known neurotrophic factors and their receptors (trk: tyrosine kinase receptors) have been found in developing and adult spinal cords. The possibility of applying neurotrophic factors such as glial-derived neurotrophic factor or BDNF to facilitate spinal cord repair is showing promise in animal models. A variety of cell adhesion, extracellular matrix, and guidance molecules that are axonal-growth promoting are found both in vitro and in the developing spinal cord. The concept that adhesion is the main determinant for neurite outgrowth has been replaced by the suggestion that axonal growth depends on intracellular secondary messenger events triggered by specific interactions at the cell surface.

Antagonism of Nerve Growth Inhibitors

In addition to the use of growth facilitators, the neutralization of neurite growth inhibitors is also receiving much attention. Oligodendrocytes are believed to play a key role in mediating inhibitory signals of axonal growth. The myelin proteins NI-35 and NI-250, as well as myelin-associated glycoprotein, have all been implicated. These are associated with the myelin of central, but not peripheral axons. A monoclonal antibody (IN-1) raised against IN-220/250, a myelin protein that is a potent inhibitor of neurite growth, promoted axonal regeneration and compensatory plasticity following CNS lesions. The *nogo-A* gene is the rat complementary DNA encoding NI-220/250, and it encodes at least three major protein products (Nogo-A, -B and -C). Recombinant Nogo-A is recognized by monoclonal antibody IN-1 and inhibits outgrowth from dorsal root ganglia. Antibodies against Nogo-A stain CNS myelin and oligodendrocytes and allow dorsal root ganglion cells to grow onto CNS myelin and into optic nerve. Nogo-A is a potent neurite growth inhibitor and an IN-1 antigen produced by oligodendrocytes, and it may allow for the production of new reagents to aid in CNS regeneration. Despite these results, it may still come to pass that the strategies for spinal cord restoration will need to focus on augmentation of growth factor effects, rather than antagonism of potential growth inhibitors.

Stem Cells

An exciting area of possible future clinical implication for spinal cord restoration is the use of stem cells to mitigate partial recovery after spinal cord injury. At this stage only experimental animal studies have been performed. In a rat spinal cord injury model, embryonic stem cells are injected into the injured spinal cord some time after the initial insult. Using fluorescent antibody techniques, it is demonstrable that in time these stem cells differentiate to form neurons and glial cells. Within months, the animals exhibit some motor function recovery, which is not seen in control animals. The possible mechanisms underlying these observations are specula-

tive. The newly acquired neurons may rewire severed connections. The new oligodendrocytes may form myelin sheaths around previously injured neurons, aiding recovery of conducive properties; they may reduce scar tissue formation at the host-graft interface; or the stem cell derivatives may provide trophic factors to prevent cell death and aid recovery of damaged neurons.

Olfactory Glial Cell Grafts

Olfactory mucosa neurons are the only neurons that retain the ability to divide and replicate in adult life. Olfactory glial cells also are unique in that they can cross the boundary between the peripheral nervous system and CNS. They also have been shown to bridge across scar tissue rather than migrate around it. To date, only rat studies have been reported. If human applications do develop, one advantage of this autograft for spinal cord injury would be elimination of problems of rejection or immunosupression.

Electrical Stimulation

The role of electrical stimulation in recovery from spinal cord injury is an interesting area of research. The effect of an electric field in promoting neurite growth in culture is well-established, with proliferation and faster growth occurring toward the cathode. Improved recovery has been demonstrated in rats that have sustained an experimental spinal cord injury at the T1 level and are exposed to direct-current field (cathode distal). The mechanisms are not clear. Electrical fields have a direct effect on receptors within the neurite and are associated with increased calcium ion entry into the growing tip. It may also be that changes in the extracellular matrix molecules and their interactions with the growing axons, alterations in glial orientation, changes to posttraumatic spinal cord blood flow, or parenchymal edema are all modulated by electrical fields.

Modification of Fiber Tracts

Axonal Sprouting

Elongation of lesioned axons after acute experimental spinal cord injury is a rare spontaneous phenomenon in the CNS. Neutralization of the myelin-associated proteins with the antibody IN-1 can restore this function. Sprouting of spared descending fibers occurs in the spinal cord caudal to lesions. Plastic rearrangement of neuronal circuits is believed to occur with physiologic changes in the existing synaptic connections. These changes can be either beneficial or maladaptive and are modulated by factors governing synapse formation and stabilization. The precise details of the cellular mechanisms regulating the formation of new connections is poorly understood; however, a significant potential for reorganization exists in the lesioned spinal cord.

Computer Interfaces

The potential establishment of functional contacts between axons and implanted electronic computer microchips is relatively new. In rat studies, microchip implants composed of a silicone chamber capped with two nerve segments, with a microchip wafer between them, attracted central axons when attached above a minimal lesion of the spinal cord. These axons not only entered the tube implant but also grew through the holes in the microchip wafer. So far, such studies have been performed only in rats, and the precise applicability to humans is yet to be defined.

Potassium Channel Blockade

After acute spinal cord injury, transection is rare, and characteristically, survival of a small population of thinly myelinated, small-diameter axons in the subpial rim may occur. There is evidence that demyelination of these surviving axons with exposure of paranodal "fast" potassium channels contributes to axonal dysfunction and neurologic deficits. In the clinical scenario, the potassium channel blocker 4-AP is associated with improved neurologic function in about one third of patients with chronic spinal cord injury. The beneficial effects of 4-AP are believed to be a result of (1) the blockage of fast A-type potassium channels that increase the safety factor of conduction across demyelinated or thinly remyelinated internodes and (2) increased calcium influx at presynaptic terminals, leading to improved transmission across CNS synapses or at the neuromuscular junction. The dosage of 4-AP is limited by its potential to induce seizures. The drug is most effective in patients with incomplete injuries (American Spinal Injury Association grade B to D); however, the functional significance of the neurologic changes, which are modest, remain unproven.

Conclusion

Although the ultimate aim of clinicians is complete restoration of both motor and sensory function after acute spinal cord injury, at the start of the new millenium, the main therapeutic interventions are still prevention and pharmacotherapy with corticosteroids, which provides modest gains. The understanding of primary and secondary spinal cord injury has improved, and limitation of the acute injury and amelioration of the early cascades is being intensively targeted; however, recovery of the intermediate and chronic injury

still remains elusive. Long-distance regeneration is slowly becoming a realization, and the barrier effect of scar tissue is being overcome slowly through the use of maneuvers such as stem cell transplants or Schwann cell bridges. Much effort is being focused on the factors that control and inhibit neurite growth. Fully understanding the scenario in the developing spinal cord is likely to be the key toward solving the scenario of injury to the adult spinal cord. It seems likely that combination therapies addressing multiple mechanisms will be required to have meaningful clinical impact.

Annotated Bibliography

Bracken MB, Shepard MJ, Holford TR, et al: Administration of methylprednisolone for 24 or 48 hours or tirilazad mesylate for 48 hours in the treatment of acute spinal cord injury: Results of the Third National Acute Spinal Cord Injury Randomized Controlled Trial. National Acute Spinal Cord Injury Study. *JAMA* 1997; 277:1597-1604.

This is the latest study supporting the efficacy of pharmacotherapy in promoting recovery in the clinical scenario of acute spinal cord injury.

Bregman BS, McAtee M, Dai HN, Kuhn PL: Neurotrophic factors increase axonal growth after spinal cord injury and transplantation in the adult rat. *Exp Neurol* 1997;148:475-494.

This study suggests that BDNF and NT-3 are both capable of influencing axotomized neurons, and that when applied in combination, transplants and neurotropins have an additive influence in preserving cell morphology.

Chen MS, Huber AB, van der Haar ME, et al: Nogo-A is a myelin-associated neurite outgrowth inhibitor and antigen for monoclonal antibody IN-1. *Nature* 2000;403: 434-439.

This study describes the *nogo-A* gene, a rat complementary DNA encoding NI-220/250. Recombinant Nogo-A is recognized by monoclonal IN-1 and inhibits outgrowth from dorsal root ganglia. Antibodies against Nogo-A stain CNS myelin and oligodendrocytes and allow dorsal root ganglion cells to grow onto CNS myelin and into optic nerve.

Diener PS, Bregman BS: Fetal spinal cord transplants support the development of target reaching and coordinated postural adjustments after neonatal cervical spinal cord injury. *J Neurosci* 1998;18:763-778.

This study was the first to demonstrate that fetal spinal cord transplants into damaged neonatal spinal cord induce anatomic remodeling. This remodeling supports the recovery of complex postural adjustments and skilled forelimb reaching, both of which were carefully assessed.

Fehlings MG, Tator CH: An evidence-based review of decompressive surgery in acute spinal cord injury: Rationale, indications, and timing based on experimental and clinical studies. *J Neurosurg* 1999;91(suppl 1): 1-11.

This is a comprehensive review on the timing of surgery in acute spinal cord injury. As of yet, only experimental evidence supports early decompression, except, perhaps, in the case of bilateral jumped facet joints.

McDonald JW, Liu XZ, Qu Y, et al: Transplanted embryonic stem cells survive, differentiate and promote recovery in injured rat spinal cord. *Nat Med* 1999;5:1410-1412.

The authors of this study transplanted neural differentiated mouse embryonic stem cells into a rat spinal cord 9 days after traumatic injury. Histologic analysis 2 to 5 weeks later showed that transplant-derived cells survived and differentiated into astrocytes, oligodendrocytes, and neurons, and migrated as far as 8 mm away from the lesion edge. Furthermore, gait analysis demonstrated that transplanted rats showed hindlimb weight support and partial hindlimb coordination not found in 'sham-operated' controls or control rats transplanted with adult mouse neocortical cells.

Ramon-Cueto A, Plant GW, Avila J, Bunge MB: Long-distance axonal regeneration in the transected adult rat spinal cord is promoted by olfactory ensheathing glia transplants. *J Neurosci* 1998;18:3803-3815.

This study clearly demonstrates that olfactory ensheathing glial cells, transplanted into a region of spinal cord injury, can migrate and overcome the inhibitory effects of CNS myelin. Consequently, it was shown that these cells allowed for regrowth of axons over long distances within the spinal cord and facilitated spinal cord regeneration after acute injury.

Segal JL, Pathak MS, Hernandez JP, Himber PL, Brunnemann SR, Charter RS: Safety and efficacy of 4-aminopyridine in humans with spinal cord injury: A long-term, controlled trial. *Pharmacotherapy* 1999;19: 713-723.

Twenty-one patients were treated with 4-AP. Long-term oral administration of immediate-release 4-AP was associated with improvement in and recovery of sensory and motor function, enhanced pulmonary function, and diminished spasticity in patients with long-standing spinal cord injury. The 4-aminopyridine appears to be safe and relatively free from toxicity when administered orally over 3 months.

Stichel CC, Müller HW: Experimental strategies to promote axonal regeneration after traumatic central nervous system injury. *Prog Neurobiol* 1998;56:119-148.

This excellent review article covers spinal and brain regeneration, particularly the role of grafting.

Classic Bibliography

Amar AP, Levy ML: Pathogenesis and pharmacological strategies for mitigating secondary damage in acute spinal cord injury. *Neurosurgery* 1999;44:1027-1040.

Emery E, Aldana P, Bunge MB, et al: Apoptosis after traumatic human spinal cord injury. *J Neurosurg* 1998; 89:911-920.

Geisler FH, Dorsey FC, Coleman WP: Recovery of motor function after spinal-cord injury: A randomized, placebo-controlled trial with GM-1 ganglioside. *N Engl J Med* 1991;324:1829-1838.

Lu J, Waite P: Advances in spinal cord regeneration. *Spine* 1999;24:926-930.

Lundborg G, Drott J, Wallman L, Reimer M, Kanje M: Regeneration of axons from central neurons into microchips at the level of the spinal cord. *Neuroreport* 1998;9:861-864.

Schwab ME, Bartholdi D: Degeneration and regeneration of axons in the lesioned spinal cord. *Physiol Rev* 1996;76:319-370.

Tatagiba M, Brosamle C, Schwab ME: Regeneration of injured axons in the adult mammalian central nervous system. *Neurosurgery* 1997;40:541-547.

Tator CH, Fehlings MG: Review of clinical trials of neuroprotection in acute spinal cord injury. *Neurosurgery Focus* 1999;6(1):Article 8. (www.neurosurgery.org)

Ye JH, Houle JD: Treatment of the chronically injured spinal cord with neurotrophic factors can promote axonal regeneration from supraspinal neurons. *Exp Neurol* 1997;143:70-81.

Chapter 50

Developing and Future Methods for Spine Care: Miscellaneous Trends, Materials, and Techniques

David F. Fardon, MD

Introduction

Rapid advances in biomedical engineering, molecular cell biology, and genetics have led to the introduction of exciting new possibilities for the care of spinal disorders at a rate that exceeds the abilities of physicians to evaluate their efficacies. Relatively new methods are widely accepted with uncertain confidence even as their obsolescence is threatened. This chapter provides a brief overview of some relatively new procedures, not detailed elsewhere in this text, which are widely but not universally accepted, and considers the spectrum of possibilities for future development.

Diagnostics

Technological advances, applied to noninvasive measurement of clinical integrity and performance of the spine, help refine treatment needs and outcomes, biomechanical research, and judgments of impairment. The scoliometer and Adams forward bend tests have been shown to have roles in scoliosis care. Stereovideographic analysis of skin markers noninvasively measures sagittal alignment of the scoliotic spine. Rasterstereographic surface topography images of the back provide quantifiable images of scoliotic deformity. A computerized inclinometer provides reliable measurements of lumbar range of motion (ROM). Another device, the lordosimeter, measures lumbar and thoracic ROM along with changes in lumbar length and curvature. Measurement of cervical ROM, assessed by goniometers, inclinometers, and by a computerized tracking system, has been shown to be reliable, at least in healthy volunteers.

Novel applications of standard imaging techniques have been applied to specific spinal disorders. Radiostereometric analysis has been used to assess sacroiliac motion and to determine stability after spinal fusion. Refinements of MRI techniques brought MRI closer to simulation of the few types of images previously unique to discography (see Chapter 8) and myelography. MRI

spectroscopy has been used to study cerebrospinal fluid in patients with lumbar disorders. Positron emission tomography (PET) scans have been used to evaluate destructive diseases of the spine. Imaging technology is being extended to interface with surgical techniques and to adapt spine care to the changes anticipated from the revolution in genetics and molecular biology. Integration of information from the various imaging modalities will facilitate molecular imaging of biologic processes in vivo and visualization of targets for treatment at the molecular level. In vivo imaging of genetic and molecular markers will be one of the means by which data become available to provide for very early recognition of and treatment for spinal diseases.

Nonsurgical Care

Work with new technology, such as transcript profiling, used for mapping genomes allows examination of complex systems of proteins and pathways relevant to cellular physiology. Such knowledge facilitates gene therapy, treatment derived from genetic modification of cells to induce a therapeutic effect. Gene therapy may involve replacement of a defective gene with a normal copy in patients with a single gene disorder such as Duchenne dystrophy. For disorders of more complex etiology, gene therapy may add important benefits, even if the genetics of the disorder are incompletely understood, by delivery of an efficacious gene or nucleic acid (DNA) requiring a delivery vector. The early application of such knowledge to the spine has included transfer of genes to rabbit and human chondrocytic cells of the intervertebral disc in vitro and the stimulation of proteoglycan synthesis from adenovirus-mediated transfer of a gene to animal intervertebral discs in vivo. The potential use of stem cells for the treatment of spinal disorders has been explored since the recognition (1) that stem cells exist in neurologic and musculoskeletal tissues not formally known to contain them and (2) that stem cells of various origins, particularly embryonal cells, can differentiate into diverse mature cells. Applications of gene therapy to spinal fusion and to restoration of spinal cord function are discussed in Chapters 46 and 49.

Genetics research also promises to provide revolutionary acceleration in the development of pharmacologic agents. Knowledge of the genetic background of disease and of individual vulnerability permits identification of pharmacologic targets in the newly mapped molecular pathways embedded in the genome. Future drugs should have highly specific pathways as opposed to those with multiple pathways and accompanying undesirable effects.

Some invasive procedures blur the distinctions between surgical and nonsurgical care. Three models of treatment—accelerating the degradation of nuclear disc material, bolstering the strength of the disc anulus, and rapidly stabilizing osteoporotic vertebral fractures—are undergoing widespread clinical trial and ongoing refinement of technique.

Chemonucleolysis with chymopapain, introduced in 1963, is still used for certain types of disc herniations. Concerns over neural toxicity and late spondylotic degenerative effects continue to stimulate the search for a better proteolytic agent. Cathepsin L, stromelysin-1, and chondroitinase ABC have been tested recently in animal and in vitro models.

Recently, attempts have been made to address the problem of painful radial tears and incompetency of the anulus using a flexible electrode passed to the interior of the disc for electrothermal coagulation of the anulus and of nociceptive pain fibers within the anulus. The procedure has been called intradiscal electrothermal anuloplasty (IDTA) and intradiscal electrothermal therapy. Proponents cite the need to deliver to the interior of the anulus an adequate range of thermal energy, which may not be delivered with other means of disc thermocoagulation, such as radiofrequency delivered through a needle. Optimal temperatures and application times, correlation with in vivo biologic effects, and outcomes for various permutations of disc disorders and clinical syndromes are under investigation as clinical experience with the procedure is accumulating.

The problem of painful compression fractures caused by osteoporosis or vertebral osteonecrosis has been addressed with increasing frequency by rapid stabilization, with or without attempts to reconstitute vertebral body height, since the method was introduced in France in 1984. Injection of polymethylmethacrylate (PMMA) into the compressed vertebral body (vertebroplasty) results in immediate stabilization and rapid pain relief for many patients. Development of an inflatable bone tamp has improved the capacity to reduce the fracture by reconstituting the height of the vertebral body (kyphoplasty) before injection of PMMA and may provide additional safety because it permits injection of cement at lower pressures. Data from larger and better-controlled series are accumulating, but diversity of fracture types and medical comorbidities challenge meaningful outcomes information. The debate over the value of fracture reduction hinges on evaluation of the role of kyphosis in the morbidity related to compression fractures and on whether the procedures reduce the incidence of compression fractures at other vertebrae. It is likely that biodegradable, osteoconductive, and osteoinductive materials will be introduced before there are clear patient-selection guidelines for the two currently used procedures. A variety of techniques are available for treatment of these extremely common fractures, which usually are self-limited with regard to pain. Therefore, more data are needed to determine which patients should be treated noninvasively and which patients would be better treated using kyphoplasty or vertebroplasty.

Surgical Care: Techniques

Spine surgery of the future will evolve to incorporate robot-mediated extensions of minimally invasive surgical techniques, guided by data from increasingly sophisticated imaging. Robots have been used to refine some surgical techniques that demand skill beyond that of the human hand. Currently, advanced imaging is used intraoperatively to enhance conventional surgical skills.

Data from CT, transferred to a tracking and navigation system, have been shown to be valuable in probing the pedicles of all parts of the spine. Virtual fluoroscopy has been shown in vitro to reduce radiation exposure and improve localization skills with spinal probes while using a single C-arm. Construction of individual three-dimensional templates has been used as an alternative to navigational systems. Use of a persistently electrified pedicle probe, following the principle of electrical stimulation of guide wires and screws, has been tested as a further check on intraoperative accuracy of pedicle boring. Intraoperative ultrasound has been refined as a technique to test the adequacy of spinal decompression from anterior as well as posterior approaches. A few centers have MRI scanners in their operating rooms.

Electrical stimulation as an adjunct to achieve fusion continues to be tested in a variety of clinical and laboratory circumstances. In one controlled, prospective study of high-risk patients undergoing pedicle-screw-supported lumbar fusion there was a higher fusion rate in those who received implanted direct-current electrical stimulation. In another study there was no difference in fusion rates among three groups of patients in whom instrumented posterolateral fusions were enhanced by implanted direct current, external pulsed electromagnetic field therapy, or no electrical adjunct. In yet another study the fusion rate of lumbar-cage-supported fusions in sheep was improved by addition of implanted direct current stimulation. Coralline-hydroxy-apatite-conducted fusion in rabbits was improved by addition of implanted direct current. Stress-shielding-induced osteopenia in beagles was reduced by addition of externally applied pulsed electromagnetic fields. Fusion stiffness and load-to-failure of the fusion mass of rabbits were enhanced by external fields. Another rabbit study showed that ultrasound increased the lumbar fusion rate. All of these adjuncts require careful validation before their additive effects are known.

Surgical Care: Materials

Numerous permutations of screw, wire, hook, rod, plate, and cage fixation systems continue to undergo testing and add to accumulated clinical experience. Most of these devices are constructed of steel or titanium alloys. Tantalum and vitreous carbon, carbon fiber, and silicone implant testing in vitro have been reported. Anchoring devices and biocompatible cement materials have been used to augment screw fixation. Future technology is likely to include use of materials that are bioabsorbable or bioincorporable so they no longer present an obstacle to imaging or potential for implant-related complications after their purpose has been served. Bioabsorbable poly-L-lactide pins have been tested for facet joint fixation in sheep. Tissue engineering of bone composites to suit individual needs probably will supersede many current uses for spacers and fixation devices, so that future implants are more likely to be cell-based than constructed of metals or plastics.

Improved stability without fusion would be an advantage for many patients. Direct repair of annular defects, with or without local tissue grafts, has been shown to have no advantage in the sheep model. Posterior stabilization by using nonrigid artificial ligaments has been tested successfully in vitro in pigs. Results were disappointing in a series of patients treated by implantation of a composite of braided polyester bands looped over titanium pedicle screws to provide nonrigid stability of the lumbar spine. A silicone implant inserted between spinous processes has been tested in vitro for increasing lumbar stability by limiting lordosis.

The desirability of an ideal interposition membrane to protect dura and neural tissues from postoperative epidural fibrosis is balanced by the need for the healing of incidental durotomies, which may be more common than has been recognized clinically. A resorbable, flowable gel used clinically as an interposition membrane has been implicated as a factor in clinically significant postoperative cerebrospinal fluid leak. Muscle or fat grafts, autologous fibrin patches, and homologous fibrin glues have been clinically useful means of dealing with recognized durotomies.

Conclusion

Computer technology and universal access to the Web foster presentation of topics in depths heretofore undreamed of, stimulating a proliferation of new information and cross-referencing. This abundance of data and access to it make the public hungry for miraculous cures, quick and simple. The stepwise progression of formulation of an idea, preclinical testing, prospective randomized studies, multicenter studies, and register studies cannot be rushed with the speed the public demands or to satisfy the hunger for answers to newly developed questions. Before one idea can be tested, what appears to be a better solution for the same problem comes along. The revolution under way in genetics research at the turn of the millennium will shift the paradigm for spine care, as it does for the rest of medical science, further straining the performance of orderly testing. The difficulties imposed on advances in spine care by this conundrum, as of the end of the last millennium, are addressed in a series of editorial comments in the December 1, 1999, issue of the journal *Spine*.

Annotated Bibliography

Diagnostics

Cote P, Kreitz BG, Cassidy JD, Dzus AK, Martel J: A study of the diagnostic accuracy and reliability of the Scoliometer and Adams forward bend test. *Spine* 1998; 23:796-803.

The scoliometer and Adams forward bend test have adequate interexaminer reliability for thoracic curves, but the scoliometer is a less reliable test of lumbar curves and is less sensitive than the Adams forward bend test.

Goldberg CJ, Kaliszer M, Moore DP, Fogorty EE, Dowling FE: Surface topography, Cobb angles, and cosmetic change in scoliosis. *Spine* 2001;26:E55-E63.

Surface topography was found useful in measuring scoliosis, but does not measure the same aspects of the deformity and, therefore, does not supersede the use of Cobb angle measurements in many situations.

Gracovetsky SA, Newman NM, Richards MP, Asselin S, Lanzo VF, Marriott A: Evaluation of clinician and machine performance in the assessment of low back pain. *Spine* 1998;23:568-575.

A prospective study compared the findings of two examiners and a machine that measured skin marker kinematics and surface electromyography during lifting and bending. The examiners more accurately assessed honest subjects, whereas the machine more accurately assessed simulators and dissimulators.

Leroux MA, Zabjek K, Simard G, Badeaux J, Coillard C, Rivard CH: A noninvasive anthropometric technique for measuring kyphosis and lordosis: An application for idiopathic scoliosis. *Spine* 2000;25:1689-1694.

Stereovideographic collection of coordinate data from skin markers placed over the spinous processes correlated with radiographic measurement of kyphosis and lordosis of scoliosis patients with curves ranging from 4° to 66°.

Mayer TG, Kondraske G, Beals SB, Gatchel RJ: Spinal range of motion: Accuracy and sources of error with inclinometric measurement. *Spine* 1997;22:1976-1984.

Tests of lumbar motion of healthy volunteers with a computerized inclinometer showed device inaccuracy to be insignificant but highly dependent on the test administrator.

McGorry RW, Hsiang SM: A method for dynamic measurement of lumbar lordosis. *J Spinal Disord* 2000;13:118-123.

A device, the lordosimeter, measured trunk flexion and extension while tracking lumbar length and curvature statically and dynamically during a lifting task. Measurements correlated with thoracic and pelvic angular displacement during lifting.

Ordway NR, Seymour R, Donelson R, Hojnowski LS, Edwards WT: Cervical sagittal range-of-motion analysis using three methods: Cervical range-of-motion device, 3 space, and radiography. *Spine* 1997;22:501-508.

Sagittal motions of the cervical spines of healthy volunteers measured with a simple compass goniometer and with a double inclinometer with computerized tracking system were compared to radiographs. All three methods produced reliable measurements, including those of protrusion and retraction, but the computerized double inclinometer better isolated cervical from upper thoracic motion.

Pape D, Adam F, Fritsch E, Muller K, Kohn D: Primary lumbosacral stability after open posterior and endoscopic anterior fusion with interbody implants: A roentgen stereophotogrammetric analysis. *Spine* 2000;25:2514-2518.

Roentgen stereophotogrammetric analysis is sensitive to the difference in stability created when anterior interbody fusion is added to posterior fixation for fusion.

Paassilta P, Lohiniva J, Goring HHH, et al: Indentification of a novel common genetic risk for lumbar disk disease. *JAMA* 2001;285:1843-1849.

A Finnish study of 171 individuals with lumbar disc disease compared coding sequences and exon boundaries of collagen IX genes to those of 321 patients, including 186 healthy, 83 with osteoarthritis, 31 with rheumatoid arthritis, and 21 with chondrodysplasias. Genetic configuration unique to those with lumbar disc disease was found to be highly significant ($P = 0.000013$).

Schmitz A, Kalicke T, Willkomm P, Grunwald F, Kandyba J, Schmitt O: Use of fluorine 18 fluoro-2-deoxy-D-glucose positron emission tomography in assessing the process of tuberculous spondylitis. *J Spinal Disord* 2000;13:541-544.

A case demonstrates use of PET scanning to image tuberculous infection of the spine. PET scanning is sensitive to inflammation, can distinguish bone from soft-tissue involvement, and is not degraded by the presence of metal.

Suzuki S, Inami K, Ono T, et al: Analysis of posterior trunk symmetry index (POTSI), in Stokes IAF (ed): *Scoliosis: Part 1. In Research Into Spinal Deformities 2.* Amsterdam, The Netherlands, IOS Press, 1999, pp 81-84.

A composite index of six dimensionless numbers reflecting mediolateral asymmetry at C7, axillae, and waist and vertical asymmetry at the shoulders, axillae, and waist, termed the posterior symmetry index, describes surface topography for scoliosis patients.

Tempany CM, McNeil BJ: Advances in biomedical imaging. *JAMA* 2001;285:562-567.

The scientific foundation of current new technologies and the prospects for research activities in the field of biomedical imaging, as of the beginning of 2001, are discussed in an overview accompanied by current references.

Tousignant M, de Bellefeuille L, O'Donoughue S, Grahovac S: Criterion validity of the cervical range of motion (CROM) goniometer for cervical flexion and extension. *Spine* 2000;25:324-330.

The CROM goniometer was found to be reliable for measurement of flexion and extension when compared to radiographs of healthy volunteers.

Nonsurgical Care

Bai B, Jazrawi LM, Kummer FJ, Spivak JM: The use of an injectable, biodegradable calcium phosphate bone substitute for the prophylactic augmentation of osteoporotic vertebrae and the management of vertebral compression fractures. *Spine* 1999;24:1521-1526.

Fresh cadaveric osteoporotic vertebral bodies, whole and fractured in vitro, were injected with biodegradable calcium phosphate and PMMA. No difference in strength, stiffness, or restoration of height was noted on comparison of the two materials.

Barendse GA, van den Berg SG, Kessels AH, Weber WE, van Kleef M: Randomized controlled trial of percutaneous intradiscal radiofrequency thermocoagulation for chronic discogenic back pain: Lack of effect from a 90-second 70C lesion. *Spine* 2001;26:287-292.

A randomized, controlled group of 28 patients with discogenic low back pain underwent thermocoagulation at 70° for 90 s versus no current. No significant difference between the two groups was found 8 weeks later.

Barr JD, Barr MS, Lemley TJ, McCann RM: Percutaneous vertebroplasty for pain relief and spinal stabilization. *Spine* 2000;25:923-928.

Significant pain relief was obtained by injection of PMMA into osteoporotic compression fractures for 95% of 38 consecutive patients studied retrospectively. Four of eight patients with fractures of vertebrae affected by malignant disease obtained significant relief.

Cunin G, Boissonnet H, Petite H, Blanchat C, Guillemin G: Experimental vertebroplasty using osteoconductive granular material. *Spine* 2000;25:1070-1076.

Coral granules were injected into cadaveric human osteoporotic vertebrae and into cavities created in sheep vertebral bodies. The coral granules were distributed homogeneously in the injected human bone, and were osteoconductive when injected into the sheep vertebral bodies.

Deramond H, Depriester C, Galibert P, LeGars D: Percutaneous vertebroplasty with polymethylmethacrylate: Technique, indications, and results. *Radiol Clin North Am* 1998;36:533-546.

The authors review the international experience with vertebroplasty, citing success rates as high as 92%. Complications included bleeding, infection, cement embolus, pneumothorax, fracture, neurologic injury, and death; all of these complications were infrequent.

Haro H, Murakami S, Komori H, Okawa A, Shinomiya K: Chemonucleolysis with human stromelysin-1. *Spine* 1997;22:1098-1104.

Stromelysin-1, an enzyme previously identified in degrading herniated disc tissues, was shown to have in vitro activity in degrading surgical specimens of human disc and in vivo activity in degradation of transplanted rat nucleus pulposus.

Jensen ME, Garfin SR: Vertebroplasty vs. kyphoplasty. *Spine Line* 2001;2:11-13.

The authors debate the merits of vertebroplasty and kyphoplasty based on current information.

Kaji EH, Leiden JM: Gene and stem cell therapies. *JAMA* 2001;285:545-550.

The authors provide an overview of the current and future applications of gene therapy to medical care in general.

Karasek M, Bogduk N: Twelve-month follow-up of a controlled trial of intradiscal thermal anuloplasty for back pain due to internal disc disruption. *Spine* 2000; 25:2601-2607.

A 12-month follow-up of 53 patients treated by IDTA compared the treatment group favorably with a control group treated with conventional rehabilitation methods. The authors state that the success of IDTA may be as low as 23% or as high as 60%, depending on the stringency of the criteria used.

Kubo S, Tajima N, Katunuma N, Fukuda K, Kuroki H: A comparative study of chemonucleolysis with recombinant human cathepsin L and chymopapain: A radiologic, histologic, and immunohistochemical assessment. *Spine* 1999;24:120-127.

Cathepsin L injected into rabbit disc spaces resulted in chemonucleolysis by a pathway that differed from that occurring after injection of chymopapain.

Lu DS, Shono Y, Oda I, Abumi A, Kaneda K: Effects of chondroitinase ABC and chymopapain on spinal motion biomechanics: An in vivo biomechanical radiologic, and histologic canine study. *Spine* 1997;22:1828-1835.

Chondroitinase ABC caused less segmental instability and disc-space narrowing than did chymopapain after chemonucleolysis in beagles.

Moon SH, Gilbertson LG, Nishida K, et al: Human intervertebral disc cells are genetically modifiable by adenovirus-mediated gene transfer: Implications for the clinical management of intervertebral disc disorders. *Spine* 2000:25;2573-2579.

Using an adenovirus vector, lacZ genes and luciferase genes were successfully transduced into human intervertebral disc tissue removed at surgery.

Nishida K, Gilbertson LG, Evans CH, Kang JD: Potential applications of gene therapy to the treatment of spinal disorders. *Spine* 2000;25:1308-1314.

The authors review the progress made and potential for applications of gene therapy to spinal disorders.

Nishida K, Kang JD, Gilbertson LG, et al: Modulation of biologic activity of the rabbit intervertebral disc by gene therapy: An in vivo study of adenovirus-mediated transfer of human transforming growth factor beta-1 encoding gene. *Spine* 1999;24:2419-2425.

This article describes the successful transfer of a human gene to a rabbit disc using an adenovirus vector.

Ohlstein EH, Ruffolo RR Jr, Elliott JD: Drug discovery in the next millennium. *Ann Rev Pharmacol Toxicol* 2000;40:171-191.

The authors review the changes anticipated in 21st century pharmacology, including the role of genetics research in accelerating those advances.

Saal JA, Saal JS: Intradiscal electrothermal treatment for chronic discogenic low back pain: A prospective outcome study with minimum 1-year follow-up. *Spine* 2000;25:2622-2627.

A cohort of 62 patients who had not improved with aggressive noninvasive care achieved a statistically significant and clinically meaningful improvement 1 year after IDET. The authors state the need for placebo-controlled, randomized trials and comparisons with alternative treatments.

Wehling P, Schulitz KP, Robbins PD, Evans CH, Reinecke JA: Transfer of genes to chondrocytic cells of the lumbar spine: Proposal for a treatment strategy of spinal disorders by local gene therapy. *Spine* 1997;22:1092-1097.

LacZ and a complementary DNA of human interleukin-1 receptor antagonist genes were successfully transferred to bovine end-plate cartilage cells in vitro, supporting the concept of introducing therapeutic agents to counteract degenerative disease.

Surgical Care: Techniques

Birnbaum K, Schkommodau E, Decker N, Prescher A, Klapper U, Radermacher K: Computer-assisted orthopedic surgery with individual templates and comparison to conventional operation method. *Spine* 2001;26:365-370.

Three-dimensional models created from CT data were used in human cadaver specimens to guide pedicle screw placement with greater accuracy than achieved by conventional methods. The authors suggest the method may be a less costly and time-consuming method than intraoperative computer-assisted techniques.

Bozic KJ, Glazer PA, Zurakowski D, Simon BJ, Lipson SJ, Hayes WC: In vivo evaluation of coralline hydroxyapatite and direct current electrical stimulation in lumbar spinal fusion. *Spine* 1999;24:2127-2133.

Implanted direct-current electrical stimulation increased the fusion rate in rabbits fused with coralline hydroxyapatite.

Carl AL, Khanuja HS, Gatto CA, et al: In vivo pedicle screw placement: Image-guided virtual vision. *J Spinal Disord* 2000;13:225-229.

Near real-time frameless stereotaxy was used for intraoperative navigation in placement of 32 lumbar pedicle screws in eight patients. Overall accuracy was ± 2mm.

Foley KT, Simon DA, Rampersaud YR: Virtual fluoroscopy: Computer-assisted fluoroscopic navigation. *Spine* 2001;26:347-351.

Computerized data from fluoroscopically examined in vitro vertebrae were used to construct a virtual image and subsequently to guide a surgical probe tracked by a single, stationary C-arm, limiting surgical radiation exposure and repositioning problems.

Glaser PA, Heilmann MR, Lotz JC, Bradford DS: Use of electromagnetic fields in a spinal fusion: A rabbit model. *Spine* 1997;22:2351-2356.

Externally applied pulsed electromagnetic fields applied to rabbits fused by posterolateral noninstrumented technique decreased the pseudarthrosis rate insignificantly, but provided significant increases in stiffness, area under the load displacement curve, and load to failure.

Glaser PA, Heilmann MR, Lotz JC, Bradford DS: Use of ultrasound in spinal arthrodesis. *Spine* 1998;23:1142-1148.

Externally applied ultrasound statistically increased the noninstrumented lumbar fusion rate, stiffness, area under the load displacement curve, and load to failure of rabbits.

Ito M, Fay LA, Ito Y, Yuan MR, Edwards WT, Yuan HA: The effect of pulsed electromagnetic fields on instrumented posterolateral spinal fusion and device-related stress shielding. *Spine* 1997;22:382-388.

In beagles with fusions stress-shielded by anterior plate and screw fixation, an external pulsed electromagnetic field reduced the degree of stress-shield induced osteopenia.

Jenis, LG, An HS, Stein R, Young B: Electrical stimulation in instrumented posterolateral lumbar arthrodesis. *J Spinal Disord* 2000;13:290-296.

Jenis LG, An HS, Stein R, Young B: Prospective comparison of the effect of direct current electrical stimulation and pulsed electromagnetic fields on instrumented posterolateral lumber arthodesis. *J Spinal Disord* 2000; 13:290-296.

Sixty-one patients undergoing instrumented posterolateral arthrodesis were prospectively randomized to three groups: one in which no electrical adjunct was applied, another in which direct current was applied through an implanted device, and one in which electrical stimulation was applied externally. There were no significant differences in fusion rates.

Kamimura M, Ebara S, Itoh H, Tateiwa Y, Kinoshita T, Takaoka K: Cervical pedicle screw insertion: Assessment of safety and accuracy with computer-assisted image guidance. *J Spinal Disord* 2000;13:218-224.

In nine plastic cervical spine models, 2-mm drills guided into 108 pedicles resulted in perforation of 25 pedicles. Clinically, 36 pedicle screws were guided into the cervical spines of patients with 100% accuracy by clinical and postoperative CT assessment.

Kim KD, Johnson JP, Bloch O, et al: Computer-assisted thoracic pedicle screw placement. *Spine* 2001;26: 360-364.

A computer-assisted navigation system was found to guide accurately screw placement in the pedicles of the thoracic spines of human cadavers.

Kucharzyk DW: A controlled prospective outcome study of implantable electrical stimulation with spinal instrumentation in a high-risk spinal fusion population. *Spine* 1999;24:465-469.

Comparison of 65 instrumented lumbar fusion patients to a later series of 65 instrumented lumbar fusion patients with implanted electrical stimulators revealed a fusion success rate of 95.6% in the electrically stimulated group compared with 87% in the nonstimulated and a clinical success rate of 93% in the electrically stimulated group compared with 81% in the nonstimulated group.

Laine T, Schlenzka D, Makitalo K, Tallroth K, Nolte LP, Visarius H: Improved accuracy of pedicle screw insertion with computer-assisted surgery: A prospective clinical trial of 30 patients. *Spine* 1997;22:1254-1258.

CT data were transferred to a navigation system to guide a pedicle awl and probe in placement of 139 lumbar pedicle screws. The misplacement rate was 4.3% for computer-guided screws, compared with 14.3% for those not inserted with computer guidance.

Mack MJ: Minimally invasive and robotic surgery. *JAMA* 2001;285:568-572.

Advanced techniques of imaging and minimally invasive surgery will come together to facilitate voice control over networked operating rooms, enhanced dexterity for microprocedures, and virtual simulation.

Raynor RB: Intraoperative ultrasound for immediate evaluation of anterior cervical decompression and discectomy. *Spine* 1997;22:389-395.

Usefulness of ultrasound to assess decompression, previously documented for laminectomy exposures, was demonstrated for anterior cervical decompressions.

Rose RD, Welch WC, Balzer JR, Jacobs GB: Persistently electrified pedicle stimulation instruments in spinal instrumentation: Technique and protocol development. *Spine* 1997;22:334-343.

A persistently electrified pedicle probe may facilitate early detection of breach of the cortex of the pedicle.

Toth JM, Seim HB III, Schwardt JD, Humphrey WB, Wallskog JA, Turner AS: Direct current electrical stimulation increases the fusion rate of spinal fusion cages. *Spine* 2000;25:2580-2587.

Sheep implanted with autograft and interbody lumbar cages and direct current electrical stimulators achieved more rapid fusions by histologic examination and stiffness testing than did those similarly treated without electrical stimulation.

Surgical Care: Materials

Ahlgren BD, Lui W, Herkowitz HN, Panjabi MM, Guiboax JP: Effect of anular repair on the healing strength of the intervertebral disc: A sheep model. *Spine* 2000; 25:2165-2170.

In the sheep model, direct repair, with or without local tissue graft supplements, had no effect on the strength of various types of anulotomy for discectomy.

Boskey AL: Musculoskeletal disorders and orthopedic conditions. *JAMA* 2001;285:619-623.

Among the topics discussed in this overview of the future of musculoskeletal and orthopaedic care is a presentation of the research needed to effect tissue-engineered, individualized bone composite implants.

Cammisa FP, Girardi FP, Sangani PK, Parvataneni HK, Cadag S, Sondhu HS: Incidental durotomy in spine surgery. *Spine* 2000;25:2663-2667.

A retrospective review of 2,144 patients showed a 3.1% incidence of recognized incidental durotomy at the time of surgery. The incidence of unrecognized durotomies that became clinically significant was 0.28%.

Deguchi M, Cheng BC, Sato K, Matsuyama Y, Zdeblick TA: Biomechanical evaluation of translaminar facet joint fixation: A comparative study of poly-L-lactide pins, screws, and pedicle fixation. *Spine* 1998;23: 1307-1313.

Poly-L-lactide pins, which are bioabsorbable, implanted as translaminar facet joint fixation, significantly reduced intervertebral and facet joint motion but were not as stiff as metal screws.

Hadlow SV, Fagan AB, Hillier TM, Fraser RD: The Graf ligamentoplasty procedure: Comparison with posterolateral fusion in the management of low back pain. *Spine* 1998;23:1172-1179.

A soft-tissue stabilization procedure using braided polyester bands looped over pedicle screws to hold the spinal segments in extension compared unfavorably to posterolateral fusion when evaluated at 1 year and required a higher revision rate in the first 2 years.

Hodges SD, Humphreys SC, Eck JC, Covington LA: Management of incidental durotomy without mandatory bed rest: A retrospective review of 20 cases. *Spine* 1999;24:2062-2064.

Incidental durotomies were repaired with suture, a fibrin glue made from topical thrombin and calcium carbonate, and a cryoprecipitate. Twenty patients so treated were allowed immediate ambulation without adverse effect.

Korovessis PG, Deligianni D, Stamatakis M, Missirlis Y: Augmentation of anterior transvertebral screws using threaded Teflon anchoring. *J Spinal Disord* 1998;11: 300-306.

Teflon anchors were shown in vitro in pigs to increase the anchorage and stability of Zielke screws.

Le AX, Rogers DE, Dawson EG, Kropf MA, DeGrange DA, Delamarter RB: Unrecognized durotomy after lumbar discectomy: A report of four cases associated with the use of ADCON-L. *Spine* 2001;26:115-118.

An increased incidence of postoperative spinal fluid leak as a result of unrecognized durotomy was attributed to a greater than previously reported incidence of unrecognized durotomy with failure of spontaneous resolution because a resorbable, flowable gel was implanted for the purpose of retarding epidural fibrosis.

Levi AD, Choi WG, Keller PJ, Heiserman JE, Sonntag VK, Dickman CA: The radiographic and imaging characteristics of porous tantalum implants within the human cervical spine. *Spine* 1998;23:1245-1251.

Implants of a composite of tantalum with 2% vitreous carbon were compared with titanium when used as a spacer in human cadaveric cervical spines. Tantalum was superior for imaging with several MRI sequences but inferior for CT.

Lotz JC, Hu SS, Chiu DF, Yu M, Colliou O, Poser RD: Carbonated apatite cement augmentation of pedicle screw fixation in the lumbar spine. *Spine* 1997;22: 2716-2723.

Testing of 43 cadaver lumbar vertebral bodies showed that pedicle screw fixation augmented by injectable, biocompatible carbonated apatite cancellous bone cement had 68% greater pull-out strength and 30% to 63% improvement in measures of performance in response to cyclic loading. These data suggest that such material might be an acceptable alternative to polymethylmethacrylate for augmentation of pedicle screw purchase.

Minns RJ, Walsh WK: Preliminary design and experimental studies of a novel soft implant for correcting sagittal plane instability in the lumbar spine. *Spine* 1997; 22:1819-1827.

A soft, silicone implant placed between the spinous processes to reduce spinal instability by a minimal procedure and without the consequences of fusion was designed and tested in vitro.

Suzuki K, Mochida J, Chiba M, Kikugawa H: Posterior stabilization of degenerative lumbar spondylolisthesis with a Leeds-Keio artifical ligament: A biomechanical analysis in a porcine vertebral model. *Spine* 1999;24: 26-31.

In vitro testing in pigs of an artificial ligament to posteriorly stabilize a spondylolisthetic lumbar segment resulted in an initial stabilizing effect that was maintained during cyclic loading.

Chapter 51

Statistical Relevance

Kevin F. Spratt, PhD

Introduction

As a methodologist and statistician trained in experimental design and measurement, I have focused primarily on designing studies, analyzing data, and assessing factors associated with problems of the lumbar spine. After doing this work for almost 20 years, I believe that, although the number of treatment options and diagnostic tests have grown substantially, patients with many forms of low back troubles are no better off in terms of likelihood of cure or long-term symptom relief than they were 20 years ago. Why not?

Overviews of statistics and references that could be used to learn more about statistical methods are not very interesting to clinicians, probably because this information does not provide them with tools needed to investigate and better understand their clinical practices. However, when I give talks related more directly to issues that arise when attempting to conduct and review research, audiences ask for references about these issues. Unfortunately, I know of no references that specifically speak to clinicians about the nuts and bolts of measurement, methods, and statistical reasoning as those things apply to the experimental design of clinical studies.

Therefore, this chapter contains some insights into measurement and methodologic and statistical reasoning, which are necessary for would-be researchers to isolate good clinical questions to investigate. The purposes of this chapter are to provide the clinical researcher with a basic overview of some of the measurement, methodologic, and statistical issues involved in conducting clinically-oriented medical research, and to increase the critical acumen of readers of the published results of clinical studies.

Good research, clinical or otherwise, must involve collaboration between the various disciplines that have knowledge of the topic. For clinical issues associated with the spine, input from both the clinician and the methodologist/statistician are vital. Depending on the topic, biomedical engineers, radiologists, biochemists, psychologists, and others may be important participants in carefully crafting the questions of interest. Those questions, in turn, focus the information that must be gathered if reasonably accurate answers are to be forthcoming. Hopefully, this chapter will lead to more informative research, at least partly because it will help clinicians better communicate with the other members of the research team.

Better clinical research should result in significant improvement in the treatment of patients with spine-related problems. Clinicians should understand that their goals should not be to become methodologists or statisticians, but to gain sufficient understanding to communicate better their clinical problems to the methodologists and statisticians.

Why is Statistical Relevance Important?

Patients, physicians, and medical researchers are interested ultimately in treatment efficacy for the individual patient. Payers, although interested in treatment efficacy (they do not want to pay for treatments that do not work), take a wider view by considering the effectiveness of a given treatment for broad classes of patients. For payers, the issue becomes how much benefit and risk a particular treatment offers a group of patients. They want to know how much a treatment will cost, relative to how much and what types of outcomes (positive and negative) the population of treated patients will experience.

The debate about treatment efficacy versus treatment efficiency is at the heart of debates about health care and costs and has generated a number of interesting opinions. At the end of the day, however, the debates are marred by the fact that data supporting both positions are essentially flawed because, in many instances (eg, spine care), the links between diagnosis, treatment, and outcome are not well established. Thus, the debates are powered by opinion, which often and perhaps inherently is biased and, therefore, not easily changed. Empiric evidence is the best weapon for combating opinion-based argument. If treatment efficacy rather than treatment efficiency is to carry the day, then the arguments to support efficacy must be fueled by evidence, which means improved clinical trials must be conducted. For improved clinical trials, methodologic and statistical relevance must play larger roles.

The Clinical Model for Patient Care

The clinical model for patient care traditionally has been a diagnosis-treatment model, ie, a diagnosis is determined and from that diagnosis a treatment is prescribed. The full model should involve two other major components—assessment and outcomes. Thus, evaluating treatment efficacy and/or efficiency requires establishing the validity of an assessment-diagnosis-treatment-outcome model. At its core, statistical relevance, as it applies to clinical care, concerns the measurement, methodologic, and statistical implications associated with evaluating this model.

Establishing the validity of an assessment-diagnosis-treatment-outcome model requires a clear understanding of the theory behind assessment. For spine care, in which there has been a lack of explicit rules linking assessment to diagnosis, linking diagnosis to treatment, and linking treatment to outcome, the problems of establishing validity are immense. When a problem is too complex, one scientific approach is to isolate some aspect of the problem, work to solve that, then move on to another aspect of the problem, hopefully in a hierarchical way so as to build toward a coherent structure or theory. This iterative approach is probably the best, if not the only, way for the spine community to establish a sound basis for evaluating the efficacy of treatment.

To illustrate the issues associated with establishing validity, a narrow scenario will be considered. The focus will be on a single diagnosis (D) that is unambiguously derived from a well-defined assessment (A), for which there is consensus for a single specific treatment (T), and where specific outcomes of treatment (O) are specified. To my knowledge, this situation does not exist for any spine-related diagnosis; however, points to be made based on these assumptions are important and the difficulties encountered, even in this best of all possible worlds, are useful in making clear just how difficult validating efficacy of treatment can be. If it were easy, it would have been done.

As a specific example, suppose a patient of type X presents to clinician C. C conducts an assessment (A) and, as a result, determines that the patient has diagnosis D. Based on D, the clinician prescribes treatment T, for which outcomes (O) must be measured. To validate

adequately this very narrow situation, three basic requirements or imperatives must be accepted.

Imperative I: The Assessment-Diagnosis Link

Establishing the Reliability and Validity of a Diagnosis

To establish the reliability of D, the extent must be determined to which, for a patient of type X, a randomly selected clinician from a well-defined cohort of clinicians (any clinician C1 through Cxxx) would generally and repeatedly agree that the assessment indicates that the diagnosis is D.

The Quebec Task Force Report stated, "There is so much variability in making a diagnosis that this initial step routinely introduces inaccuracies which are then further confounded with each succeeding step in care," adding that the resulting terminology used for diagnosis "is the fundamental source of error.... Faced with uncertainty, physicians become inventive." Among many possibilities, inventiveness could mean unique diagnoses and/or unorthodox treatment. Variability in diagnosis is caused by invalid assessment. Assessment may be invalid because interpretation of the way the assessment is conducted or how the information obtained lacks stability (unreliability), because of failure to look for enough of the right things (lack of accuracy), or some combination of these errors. There has been a multitude of studies evaluating the reliability of clinicians in interpreting diagnostic tests such as radiographs, MRI studies, and results of physical examination. However, the end points of these studies generally have been the consistency of the raters in making specific evaluations, not the final diagnosis, primarily because, in many instances in spine care, the final diagnosis is based on a variety of information sources, including self-report, physical examination, and diagnostic tests. The basis of the clinical diagnosis generally is not standardized, which, in conjunction with the known levels of reliability of components of the clinical information, makes it quite likely that clinician-to-clinician variability in an overall diagnosis requiring multiple sources of information is quite high.

In an assessment-diagnosis link in which a clear algorithm has been established, agreement in diagnosis is a final step, but agreement at each choice point in the algorithm defining the assessment-diagnosis link and agreement in correctly navigating the algorithm are indicators of validity. Only when agreement at each choice point and agreement in the overall classification are documented can it be argued that the assessment process was both reliable and valid. It has been found that some raters who agreed on each choice point in an algorithm, on some occasions, classified the patients differently, thus illustrating how fragile diagnosis reliability and validity can be.

Consider the following parable. Suppose Doctor N developed a nitroglycerin tablet for treating people with chest pain. Suppose further, that at this point in time, the medical profession has no useful diagnostic tests beyond self-report of symptoms to determine who may have heart trouble, and therefore, every patient with complaints of chest pain is considered a candidate for nitroglycerin therapy. Suppose further, that the incidence of heart problems in a population of chest pain patients is 10%, with the remaining 90% having chest pains from a variety of other causes. If the nitroglycerin is effective in 90% of the heart patients, it would be only 9% effective in the at-large population of patients with chest pain and would therefore be discredited. Poor diagnostic methods would have resulted in a therapy with 90% efficacy for the specific subgroup to be have been incorrectly estimated to be only 9% effective.

To extend the above example, further suppose that, during this same era of no tests to diagnose accurately the causes of chest pain, Doctor W developed a thick, white, antacid liquid that, when consumed, relieved the chest pains of some patients. A randomized trial comparing nitroglycerin with the antacid found that both were effective in a small percentage of the overall group, with many patients responding to neither. Neither treatment would be effective in large enough percentage to be recommended for treatment of the unrefined diagnosis of chest pain.

Of course, the above examples are easily dismissed when applied to nonspecific chest pain, because it is obviously false that there are no tests to provide more specific diagnoses. Even from self-report evidence alone, if those conducting the study learned to create subgroups, such as (1) those with pain referred into the arm, (2) those with a substernal burning sensation, and (3) those with additional distinguishing symptoms, a group-by-treatment interaction may have been detected, resulting in the effectiveness of nitroglycerin soaring to 90% for the subgroup with arm pain. Similarly, the effectiveness of antacid might have been substantial for those with substernal burning. Perhaps most importantly, from the viewpoints of efficacy and efficiency, now that effective treatments for groups 1 and 2 have been established, more efforts can be focused on the remaining subgroup.

The above example of nonspecific chest pain, when applied to patients with nonspecific low back pain, coupled with the inability to define specific diagnoses and the potential for inaccurate assessment of treatment efficacy is, unfortunately, not so far fetched. Although clinicians treating low back pain have at their disposal a myriad of diagnostic tests and many specific and non-specific diagnostic categories, the lament that as many as 85% of patients with low back complaints have no clear diagnosis is considered by many to be as true today as it was in 1976. It seems quite likely that multiple underlying conditions having different treatment needs contribute to low back pain. Consequently, determining efficacy for many treatments of low back pain remains controversial. As illustrated in the chest-pain analogy, results of randomized controlled trials will continue to be frustrating, meaningless, and even misleading. Perhaps more importantly, development of new treatments or refinements of current treatments are greatly hindered.

Forging the Assessment-Diagnosis Link: What Must be Done?

Strong protocols for establishing specific diagnoses must be developed. Patients, as they progress within their treatment regimen, must be monitored continually for evidence that additional factors could further define subgroups with special treatment needs. It always must be assumed that the classification protocols need further refinement.

Imperative II: The Diagnosis-Treatment Link

Establish That, for Patients of Type X With D, the Appropriate Treatment Plan Within the Assessment-Treatment Paradigm is T

Agreement between clinicians (C1 through Cxxx) concerning what treatment should apply to a given diagnosis for patients of Type X and consistency in treatment assignment by appropriate adherence to a model paradigm are primary factors that can be viewed as issues of reliability and validity.

A key phrase in both Imperative I and Imperative II is patients of Type X, which implies that there are defining characteristics from the assessment that place the patients in an appropriate subgroup within a diagnostic category. For example, perhaps patients with herniated discs who are in their teens should not be grouped with patients in their 40s, 50s, and 60s who have the same problem.

The notion of forming subgroups or looking for subgroups of patients within a single diagnostic classification (eg, cardiac pain versus reflux esophagitis within the overall group of patients with chest pain) that might be better treated with differential approaches has not gained sufficient attention, although research often supports the notion of differential effectiveness of treatment depending on age and other demographics, such as marital status. The lack of interest in restricting patients cohorts based on personal demographics or, at least, focusing on these demographics as explanatory variables when evaluating treatment effects was reported by authors who randomly selected four studies from a randomly selected issue of *Spine* (vol 10, no 4, 1985) and summarized the patient cohorts. The age ranges were 15 to 70, 28 to 62, 17 to 74, and 22 to 74 years, respectively. In none of these studies was age considered as an explanatory factor of outcome or as a defining factor for the diagnostic cohort. To the extent that age and its correlates of general health status can strongly affect treatment decisions and outcomes, it would seem that the spine community, at least in 1985, was less concerned about a clearly defined cohort of patients with a given diagnosis than they may have been about obtaining a sufficiently large number of patients to warrant publication.

This notion of sacrificing integrity of a cohort to increase sample size, which will increase statistical power and thereby increase the likelihood of obtaining a statistically significant result is seriously flawed logic. First, to the extent that broadening the cohort definition results in a less optimal treatment for some patients, the aggregated treatment effect will be diminished, which usually deflates power more than increased sample size will increase it. Perhaps more importantly, the broadening of the cohort in the name of increasing statistical power effectively breaks the assessment-diagnosis and diagnosis-treatment links, thereby providing critics a large number of rival interpretations for treatment efficacy.

For many conditions of the spine, the diagnosis-treatment link is not isomorphic (ie, a one-to-one relationship), meaning that a given diagnosis may result in a wide range of different treatments. For example, symptomatic herniated discs have been treated nonsurgically with exercise, manipulation, and/or steroid injections, and surgically with open discectomy, microdiscectomy, laser surgery, and many other approaches. These differences in treatments reflect, among other things, differences in the patients' wishes, the patients' general health status, the clinicians' comfort level and expertise, and the facilities available. By and large, the details or caveats that mediate the diagnosis-treatment link, as with the assessment-diagnosis link, are implicit. There is no standard protocol followed that would result in different clinicians arriving at the same treatment for a given diagnosis for a given patient of type X. This both follows from and leads to the fact that, for most diagnoses, no treatment has been demonstrated clearly to be the most effective. The implications are similar to those summarized for the assessment-diagnosis link. The factors that affect choice of treatment (eg, patients' wishes or comorbidities, clinicians' expertise or preference) other than the diagnosis itself may better predict the outcome than the treatment itself. Thus, studies that attempt to evaluate efficacy of treatment for a given diagnosis may not generalize well because the patients included in the study are self-selected based on their treatment preference and their clinicians' perceptions of the appropriateness of treatment. These perceptions likely vary from clinician to clinician and patients' wishes may depend, at least in part, on their clinicians' perceptions.

Forging the Diagnosis-Treatment Link: What Must be Done?

The goal should be to establish isomorphic relationships between specific diagnoses and specific treatments. The basis of isomorphism probably will be the extenuating circumstances of the patients, such as personal and health demographics and preferences for the outcome of greatest value to them. For example, the signs and symptoms for a specific type of herniated disc might generate four distinct diagnostic categories based on age and outcome needs. For young athletes, where concern is speed of recovery, the treatment of choice might be a minimally invasive injection technique. For patients of middle age who are in good health and for whom rapid recovery is a secondary concern, an open discectomy might be preferable. Such examples are, of course, not meant as specific guidelines, but do illustrate how patients' personal health and preference factors could drive a diagnosis-treatment link.

Once established, evidence of the effectiveness of diagnosis-treatment links must be evaluated. In the long run, this evidence must be used to help redefine and refine the links and to inform the patient and the clinician of possible side effects or problems with the established links. For example, if the long-term prognosis for the young athlete with a specific type of disc herniation, who undergoes injection therapy to speed recovery, is poor, either because the recovery is not sufficiently quick or because the long-term health consequences of a quick return to sport are deleterious, then these factors would argue against the validity of that particular diagnosis-treatment link. Perhaps further research would support that link for athletes in some sports but not for athletes in other sports. In this process, more fully refined cohorts and subgroups for which particular diagnosis-treatment links are effective would be established. The extent that these links are found to be idiosyncratic to a particular clinician, department, care facility, state, area of the country, or region of the world begs additional questions concerning the validity of both the assessment-diagnosis and the diagnosis-treatment links. Potential sources of inconsistencies could include differences between patients' attitudes about the possible outcomes from therapies. Many of these questions also are related directly to the treatment-outcome link.

Imperative III: The Treatment-Outcome Link

Once Imperatives I and II Are Established, Alternative Explanations for the Change in Status Across Time of Patients Experiencing Treatment Must Be Ruled Out
If patients of type X are reliably diagnosed as having D, and it is a tenet of the assessment-diagnosis-treatment-outcome model that patients of type X diagnosed with D should be treated with T, then what other factors might influence the success of this treatment for these patients? There are three general classes of factors that can lead to an unsuccessful outcome: the treatment itself is not effective; the treatment is not appropriately and/or effectively applied; and the outcomes selected to evaluate the treatment are not valid.

The Treatment Itself Is Not Effective An obvious, but often overlooked reason that T is found to be ineffective is because the approach does not work for patients of type X with D, even when T is appropriately implemented. The patient could get worse if the treatment is detrimental or has no effect on the natural progression of the symptoms associated with D. It is not hard to detect when this happens, although distinguishing between deleterious effects and worsening due to natural progression can be difficult.

Another possible result is that patients of type X with D, treated by T, get better independent of T. This natural history hypothesis is familiar to clinicians who treat back pain. The question becomes, "how do we know that T was responsible for the recovery when 80% to 90% of some type X patients with D (eg, nonspecific acute low back pain) recover spontaneously?"

Effectively ruling out rival hypotheses usually requires randomization of patients to different treatment modalities, some of which are, by the theory guiding the research, less effective than the active treatment under consideration. One particularly effective approach would be to include as alternative treatments: (1) placebo (same amount of clinical interaction, but no therapeutic input); (2) partial treatments, in which various components of the treatment are eliminated or inactivated; and (3) detrimental treatments, in which a treatment regimen is designed to actually exacerbate the patient's condition.

An example of alternative treatment was reported in a study in which two different bracing regimens were crossed with two different spinal disorders, so that the different bracing regimens were applied to the diagnoses both in ways hypothesized to improve and to exacerbate the patients' conditions. Ethical issues abound when considering how to compare various treatments and necessarily modulate the application of ideal methodologic/statistical design.

The Treatment Was Not Applied Appropriately and/or Effectively Reasons for inappropriate implementation generally fall into three classes: (1) clinician-centered factors, (2) patient-centered factors, and (3) clinician-patient-environmental factors.

A surgeon who had pioneered a surgical technique responded to another surgeon who suggested that the technique was flawed because the questioning surgeon had not had much success with it, "Well, not all piano players are pianists." That this response may have been unkind, does not mean it is not true. Clearly, for any given procedure, some clinicians are more skilled than others. These differential skills, be they surgical or interpersonal, affect treatment outcome.

The extent to which there is clinician to clinician variation in results must be considered. Assuming an adequate assessment-diagnosis and diagnosis-treatment link, to the extent that there is large variation in patient outcomes across clinicians, the argument for differential skill in applying the treatment is strengthened. A corollary point would be to investigate what factors about the treating clinicians might predict patient outcomes. For example, are more experienced clinicians more or less successful? Audits of treatment implementations also provide a potential area for distinguishing between clinicians. For example, in surgical cases, differences in blood loss, surgical time, and other related factors may be predictive of patient outcome. In nonsurgical cases, clinician contact time, number of visits, and inclusion of nonstandard procedures or adjunct therapies not normally associated with the treatment regimen might be predictive. Of course, evaluating these issues requires careful documentation of the clinical process associated with each patient. Differential detail in this documentation (not all doctors document their contacts with the same level of detail) can make this level of analysis problematic.

Evaluating, documenting, and publicizing clinician-centered sources of error in understanding treatment efficacy, perhaps understandably has not been popular among treating clinicians, and unless or until a system is established that accurately tracks clinicians' statistics, this area of explanation for differential treatment efficacy is not likely to be fruitful.

Patient-Centered Factors Affected Treatment Outcome Although specific ways in which patients might influence efficacy of therapy are myriad, a few common themes recur when evaluating clinical trials. One of the greatest is compliance.

Although compliance problems have been documented even when the therapy is as simple as taking a medicine, and generally are considered more problematic as involvement of patients with their therapy increases as with reconditioning, there is a paucity of research that investigates mechanisms to increase compliance with spine care. One explanation might be that compliance is generally thought to be good for surgical patients because their roles are passive once they arrive at the operating room. Postsurgical compliance with following the recommended regimen is likely no better than that with many nonsurgical therapies and likely affects treatment outcomes. Approaches for evaluating compliance include frequent follow-up assessments of improvements promoted by therapy, tracking medication usage by laboratory assessment or simply asking that patients bring their medications to their clinic visits, use of pedometers or other activity tracking devices, maintenance of an activity log, and reports from family. Of course, the ingenious patient can find ways to thwart most efforts to estimate compliance.

The propensity of some patients to engage simultaneously in other treatments is a second factor that can confound evaluation of the efficacy of a treatment under study. Patients with multiple medical issues are often involved in multiple treatment regimens such as medications, therapies, counseling, and so forth. Determining the extent of these confounding issues can be especially difficult because some patients do not readily volunteer information about supplemental treatments.

A third, patient-centered factor relates to latent variables, meaning aspects of the patient that are not known or not considered relevant when the assessment-diagnosis, diagnosis-treatment, or treatment-outcome links of the model are determined. Latent variables can be an integral part of the notion indicated by the phrase patients of type X. If a latent variable is discovered that has a significant impact on treatment efficacy, a modification in the assessment-diagnosis and the diagnosis-treatment links must be made to accommodate this knowledge. For example, a concomitant spine condition, such as disc herniation at an adjacent level, might make the treatment for the primary diagnosis ineffective. An important goal of treatment efficacy research should be identification of subgroups for whom the treatment is ineffective, in hope of refining the assessment-diagnosis and diagnosis-treatment links by establishing explicit criteria for excluding some patients from the standard treatment because known problems with the treatment apply to their specific diagnoses.

Patient/Clinician/Environmental Factors Perhaps most of the time, it is difficult to isolate factors that influence treatment efficacy to just clinician or just patient factors. It is not uncommon for the treatment efficacy to be influenced, both positively and negatively, based on the relationship between the clinician and the patient and the environment that they establish.

Treatment efficacy is likely to suffer to the extent that the patient is not capable of performing and/or the clinician is unable to effectively explain, teach, or implement the treatment. As discussed previously, this could be considered noncompliance or lack of the clinician's ability to motivate the patient to participate in recovery.

Secondary gain or incentives to patients to remain ill can be problems for those performing outcomes assessment if the treatment is effective but the patients will not perform to their capability, are noncompliant with therapy, or understate their true progress. Common factors contributing to secondary gain include job-related issues, family influences, and dependency on the relationship with clinicians and other caregivers.

Perhaps the most discussed factors that can mediate treatment efficacy are history and maturation variables. Factors external to treatment can superimpose themselves and affect the health status of patients. Many things are difficult to control, but the information system tracking the patient should be sensitive to these issues for there to be control. Examples of physical and/or psychological factors that might improve or worsen the health status of patients, independently from the treatment under evaluation, include loss or gain of weight, marriage or divorce, financial fortune or misfortune, job loss or gain, addition of or separation from children, and the occurrence or remission of concurrent injury or illness. Especially influential can be the course of concomitant injuries unrelated to the spine.

The Outcomes Measurement Method Selected to Evaluate the Treatment Is Not Valid for the Purpose

Outcomes measurements typically used to evaluate the efficacy of treatments prescribed for patients diagnosed with spine-related injuries too often have not been linked specifically to the treatment. Although several outcomes instruments, such as the Million Visual Analogue Scale, the Roland and Morris Disability Inventory, and the Oswestry Inventory, have been specifically devised as condition-specific instruments to assess the symptom and health status of patients, they were not designed as treatment-specific instruments. Because, within the logic of the assessment-diagnosis-treatment-outcome model described in this chapter, the treatment is directly related to patients of type X with a given diagnosis, the specified treatment is bound with related preferences and outcomes of interest to the patients. It follows that outcomes measures of particular interest should be treatment-specific. The basis for evaluating treatment, then, should be directly related back to the assessment model used to establish the diagnosis, with additional information, if necessary, to specifically evaluate the ability of the treatment to establish the outcomes the treatment was expected to effect.

To illustrate, consider Figure 1, which summarizes two patient types, X1 and X2, associated with a specific diag-

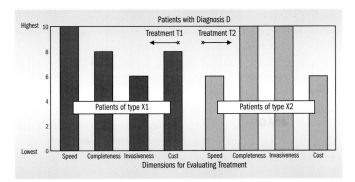

Figure 1 Illustration showing two different types of patients with the same diagnosis who, based on their preference profile for treatment characteristics and outcomes, have different diagnosis-treatment links. Given their different preference profiles and treatments that reflect these differences, different outcomes should be assessed to validly evaluate treatment efficacy.

nosis. The differences between the two patient types is depicted in terms of preferences for treatment with outcomes defined on the four dimensions of speed of recovery, completeness of recovery, invasiveness of treatment, and treatment cost. The point is that differences in these perceptions form the basis for considering these patients, all with D, as two separate subgroups of patients, with type X1 linked to T1 and type X2 linked to T2. The main point is that the outcome measures used to evaluate these patients should be tailored to reflect the differential goals of the two treatments. Treatment efficacy for treatments T1 and T2 may not be reasonably compared with a common set of outcomes.

A frequent misconception associated with the concepts of reliability and validity is that these constructs are attributes of the instruments themselves. One often reads that the instrument is reliable and valid. In fact, reliability and validity do not apply to the instrument, but rather to the decisions or interpretations based upon the instrument. Thus, an instrument produces a score and the score is used to make a decision. To the extent that the score is stable (reliable) and the decision that is made is correct (valid), then, for that person who completed the instrument, the resultant score was reliable and valid for the purpose of making the specified decision.

An instrument that produces a score that is reliable and valid for a person of type X1 relative to a specific decision about treatment efficacy may produce a score that is not reliable or valid for a person of type X2 relative to the same specific decision. To further clarify this point, consider a simple example of a math test designed to assess the ability of third graders' math skills. Such a test might produce scores that are reliable and valid for third graders, but the same instrument would be of little value if used to assess the mathematical abilities of college students, even though the instrument would pro-

duce reliable and stable scores for either group. The instrument does not possess the attributes of reliability and validity—the interpretation of the score does.

Suppose a patient with low back pain and a herniated disc is treated by discectomy. The outcome measure used to assess the success of the surgery is a range-of-motion test (ROM), which was judged appropriate because ROM was considered a good indicator of flexibility and general functional status. Before surgery, flexion was 30°. Two weeks postoperatively flexion was 25°. Based on these measurements, the surgeon concludes that the surgery was unsuccessful. Unhappy with this result, the surgeon retests the patient and finds that, on six consecutive evaluations the ROM in flexion was 25°, 24°, 25°, 26°, 25°, and 24°. The surgeon now believes that the original postoperative measurement was not a fluke, but, in fact, a reliable and accurate estimate of the patient's ROM in flexion. But does this test provide a score that is valid for inferring the success of the treatment? The validity of the ROM score in evaluating treatment success must be based on the predicted outcome of the treatment. If the discectomy is predicted to return the patient to a complete state of wellness after 2 weeks, and a complete state of wellness should result in an increased ROM, then the ROM test result should be considered a valid measure of outcome. However, the assumptions that the patient had flexion greater than 30° before the disc herniation occurred and that recovery should occur within 2 weeks of surgery are not necessarily valid. The former, being somewhat likely, is considered a weak assumption, whereas, the latter, being unlikely, is a strong assumption. The latter assumption is easily tested by repeating the ROM evaluations across time to determine the extent to which flexion changes with longer recovery times.

Forging the Treatment-Outcome Link: What Must be Done?

When surveying spine-related clinical literature, the most common study designs attempt to relate treatment to outcomes. Unfortunately, these studies typically assume reliable and valid assessment-diagnosis and diagnosis-treatment links rather than explicitly evaluating these links prior to assessing the treatment-outcome link. The single most important thing that should result from a careful reading of this chapter is the understanding that the three imperatives for evaluating the assessment-diagnosis-treatment-outcome model, the assessment-diagnosis, the diagnosis-treatment, and the treatment-outcome links, are strictly hierarchical. Therefore, establishing the validity of any one link requires that the validity of all previous links has been established. Further, because each link does not generalize beyond patients of type X, previous studies that did not explicitly consider the same population do not lend strong support for the reliability and validity of these links. Thus, forging the treatment-outcome link first and foremost requires a strong commitment to establishing the reliability and validity of the assessment-diagnosis and diagnosis-treatment links. Subsequent to this, careful consideration of rival hypotheses for the effects of treatment, including clinician-based, patient-based, and clinician-patient-environment-based factors need to be carefully documented as part of the medical record. Finally, outcomes specific to the treatment, which should be closely tied to the assessments used to diagnose the condition and to the patient-based factors that influence the diagnosis-treatment link in the model must become a priority. I believe that failing to move in these directions will result in articles written in another 25 years that suggest that the lament that 85% of patients with low back pain have no specific diagnosis remains as true then as it was 50 years before.

Summary

For the simple situation described, patients of type X with D, the issues in establishing the validity of an assessment-diagnosis-treatment model are several: (1) establish Imperative I, the reliability and validity of the assessment-diagnosis link; (2) establish Imperative II, the reliability and validity of the diagnosis-treatment link; and (3), assuming the reliability of those links, establish Imperative III, the reliability and validity of the treatment-outcome link by demonstrating treatment efficacy. If the patient experienced a positive change, in combination with few and/or weak evidences supporting rival hypotheses, then the conclusion that the treatment is efficacious is suggested and, in turn, the assessment-diagnosis-treatment-outcome paradigm is supported. Obviously, if the patient's change was negative, with few and/or weak evidences supporting rival hypotheses, then the conclusion that the treatment is not efficacious is suggested and, in turn, the assessment-diagnosis-treatment outcome paradigm is not supported. Regardless of the patient's outcome, good or bad, to the extent that there are many and/or strong evidences supporting rival hypotheses for change in the patient, the research can neither reject nor support the assessment-treatment paradigm.

In addition, to paraphrase the Heisenberg principle, the act of studying a phenomenon affects the phenomenon. Relative to this discussion, conducting a study of an assessment-diagnosis-treatment-outcome paradigm may affect the reliability and validity characteristics of the paradigm. It is well accepted that reliability obtained in reliability studies of clinical decision-making is generally higher than that observed in practice. When retrospec-

tively evaluating the reliability of clinical judgments, the consistency in classification is typically lower than obtained when it is studied prospectively.

Because validity often depends on reliability, validity evidence may not generalize well. These issues argue the need for validity studies to be as unobtrusive as possible to maximize the external validity and for the ability of the obtained results to be generalizable to the clinical setting. However, it is challenging to gather all the information needed to rule out the many rival explanations for outcomes without simultaneously changing the nature of the tasks being performed in the clinic.

To the extent that the assessment-diagnosis-treatment-outcome model is more complicated, the number of threats to the internal and external validity of a study of treatment efficacy increase—exponentially more than linearly. In other words, an increase of one level of complexity in the assessment-diagnosis-treatment-outcome model is likely to suggest a substantially larger number of rival hypotheses to explain the outcomes, which in turn will necessitate a much more comprehensive study design in an attempt to control or discount the rival hypotheses.

The potential classes of rival, relevant hypotheses, when considering study of treatment efficacy derived from the simple assessment-diagnosis-treatment-outcome model used in this example (a single diagnostic category and a single treatment considered for patients of a specific type), suggest that a relatively complex information system that tracks the clinicians' actions, compliance of patients, longitudinal influences from the clinician, and the patients' environment would be needed to reasonably evaluate rival explanations for the course of the patients. Current clinical practice does not routinely gather much of this information. The computer age and the increasing implementation of electronic medical records, in conjunction with the rapidly developing areas of data warehousing and data mining, are ushering in the day when the infrastructure will be available to develop studies with information systems that have sufficient scope to effectively evaluate many rival hypotheses for explanations of response to treatment. The stumbling blocks are formidable, however, including issues of patient privacy and concern of clinicians that their track records will be misinterpreted or misused.

This chapter used the assessment-diagnosis-treatment-outcome model to illustrate some of the multitude of measurement, methodologic, and statistical issues to consider when attempting to understand what treatments work for which patients. The things that make a difference all involve proper selection of a reliable and valid diagnostic cohort, of an appropriate treatment for that cohort, and of the appropriate means of measuring the outcome. Classic randomized clinical trial (RCT) studies, which generally focus on the treatment-outcome link without carefully and explicitly establishing the assessment-diagnosis and diagnosis-treatment links, are doomed because they fail to establish all three links and thus leave too many alternative explanations or rival hypotheses for interpreting the results. New-age RCTs must begin with a very narrow focus, a single diagnostic group that can be reliably and validly determined, and for which a small number of standardized treatments can be justified. From this narrow base, with outcomes derived from both a patient-specific and treatment-specific basis, the opportunity to establish strong assessment-diagnosis-treatment-outcome models can begin. Hopefully, from successful small projects, the information infrastructure will develop that will allow consideration of more comprehensive models.

Acknowledgment

The author acknowledges, with gratitude, the contributions of Ron Donelson, MD, MS to this chapter.

Annotated Bibliography

Neyt JG, Weinstein SL, Spratt KF, et al: Stulberg classification system for evaluation of Legg-Calve-Perthes disease: Intra-rater and inter-rater reliability. *J Bone Joint Surg Am* 1999;81:1209-1216.

   What began as a relatively straightforward study designed to assess the reliability of the Stulberg classification system became a classic example of the problems in establishing reliable clinical assessment. This study found that: (1) overall clinical impressions may vary between raters, even when there is

agreement on the constituent parts of the evaluation used to make the overall evaluation; (2) greater experience does not result in more consistent evaluations; and (3) formal training, after less than satisfactory initial efforts to establish reliability, can have deleterious effects on reliability.

Classic Bibliography

Fairbank JC, Couper, J, Davies JB, O'Brien JP: The Oswestry low back pain disability questionnaire. *Physiotherapy* 1980;66:271-273.

Million R, Hall W, Nilsen KH, Baker RD, Jayson MI: Assessment of the progress of the back-pain patient. *Spine* 1982;7:204-212.

Nachemson AL: The lumbar spine: An orthopaedic challenge. *Spine* 1976;1:59-71.

Report of the Quebec Task Force on Spinal Disorders: Scientific approach to the assessment and management of activity-related spinal disorders: A monograph for clinicians. *Spine* 1987;12(suppl):1-59.

Roland M, Morris R: A study of the natural history of back pain: Part I. Development of a reliable and sensitive measure of disability in low-back pain. *Spine* 1983; 8:141-144.

Spratt KF, Weinstein JN: Measuring clinical outcomes, in Weisel SW, Weinstein JN, Herkowitz HN, Dvorak J, Bell GR (eds) *The Lumbar Spine*, ed 2. Philadelphia, PA, WB Saunders Co, 1996, pp 1313-1338.

Spratt KF, Weinstein JN, Lehmann TR, Woody J, Sayre H: Efficacy of flexion and extension treatments incorporating braces for low-back pain patients with retrodisplacement, spondylolisthesis, or normal sagittal translation. *Spine* 1993;18:1839-1849.

Chapter 52

Knowledge Access and Dissemination

Tamara A. Shawver, MA

James N. Weinstein, DO, MS

We hear frequently that we are in the midst of an information revolution, an explosion of technology that makes finding information about virtually any topic almost instantaneous. At first, this revolution was considered to have the potential to make print media obsolete: physicians would be reading their journals on line from their personal digital assistants, or at least downloaded from the journal's Website. The flow of information would be likened to the cartoon in which a student was having liquid "knowledge" pumped into his ear via syringe and just sat there grinning as his head, and presumably his intelligence, expanded. Physicians would have swifter access to the latest practice guidelines through specialty society and governmental Websites, and would read cutting-edge research almost as soon as the manuscript was e-mailed to the online journal. Continuous improvement of every physician's practice, according to the latest information available, would become easy and commonplace. Better medicine through technology was at hand.

But we'll bet there are many physicians who hear a little voice whispering "I didn't get into medicine to become a computer hacker!" Surfing the Web may be easy for today's children, or surgical interns and residents, representing Generation X. For other mere mortals it can be a bit intimidating, and especially frustrating if they have high expectations of how easy it's going to be. We've all probably seen at least one commercial, magazine ad, or cartoon in which a frustrated person is trying to physically harm his or her computer, or is performing mystical incantations in hopes that spells will work better than the manual's instructions, which didn't work no matter how often the various key combinations were pressed.

Access to this information is not just a matter of figuring out which new key opens what lock, either. The sheer volume of the information itself is overwhelming. A study has shown that "[A] Sunday edition of the NY Times carries more information than the average 19th-century citizen accessed in his entire life." How on earth can any one individual hope to keep up, especially an extremely busy clinician? Physicians already have full-time jobs, and keeping up with the latest developments in their fields can amount to a second career. Even patients, having surfed the Web, are coming to their physicians with information the physician has never heard about. Patients are being bombarded with print and television ads for drugs about which they are told to "ask your doctor." Some of the ads don't even articulate, in any meaningful way, what ailment the particular drug is meant to alleviate or improve, they just say to "ask." And it's not just patients who bring physicians news of new drugs. The outright attempts to influence clinical decision-making go beyond the Internet and television advertising and go right into the doctor's office. The use of the Internet has not eliminated any of the traditional information highways but has exponentially increased access and suffers from lack of appropriate censoring and/or monitoring, the "Good Housekeeping Seal of Approval," so to speak. After a while, this information explosion becomes an assault on our senses, and we have to just shut our eyes, put our hands over our ears, curl up in a ball and rock in the corner, humming a little tune, "don't worry be happy," to keep our sanity.

Keeping up does not necessitate a degree in computer science (or psychotherapy!), but does require awareness of where the best information can be found and the acquisition of some skills in accessing and assessing that information. Finally, many physicians may find themselves involved in research. For research purposes it's important to know the current options for disseminating the results of research, and again, how to assess the worthiness of the vehicle(s) by which that work is disseminated. Generally, a trusted source of information can be trusted to be conscientious in publishing research results. Sources relating to how to analyze information include "Guidelines for Medical and Health Information Sites on the Internet: Principles Governing AMA

Websites" and "Critical Appraisal of the Literature: How to Assess an Article and Still Enjoy Life."

The following tables provide information about journals, societies, databases, Websites, and other sources of information from which orthopaedists may reliably gather and disseminate the rich wealth of information that has become the ocean we must navigate if we are to make a successful voyage through the world of spine and its many associated disciplines of study.

TABLE 1 | Journals

Journal/Editor-in-Chief/Website address	Scope
Journal of Bone & Joint Surgery Am James D. Heckman, MD **Journal of Bone & Joint Surgery Br** Frank Horan http://www.jbjs.org	Manuscripts are subjected to blinded peer review by experts and a final decision by the editor. Papers are judged by the quality and relevance of the work, not by the country of origin, the reputation of the author, or the fame of the department. The journal claims, "Our aim is to publish the best material available from anywhere in the world." The American and British volumes function independently. They cooperate in matters of general policy such as finance, advertising, printing, and distribution, but do not discuss individual papers. Methods of editing and styles differ to some extent, and the content is totally different. The American volume is published monthly and the British volume is published six times a year.
European Spine Journal Max Aebi, MD http://link.springer.de/link/service/journals/00586/index.htm	The *European Spine Journal* is a publication founded in response to the increasing trend toward specialization in spinal surgery. The *Journal* is devoted to spine surgery and all related disciplines, including functional and surgical anatomy of the spine, biomechanics and pathophysiology, diagnostic procedures, and neurology. The aim of the *Journal* is to support the further development of highly innovative European spine surgery and to provide an integrated and balanced view of diagnostic, research, and treatment procedures that will enhance effective collaboration among specialists worldwide.
Journal of the American Academy of Orthopaedic Surgeons Alan M. Levine, MD http://www.jaaos.org	The official journal of the American Academy of Orthopaedic Surgeons, *JAAOS* invites highly qualified authors to write the majority of its reviews of current knowledge and developments in the diagnosis and treatment of musculoskeletal conditions affecting people of all ages. It is a peer-reviewed journal and does accept unsolicited manuscripts for review. The *Journal* is published six times a year.
Acta Orthopaedica Scandinavica (English) Anders Rydholm http://www.lise.se/scup/gb/474.htm	*Acta Orthopaedica* is the official publication of the Nordic Orthopaedic Federation and the Netherlands Orthopaedic Society and publishes original papers from all parts of the world. Articles requiring extensive space, such as monographs, doctoral theses, and congress transactions, are published as supplements. Over the years, *Acta Orthopaedica Scandinavica* has issued more than 250 supplements. Geographic distribution: Scandinavia: 36%; Europe: 36%; USA: 15%; Japan: 9%.
Archives of Physical Medicine & Rehabilitation http://www.archives-pmr.org	This is the official journal of the American Congress of Rehabilitation Medicine and the American Academy of Physical Medicine & Rehabilitation.
Journal of Orthopaedic Research Joseph A. Buckwalter, MD Timothy M. Wright, Ph.D. http://www.ors.org/jor/index.html	The *Journal of Orthopaedic Research* provides a forum for rapid publication of high-quality manuscripts and short communications reporting new information on experimental, theoretical, and clinical aspects of orthopaedic research, including prospective clinical studies, especially when multidisciplinary approaches are used to provide methods and standards for diagnosis, treatment, and evaluation of clinical results.
The Back Letter Sam W. Weisel, MD http://news.medscape.com/LWW/BL/public/BL-journal.html	*The Back Letter* endeavors to deliver in-depth information on the latest thinking and research that affects the diagnosis and treatment of spinal problems and back pain, by reporting on new trends in the field, examining new research, and providing extensive referencing in each of the 12 issues.

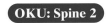

TABLE 1 | Journals *(continued)*

Journal/Editor-in-Chief/Website address	Scope
Clinical Orthopedics & Related Research Carl T. Brighton, MD, Ph.D. http://www.corronline.com	Sponsored by the Association of Bone & Joint Surgeons, this is the official publication of: The Academic Orthopedic Society, The Hip Society, The Musculoskeletal Tumor Society, The Knee Society, The International Cartilage Repair Society, and The Limb Lengthening and Reconstruction Society.
Current Opinion in Orthopedics James H. Herndon, MD Vincent D. Pellegrini, Jr, MD http://www.co-orthopedics.com/	In these bimonthly reviews of articles encompassing the entire field of orthopaedics, "specialists express their frank opinions on developments during the previous year."
Contemporary Spine Surgery Gunnar J.B. Andersson, MD, Ph.D.	This newsletter covers a single topic in spine surgery per issue. Physicians can gain up to 18 hours of CME credits through taking the multiple-choice tests in each issue.
Internet Medicine Louis G. Pareras, MD Barbara Ward http://www.internetmedicine.com	Published monthly, this 12-page newsletter endeavors to provide physicians with critical reviews of Websites and databases of interest to those in the medical professions. In addition, it supplies techniques and suggestions for navigating the Internet, as well as articles focusing on the use of the Internet in medicine, including technologies and strategies such as online research, telemedicine, and imaging. This is not a peer-reviewed publication.
Journal of Neurosurgery http://www.thejns-net.org	Founded in 1944 as an international journal devoted to the study of neurosurgery, *JNS* is a monthly journal that has recently extended itself to a subspecialty journal, *JNS: Spine*, which comes out quarterly. Both are peer-reviewed. In 1995, *JNS* was the most widely referenced neurosurgical journal and had an impact factor that ranked it number 6 among 107 surgical journals.
American Journal of Neuroradiology http://www.asnr.org/ajnr	This is the official journal of the American Societies of Neuroradiology, Head and Neck Radiology, Interventional and Therapeutic Radiology, Pediatric Neuroradiology, and Spine Radiology. It publishes original peer-reviewed articles on a broad range of issues pertaining to neuroradiology on a monthly basis (except for July and December).
Journal of Orthopaedic Trauma Roy W. Sanders, MD http://www.jorthotrauma.com	This is the official journal of the Orthopaedic Trauma Association, the American Fracture Society, the International Society for Fracture Repair, the Belgian Orthopaedic Trauma Association, the Japan Fracture Society, the Canadian Orthopaedic Trauma Society, and the American Fracture Association. This peer-reviewed journal is devoted exclusively to the diagnosis and management of hard- and soft-tissue trauma, including injuries to bone, muscle, ligament, and tendons, as well as spinal cord injuries. It is published eight times a year.
Journal of Pediatric Orthopaedics Lynn T. Staheli, MD Robert N. Hensinger, MD http://www.pedorthopaedics.com	The *Journal of Pediatric Orthopaedics* publishes peer-reviewed papers from around the world on the diagnosis and treatment of pediatric orthopaedic disorders. It is the official journal of the Pediatric Orthopaedic Society of North America and the European Orthopaedic Society; it is published quarterly.
Journal of Prosthetics and Orthotics Thomas M. Gavin, CO	Published quarterly by the American Academy of Orthotists and Prosthetists, the *Journal* provides information on new devices, fitting and fabrication techniques, and patient management experiences. Each issue contains research-based articles reviewed and approved by an editorial board and an Academy self-study quiz offering two PCEs.
Journal of Spinal Disorders Dan M. Spengler, MD Thomas B. Ducker, MD http://www.jspinaldisorders.com	The *Journal of Spinal Disorders* is published bimonthly and features peer-reviewed, original articles on diagnosis, management, and surgery for spinal problems.

TABLE 1 | Journals (continued)

Journal/Editor-in-Chief/Website address	Scope
Medicine & Science in Sports & Exercise Peter B. Raven, PhD, FACSM http://www.acsm-msse.org/	This is the official journal of the American College of Sports Medicine. It provides exercise physiologists, physiatrists, physical therapists, team physicians, and athletic trainers a vital exchange of information from basic and applied science, medicine, education, and allied health fields. Its original articles report monthly on new educational developments as well as sound physical fitness practices and the treatment of sports injuries. The journal helps readers enhance their basic understanding about the role of physical activity in human health and function.
Neurology http://www.neurology.org	*Neurology* is the official journal of the American Academy of Neurology. The leading clinical neurolgy journal worldwide, *Neurology* is directed at physicians concerned with diseases and conditions of the nervous system. The *Journal* presents new basic and clinical research with emphasis on knowledge that will influence the way neurology is practiced. The journal is peer-reviewed and is published biweekly.
Neurology & Clinical Neurophysiology Keith H. Chiappa http://www.mit.edu (Search "mit press" and choose "Journals" then "Science & Technology."	*Neurology & Clinical Neurophysiology*, the official journal of the American Academy of Clinical Neurophysiology, is an electronic peer-reviewed journal publishing both clinical and research articles about human neurology, neuroscience, and related fields, and studies of other species that relate to the human nervous system. It formerly was titled *Journal of Contemporary Neurology*. Articles are published online as they are accepted and in an annual print volume.
Neurosurgery Michael L. J. Apuzzo, MD http://www.neurosurgery-online.com	*Neurosurgery* is the official journal of the Congress of Neurological Surgeons. Its goal is to provide a medium for prompt publication of peer-reviewed scientific papers dealing with clinical or experimental neurosurgery. It is published monthly.
Spine James N. Weinstein, DO, MS	*Spine* is the official journal of the Cervical Spine Research Society, European Spine Society (Affiliate), International Society for the Study of the Lumbar Spine, Japan Spine Research Society, Korean Society of Spine Surgery, North American Spine Society, Scoliosis Research Society, Spine Society of Australia, and The Western Pacific Orthopaedic Association–Spinal Section. The leading journal in its field, *Spine* is a bimonthly journal that publishes peer-reviewed articles and selected abstracts from international journals. Special issues contain papers from meetings of the North American Spine Society, Scoliosis Research Society, International Society for the Study of the Lumbar Spine, and the Cervical Spine Research Society.
Spine Line Stuart M. Weinstein, MD http://www.towne@spine.org	This newsletter, published six times a year by the North American Spine Society, contains invited review articles and updated information about educational, social, political, and practice management issues as related to spine care.
The Spine Journal Tom G. Mayer, MD http://www.kenyon@spine.org	*The Spine Journal*, the scientific journal of the North American Spine Society, publishes peer-reviewed clinical and basic science articles emphasizing multidisciplinary approaches to spine care.
Strategic Orthopaedics Thomas J. Grogan, MD Patricia L. Brewster, FACMPE http://www.lww.com (you can search for a description of the newsletter from here)	This monthly newsletter is the first of its kind to cover the practice management and clinical issues specific to orthopaedics. Regular areas covered include managed care, business management, cost-effectiveness studies, clinical issues, and physician compensation—all specific to the orthopaedic practice.
Techniques in Orthopaedics Bruce D. Browner, MD Courtland G. Lewis, MD Clarence L. Shields, MD http://www.techortho.com	*Techniques in Orthopaedics* provides quarterly information on new and established surgical techniques as well as comprehensive management and treatment guidelines. Each issue is guest-edited and deals with a single topic in the field, allowing for focused, in-depth coverage of important issues and clinical problems.

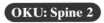

TABLE 2 | Societies and Meeting Schedules

Society	Meetings	Website URLs
American Academy of Orthopaedic Surgeons (AAOS)	Annual	http://www.aaos.org
American Orthopaedic Association (AOA)	Annual	http://www.aoassn.org
North American Spine Society (NASS)	Annual	http://www.spine.org
International Society for the Study of the Lumbar Spine (ISSLS)	Annual	http://www.issls.org
Scoliosis Research Society (SRS)	Annual	http://www.srs.org
Cervical Spine Research Society (CSRS)	Annual	http://www.csrs.org
Orthopaedic Research Society (ORS)	Annual	http://www.ors.org
Orthopaedic Research & Education Foundation (OREF)	N/A	http://www.oref.org
Clinical Orthopaedic Society	Annual	http://www.cosociety.org
American Academy of Clinical Neurophysiology (AACN)	Annual	http://aacn.mit.edu
American Academy of Neurology	Annual	http://www.aan.com
American Academy of Physical Medicine & Rehabilitation	Annual	http://www.aapmr.org
American Association of Neurological Surgeons		http://www.aans.org
Arthritis Foundation	N/A	http://www.arthritis.org/
Academic Orthopedic Society	Annual	http://www.a-o-s.org
Congress of Neurological Surgeons	Annual	http://www.neurosurgery.org/cns
Musculoskeletal Tumor Society	Annual	http://www.msts.org
Hip Society/AAHKS	Annual	http://www.aahks.org
Pediatric Orthopaedic Society of North America	Annual	http://www.posna.org
International Society of Arthroscopy, Knee Surgery and Orthopaedic Sports Medicine	Biannual	http://www.isakos.com
American Orthopaedic Society of Sports Medicine	Annual	http://www.sportsmed.org
American Academy for Cerebral Palsy and Developmental Medicine (AACPDM)	Annual	http://www.aacpdm.org
American Society of Neuroradiology and the American Society of Spine Radiology	Annual	http://www.asnr.org

Research Meets the Internet

Librarians at institutions, and even at some well-funded public libraries, have access to databases that a private individual would not necessarily want to buy. For example, at Dartmouth, we have Ovid, a medical/scientific database search engine described below, with certain databases available to everyone at Dartmouth. However, our reference librarians also have access to many more databases offered by Ovid on a pay-as-you-go basis. Therefore, physicians should not hesitate to use the old-fashioned librarian's help, because many of them are on the cutting edge of information technology and can be great sources of help and information.

Spine Websites

Web searching is an art, based partly on logic and partly on the intuitive hunch. The following is an example of how different the results from two search engines can be. First, using Lycos and the word "orthopedic," we got four "popular" websites (based on user traffic) and 146,047 hits in general. Then, using Yahoo and the word "orthopedic," we got 57 categories, 365 sites, 233 news headline matches, two "net events" (live chats or film archives), and 103,995 pages on which the word "orthopedic" appears. Tom Meade, a reference librarian here at Dartmouth, says he thinks of most Websites as indexes, which provide everything in a somewhat enig-

TABLE 3 | Online Sources of CME Credits

Source	Website	Comments
American Academy of Orthopaedic Surgeons	http://www.aaos.org	There is a section on the AAOS home page devoted to Medical Education. One link brings you to a calendar of CME events, the other to their library of online and CD-ROM-based tutorial exams.
Medscape Orthopaedics	http://orthopedics.medscape.com	Click on "CME Center" for their offerings. They also make very clear whether there are CME opportunities at any of the links they provide to meetings, conferences, online tutorials, and the like.
CME Unlimited	http://www.audio-digest.org/cgi-bin/start/cmeu/index.htm	This is an online store of audio, video, CD, and online tutorials and lectures for CME credit.
North American Spine Society	http://www.spine.org	On the NASS homepage, members can enroll in online courses for CME credit.

matic order, and thinks of Yahoo as a table of contents, which arranges that information in a clearer fashion. Understanding the criteria by which individual search engines both find and organize the results of their searches cuts down on research time. Many of the orthopaedic sites found using any search engine are the home pages of orthopaedic clinics throughout the United States and the world, while others are links to device manufacturers. Another large segment of hits are news stories that have the word "orthopedic" somewhere in the first part of the page's text.

Table 4 is a sampling of some of the better Internet sources for orthopaedic information. Some of the Websites are subscription-based; often, if you are affiliated with an institution, they will have a group subscription available.

Acknowledgment

This chapter was partially funded by the National Institutes of Arthritis and Musculoskeletal and Skin Diseases (AR45444-01A1), the Office of Research on Women's Health, National Institutes of Health, and the National Institute of Occupational Safety and Health of the Centers for Disease Control and Prevention.

Annotated Bibliography

Miser WF: Critical appraisal of the literature: How to assess an article and still enjoy life. *J Am Board Fam Pract* 1999;12:315-333.

The author gives practical advice on how to determine a journal article's relevance and quality.

Winker MA, Flanagin A, et al: Guidelines for medical and health information sites on the internet: Principles governing AMA Web sites. *JAMA* 2000;283:1600-1606.

These are the American Medical Association's guidelines for Website content, advertising and sponsorship, and privacy and confidentiality.

Winkle WV: Information overload. *Computer Bits* 1998;8

This article provides an entertaining look at how much information we are bombarded with, with tips on how to keep our sanity in the information age.

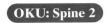

TABLE 4 | Internet Sources for Spine Information

Orthopaedic Websites/ Search Engines/Databases URL	Comments
AAOS http://www.aaos.org	Besides an online store, an "Orthopaedic Yellow Pages," and various links to AAOS-specific sites, this home page links to other medical sites, such as those of state medical societies and college/university medical schools. It also links to the National Library of Medicine home page with links to PubMed and two Medline search engines.
Medline/PubMed http://www.ncbi.nlm.nih.gov/PubMed	Medline is a database maintained by the National Library of Medicine, a branch of the National Institutes of Health. PubMed is the interface for Medline that is provided free by the government to the public.
Ovid n/a	This search engine can be purchased by individuals or institutions and configured to access those medical/ scientific databases that the purchaser deems most useful. For example, Dartmouth accesses the Medline, CINAHL, BIOSIS, HealthSTAR, and Evidence-Based Medicine Reviews databases. Ease of access might also differ from institution to institution; some require passwords to access certain information.
Medscape Orthopaedics http://orthopedics.medscape.com/ Home/Topics/orthopedics/ orthopedics.html	Medical professionals are provided free access to Medline and other databases to search for research information. It is also full of links to other resources ranging from free e-mail to stock quotations. It also provides news, conference summaries, etc. It had last been updated on the day we visited (an important criterion of judging a site's quality).
MD Consult http://home.mdconsult.com	This is a partially open, partially subscription-based Website. It contains a lot of information, including a library of textbooks, access to practice guidelines, printable patient education handouts (very text-heavy, however), and features such as "Today in Medicine," "What Patients are Reading," and "Drug Updates." It appears that the primary function provided to a personal edition is the CME Center, which offers over 450 on-line tests for Category 1 credits in 25 specialties.
National Academy Press http://search.nap.edu	This site contains over 1,500 books published by the NAP in fully browsable format. It states, "the Open Book page image presentation framework is not designed to replace printed books, nor emulate HTML. Rather, it is a free, browsable, nonproprietary, fully and deeply searchable version of the publication which we can inexpensively and quickly produce to make the material available worldwide."
MedNav.com http://www.medsitenavigator.com	This is essentially an index of links to medically related sites, such as "Companies," "Disabilities," "Emergencies," "Organizations," "Research," etc. It is very easy to navigate for patients or professionals.
The Cochrane Collaboration http://www.cochrane.org	The ad copy says, "Preparing, maintaining and promoting the accessibility of systematic reviews of the effects of health care interventions." Abstracts of these reviews are available to anyone and include several from orthopaedic review groups. A subscription gains access to the extensive full text library.
Aunt Minnie http://www.auntminnie.com	AuntMinnie.com provides the first comprehensive community Internet site for radiologists and related professionals in the medical imaging industry. AuntMinnie provides a forum for radiologists, business managers, technologists, members of organized medicine, and industry to meet, transact, research, and collaborate on topics within the field of radiology.
NASS http://www.spine.org	The NASS Website has three sections: information and services for members; links and services for health care professionals who are not NASS members; and spine care information for the general public.

Index